Basic Ophthalmology

UMBREEN

Published by
Jitendar P Vij
Jaypee Brothers Medical Publishers (P) Ltd

Corporate Office
4838/24 Ansari Road, Daryaganj, **New Delhi** - 110002, India, Phone: +91-11-43574357

Registered Office
B-3 EMCA House, 23/23B Ansari Road, Daryaganj, **New Delhi** - 110 002, India
Phones: +91-11-23272143, +91-11-23272703, +91-11-23282021, +91-11-23245672
Rel: +91-11-32558559, Fax: +91-11-23276490, +91-11-23245683
e-mail: jaypee@jaypeebrothers.com, Website: www.jaypeebrothers.com

Branches

- 2/B, Akruti Society, Jodhpur Gam Road Satellite
  Ahmedabad 380 015, Phones: +91-79-26926233, Rel: +91-79-32988717
  Fax: +91-79-26927094, e-mail: ahmedabad@jaypeebrothers.com
- 202 Batava Chambers, 8 Kumara Krupa Road, Kumara Park East
  Bengaluru 560 001, Phones: +91-80-22285971, +91-80-22382956, 91-80-22372664
  Rel: +91-80-32714073, Fax: +91-80-22281761, e-mail: bangalore@jaypeebrothers.com
- 282 IIIrd Floor, Khaleel Shirazi Estate, Fountain Plaza, Pantheon Road
  Chennai 600 008 Phones: +91-44-28193265, +91-44-28194897, Rel: +91-44-32972089
  Fax: +91-44-28193231, e-mail: chennai@jaypeebrothers.com
- 4-2-1067/1-3, 1st Floor, Balaji Building, Ramkote Cross Road
  Hyderabad 500 095, Phones: +91-40-66610020, +91-40-24758498, Rel: +91-40-32940929
  Fax:+91-40-24758499, e-mail: hyderabad@jaypeebrothers.com
- No. 41/3098, B and B1, Kuruvi Building, St. Vincent Road
  Kochi 682 018, Kerala, Phones: +91-484-4036109, +91-484-2395739, +91-484-2395740
  e-mail: kochi@jaypeebrothers.com
- 1-A Indian Mirror Street, Wellington Square
  Kolkata 700 013, Phones: +91-33-22651926, +91-33-22276404, +91-33-22276415
  Rel: +91-33-32901926, Fax: +91-33-22656075, e-mail: kolkata@jaypeebrothers.com
- Lekhraj Market III, B-2, Sector-4, Faizabad Road, Indira Nagar
  Lucknow 226 016, Phones: +91-522-3040553, +91-522-3040554, e-mail: lucknow@jaypeebrothers.com
- 106 Amit Industrial Estate, 61 Dr SS Rao Road, Near MGM Hospital, Parel
  Mumbai 400 012, Phones: +91-22-24124863, +91-22-24104532, Rel: +91-22-32926896
  Fax: +91-22-24160828, e-mail: mumbai@jaypeebrothers.com
- "KAMALPUSHPA" 38, Reshimbag, Opp. Mohota Science College, Umred Road
  Nagpur 440 009 (MS), Phone: Rel: +91-712-3245220, Fax: +91-712-2704275, e-mail: nagpur@jaypeebrothers.com

USA Office
1745, Pheasant Run Drive, Maryland Heights (Missouri), MO 63043, USA, Ph: 001-636-6279734
e-mail: jaypee@jaypeebrothers.com, anjulav@jaypeebrothers.com

Basic Ophthalmology

© 2009, Renu Jogi

All rights reserved. No part of this publication should be reproduced, stored in a retrieval system, or transmitted in any form or by any means: electronic, mechanical, photocopying, recording, or otherwise, without the prior written permission of the author and the publisher.

This book has been published in good faith that the material provided by author is original. Every effort is made to ensure accuracy of material, but the publisher, printer and author will not be held responsible for any inadvertent error(s). In case of any dispute, all legal matters are to be settled under Delhi jurisdiction only.

First Edition: 1994
Second Edition: 1999
Third Edition: 2003
Fourth Edition: **2009**

ISBN 978-81-8448-451-9

Typeset at JPBMP typesetting unit
Printed at Gopsons Papers Ltd., Noida

Dedicated to
our beloved
Anusha

Preface to the Fourth Edition

The eye is the lamp of the body. If your eyes are good, your whole body will be full of light.
                                                                                              The Bible

The need for a textbook for undergraduate medical students in ophthalmology dealing with the basic concepts and recent advances has been felt for a long-time. Keeping in mind the changed curriculum this book is intended primarily as a first step in commencing and continuing the study for the fundamentals of ophthalmology which like all other branches of medical sciences, has taken giant strides in the recent past.

While teaching the subject I have been struck by the avalanche of queries from the ever inquisitive students and my effort therefore has been to let them find the answers to all their interrogatories.

It is said that revision is the best testimony to the success of a book. In the competitive market of medical text publishing, only successful books survive.

Any textbook, more so, a medical one such as this, needs to be updated and revised from time to time. Yet the very task of revising *Basic Ophthalmology* presents a dilemma: how does one preserve the fundamental simplicity of the work while incorporating crucial but complex material lucubrated from recent research, investigations and inquiries in this ever expanding field.

In essence, Basic Ophthalmology is both a 'textbook' and a 'notebook' that might as well have been written in the student's own hand. The idea is for the student to relate to the material; and not merely to memorize it mechanically for reproducing it during an examination. It is something I wish was available to me when I was an undergraduate student not too long ago.

The past few years have witnessed not only an alarming multiplication of information in the field of ophthalmology, but more significantly, a definite paradigmatic shift in the focus and direction of ophthalmic research and study. The dominant causes of visual disabilities are no longer pathological or even genetic in nature, but instead a direct derivative and manifestation of contemporary changes in predominantly modern urban lifestyles. The student will thus find a new section devoted to a discussion on Visual Display Terminal Syndrome (VDTS) that is an outcome of excessive exposure of the eyes to the computer monitor as well as the use of contact lenses. Two additional sections deal with the Early Treatment for Diabetic Retinopathy Study (ETDRS) classification and Scheie's classification for hypertensive retinopathy that replaces the pre-existent taxonomy prevalent for little less than seven decades. With posterior chamber intraocular lenses establishing themselves as the primary modality in the optical rehabilitation of patients undergoing cataract surgery, the emphasis has shifted from just visual rehabilitation to an early, perfect optical, occupational and psychological rehabilitation.

When I initiated this project I scarcely realized that it only had toil, sweat and hard work to offer. Whenever anyone reminded me that I was working hard, my answer always was; I am trying to create something very enduring.

To conclude, for me, this has really been a *trabalho do coracao* a phrase which does not have a correct synonym in English but when literally translated from Portuguese would mean "a work of the heart". In truth, it is a vivid reflection of my long lasting concern and affection for my students.

All books are collaborative efforts and I would like to take this opportunity to thank all the people who have advised and encouraged me in this project: specially my husband Shri Ajit Jogi, my son Aishwarya, Amit and Dr Nidhi Pandey.

I offer special thanks to my publisher Shri JP Vij, Chairman and Managing Director of M/s Jaypee Brothers Medical Publishers (P) Ltd., Mr Tarun Duneja, Director (Publishing) and his staff namely Mrs Yashu Kapoor, Mr Manoj Pahuja, Mr Arun Sharma, Mr Akhilesh Kumar Dubey and Mrs Seema Dogra.

By the grace of the Almighty God and with the continuing support of the teachers, I am happy to present the fourth updated edition of my book.

ग्राह्यं च रूपस्य मुखस्य शोभा,
प्रत्यक्षबोधस्य च हेतु भूतम्!
तमिस्त्र-दिक्-कर्मसु मार्गदर्शि,
नेत्रं प्रधानं सकलेन्द्रियाणाम्।

An eye can perceive forms,
it adorns the face;
it is a source of direct knowledge;
it is a guide to avoid wrong deeds;
hence the eye is most important
of all the sense organs.

Renu Jogi

Contents

1. Embryology and Anatomy *1*
2. Physiology of Vision *9*
3. Neurology of Vision *15*
4. Examination of the Eye *22*
5. Errors of Refraction *47*
6. The Conjunctiva *71*
7. The Cornea *107*
8. The Sclera *153*
9. The Uveal Tract *161*
10. The Lens *205*
11. The Vitreous *246*
12. Glaucoma *258*
13. The Retina *300*
14. The Optic Nerve *341*
15. Injuries to the Eye *361*
16. The Ocular Motility and Squint (Strabismus) *375*
17. The Lids *403*
18. The Lacrimal Apparatus *424*
19. The Orbit *437*
20. General Therapeutics *448*
21. The Causes and Prevention of Blindness *458*
22. Ophthalmic Instruments *469*

Index *489*

CHAPTER 1
Embryology and Anatomy

EMBRYOLOGY

The central nervous system develops from the neural tube. A thickening appears on either side of the neural tube in its anterior part, known as the *optic plate*. The optic plate grows towards the surface to form the *optic vesicle*. The two eyes develop from these optic vesicles and the ectoderm and mesoderm coming in contact with the optic vesicles.

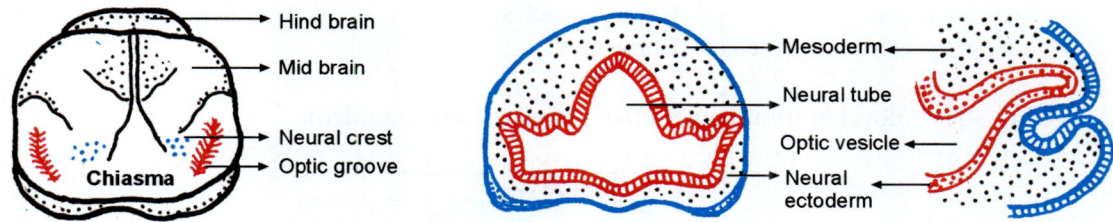

The optic vesicle invaginates from in front and below to form the *optic cup*. The line of invagination remains open for sometime as the *embryonic fissure*. The hyaloid artery enters through the fissure to provide nutrition to the developing structures. Later it atrophies and disappears.

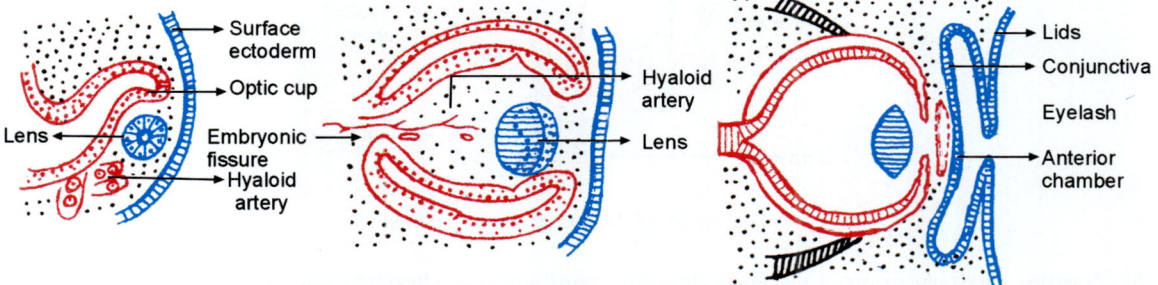

The inner layer of the optic cup forms the inner nine layers of the *main retina* and the outer layer develops into the *pigment epithelium*. The neural ectoderm secretes jelly-like structure, *the vitreous* which fills the cavity.

The *ciliary body and iris* are formed by the anterior portion of the optic cup and mesoderm. The mesoderm around the cup differentiates to form the *coats of eye, orbital structures, angle of anterior chamber* and *main structure of cornea*.

Meanwhile the surface ectoderm invaginates and later separates to form the *lens*. The surface ectoderm remains as the *corneal* and *conjunctival epithelium*. The mesoderm in front of the cornea grows in folds, unites and separates to form the *lids*.

PRIMORDIA OF OCULAR STRUCTURES

The eye originates from neural ectoderm, surface ectoderm and mesoderm.

SURFACE ECTODERM	MESODERM	NEURAL ECTODERM
1. Conjunctival epithelium	1. Corneal stroma	1. Sensory retina
2. Corneal epithelium	2. Corneal endothelium and Descemet's membrane	2. Retinal pigment epithelium
3. Crystalline lens	3. Iris stroma	3. Pigment epithelium of iris
4. Eyelash	4. Choroid	4. Ciliary body epithelium
5. Epithelium of	5. Sclera	5. Sphincter pupillae
— meibomian glands	6. Vitreous	6. Dilator pupillae
— glands of Moll	7. Extraocular muscles	7. Melanocytes
— lacrimal gland	8. Ciliary muscles	8. Neural part of optic nerve
— accessory lacrimal glands	9. Bony orbit	

1. Eyelids—They develop from both surface ectoderm and mesoderm

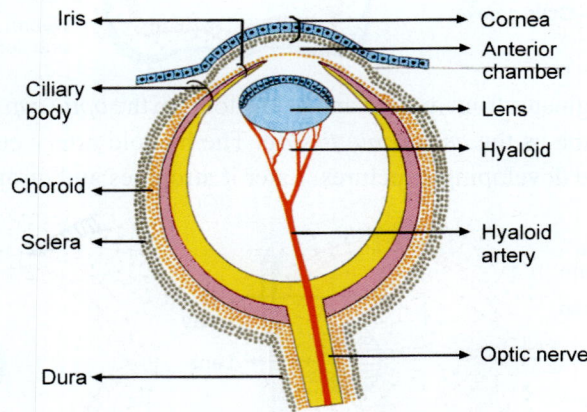

Derivation of various ocular structures

2. Zonules (tertiary vitreous)—They develop from surface ectoderm and mesoderm
3. Bruch's membrane—It develops from neural ectoderm and mesoderm

The Eye at Birth

1. Orbit is more divergent (50°) as compared to an adult (45°).
2. Eyeball is about 70% of adult length. It is fully developed at the age of 8 years.
3. The newborn is hypermetropic by +2.5 D.
4. Cornea is approximately 80% of its adult size, being fully grown at the age of 3 years.
5. Anterior chamber is shallow and the angle is narrow.

ANATOMY

The eye is the organ of sight situated in the orbital cavity. It is almost spherical in shape and is about 2.5 cm in diameter. The volume of an eyeball is approximately 7 cc. The space between the eye and the orbital cavity is occupied by fatty tissue. The bony wall of the orbit and the fat helps to protect the eye from injury.

Structurally the two eyes are separate but they function as a pair. It is possible to see with only one eye, but three-dimensional vision is impaired when only one eye is used specially in relation to the judgement of distance.

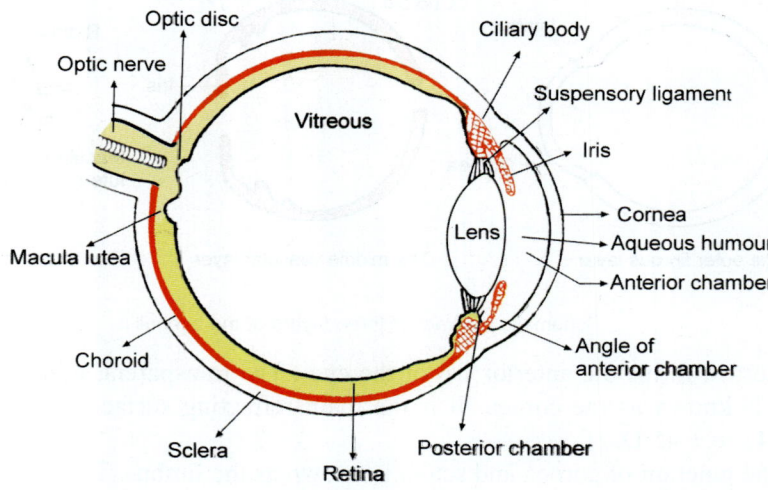

Structure of the eye

Structure of the Eye
The eyeball has three layers namely:
1. *The outer fibrous layer—Sclera and cornea*
2. *The middle vascular layer—Iris, ciliary body and choroid*
3. *The inner nervous tissue layer—Retina.*

Interior of the Eyeball
The structures inside the eyeball are:
1. *Aqueous humour*
2. *Lens*
3. *Vitreous.*

Accessory Structures of the Eye
1. *Eyebrows*
2. *Eyelids and eyelashes*
3. *Lacrimal apparatus*
4. *Extraocular muscles of the eye.*

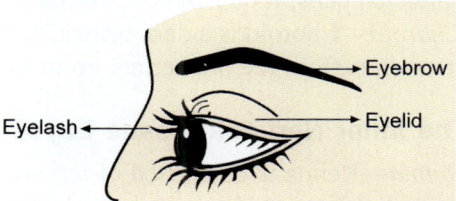

Side view of some structures which protect the eye

STRUCTURE OF THE EYE

1. The Outer Fibrous Layer

1. *Sclera*—The sclera or white of the eye forms the firm, fibrous outermost layer of the eye. It maintains the shape of the eye and gives attachment to the extraocular muscles. It is about 1 mm thick. The sclera becomes thin (seive-like membrane) at the site where the optic nerve pierces it. It is called *Lamina cribrosa*.

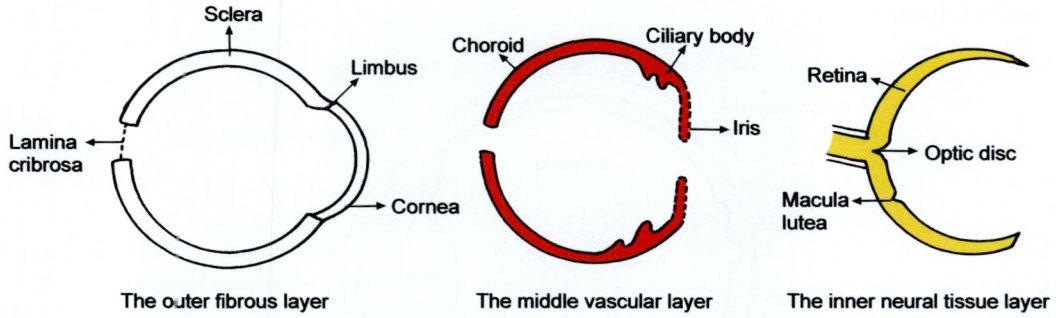

Schematic diagram of three layers of the eyeball

2. *Cornea*—Cornea forms the anterior 1/6 of the eye. The transparent, ellipsoid, anterior part of the eyeball is known as the cornea. It is the main refracting surface of the eye. The dioptric power is + 43 to + 45 D.
3. *Limbus*—The junction of cornea and sclera is known as the limbus. There is a minute arcade of blood vessels about 1 mm broad present at the limbus.

2. The Middle Vascular Layer

1. *Iris*—Iris is a coloured, free, circular diaphragm with an aperture in the centre—*the pupil*. It divides the anterior segment of the eye into anterior and posterior chambers which contain aqueous humour secreted by the ciliary body. It consists of endothelium, stroma, pigment cells and two groups of plain muscle fibres, one circular (sphincter pupillae) and the other radiating (dilator pupillae).
2. *Ciliary body*—Ciliary body is triangular in shape with base forwards. The iris is attached to the middle of the base. It consists of non-striated muscle fibres (ciliary muscles), stroma and secretory epithelial cells. It consists of two main parts, namely pars plicata and pars plana.
3. *Choroid*—Choroid is a dark brown, highly vascular layer situated between the sclera and retina. It extends from the ora serrata up to the aperture of the optic nerve in the sclera.

3. The Inner Nervous Tissue Layer

1. *Retina*—Retina is composed of ten layers of nerve cells and nerve fibres lying on a pigmented epithelial layer. It lines about 3/4 of the eyeball. Macula lutea is a yellow area of the retina situated in posterior part with a central depression called *fovea centralis*. It is the most sensitive part of retina.

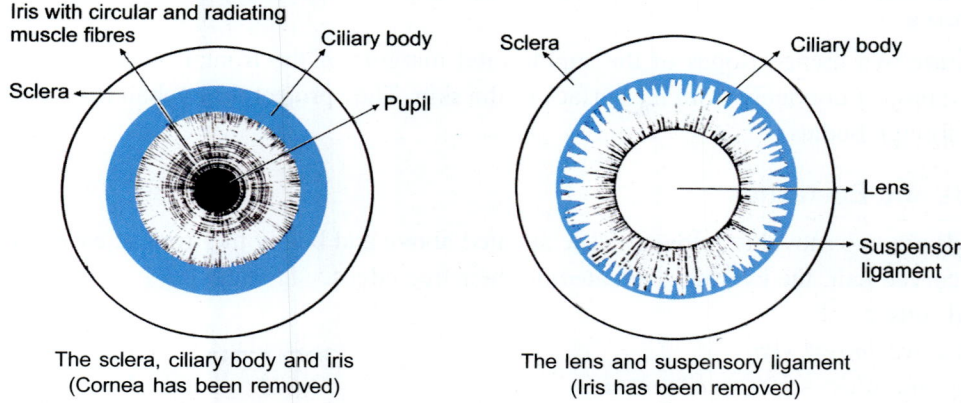

The sclera, ciliary body and iris (Cornea has been removed)

The lens and suspensory ligament (Iris has been removed)

2. *Optic disc*—Optic disc is a circular, pink coloured disc of 1.5 mm diameter. It has only nerve fibre layer so it does not excite any visual response. It is known as the *blind spot*.
3. *The optic nerve*—The optic nerve extends from the lamina cribrosa up to the optic chiasma. The total length of the optic nerve is 5 cm. It has four parts namely,

Intraocular — 1 mm
Intraorbital — 25 mm
Intraosseous — 4-10 mm
Intracranial — 10 mm (Duke–Elder).

INTERIOR OF THE EYEBALL

1. Aqueous Humour

Both anterior and posterior chambers contain a clear aqueous humour fluid secreted into the posterior chamber by the ciliary epithelium. It passes in front of the lens, through the pupil into the anterior chamber and returns to the venous circulation through the canal of Schlemm situated in the angle of anterior chamber.

2. Lens

Lens is a transparent, circular, biconvex structure lying immediately behind the pupil. It is suspended from the ciliary body by the suspensory ligament or zonule of Zinn. It is enclosed within a transparent capsule.

3. Vitreous

Vitreous is a transparent, colourless, inert gel which fills the posterior 4/5 of the eyeball. It contains few hyalocytes and wandering leucocytes. It consists of 99% water, some salts and mucoproteins.

ACCESSORY STRUCTURES OF THE EYE

The eye is a delicate organ which is protected by several structures such as eyebrows, eyelids, eyelashes and extraocular muscles.

6 Basic Ophthalmology

1. Eyebrows

Eyebrows are two arched ridges of the supraorbital margins of the frontal bone. Numerous hair (eyebrows) project obliquely from the surface of the skin. They protect the eyeball from sweat, dust and other foreign bodies.

2. Eyelids and Eyelashes

The eyelids are two movable folds of tissue situated above and below the front of each eye. There are short curved hair, the eyelashes situated on their free edges.
The eyelid consists of:
- *A thin covering of skin*
- *Three muscles—the orbicularis oculi, levator palpebrae superioris and Müller's muscles*
- *A sheet of dense connective tissue, the tarsal plate*
- *A lining of the conjunctiva.*

3. Lacrimal Apparatus

Lacrimal apparatus consists of:
- *Lacrimal gland and its ducts*
- *Accessory lacrimal glands*
- *Lacrimal canaliculi*
- *Lacrimal sac*
- *Nasolacrimal duct*

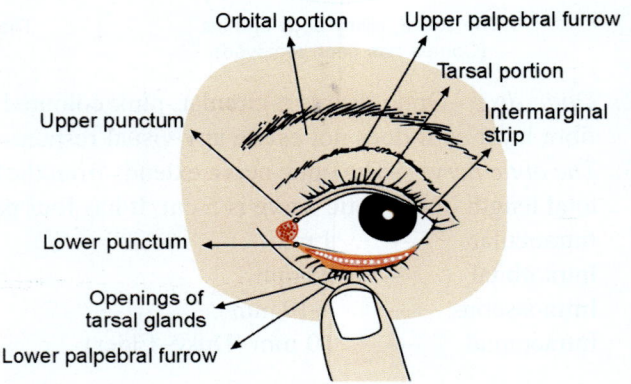

Gross anatomy of the eyelid

The tears are secreted by the lacrimal gland and accessory lacrimal glands. They drain into the conjunctival sac by small ducts. The tears then pass into the lacrimal sac (via the two canaliculi), nasolacrimal duct and finally into the nasal cavity (inferior meatus).

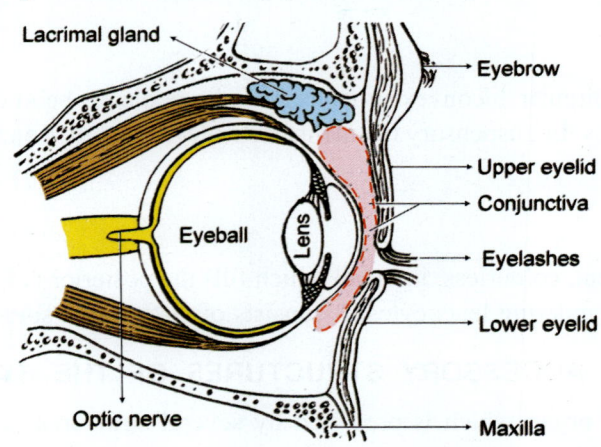

Section of the eye and its accessory structures

4. Extraocular Muscles of the Eye

The eyeballs are moved by six extrinsic muscles, attached at one end to the eyeball and at the other to the walls of the orbital cavity. There are four straight and two oblique muscles.

They consist of striated muscle fibres. Movement of the eyes to look in a particular direction is under voluntary control but co-ordination of movement needed for convergence and accommodation to near or distant vision, is under autonomic control.

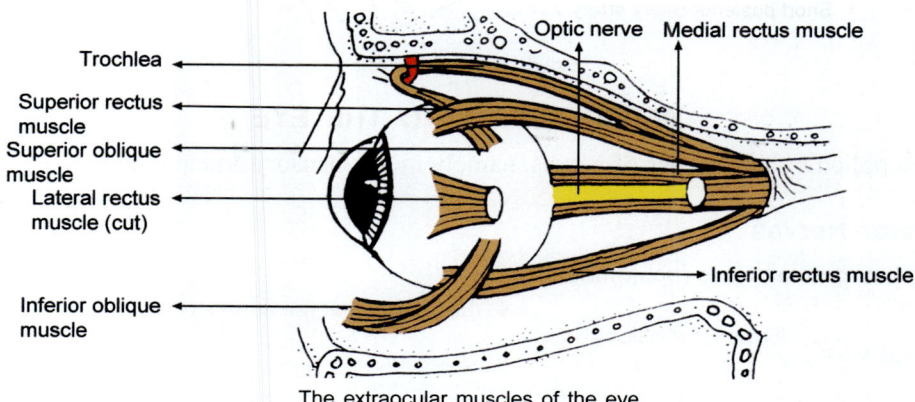

The extraocular muscles of the eye

The medial rectus rotates the eyeball inwards.
The lateral rectus rotates the eyeball outwards.
The superior rectus rotates the eyeball upwards.
The inferior rectus rotates the eyeball downwards.
The superior oblique rotates the eyeball so that the cornea turns in a downward and outward directions.
The inferior oblique rotates the eyeball so that the cornea turns upwards and outwards.

BLOOD SUPPLY TO THE EYE

Arterial Supply

The eye is supplied by the short (about 20 in number) and long ciliary (2 in number) arteries and the central retinal artery. These are branches of the ophthalmic artery, which is one of the branch of the internal carotid artery.

Venous Drainage

Venous drainage is done by the short ciliary veins, anterior ciliary veins, 4 vortex veins and the central retinal vein. These eventually empty into the cavernous sinus.

8 Basic Ophthalmology

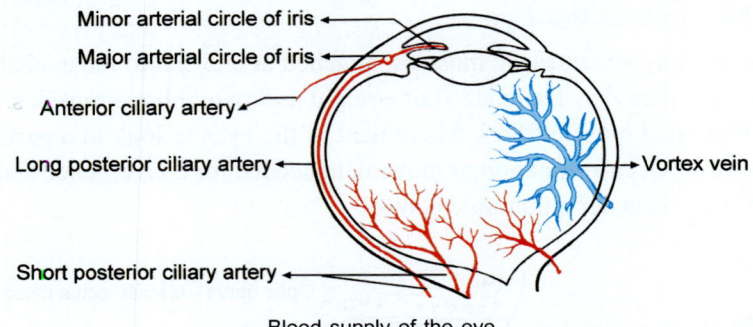

Blood supply of the eye

NERVE SUPPLY TO THE EYE

The eye is supplied by three types of nerves, namely motor, sensory and autonomic.

1. The Motor Nerves
   i. The third cranial nerve (oculomotor)

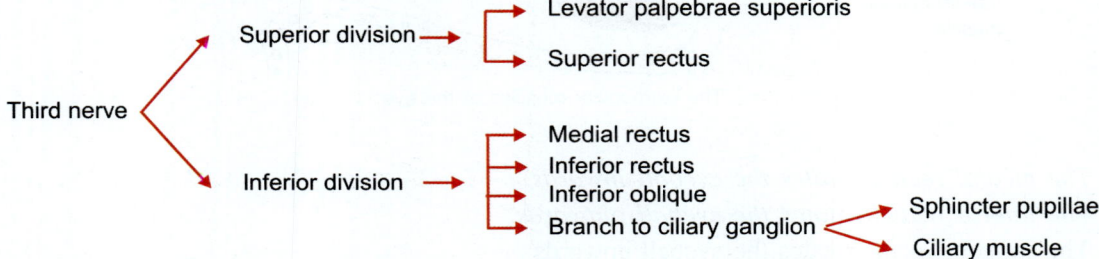

   ii. The 4th cranial nerve [trochlear]—It supplies the superior oblique muscle.
   iii. The 6th cranial nerve [abducens]—It supplies the lateral rectus muscle.
   iv. The 7th cranial nerve [facial]—It supplies the orbicularis oculi muscle.

2. The Sensory Nerve
The 5th cranial nerve [trigeminal]—The ophthalmic division supplies the whole eye.

3. The Autonomic Nerves
1. The sympathetic nerve supply is through the cervical sympathetic fibres to:
   i. *Iris—Dilator pupillae muscle*
   ii. *Ciliary body*
   iii. *Müller's muscle in the lids*
   iv. *Lacrimal gland.*
2. The parasympathetic nerve supply originates from the nuclei in the midbrain. It gives branches to:
   i. *Iris—Sphincter pupillae muscle*
   ii. *Ciliary body*
   iii. *Lacrimal gland.*

CHAPTER 2
Physiology of Vision

Light waves travel at a speed of 300,000 kilometres per second. Light is reflected into the eyes by objects within the field of vision. White light is a combination of all the colours of the visual spectrum, i.e. red, orange, yellow, green, blue, indigo, and violet. This can be demonstrated by passing white light through a glass prism which refracts or bends the rays of the different colours to a greater or lesser extent, depending on their wavelengths. Red light has the longest wavelength and violet the shortest. This range of colours is the spectrum of visible light. In a rainbow, white light from the sun is broken up by raindrops which act as prisms and reflectors.

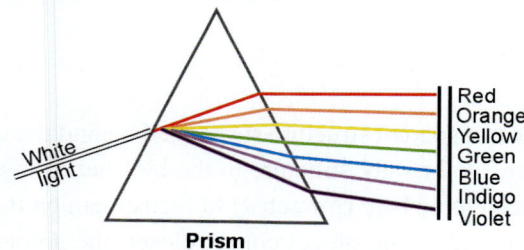

White light broken into the colours of the visible spectrum when passed through a prism

The Spectrum of Light

The spectrum of light is broad but only a small part is visible to the human eye. The visible spectrum extends from 723 nm at the red end to 397 nm at the violet end or roughly 700 to 400 nm. Beyond the long end there are infrared (heat), radar and radio waves. Beyond the short end there are ultraviolet (UV), X-ray and cosmic waves. UV light is not normally visible because it is absorbed by a yellow pigment in the lens. Following removal of the lens (cataract operation), UV light is visible and it has been suggested that long-term exposure may damage the retina.

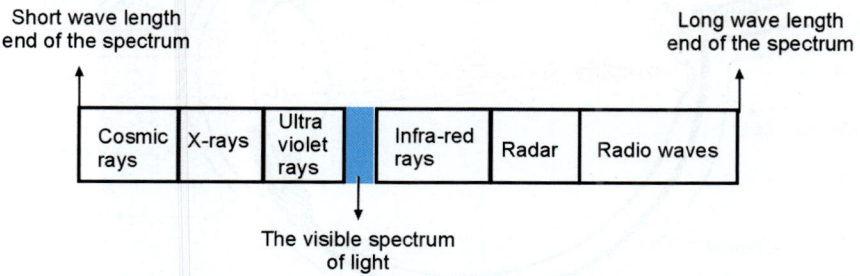

A specific colour is perceived when only one wavelength is reflected by the object and all the others are absorbed, e.g. an object appears red when only the red wavelength is reflected. Objects appear white when all wavelengths are reflected, and black when they are all absorbed.

PHYSIOLOGY OF VISION

In order to achieve clear vision, light reflected from objects within the visual field is focused on to the retina of both eyes. The processes involved in producing a clear image are:
1. Refraction of the light rays
2. Accommodation of the eyes to light.

Although these may be considered as separate processes, effective vision is dependent upon their coordination.

1. REFRACTION OF THE LIGHT RAYS

When light rays pass from a medium of one density to a medium of a different density they are refracted or bent. This principle is used in the eye to focus light on the retina. Before reaching the retina light rays pass successively through the conjunctiva, cornea, aqueous fluid, lens and vitreous. They are all more dense than air and with the exception of the lens, they have a constant refractory power similar to that of water.

Lens

The lens is a biconvex elastic transparent structure suspended behind the iris from the ciliary body by the suspensory ligament. Lens is the only structure in the eye that changes its refractive power. All light rays entering the eye need to be bent (refracted) to focus them on the retina. Light from distant objects needs least refraction and as the object comes closer, the amount needed is increased. To increase the refractive power the ciliary muscle contracts, releasing its pull on the suspensory ligament and the anterior surface of the lens bulges forward, increasing its convexity. When the ciliary muscle relaxes it slips backwards, increasing its pull on the suspensory ligament, making the lens thinner.

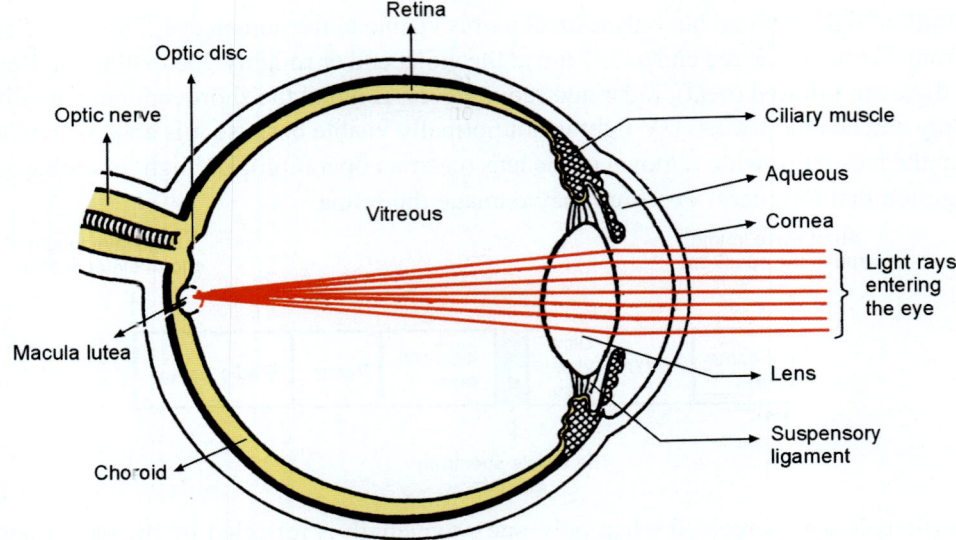

Section of the eye showing the focussing of light rays on the retina

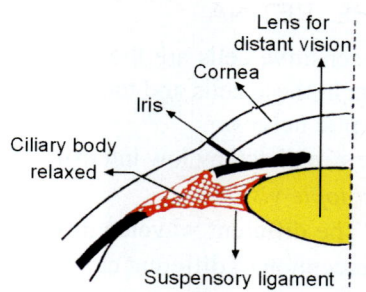 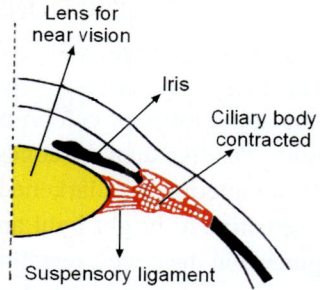

Diagram of the difference in the shape of the lens for distant and near vision

Looking at near objects 'tires' the eyes more quickly due to the continuous use of the ciliary muscle.

2. ACCOMMODATION OF THE EYES TO LIGHT

There are three factors which are involved in accommodation
1. Pupil
2. Movement of the eyeballs-convergence
3. Lens.

1. Size of the Pupil

Pupil size influences accommodation by controlling the amount of light entering the eye. In a bright light the pupils are constricted. In a dim light they are dilated.

If the pupils were dilated in a bright light, too much light would enter the eye and damage the retina. In a dim light, if the pupils were constricted, insufficient light would enter the eye to activate the photosensitive pigments in the rods and cones which stimulate the nerve endings in the retina.

The iris consists of one layer of circular and one of radiating smooth muscle fibres. Contraction of the circular fibres constricts the pupil, and contraction of the radiating fibres dilates it. The size of the pupil is controlled by the nerves of the autonomic nervous system. Sympathetic stimulation dilates the pupil and parasympathetic stimulation causes contraction of the pupil.

2. Movements of the Eyeballs-convergence

Light rays from objects enter the two eyes at different angles and for clear vision they must stimulate corresponding areas of the two retinae. Extraocular muscles move the eyes and to obtain a clear image they rotate the eyes so that they converge on the object viewed. This co-ordinated muscle activity is under autonomic control. When there is voluntary movement of the eyes both eyes move and convergence is maintained. The nearer an object is to the eyes the greater the eye rotation needed to achieve convergence. If convergence is not complete there is double vision, i.e. diplopia. After a period of time during which convergence is not possible, the brain tends to ignore the impulses received from the divergent eye.

FUNCTIONS OF THE RETINA

The retina is the photosensitive part of eye. The light sensitive cells are the rods and cones. Light rays cause chemical changes in photosensitive pigments in these cells and they emit nerve impulses which pass to the occipital lobes of cerebrum via the optic nerves.

The rods are more sensitive than the cones. They are stimulated by low intensity or dim light, e.g. by the dim light in the interior of a darkened room *(scotopic vision)*.

The cones are sensitive to bright light and colour. The different wavelengths of light stimulate photosensitive pigments in the cones, resulting in the perception of different colours. In a bright light the light rays are focused on the macula lutea *(photopic vision)*.

The rods are more numerous towards the periphery of the retina. Visual purple (rhodopsin) is a photosensitive pigment present only in the rods. It is bleached by bright light and when this occurs the rods cannot be stimulated. Rhodopsin is quickly reconstituted when an adequate supply of vitamin A is available. When the individual moves from an area of bright light to one of dim light, there is variable period of time when it is difficult to see. The rate at which dark adaptation takes place is dependent upon the rate of reconstitution of rhodopsin. In dim evening light different colours cannot be distinguished because the light intensity is insufficient to stimulate colour sensitive pigments in cones.

VISUAL PERCEPTIONS

Visual perceptions are of four types namely,

1. Light Sense

Light sense is the faculty which permits us to perceive light as such and in all its gradation of intensity.

Light Minimum

Light minimum is the minimum intensity of light appreciated by the retina. If the light which is falling on the retina is gradually reduced in intensity, a point comes when light is no longer perceived.

Dark Adaptation

Dark adaptation is the ability of the eye to adapt itself to decreasing illumination. If one goes from a bright light into a dimly lit room, one cannot perceive the objects in the room until sometime has elapsed. This time interval is known as dark adaptation.

2. Form Sense

Form sense is the faculty which enables us to perceive the shape of objects. Visual acuity is a record of form sense.

3. Sense of Contrast

Sense of contrast is the ability to perceive slight changes in luminance between regions which are not separated by definite borders.

4. Colour Sense

Colour sense is that faculty which helps us to distinguish between different colours as excited by light of different wavelengths. Three important factors influence colour vision:
  i. Wavelength
  ii. Brightness or luminosity
  iii. Saturation or calorimetric purity

The normal colour vision is called "trichromatic" (red, green, blue) and it is the basis of the Young-Helmholtz theory. When red, green, and blue portion of spectrum mix together, they produce white colour. Thus red, green, and blue are known as primary colours. The exact nature of the defect is tested by:

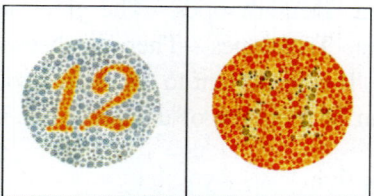

Ishihara isochromatic plates

1. *Isochromatic chart*—These are coloured lithographic plates in which bold numbers are represented in dots of various colours, e.g. Japanese Ishihara lithographic plates, American H-R-R test, Swedish-Bostrom test. Colour blind person finds it difficult to identify the bold numbers.
2. *The lantern test*—Various colours are shown by a lantern, e.g. Edridge-Green's lantern. He is judged by the mistakes he makes.
3. *Holmgren's wools*—This consists of a selection of skeins of coloured wools from which the candidate is required to make a series of colour matches.
4. *Nagel's anomaloscope*—A bright disc coloured yellow, red, and green is used.
5. *The Farnsworth-Munsell 100 hue test*—This represents hue discrimination by an error score. Patients with toxic optic neuropathy show a characteristic pattern.

COLOUR BLINDNESS [ACHROMATOPSIA]

It is an inability to recognise colour. Defective colour vision is seen in 1% males and 0.4% females.

Etiology

1. *Congenital*—There is absence of red, green or blue pigments in the cones. It can be either partial or complete. It is an inherited condition being transmitted through females. It is bilateral and incurable.

   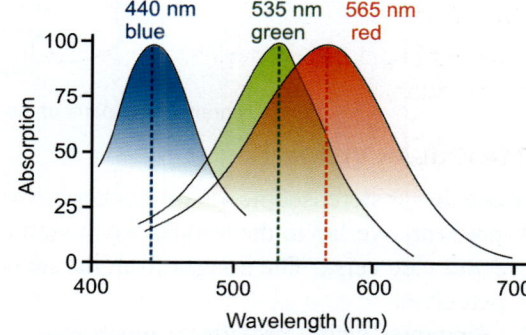

   Absorption spectrum of three cone pigments

    i. *Partial colour blindness*—A person cannot recognise green, red or blue colours. Green blindness is most common. There is absence of one or two of the photopigments normally found in foveal cones.
    ii. *Total colour blindness*—A person cannot recognise any colour and sees everything grey. It is rare and is associated with nystagmus and central scotoma.
2. *Acquired*—This is due to the diseases of the macula and optic nerve, e.g. macular degenerations, toxic amblyopias. Blue blindness occurs in sclerosing black cataracts which is said to affect the paintings of artists in old age.

14 Basic Ophthalmology

Types

In most cases red and green colours are confused.
  i. Protanopes—The red sensation is defective.
  ii. Deuteranopes—The green sensation is defective.
  iii. Tritanopes—There is absense of blue sensation. It is very rare.

It is important to test colour vision in certain occupations like drivers, pilots, sailors, etc. as they can be a source of danger to the society.

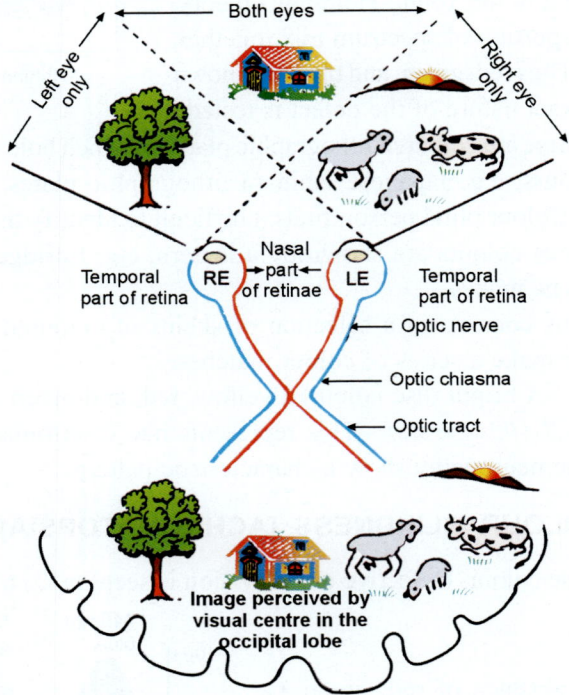

Diagram of the parts of the visual field monocular and binocular

BINOCULAR VISION

Binocular or stereoscopic vision has certain advantages. Each eye 'sees' a scene slightly differently. There is an overlap in the middle but the left eye sees more on the left than can be seen by the other eye and vice versa. The images from the two eyes are fused in the cerebrum so that only one image is perceived.

Binocular vision provides a much more accurate assessment of one object relative to another, e.g. its distance, depth, height and width. This is done by mechanisms of:
1. Simultaneous macular perception
2. Fusion
3. Stereopsis.

Some people with monocular vision may find it difficult to judge the speed and distance of an approaching vehicle.

CHAPTER 3
Neurology of Vision

THE VISUAL PATHWAY AND ITS LESIONS

The visual pathway consists of:
1. *The optic nerves*
2. *The optic chiasma*
3. *The optic tracts*
4. *The lateral geniculate bodies*
5. *The optic radiations*
6. *The occipital cortex.*

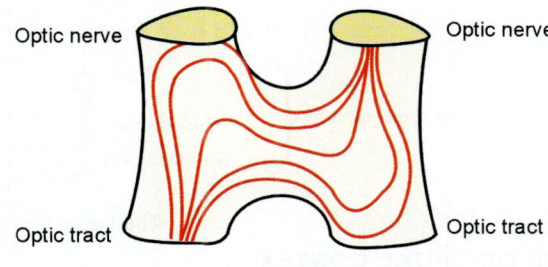

The optic chiasma

1. THE OPTIC NERVES

The fibres of the optic nerve originate in the retina. The retina is divided into the temporal and nasal halves at the level of the fovea centralis. The optic nerves join the optic chiasma at the anterolateral angle.

2. THE OPTIC CHIASMA

It is a flat band-like structure lying above the pituitary fossa. In the optic chiasma there is semi-decussation of the nerve fibres.
   i. The nerve fibres from the nasal side of each retina cross-over to the opposite side.
   ii. The nerve fibres from the temporal side do not cross but pass into optic tracts of the same side.

3. THE OPTIC TRACT

The optic tracts originate from the postero-lateral angle of the optic chiasma. They are cylindrical bands running outwards and backwards to end in the lateral geniculate bodies. They consist of the temporal fibres of the same side and the nasal fibres of the opposite side.

4. THE LATERAL GENICULATE BODIES

These are oval structures situated at the posterior end of the optic tracts. The fibres of the optic tracts end in the lateral geniculate bodies and new fibres of the optic radiations originate from them.

5. THE OPTIC RADIATIONS

The nerve fibres proceed backwards and medially as the optic radiations to terminate in the visual centres situated in the occipital lobes.

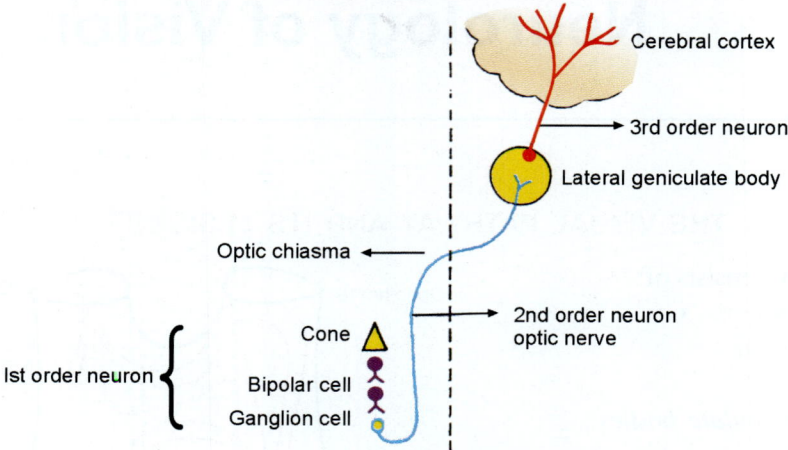

The visual nerve pathway

6. THE OCCIPITAL CORTEX

It is situated above and below the calcarine fissure in the occipital lobes extending up to the occipital pole.

The visual nerve pathway can be divided into three parts:

1. *The neuron of the first order* is the bipolar cell in the retina. The rods and cones are the sensory end organs.
2. *The neuron of the second order* is the ganglion cell in the retina, the process of which pass along the optic nerve, optic chiasma and optic tract to the lateral geniculate body.
3. *The neuron of the third order* takes up the impulses via the optic radiations to the occipital lobe (visual centre).

LESIONS OF THE VISUAL PATHWAY

Lesions of the visual pathway usually cause defects in the visual fields and diminution of visual acuity depending on the site of lesion.
1. Hemianopia
2. Amblyopia
3. Amaurosis.

1. HEMIANOPIA

Hemianopia is a condition of loss of half the field of vision of both eyes.

Etiology

Lesions in the visual pathway may be commonly due to:
  i. *Trauma,* e.g. injury by the falls on the back of the head, gun shot wounds.
 ii. *Tumour,* e.g. cerebral tumour, pituitary gland tumour.

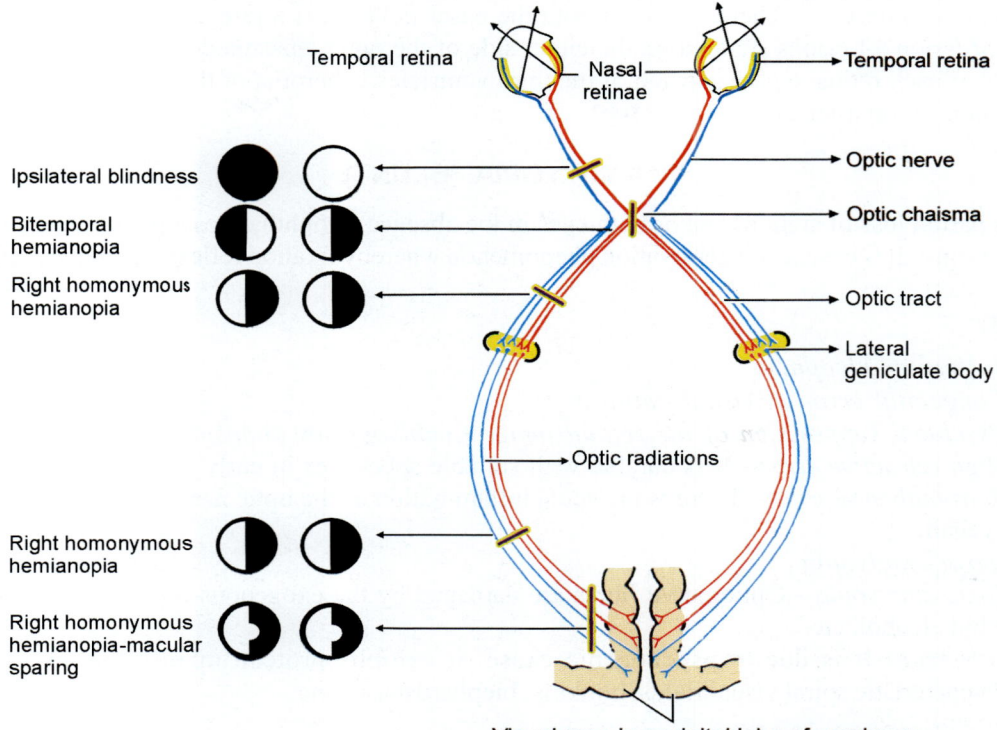

iii. *Vascular lesion,* e.g. aneurysms, atheroma of carotids, cerebral thrombosis.
iv. *Inflammation,* e.g. meningitis, chronic arachnoiditis, encephalitis.
v. *Degeneration,* e.g. multiple sclerosis.

Types

1. *Homonymous hemianopia*—There is loss of right or left half of binocular field of vision. Lesions of the occipital lobe often result in homonymous hemianopia with sparing of the fixation area.
   Site of lesion—Optic tract, optic radiations and occipital lobe, e.g. vascular lesions.

2. *Bitemporal hemianopia*—There is loss of both the temporal fields.
   Site of lesion—Lesions of the central part of optic chiasma, e.g. pituitary tumour, aneurysms.

3. *Binasal hemianopia*—There is loss of both the nasal fields. It is a rare condition.
   Site of lesion—Lesions situated on the either side of the optic chiasma destroying the temporal fibres of each retina, e.g. distension of the third ventricles, atheroma of the carotids or posterior communication arteries.

2. AMBLYOPIA (BLUNT)

There is partial loss of sight in one or both eyes in the absence of ophthalmoscopic or other marked objective signs. It is basically a deprivation phenomenon whereby fixation reflexes are not developed.

Etiology

1. *Unilateral amblyopia*
   i. *Congenital error in visual pathway*
   ii. *Psychical suppression of the retinal image (amblyopia ex anopsia)*
   iii. *High refractive error*—It is curable with suitable spectacles in early life.
   iv. *Retrobulbar neuritis*—There is the acute inflammation of the optic nerve situated behind the eyeball.
2. *Bilateral amblyopia*
   i. *Toxic amblyopia*—Optic nerve fibres are damaged by the exogenous poisons, e.g. tobacco, ethyl alcohol, etc.
   ii. *Hysteria*—It is due to psychogenic cause. It exhibits protean manifestations such as characteristic spiral visual fields, blinking, blepharospasm, etc.

3. AMAUROSIS (DARK)

There is complete loss of sight in one or both eyes in the absence of ophthalmoscopic or other marked objective signs.

Etiology

1. *Unilateral amaurosis*
   i. *Amaurosis fugax*—There is sudden loss of vision due to embolisation of retinal circulation. The episode lasts for few minutes.
   ii. *Cardiovascular abnormalities* such as valvular defect, arrhythmias.
   iii. *Migraine*—There may be vasospasm of retinal vessels.
   iv. *Gaze-evoked amaurosis*—Transient loss of vision occurs in a particular direction of eccentric gaze.
2. *Bilateral amaurosis*
   i. *Uraemia*—It occurs in acute nephritis and chronic renal disease due to circulation of toxins, which act on visual centres.
   ii. *Meningitis, encephalitis*—The visual pathway and centre are affected.
   iii. *Hysteria*—Psychogenic aspect of the disease is often treated but great care is taken to eliminate any organic disease.
   iv. *Lebers congenital amaurosis (retinal aplasia)*—It is characterised by reduced visual acuity, head nodding and nystagmus.

MULTIPLE CHOICE QUESTIONS

1. Lens develops from
   a. neural ectoderm
   b. surface ectoderm
   c. optic vesicle
   d. all of the above
2. Retina develops from
   a. surface ectoderm
   b. mesoderm
   c. optic vesicle
   d. embryonic fissure
3. Muscles controlling pupil arise from
   a. mesoderm
   b. ectoderm
   c. endoderm
   d. none of the above
4. The avascular structure of eye is
   a. choroid
   b. lens
   c. conjunctiva
   d. ciliary body
5. Aqueous humour is secreted by
   a. angle of anterior chamber
   b. choroid
   c. ciliary body
   d. iris
6. Optic disc is also known as
   a. macula lutea
   b. blind spot
   c. fovea
   d. rods and cones
7. Superior oblique muscle is supplied by the
   a. optic nerve
   b. third cranial nerve
   c. fourth cranial nerve
   d. sixth cranial nerve
8. The sensory nerve supply of the eye is by the
   a. optic nerve
   b. third cranial nerve
   c. fifth cranial nerve
   d. seventh cranial nerve
9. Optic nerve contains
   a. pigment layer
   b. ganglion cell layer
   c. nerve fibre layer
   d. all of the above
10. The junction of cornea and sclera is known as
    a. angle of anterior chamber
    b. ciliary body
    c. pupil
    d. limbus
11. Tarsal plate is situated in
    a. eyebrow
    b. eyelid
    c. lacrimal apparatus
    d. conjunctiva
12. Between epithelium and stroma of cornea lies
    a. Bowman's membrane
    b. Descemet's membrane
    c. endothelium
    d. none of the above
13. Lamina cribrosa is present in
    a. choroid
    b. ciliary body
    c. sclera
    d. retina

14. Suspensory ligament extends between lens and
    a. iris
    b. ciliary body
    c. choroid
    d. limbus
15. Oculomotor nerve palsy features include all, *EXCEPT*
    a. facial weakness
    b. divergent squint
    c. dilated fixed pupil
    d. absent accommodation
16. The normal trichromatic colour vision consists of following colours
    a. red, blue, yellow
    b. red, blue, green
    c. red, blue, white
    d. red, green, yellow
17. The trichromatic theory of colour vision has been propounded by
    a. Schiotz
    b. von Graefe
    c. Young-Helmholtz
    d. none of the above
18. The intraorbital length of the optic nerve is
    a. 1 mm
    b. 5 mm
    c. 10 mm
    d. 25 mm
19. The total length of the optic nerve is
    a. 2.5 cm
    b. 3 cm
    c. 4.5 cm
    d. 5 cm
20. The neuron of the 1st order in the visual pathway lies in which layer of retina
    a. inner plexiform
    b. outer plexiform
    c. optic nerve fibre
    d. none of the above
21. Lesion of the optic tract causes
    a. homonymous hemianopia
    b. bitemporal hemianopia
    c. binasal hemianopia
    d. ipsilateral blindness
22. Scotopic vision is due to
    a. cones
    b. rods
    c. both
    d. none
23. Visual acuity is a record of
    a. light sense
    b. form sense
    c. contrast sense
    d. colour sense
24. Visual centre is situated in
    a. parietal lobe
    b. frontal lobe
    c. midbrain
    d. occipital lobe
25. Optic nerve extends up to
    a. optic chiasma
    b. optic tracts
    c. lateral geniculate body
    d. optic radiations
26. Visible spectrum extends from
    a. 100-300 nm
    b. 300-650 nm
    c. 400-700 nm
    d. 720-920 nm
27. Vortex vein drain
    a. iris and ciliary body
    b. sclera
    c. uveal tract
    d. retina

28. Highest visual resolution is seen in
    a. macula lutea
    b. fovea centralis
    c. optic disc
    d. ora serrata
29. Second order neurons in the optic pathway are present in
    a. superior colliculus
    b. retina
    c. medial geniculate body
    d. lateral geniculate body
30. Bitemporal hemianopia is seen with
    a. aneurysm of circle of Willis
    b. temporal SOL
    c. frontal SOL
    d. retinoblastoma

ANSWERS

1—b	2—c	3—b	4—b	5—c
6—b	7—c	8—c	9—c	10—d
11—b	12—a	13—c	14—b	15—a
16—b	17—c	18—d	19—d	20—d
21—a	22—b	23—b	24—d	25—a
26—c	27—c	28—b	29—b	30—a

CHAPTER 4
Examination of the Eye

HISTORY

Patient is encouraged to narrate his complaints but relevant enquiries are made.

PRESENT HISTORY
1. **Name, Age, Sex, Occupation**
2. **Dimness of Vision**
   - Mode of onset—It may be sudden or gradual:
     Sudden loss of vision commonly occurs in central retinal artery occlusion and central retinal vein occlusion, retinal detachment, papillitis, acute congestive glaucoma, vitreous haemorrhage, etc.
     Gradual loss of vision commonly occurs in cataract, open angle glaucoma, uveitis maculopathy, toxic amblyopia, chorioretinal degenerations, optic atrophy, etc.
   - Duration—Short or long
   - For distance or near
   - Seeing double objects—This commonly occurs in cases of paralytic squint.
   - Seeing flashes of light—It is usually due to retinal disease or high myopia.
   - Night blindness—It is common in vitamin A deficiency, liver disorders (cirrhosis), retinitis pigmentosa, congenital night blindness, extensive chorioretinitis.
   - Associated with photophobia, lacrimation, blepharospasm as in keratitis.
3. **Pain in the Eyes**
   - Mode of onset—It may be sudden or gradual
   - Severity and duration—It may be mild, moderate or severe
   - Relation to close work—It is common in refractive errors
   - Time of the day when maximum—Eye strain is maximum in the evening in refractive errors
   - Associated nausea, vomiting, photophobia, impaired vision occurs in acute glaucoma.
4. **Redness, Congestion or Inflammation**
   - Of the eyelids
   - Of the area surrounding the eye
   - Of the eyeball.
5. **Secretion**
   - Excessive normal secretion
   - Type of altered secretion (discharge), e.g. mucopurulent, purulent, ropy

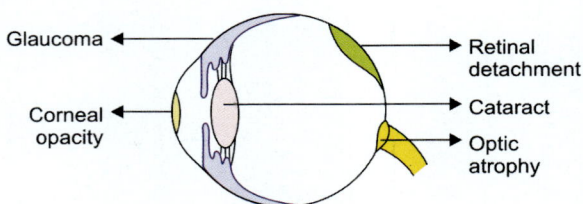

Common causes of dimness of vision

- Sticking together of lids in the morning is suggestive of acute conjunctivitis
- Associated crusts or flakes in the lid margin are seen in blepharitis.

6. Disturbances of the Eyeball

Eyelids
- Altered position—drooping of the lids below the normal position occurs in ptosis
- Altered direction of the margin, e.g. entropion, ectropion
- Disturbance in function, e.g. inability to close the lids leading to exposure

Direction • Eyes are turned out, in, up or down in squint

Fixation • Eyes "shakes" due to involuntary movements as in nystagmus.

7. Headache
- Location—frontal or occipital
- Severity and type—dull or throbbing
- Relation to near work
- Time of the day when maximum
- Factors which relieve or aggravate it
- Associated nausea, vomiting, blurred vision.

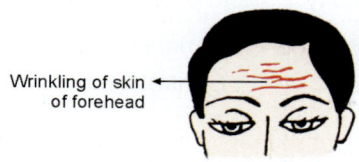

Ptosis

PAST HISTORY

Previous diseases, treatment or operation history of using glasses for distance or near.

PERSONAL HISTORY

Habits—Sleep, tobacco and alcohol intake, diet, digestion and bowel habits.
Blood pressure and diabetes mellitus.
Kidney, blood and heart diseases.
Foci of infection in teeth, tonsils, ears and sinuses.

Ocular causes of headache
1. Refractive errors
2. Poor accommodation and convergence
3. Contact lens overwear
4. Acute congestive glaucoma
5. Iritis
6. Herpes zoster
7. Orbital cellulitis
8. Superior orbital fissure syndrome

FAMILY HISTORY

Diabetes mellitus, hypertension, myopia, glaucoma, congenital cataract.

EXAMINATION OF THE EYE

1. EXAMINATION OF THE ANTERIOR SEGMENT OF THE EYE

1. Inspection
2. Palpation
3. Intraocular tension
4. Binocular loupe and slit-lamp examination
5. Gonioscope examination
6. Transillumination.

2. EXAMINATION OF THE POSTERIOR SEGMENT OF THE EYE

I. Examination of the Retinal Functions

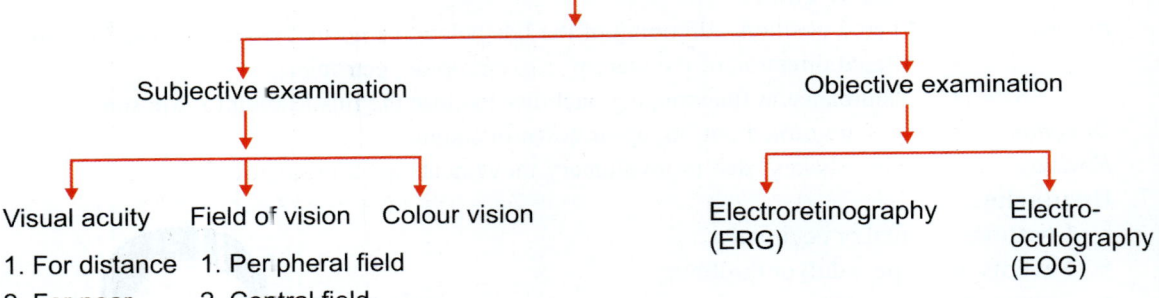

II. Examination of the Fundus Oculi

EXAMINATION OF THE ANTERIOR SEGMENT OF THE EYE

1. INSPECTION

Examination of the anterior segment of the eye is made by general inspection in good diffuse light.

1. **Head**—Position is characteristic in paralysis of extraocular muscles and ptosis.
2. **Face**—Asymmetry, facial paralysis, affections of the skin, e.g. herpes zoster.
3. **Eyebrows**—Loss of hair or depigmentation, e.g. leprosy. They are elevated due to the overaction of frontalis muscle, e.g. ptosis.
4. **Orbits**—Exophthalmos, enophthalmos, orbital cellulitis.
5. **Eyeballs**
    i. *Position and direction*—They are abnormal in cases of squint, exophthalmos, enophthalmos, phthisis bulbi, etc.
    ii. *Movements*—Involuntary oscillations are present in nystagmus.
    iii. *Size and shape*—Eyeball is small in microphthalmia
       - It is large in buphthalmos (infantile glaucoma), myopia, staphyloma.
6. **Eyelids**
    i. *Position*—Drooping of the upper lid below its normal position occurs in ptosis
       - There is outrolling of lid margin (ectropion)
       - There is inrolling of lid margin (entropion)
    ii. *Palpebral aperture*—It may be narrow, e.g. ptosis
       - It may be wide, e.g. exophthalmos, Bell's palsy
    iii. *Movement*—It is restricted in symblepharon, i.e., adhesion of the lids to the globe as in acid burn cases.
    iv. *Margins*—Crusts are seen in blepharitis, i.e., inflammation of lid margin
       - It may be thickened (tylosis) as in trachoma.
    v. *Lashes*—These are misdirected backwards and rub against the cornea (trichiasis)
       - Scanty (madarosis)

- The lashes are white in colour (poliosis)
- Multiple rows of eyelashes are present which rub against the cornea (distichiasis).

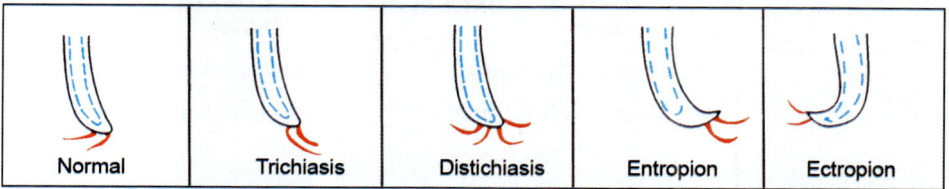

Section of the upper eyelid showing normal and abnormal position of tarsus and eyelashes

vi. *Glands*—Stye is situated at or near the lid margin
   - Chalazion is situated a little away from the lid margin.
vii. *Lacrimal puncta*—Eversion of the puncta is seen in ectropion
   - Occlusion may be present due to scarting or eyelash.

7. **Lacrimal Sac**
   - Swelling and redness (mucocele).
   - Regurgitation test—There is watery, mucoid or purulent discharge through the puncta on pressure over the sac area.
   - Fistula may be present due to repeated rupture or leakage from the infected sac with epitheliazation of the fistulous track.

8. **Conjunctiva**
   i. *Bulbar*—Congestion (conjunctival and ciliary)
      - Secretion, chemosis or oedema or subconjunctival haemorrhage may be present
      - Phlycten, growth, pterygium, cyst or Bitot's spot (vitamin A deficiency).
   ii. *Palpebral*—The upper lid is everted by asking the patient to look downwards. A gentle pull on the eyelashes and simultaneous pressure over the skin of the upper lid by index finger or glass rod is given to evert the upper lid. The lower palpebral conjunctiva and fornix are exposed by pulling the lower lid downwards. Both upper and lower lids are examined for,
      - Congestion as in conjunctivitis.
      - Follicles, papillae, foreign body, concretions
      - Scarring, e.g. trachoma, chemical burn
      - Membrane as in diphtheria, streptococcal conjunctivitis
      - Symblepharon, i.e. adhesion of the lids to the globe, e.g. chemical burn.

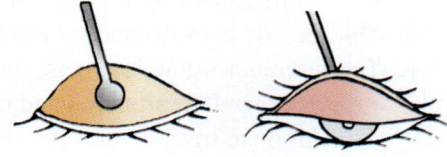

Eversion of upper eyelid

   iii. *Plica semilunaris*—It may be displaced by pterygium growth.
   iv. *Caruncle*—There may be inflammation or growth.

9. **Cornea**—In children and in marked blepharospasm, lid retractor may be used for examination after instillation of local anaesthetic.
   i. *Size*—Normal vertical diameter is 11 mm and horizontal diameter is 12 mm.

DIFFERENCES BETWEEN CONJUNCTIVAL AND CILIARY CONGESTION

	CONJUNCTIVAL CONGESTION	CILIARY CONGESTION
1. *Site*	Most marked in fornix	Most marked around the limbus
2. *Colour*	Bright red, well-defined	Greyish red (violet), ill-defined
3. *Vessels and branches*	• Superficial vessels (anterior and posterior conjunctival) • Branch dichotomously forming arborescent pattern	• Deep vessels (anterior ciliary) • Branches are parallel or radially arranged
4. *Pressure effect*	After emptying the vessels by pressure, (glass rod) they fill from the fornix	• Vessels fill from the limbus
5. *Common causes*	Acute conjunctivitis	Keratitis Acute and chronic iridocyclitis Acute congestive glaucoma

- It is measured by the keratometer.
- It is small in microphthalmos.
- It is large in buphthalmos, megalocornea and myopia.

ii. *Curvature*—Normal radius of curvature is 7.8 mm.
- It is measured by the keratometer—It may be conical, globular or flat.

iii. *Surface*—It is examined by the Placido's disc (keratoscope) or window reflex.

iv. *Transparency*—Facet, ulcers, opacities (nebula, macula, leucoma) may be present.
- Position—The situation and extent of the opacity is noted in relation to iris.
- Pigmentation over the opacity is seen in adherent leucoma
- Any iris adhesion or anterior synechia.
- Pannus or vascularisation
- Striate keratitis (postoperative) are noted.

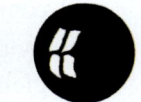

Corneal ulcer

Normal   Abnormal

v. *Sensation*—It is tested by touching the cornea with a wisp of cotton wool. Normally there is a brisk reflex closure of the lids. This is known as the corneal reflex.

Examination of the Eye

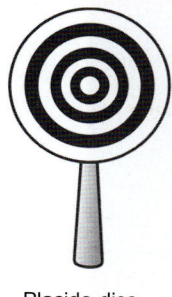
Placido disc

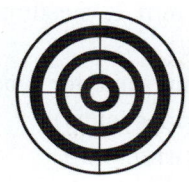
Normal corneal reflex

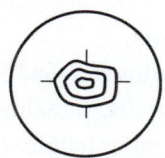
Irregular corneal reflex in keratoconus

Placido's disc (Keratoscope)

Common causes of loss or diminished corneal sensation
1. Herpes simplex
2. Herpes zoster
3. Acute congestive glaucoma
4. Absolute glaucoma
5. Leucomatous corneal opacity
6. Leprosy
7. Following alcohol injection in the Gasserian ganglion (Trigeminal neuralgia)

  vi. *Thickness*—The thickness of the periphery of the cornea is 0.67 mm. It is 0.52 mm thick in the centre. It is measured by the pachymeter.

  vii. *Staining of the cornea by vital stains*
    a. *Fluorescein 2%*—It is the most useful and commonly used vital stain. It marks the areas of denuded epithelium due to abrasions, corneal ulcer, etc. It is available as drops or disposable strips.
      i. *Superficial staining*—A drop of fluorescein is instilled in the conjunctival sac.
- Excess dye is washed with normal saline after few seconds.
- The lesion is stained bright or brilliant green.

      ii. *Deep staining*—After instilling the dye the lids are kept closed for about 5 minutes.
- The dye penetrates the intact epithelium and any infiltration in the stroma takes up the dull grass green colour.
- The defects in the endothelium appear as green-yellow dots.

    b. *Bengal rose 1%*—It is a red aniline dye. It stains the diseased or devitalized cells red, e.g. as in superficial punctate keratitis and filaments, e.g. keratoconjunctivitis sicca.
    c. *Alcian blue*—It stains only excess mucus, e.g. as in keratoconjunctivitis sicca (dry eye).

10. **Sclera**
  i. *Curvature and colour*—There is thinning, pigmentation and ectasia of the sclera in myopia, staphyloma and blue sclerotics.
  ii. *Vessels*—Ciliary injection and nodule is seen in episcleritis and scleritis.

11. **Anterior Chamber**
    i. *Depth*—The normal depth is 2.5 mm. It is estimated by the position of the cornea and plane of the iris.
        - Shallow (closed angle glaucoma, anterior synechia)
        - Deep (buphthalmos, chronic iridocyclitis)
        - Irregular (subluxation of lens, iris bomb)
    ii. *Content*—Cloudy aqueous (acute iridocyclitis)
        - Pus (hypopyon corneal ulcer)
        - Blood (hyphaema due to trauma)
        - Lens matter (following extracapsular lens extraction and trauma)
        - Foreign body.

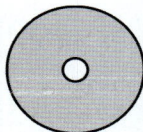 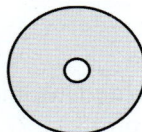

Heterochromia iridium

12. **Iris**
    i. *Colour*—Heterochromia iridium—The two irides are of different colour.

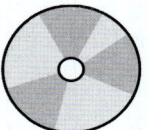 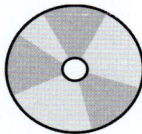

Heterochromia iridis

   - *Heterochromia iridis*—Parts of the same iris are of different colour, e.g. congenital, chronic iridocyclitis.
   - Muddy (iritis)
   - White atrophic patches (glaucoma, chronic iridocyclitis).
    ii. *Pattern*—Ill-defined or loss of pattern (chronic iridocyclitis)
    iii. *Position*—Plane of the iris is noted.
        - Anterior synechia—There is adhesion of the iris to the posterior surface of cornea.

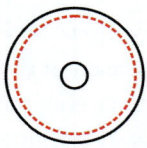 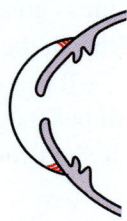

Anterior synechia

   - Posterior synechia—There is adhesion of the iris to the lens capsule.

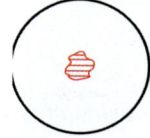 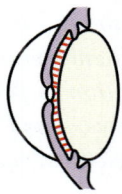

Posterior synechia

iv. *Tremulousness (Iridodonesis)*—Excessive movements or tremors of iris are seen best in a dark room (with oblique illumination) when eyes move rapidly, e.g. in aphakia or absence, shrinkage, dislocation and subluxation of lens.

13. **Pupil**
    Size—Normal size of the pupil is 2-4 mm
    Anisocoria—Unequal size of both the pupil is called anisocoria
    Miosis—The pupil is small and constricted
    Mydriasis—The pupil is dilated
    Miosis—The pupil is small and constricted due to the action of sphincter pupillae muscle.

Etiology

1. *Physiological*—Babies, old age, blue eyes
2. *Pharmacological*
   i. *Local*—Miotic, e.g. pilocarpine
   ii. *General*—Morphia
3. *Pathological*
   i. *Unilateral*—Acute iritis
      - Healed iritis
      - Horner's syndrome
   ii. *Bilateral*—Pontine haemorrhage
      - Argyll Robertson pupil

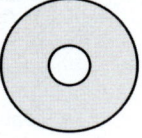 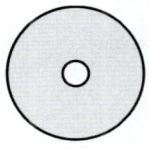 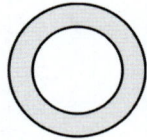

Normal   Miosis   Mydriasis

Mydriasis—The pupil is dilated due to the action of dilator pupillae muscle.

Etiology

1. *Physiological*—Myopia, nervous excitement
2. *Pharmacological*—Mydriatics, e.g. atropine, phenylephrine, cyclopentolate, tropicamide
3. *Pathological*
   i. *Retina and optic nerve diseases*
      - Optic nerve atrophy
      - Absolute glaucoma
      - Acute congestive glaucoma

ii. *Central lesion (above lateral geniculate body)*
    - Meningitis, haemorrhage, uraemia
    - The light reaction is present but the patient is blind
iii. *Third cranial nerve paralysis*—Trauma, syphilis, diphtheria, meningitis
iv. *Irritation of cervical sympathetics*, e.g. apical pneumonia, pleurisy, cervical rib.
2. Shape
   - Normally the pupil is central and circular.
   - Irregular (posterior synechia).
3. *Pupillary reactions (reflexes)*
   a. *Light reflex*
      i. Direct light reflex—If light enters an eye, the pupil of this eye contracts.
         Afferent pathway—The optic nerve
         Centre—Edinger-Westphal nucleus in midbrain (third nerve nucleus).
         Efferent pathway—The oculomotor nerve.

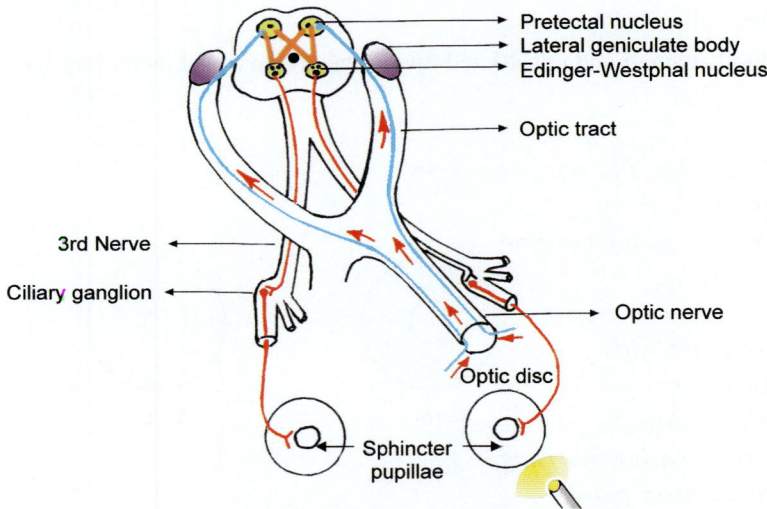

Pathway of the pupillary light reflex

   ii. Indirect (consensual) light reflex—If light enters an eye, the pupil of the other eye also contracts. The decussation of the nerve fibres in the midbrain explains the mechanism of the indirect reflex.
   b. *Near reflex (accommodation reflex)*—Contraction of the pupil occurs on looking at a near object.
   c. *Psychosensory reflex*—A dilatation of the pupil occurs on psychic or sensory stimuli, e.g. as in fear, pain, excitement, etc.
      Argyll-Robertson pupil—Accommodation reflex is retained but light reflex is lost.
      - The pupil is small.
      - There is damage to the relay path in tectum between afferent and efferent nerve pathways, e.g. in syphilis.

Horner's syndrome—*All sympathetic functions are lost on one side causing,*
- *Miosis*
- *Enophthalmos*
- *Narrow palpebral fissure*
- *Unilateral absence of sweating*

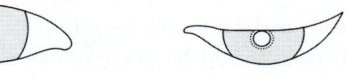

- Ptosis
- Small pupil
- Normal response to light and convergence

Horner's syndrome

Marcus-Gunn pupil—*There is ill-sustained contraction of the pupil in swinging flashlight test, e.g. as in retrobulbar neuritis.*
Adie pupil—*It presents as unilateral dilated pupil usually in young women. It is of unknown etiology.*

14. Lens

i. *Colour*—*Jet black*—Normal, aphakia
   Grey—Immature cataract
   White—Mature cataract, retinoblastoma, pseudogliomas, etc.
   Brown/black—Nuclear cataract, Morgagnian cataract

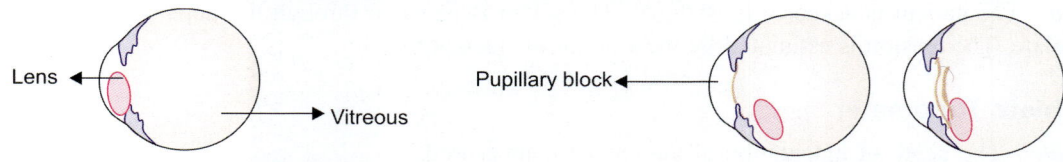

Lens ← | → Vitreous
Dislocation into anterior chamber

Pupillary block ←
Posterior dislocation

   Yellowish—Shrunken lens in hypermature cataract.
ii. *Opacity*—Central, peripheral or total.
iii. *Position*—Dislocation occurs commonly in lower part of the vitreous or in the anterior chamber due to complete rupture of the zonule as following trauma.
   - *Subluxation*—It is due to the partial rupture of the zonule. The lens is tilted causing astigmatism and uniocular diplopia (seeing double objects).
iv. *Purkinje-Sanson images*—When bright light falls obliquely on the eye (dilated pupil) in a dark room images are formed by the
   a. Anterior surface of cornea
   b. Posterior surface of cornea ⎱ → Concave surface ────→ Erect (virtual) image
   c. Anterior surface of lens ⎰
   d. Posterior surface of lens ────→ Concave surface ────→ Inverted (real) image

In clear transparent lens—There is presence of all 4 images.
In aphakia—There is absence of 3rd and 4th images.
In opaque lens—There is absence of 4th image.

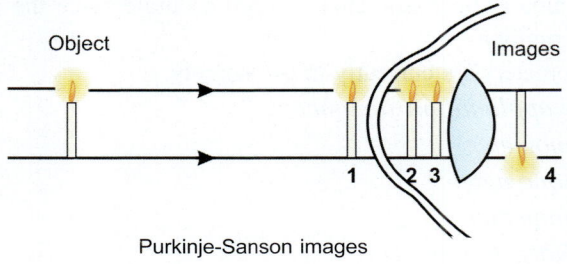

Purkinje-Sanson images

2. PALPATION

Orbit—Irregular margin, swelling growth, tenderness are noted.
Eyeball—Tenderness, pulsation are noted.
Digital tension—It is assessed by fluctuation method.
Lymph nodes—Preauricular lymph nodes may be enlarged.

3. INTRAOCULAR PRESSURE

The normal intraocular pressure is 10-20 mm Hg (Schiotz).
Suspicious cases = 20-25 mm Hg (Schiotz).
Glaucoma = above 25 mm Hg (Schiotz).

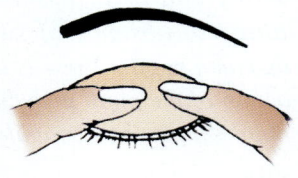

Digital tension

1. Digital Tension

Principle—The intraocular tension is estimated by palpation of the eyes with fingers.
Method—The patient is asked to look down. The sclera is palpated through the upper lid beyond the tarsal plate. The tension is estimated by the amount of fluctuation.

2. Schiotz Tonometer

Principle—The depth of indentation of the cornea is measured.
Method— The cornea is anaesthetized with suitable local anaesthetic, e.g., xylocaine 4% eyedrops.
- Lids are separated and a tonometer carrying a weight of 5.5 gm is gently placed on the cornea. (There are 3 more weights available 7.5, 10 and 15 gm)
- The deflection is measured and reading in millimeter of mercury can be read from a chart.

Advantages—It is cheap, easy to use, convenient to carry and does not require a slitlamp.
Disadvantage—There may be error due to ocular rigidity.

3. Applanation Tonometer

It is a more accurate method. The cornea is flattened by a plane surface. This is based on the principle of Imbert-Fick's law. It states that for an ideal, thin-walled sphere, the pressure inside the sphere (P) equals to force necessary to flatten its surface (F) divided by the area of flattening (A), i.e. P = F/A.

$$\text{Pressure} = \frac{\text{Force applied}}{\text{Area of flattened cornea}} \qquad P = \frac{F}{A}$$

An applanation tonometer measures the intraocular pressure by flattening (rather than indent) the cornea over a specific area (3.06 mm). This is more accurate since the pressure values recorded are uninfluenced by scleral rigidity.

Six applanation tonometers are currently in use namely,
1. The Goldmann applanation tonometer
2. The Perkins tonometer
3. The pneumatotonometer
4. The air-puff tonometer
5. The MacKay-Marg tonometer

Examination of the Eye

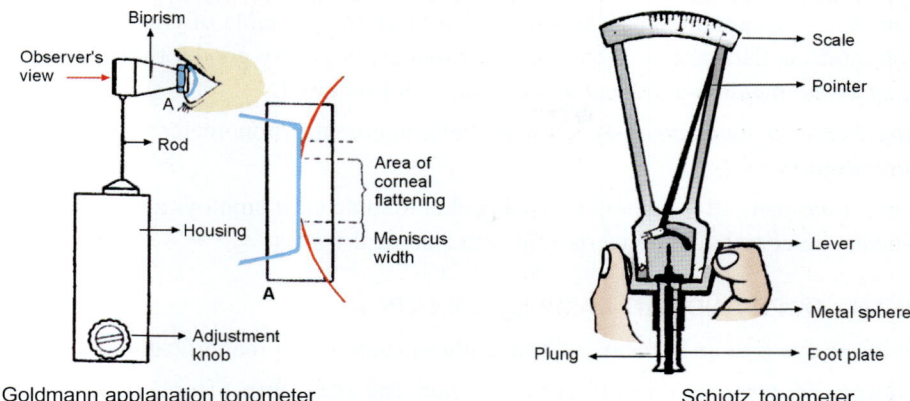

Goldmann applanation tonometer   Schiotz tonometer

6. *The Microelectronic Tono-pen*

Goldmann applanation tonometer—It is the most popular and accurate tonometer. It consists of a double prism mounted on a standard slit-lamp. The prism applanates the cornea in an area of 3.06 mm diameter. The normal IOP as measured by applanation tonometer is 15 ± 3 Hg.

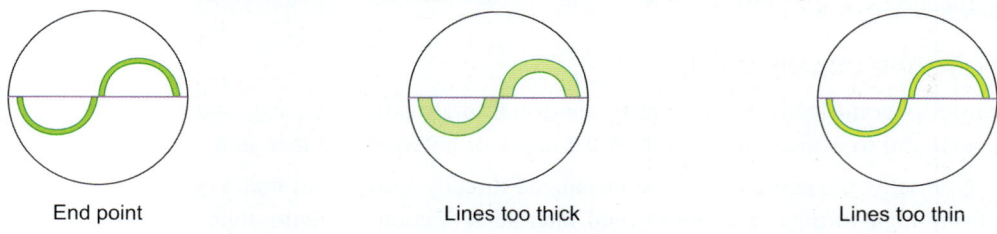

End point   Lines too thick   Lines too thin

Fluorescein stained mires of the applanation tonometer

Method

1. Anaesthetise the cornea with a drop of 2% xylocaine and stain the tear film with fluorescein.
2. Patient is seated in front of a slit-lamp. The cornea and biprisms are illuminated with cobalt blue light from the slit-lamp.
3. Biprism is then advanced until it just touches the apex of the cornea. At this point two fluorescent semicircles are viewed through the prism.
4. The applanation force against the cornea is adjusted until the inner edges of the two semicircles just touch. This is the end point.
5. The intraocular pressure is determined by multiplying the dial reading with 10.

Perkins (hand-held) applanation tonometer—It is same as above except that it does not require a slit-lamp and it can be used even in supine position. It is small and easy to carry.

Pneumatic tonometer—The cornea is applanated by touching its apex by a silastic diaphragm covering the sensing nozzle which is connected to a central chamber containing pressurised air. There is a pneumatic-to-electronic transducer which converts the air pressure to a recording on a paper-strip from where IOP is read.

Air-puff tonometer—It is a non-contact tonometer based on the principle of Goldmann tonometer. The central part of cornea is flattened by a jet of air. This tonometer is very good for mass screening as there is no danger of cross-infection and local anaesthetic is not required.

MacKay-Marg Pulse air tonometer—It is a hand held, non-contact tonometer that can be used on the patients in any position.

Microelectronic Tono-pen—It is a computerised pocket tonometer. It employs a microscopic transducer which applanates the cornea and converts IOP into electrical waves.

4. BINOCULAR LOUPE AND SLIT-LAMP EXAMINATION

Examination of the eye is done in focal or oblique illumination under magnification.

Binocular loupe—A stereoscopic effect is obtained and the depth of opacities can be assessed. Magnification = 3-4 times.

Slit-lamp examination—It is essential when minute examination of the eye is necessary. A brilliant light is brought to a focus as a slit or point by an optical system supported on a movable arm and observations are made by a binocular microscope.

Magnification = 16, 25 times.

5. GONIOSCOPE EXAMINATION

The purpose of gonioscopy is to identify abnormal angle structures, e.g. anterior synechiae, foreign body, tumour and to estimate the width of the angle of anterior chamber as in closed angle glaucoma.

Optics—Normally, the angle cannot be visualized directly through an intact cornea because light rays emitted from angle structures undergo total internal reflection. A gonioscope eliminates total internal reflection by replacing the 'cornea-air interface' by a new 'lens-air interface' that has a greater refractive index than that of the cornea and tears.

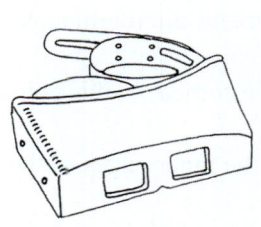

Binocular loupe

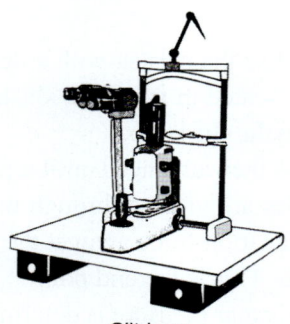

Slit-lamp

Types of Gonioscopy

 i. *Direct gonioscopy with goniolenses*—They provide a direct view of the angle. They are used both for diagnostic and operative purposes, e.g. Koeppe, Barkan goniolens, etc.
 ii. *Indirect gonioscopy with gonioprisms*—The rays are reflected by the mirror and the angle of anterior chamber is seen. They provide a mirror image of the opposite angle, and can only be used at a slit-lamp, e.g. Goldmann single mirror or three mirror gonioscope, Zeiss four mirror gonioscope, etc.

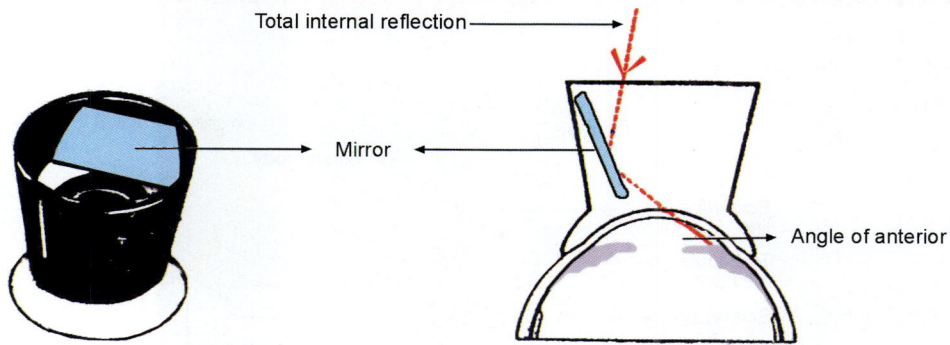

Gonioscopic examination of the angle of anterior chamber

Normal angle structures (from anterior to posterior)—Normal angle structures are:
1. Schwalbe's line—It is an opaque line which represents the peripheral termination of the Descemet's membrane.
2. Trabecular meshwork—The degree of pigmentation varies. It is a sieve-like structure with occasional visibility of the Schlemm's canal.
3. Scleral spur—It is a prominent white line which represents the most anterior projection of the sclera.
4. Ciliary band—A grey or dull brown band of ciliary body is seen at the insertion of iris root.

The presence of a narrow angle of the anterior chamber, as evident from gonioscopy, is invaluable in the diagnosis of the disease.

6. TRANSILLUMINATION

1. *Trans-scleral*—When an intense beam of light is thrown through the sclera, the pupil appears red in colour. If there is a solid mass in the path of light, the pupil remains black, e.g. as in intraocular tumour.
2. *Trans-pupillary*—When an intense beam of light is allowed to pass obliquely through the dilated pupil, the pupil becomes illuminated uniformly in the normal cases.

EXAMINATION OF THE POSTERIOR SEGMENT OF THE EYE
1. Subjective Examination of Retinal Functions

1. VISUAL ACUITY

It is a measure of smallest retinal image which can be appreciated. It tests the form sense.

Snellen's Test Type

Snellen's chart consists of a series of letters arranged in lines each diminishing in size.

The lines from above downwards should be read at 60, 36, 24, 18, 12, 9, 6, 5 m, respectively. At these distances the letters subtend a visual angle of 5' at the nodal point. It is kept at a distance of 6 m so that the rays of light are parallel for practical purpose. The minimum illumination of the test type accepted for satisfactory vision should be 15-20 foot candles.

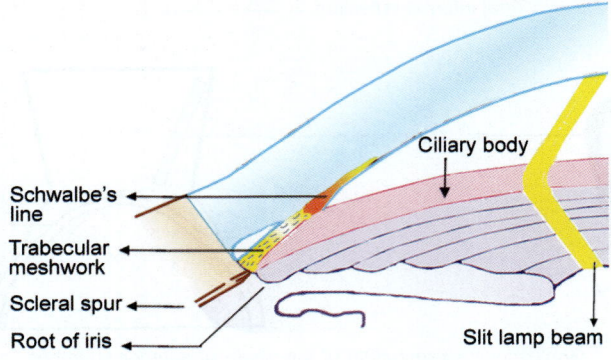

Structures forming angle of the anterior chamber

1. Recording of Visual Acuity for Distance

Each eye is tested separately. A normal person can read all the lines, i.e. up to 6 m line. Thus the normal visual acuity is = 6/6.

When the patient can only read the 18 m line, his distant vision is defective = 6/18.

When the patient cannot read the largest letter, he is asked to walk slowly towards the chart. If he can read the top most letter at 5, 4, 3 or 2 m, his visual acuity = 5/60, 4/60, 3/60, 2/60 respectively.

If the patient is unable to see the top letter when close to it, he is asked to count the surgeon's fingers held at 1 m against a dark background. If he can count the fingers, the visual acuity = 1/60. If he can count fingers only at 50 cm, the visual acuity = counting fingers at 50 cm.

If he cannot count fingers, the surgeon's hand is moved in front of the eyes close to face. If he can appreciate the movements, the visual acuity = hand movements.

In a dark room, light is concentrated on his eyes. He is asked to say when the light is on the eye or when it is off. If he tells correctly, the visual acuity = PL (perception of light).

If he gives correct indication of the direction from where the light is coming the visual acuity = PL (perception of light) and projection of rays is good.

If he fails to see the light, he is blind. The visual acuity = no PL (no perception of light).

Other Test Types

1. *Landolt's chart—'C' type—It is used for illiterate persons.*
2. *E chart—It is used for illiterate persons.*
3. *Simple picture chart—It is used for children.*

2. Recording of Visual Acuity for Near

The patient reads Snellen's test type for reading or printer's types (N series) at a distance of about 25 cm in good illumination. The normal vision is recorded as N/6.

Examination of the Eye

Snellen's chart

D.60 — H
D.36 — A V
D.24 — L T J
D.18 — V O A
D.12 — T X A L
0.9 — O A N V Z
D.6 — H Z N V T U E
D.5 — N O H X E Z A U

N.5.
The streets of London are better paved and better lighted than those of any metropolis in Europe: there are lamps are both sides of every street, in the mean proportion of one lamp to three doors. The effect pro-

cave scorn veneer succour

N.8.
Water Cresses are sold in small bunches, one penny each, or three bunches for two pence. The crier of Water Cresses frequently travels seven or eight miles

rose sauce cannon reverse

N.10.
Hearth Brooms, Brushes, Sieves, Bowls, Clothes-horses, and Lines, and almost every household article of turnery, are cried in the

noen verse runner caravan

N.12.
Strawberries, brought fresh gathered to the market in the height of their season, both morning and after noon,

nuns score severe careers

N.18.
Doors-mats of all kinds, rush and rope, from sixpence to four shillings crave savour concern

Snellen's near type

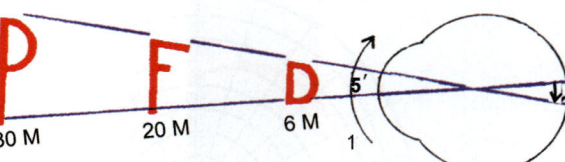

The minimum visual angle

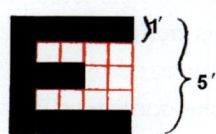

The letter of Snellen chart

2. THE FIELD OF VISION

The normal visual field is described as 'island of vision surrounded by a sea of blindness'.

The Normal Field of Vision

Upwards = 60°
Inwards = 60°
Downwards = 70°
Outwards = more than 90°

60° 60°
>90° — 60° 60° — >90°
70° 70°
Right eye Left eye

Normal visual field—The normal visual field is described by Traquair as "island of vision surrounded by a sea of blindness".

Boundary—The peripheral limits of the visual field, which normally measures from the fixation points are approximately 60° above and inwards, 70° below and more than 90° temporally.

Point of fixation—It is the area of maximum visual acuity in the normal visual field. It corresponds to the foveola of the retina.

38 Basic Ophthalmology

Blind spot—This is an area of absolute scotoma (non-seeing area) within the boundaries of normal visual field. It corresponds to the region of optic nerve head where there are no rods and cones. It is located approximately 15° temporal to the fixation point.

Scotoma—It is an absolute or relative area of depressed visual function (non-seeing area) surrounded by normal vision. It is commonly seen in cases of glaucoma, optic neuritis, papilloedema, etc.
   i. *Absolute scotoma*—All vision is lost, i.e. no perception of light (no PL)
  ii. *Relative scotoma*—A variable amount of vision remains.
 iii. *Positive scotoma*—When the patient appreciates a dark area in his field of vision.
  iv. *Negative scotoma*—It is a defect detected only when visual field is recorded.

Perimetry

The term 'perimetry' is used to describe various techniques employed to evaluate both central and peripheral visual fields using targets of various sizes and colours.

Two techniques of testing the field of vision are commonly employed:
1. *Kinetic perimetry*—A target is moved across the field to map out of the two-dimensional extent of field. It involves presentation of a moving stimulus of known luminance or intensity from periphery towards the centre till it is perceived. The point of perception is recorded along different meridians. By joining these points an isopter is plotted for that stimulus intensity. Kinetic perimetry can be performed by
   - Confrontation method
   - Listers perimeter
   - Goldmann perimeter
   - Tangent screen or Bjerrum's screen
2. *Static perimetry*—It forms the basis of modern glaucoma assessment. It is a three dimensional assessment of the height of a predetermined area of the 'hill of vision.' Non-moving stimuli of varying luminance are presented in the same position to obtain a vertical boundary of the visual field. The stimuli can be presented in two different ways

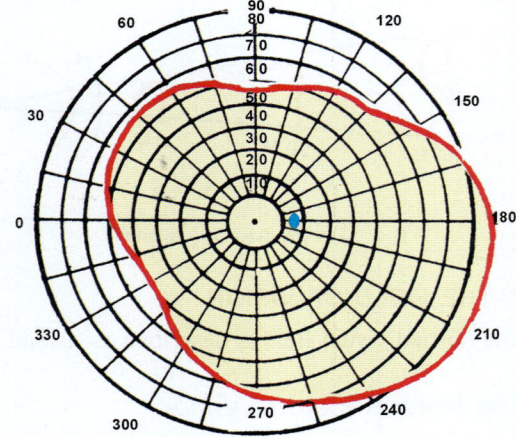
Extent of normal visual field of right eye

   a. *Suprathreshold perimetry*—It is used mainly for screening the patients. Visual stimuli are presented at luminance levels above the expected normal threshold values in various locations in the visual field. In cases of moderate to gross loss of sensitivity, the supranormal stimulus is not seen.
   b. *Threshold perimetry*—It is used for detailed assessment of the 'hill of vision'. Target of different and increasing intensities are presented at designated points in the visual fields until just visible to find out the patient's threshold for that point. This is the principle used in computerized automated perimeters.

Examination of the Eye

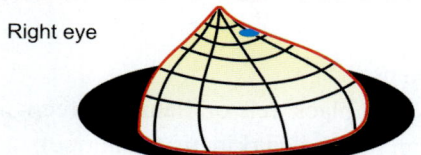

Three dimensional representation of normal field of vision—An Island of vision in sea of darkness

Right eye

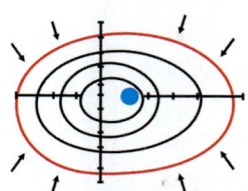 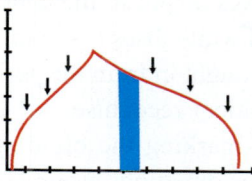

Meridional two dimensional representation of visual field (Kinetic perimetry)

Uses

Charting of the visual fields is very useful in the diagnosis of many disease conditions
- Glaucoma
- Retinal diseases e.g. retinitis pigmentosa
- Follow up of laser treatment for diabetic retinopathy
- Neurological disorders, e.g. brain tumours, head injury, multiple sclerosis, cerebral thrombosis, aneurysms.

1. Peripheral Field

i. Confrontation Method

It is a rough but very useful method. It can be done in the clinic or at the patient's bedside.

Principle—The patients field of vision is compared with that of the examiner having a normal field of vision.

Method—The surgeon stands facing the patient at a distance of about 60 cm.
- The patient covers his one eye (left) and the surgeon closes his one eye (right).
- The surgeon moves his hand from the periphery towards the centre, keeping his hand in the plane halfway between the patient and himself.
- The surgeon repeats the procedure covering the other eye.

ii. The Perimeter—(Lister's, Goldmann's)

It consists of a half sphere within which a spot of light can be moved (kinetic technique).

Method—The patient is seated with his chin supported by the chin rest.
- One eye is covered by a pad.
- The other eye fixes an object placed at the centre of the arc.
- The field is recorded first with a white object 5 mm in diameter from periphery to centre.
- At least 8 or preferably 16 meridians must be tested.

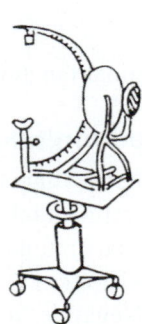

Lister's perimeter

2. Central Field (Campimetry)

It is limited to 30° from the fixation point.

i. *Bjerrum's screen*—It consists of a black felt or flannel screen, 2 m in diameter on which central 30° of the visual field can be studied (kinetic technique).

Method—The patient sits 2 m away from the screen.
- He fixes a spot in the centre of the screen.
- Small white discs (1-10 mm diameter) attached to a long rod are brought in from the periphery towards fixation point until the patient recognises the target.
- After marking the blind spot, the procedure is repeated in various directions around the fixation point. The isoptres are mapped out and labelled as 1/1000, 2/1000, 3/1000.

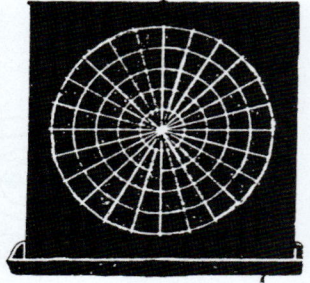

Bjerrum's screen

ii. *Automated perimeters*, e.g. Friedmann analyser, Ouplot, Auto field perimeters Field master and Humphery field analyser (static technique). In static perimetry, the visual field can be plotted by using a stationary light target of variable brightness against a background whose luminance can be adjusted.

Automated perimeters utilize computers to programme visual field sequences, e.g. Baylor visual field programmer attached to standard Goldmann perimeter. Each of them has an electronic fixation control and an automatic recording of missed points.

Advantages
1. These are more sensitive than manual perimetry.
2. Examiner bias is eliminated.
3. There is constant monitoring of fixation.
4. Visual field can be always stored and reproduced.

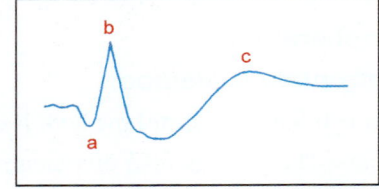

Electroretinogram

3. COLOUR VISION

The main objective of testing colour vision is:
- To find out the exact nature of the defect, e.g. red or green colour blind.
- Whether the patient is likely to be a source of danger to the society, e.g. driver, pilot, sailor.

2. Objective Examination of Retinal Functions

The retinal function can be tested objectively by:

1. Electroretinogram (ERG)

The changes induced by the stimulation of light in the resting potential of the eye are measured by electroretinography. It is extinguished or absent in complete failure of function of rods and cones, e.g. pigmentary retinal dystrophy, complete occlusion of retinal artery, complete retinal detachment, advanced siderosis, etc.

i. Negative 'a' wave represents the activity in rods and cones.
ii. Positive 'b' wave arises in inner retinal layers.
iii. Positive 'c' wave is associated with the pigmentary epithelium.

2. Electro-oculogram (EOG)
The changes in the resting current when the eyes are moved laterally are picked up by the electrodes placed at the inner and outer canthi. It is absent in retinal dystrophies and degenerations.

EXAMINATION OF THE FUNDUS OCULI
Pupil is dilated with a suitable mydriatic, e.g. phenylephrine, tropicamide, homide or cyclopentolate and the examination of the fundus oculi is done in a dark room. Atropine is preferred in children as it results in paralysis of ciliary muscle.

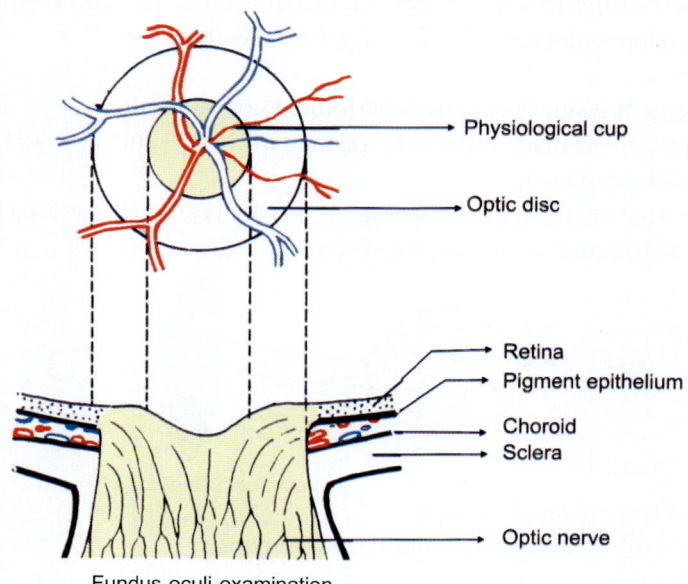

Fundus oculi examination

1. Media
Media consists of cornea, aqueous humour, lens and the vitreous. Media can be clear, hazy, partially or totally opaque.
1. *Plane mirror examination at a distance of 1 m*—Uniform red glow is seen if there are no opacities in the media.
2. *Plane mirror examination at a distance of 22 cm (distant direct ophthalmoscopy)*—The exact position of the opacities or black spots in the refractive media is determined by parallactic displacement.
3. *Direct ophthalmoscopy*—Helmholtz invented the direct ophthalmoscope.

    Method—The surgeon looks through a self-luminous ophthalmoscope and directs the light upon the pupil. A uniform red reflex or glow is seen. Examination of the fundus is done best at a close distance with accommodation relaxed.

Optical principle
   i. The convergent light beam is reflected from the ophthalmoscopic mirror
   ii. The incident rays reach the retina causing it to be illuminated.
   iii. The emergent rays from the fundus then reach the observers retina through the hole in the mirror. The image is virtual, erect and magnified (15 times in emmetrope eye).

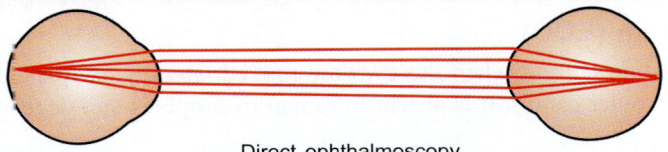

Direct ophthalmoscopy

4. *Indirect ophthalmoscopy*

Method—It is done in a dark room with a convex condensing lens (+ 30 D, + 20 D, +14 D) and a concave mirror. The lens is held in between the thumb and forefinger of the left hand. The curved surface of the lens is towards the examiner. The periphery of the retina can be seen by scleral depression with the patient in lying down position.

Optical principle
   i. The convergent beam is cast by a perforated concave mirror.
   ii. The patient's eye is made myopic by placing a +13D, +20D or +30D convex lens between the observer and the patient.
   iii. A real, inverted enlarged (5 times with +13D and 3 times with + 20D lens) image of the fundus is formed between the lens and the observer.

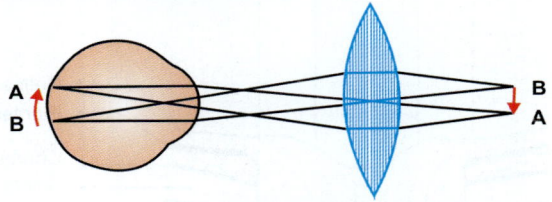

Indirect ophthalmoscopy

Advantages of indirect ophthalmoscope
1. Strong illumination, superb binocularity and stereopsis.
2. It can be used in high refractive error.
3. The beam passes through the opacities in the media.
4. Total retinal area and pars plana can be examined with the help of scleral indentation.

2. Optic Disc

It is circular or oval in shape measuring 1.5 mm in diameter. It is situated at the posterior pole of the fundus. It is pink in colour. There is a funnel-shaped depression 'the physiological cup' seen in the centre. The central retinal vessels emerge from the middle. The normal cup : disc ratio is 0.3 or 1:2
   i. *Size*—Optic disc is large in myopia and small in hypermetropia and aphakia.
   ii. *Shape*—The normal optic disc is round or oval in shape.
   iii. *Margin*—The margin is sharp and clearly defined normally and in primary optic atrophy. It is blurred in cases of secondary optic atrophy, optic neuritis, papillitis and papilloedema.
   iv. *Colour*—It is normally pink in colour. It is pale or white in cases of optic atrophy. It is waxy yellow in retinitis pigmentosa
   v. *Cupping*—Pathological cupping is seen in glaucoma. Papilloedema is seen in cases of raised intracranial tension (brain tumour) and malignant hypertension.

3. Macula Lutea

It is situated 3 mm or 2 disc diameter to the temporal side of the optic disc. It is a small circular area, deeper red than the surrounding fundus. There is a bright foveal reflex in the centre due to reflection of light from the walls of the foveal pit. Cystoid macular oedema, macular hole or macular star may be seen.

4. Retinal Vessels

These are derived from the central retinal artery and vein, which divide into two branches at or near the surface of the disc. The arteries are brighter red and narrower than veins. The normal artery: vein ratio is 2 : 3.

5. General Fundus

Normally the fundus has a uniform red appearance. In albino, the choroidal vessels are seen clearly against the white sclera. In high myopia, tesselated or tigroid fundus is seen due to degenerative changes in retina and choroid. Black pigments resembling bone corpuscles are typically seen in retinitis pigmentosa.

EXAMINATION OF THE FUNDUS BY FOCAL ILLUMINATION

The ordinary slit-lamp can only explore the eye up to the anterior parts of the vitreous. By interposing a −55 D (approximately) lens in front of the cornea, the posterior part of the vitreous and the central area of the fundus can be examined after full mydriasis.

Three types of lenses are available for biomicroscopic examination of the vitreous and fundus.
1. *Hruby's lens*—It is a plano-concave lens with a dioptric strength of −58.6 D

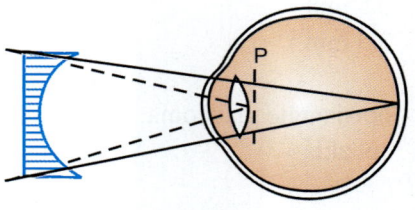
Hruby lens

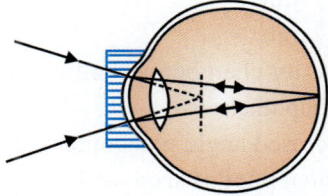
Posterior fundus contact lens

2. *Posterior fundus contact lens*—This is a modified Koeppe's lens.
3. *Goldmann three mirror contact lens*—Three mirrors are placed in a cone.
4. *Indirect slit lamp biomicroscopy* using +78D, +90D lens is presently the most commonly employed technique for biomicroscopic examination of the fundus.

MULTIPLE CHOICE QUESTIONS

1. Ciliary congestion is most marked at the
   a. sclera
   b. fornix
   c. bulbar conjunctiva
   d. limbus
2. Superficial vascularisation of cornea has all the following features, *EXCEPT*
   a. irregular and tortuous vessel
   b. rich dendritic branching
   c. vessels continuous with conjunctival vessel
   d. vessels lie deep to Bowman's membrane
3. Corneal thickness is measured by
   a. keratometer
   b. vernier scale
   c. pachymeter
   d. none of the above
4. Keratometry is used in the measurement of
   a. length of eyeball
   b. curvature of cornea
   c. diameter of cornea
   d. thickness of cornea
5. Corneal sensations are reduced in
   a. hypopyon ulcer
   b. phlyctenular keratitis
   c. herpes simplex
   d. arcus senilis
6. Corneal staining is done by following vital stains
   a. iodine
   b. fluorescein
   c. carbolic acid
   d. silver nitrate
7. All of the following result in loss of corneal sensation *EXCEPT*
   a. acute congestive glaucoma
   b. absolute glaucoma
   c. dendritic ulcer
   d. senile mature cataract
8. The normal depth of anterior chamber is
   a. 1 mm
   b. 2.5 mm
   c. 3 mm
   d. 3.5 mm
9. Anterior chamber is shallow in
   a. buphthalmos
   b. open angle glaucoma
   c. closed angle glaucoma
   d. aphakia
10. Dilated pupil is seen in all of the following *EXCEPT*
    a. pontine haemorrhage
    b. optic atrophy
    c. acute glaucoma
    d. papillitis
11. Tremulousness of iris is seen in
    a. chronic iridocyclitis
    b. closed angle glaucoma
    c. aphakia
    d. none of the above
12. Pupil is pinpoint in
    a. optic atrophy
    b. absolute glaucoma
    c. atropine
    d. iritis
13. White pupillary reflex is seen in
    a. retinoblastoma
    b. congenital cataract
    c. complete retinal detachment
    d. all of the above

14. In a frightened man, the pupil shall
    a. dilate
    b. constrict
    c. remain unaltered
    d. first dilate and then constrict
15. In aphakia there is absence of following Purkinje-Sanson's images
    a. 1st and 2nd
    b. 3rd
    c. 4th
    d. 3rd and 4th
16. The normal intraocular pressure is (Schiotz)
    a. 10-15 mm Hg
    b. 10-20 mm Hg
    c. 25-30 mm Hg
    d. less than 10 mm Hg
17. The most accurate method of measuring IOP is
    a. digital
    b. applanation
    c. Schiotz
    d. gonioscopy
18. Near vision is recorded at a distance of
    a. 10 cm
    b. 25 cm
    c. 35 cm
    d. 50 cm
19. Distant vision is recorded at a distance of
    a. 1 m
    b. 2 m
    c. 3 m
    d. 6 m
20. Normal field of vision extends on the nasal side to
    a. 40°
    b. 50°
    c. 60°
    d. 70°
21. Peripheral field of vision is tested by
    a. Bjerrum's screen
    b. Snellen's chart
    c. Lister's perimeter
    d. indirect ophthalmoscopy
22. Central field of vision is limited up to
    a. 20°
    b. 30°
    c. 40°
    d. 50°
23. Distant direct ophthalmoscopy is done at a distance of
    a. 1 m
    b. 6 m
    c. 22 cm
    d. close to the face
24. In indirect ophthalmoscopy the image is
    a. inverted, real, magnified
    b. erect, real, magnified
    c. erect, virtual, magnified
    d. none of the above
25. In direct ophthalmoscopy the image is
    a. virtual, erect, magnified
    b. virtual, inverted, condensed
    c. real, inverted, magnified
    d. real, erect, condensed
26. Periphery of retina is best visualized with
    a. direct ophthalmoscopy
    b. indirect ophthalmoscopy
    c. retinoscopy
    d. USG

27. 'A' wave in ERG corresponds to activity in
    a. rods
    b. pigment epitheluim
    c. inner retinal layer
    d. nerve bundle layer
28. Campimetry is used to measure
    a. squint
    b. angle of deviation
    c. pattern of retina
    d. field charting
29. Angle of anterior chamber is studied with
    a. indirect ophthalmoscopy
    b. gonioscopy
    c. retinoscopy
    d. amblyoscope
30. Direct ophthalmoscopy magnification of image in comparison to indirect type (+13D lens) is —— times in emmetropes.
    a. 2
    b. 3
    c. 5
    d. 6

ANSWERS

1—d	2—d	3—c	4—b,c	5—c
6—b	7—d	8—b	9—c	10—a
11—c	12—d	13—d	14—a	15—d
16—b	17—b	18—b	19—d	20—c
21—c	22—b	23—c	24—a	25—a
26—b	27—a	28—d	29—b	30—b

CHAPTER 5
Errors of Refraction

The normal eye is like a camera. The focusing elements of the eye are the cornea and the crystalline lens and the 'film' is the retina. The normal eye is so constructed that distant objects form their images upon the retina. The retinal image is inverted but it is re-inverted psychologically in the brain.

When light rays pass from a medium of one density to a medium of a different density they are refracted or bent. This principle is used in the eye to focus light on the retina. Before reaching the retina light rays pass successively through the cornea, aqueous humour, lens and vitreous which are all more dense than the air.

EMMETROPIA

It is the normal optical condition of the eye. The eye is considered to be emmetropic when incident parallel rays of light from infinity come to a focus on the retina (fovea centralis) with accommodation at rest. There is no error of refraction. An emmetropic eye will have a clear image of a distant object without any internal adjustment of its optics. The average power of a normal emmetropic eye is + 58 to + 60D.

Most emmetropic eyes are approximately 24 mm in length.

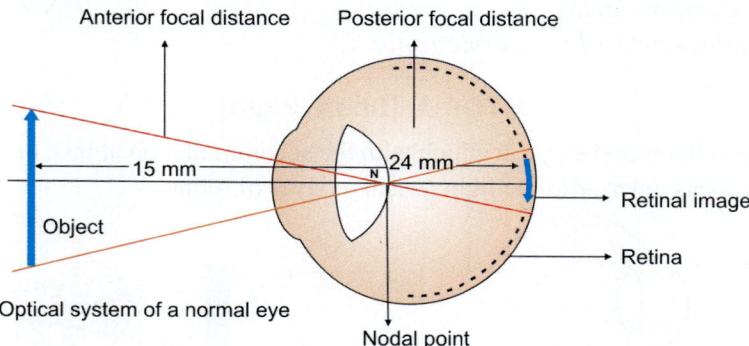

The normal schematic eye

Optic axis—The line passing through the centre of curvature of cornea and the two surfaces of the lens, meets the retina at fovea centralis.

Nodal point—The optical centre lies in the posterior part of the lens.

Anterior focal distance—It is about 15 mm in front of the cornea.

Posterior focal distance—It is about 24 mm behind the cornea.

ERRORS OF REFRACTION
[AMETROPIA]

The optical condition of the eye in which the incident parallel rays of light do not come to a focus upon the light sensitive layer of the retina, with accommodation at rest is known as ametropia.

Etiology

1. *Axial ametropia*—There is abnormal length of the eyeball.
   Too long—In myopia
   Too short—In hypermetropia.
2. **Curvature ametropia**—There is abnormal curvature of the refracting surfaces of the cornea or lens.
   Too strong—In myopia
   Too weak—In hypermetropia.
3. **Index ametropia**—There is abnormal refractive index of the media.
   Too high—In myopia
   Too low—In hypermetropia.
4. **Abnormal position of the lens**
   Forward displacement—In myopia
   Backward displacement—In hypermetropia.

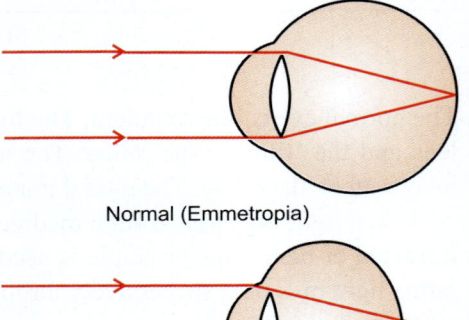
Normal (Emmetropia)

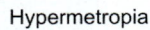
Hypermetropia

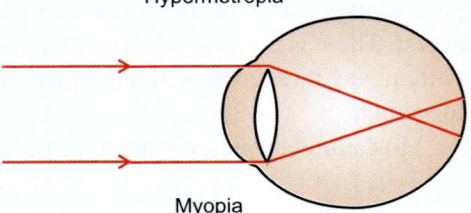
Myopia

MYOPIA [Short Sight]

It is that dioptric condition of the eye in which with the accommodation at rest, incident parallel rays of light come to a focus anterior to the light sensitive layer of retina.

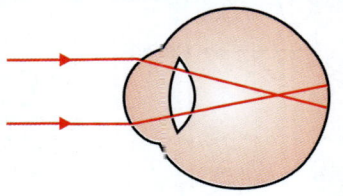
Myopic eye

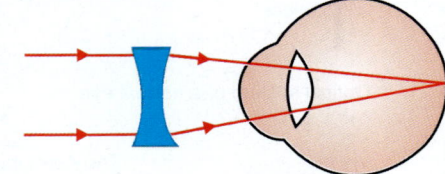
Correction with concave lens

Etiology
- It is basically a disturbance of growth on which degenerative changes are superimposed.
- The part anterior to the equator is normal.
- The increase in axial length affects the posterior pole and the surrounding area.
1. *Axial*—Increased anteroposterior diameter of the globe is the most common cause.
2. *Curvature*—Increased curvature is seen in following conditions:

i. Corneal—Conical cornea, ectasia
ii. Lens—Lenticonus.
3. *Index*—Increased refractive index of the nucleus, e.g. as in senile nuclear cataract.
4. *Forward displacement of the lens*, e.g. as in anterior dislocation of the lens.

Types

1. **Congenital [developmental] myopia**
   - It is present at birth.
   - It is stationary usually.
   - It may be unilateral or bilateral.
   - Bilateral myopia may be associated with convergent squint.
2. **Simple myopia**
   - It is the most common type of myopia.
   - There are no degenerative changes in the fundus.
   - It does not progress after adolescence when a degree of –5 or –6 D is attained.
3. **Pathological myopia**
   - It is a type of degenerative and progressive myopia.
   - It begins at the age of 5-10 years and increases steadily reaching –15 to –20 D in early adult life.
   - It is strongly hereditary.
   - It is common in women, Jews and Japanese.
   - It is associated with excessive accommodation and convergence in near work.

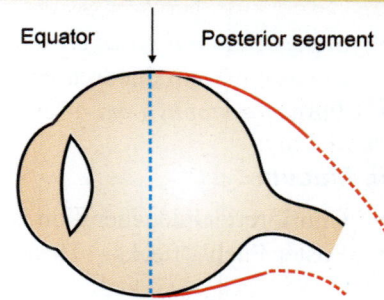

Increase in axial length

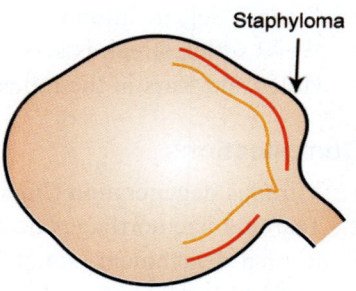

Posterior staphyloma

Symptoms

1. Indistinct distant vision is the most common symptom. Usually the young children are unable to see the blackboard clearly.
2. Black spots are seen floating before the eyes.
3. There is discomfort after near work.
4. Flashes of light may be seen.

Signs

1. Prominent eyes, large pupil and deep anterior chamber are commonly seen.
2. Apparant divergent squint may be present.
3. Fundus examination.

i. Optic Disc

- *Temporal crescent*—The retinal pigment epithelium fails to extend up to the temporal border of the disc. This leads to exposure of choroidal pigment.

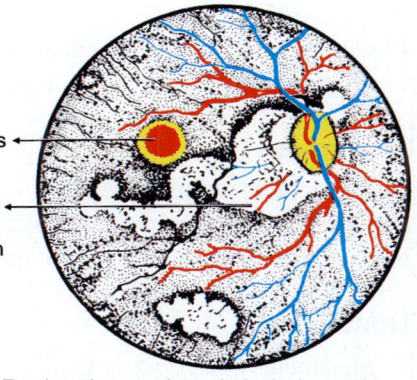

Fundus changes in pathological myopia

- *Supertractional nasal crescent*—The retina extends over the nasal disc margin causing blurring of nasal margin due to traction.
- *Posterior staphyloma*—The sclera may bulge out at the posterior pole due to thinning.

ii. Macula
- Chorioretinal degeneration is often present.
- Foster Fuch's flecks—These are dark pigmented circular areas of intrachoroidal haemorrhages.

iii. Peripheral Fundus
- Cystoid degeneration of or a serrata and tesselated (tigroid) fundus may be present.
- Weiss reflex streak is seen due to detachment of vitreous at the posterior pole.
- Holes and tears in the retina may be present peripherally.

Complications
1. Vitreous degeneration (liquefaction), opacities and detachment are commonly seen.
2. Tear and haemorrhages occur in the retina due to chorioretinal degeneration.
3. Retinal detachment (simple) is always due to break in the retina through which fluid seeps in, raising the retina from its bed.

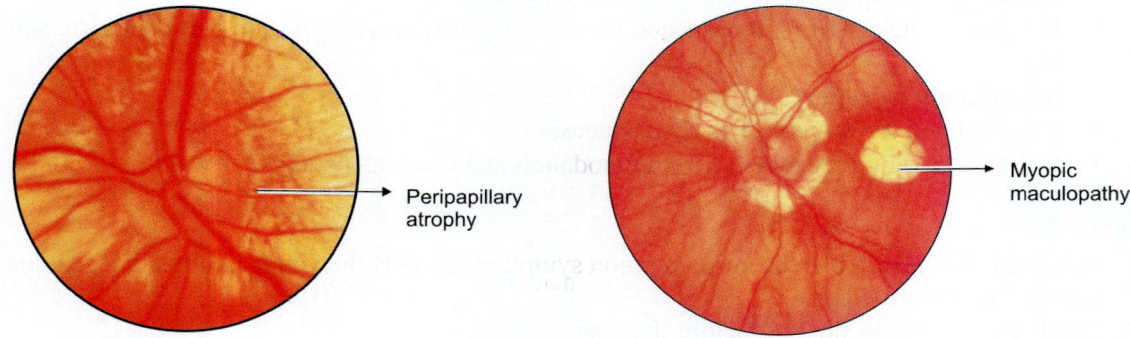

Myopic maculopathy and peripapillary atrophy   Pathological high myopia

4. Complicated cataract (posterior cortical) is due to the disturbance to the nutrition of the lens.
5. High myopia is sometimes associated with chronic simple glaucoma.

Prognosis
1. It is good in simple myopia.
2. In pathological myopia, the patient should avoid an occupation where close work is necessary.
3. Two high myopes should not get married as far as possible.

Treatment
1. Spectacles—Myopia is treated by prescribing suitable correcting spherical concave lenses for constant use. In low degree of myopia, spectacles are rarely required for near work (after the

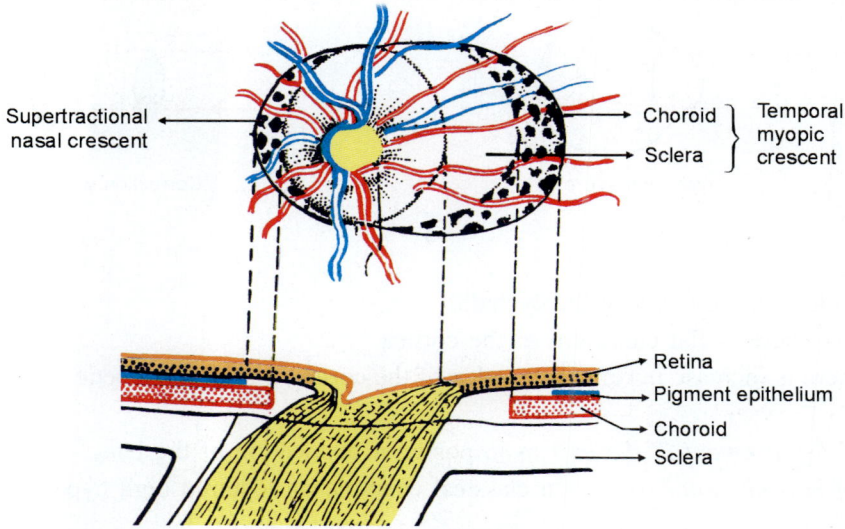

Temporal and supertractional nasal crescent

presbyopic age). In high myopia, spectacles should be made to fit closely to the eyes. Toric lense may be used. It should be undercorrected to avoid very bright and clear retinal images which are uncomfortable.
2. Hygiene of eyes—Proper position, good illumination and correct distance from the book (about 25 cm) while reading is essential.
3. Operative
   i. *Radial keratotomy*—Multiple peripheral cuts are made in the cornea in order to flatten the increased curvature of the cornea.
   ii. *Excimer laser*—It reshapes and flattens the central part of the cornea (photorefractive keratectomy)
   iii. *Epikeratophakia*—It is a procedure in which a lenticule of donor tissue of desired power is used to alter the surface topography of cornea.
   iv. *Keratomileusis*—A disc of cornea is freezed and placed on a lathe machine and keratomileusis (grinding) is performed. This alters the shape of the cornea by flattening it.
   v. LASIK—(Laser-assisted *in situ* keratomileusis) It corrects myopia of -8 to -16.

HYPERMETROPIA [Far Sight]

It is that dioptric condition of the eye in which with the accommodation at rest the incident parallel rays of light come to a focus posterior to the light sensitive layer of the retina.

Incidence

Newborns are invariably hypermetropic (average 2.5 D). The incidence decreases rapidly with age remaining at about 50% after 20 years.

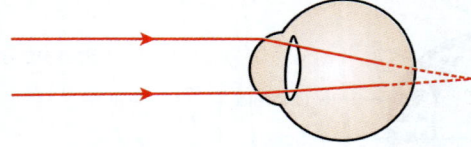
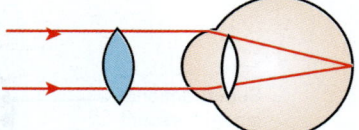

Hypermetropic eye Correction with convex lens

Etiology

1. *Axial*—There is short length of the eyeball.
2. *Curvature*—There is flat curvature of the cornea.
3. *Index*—There is increase in refractive index of the cortex, e.g. as in diabetic and senile cortical cataracts.
4. *Backward displacement of the lens* as in posterior dislocation of the lens.
5. *Absence of lens or aphakia*—It is a classical example of acquired high hypermetropia.

Types—Total hypermetropia may be divided into:
1. **Latent hypermetropia**—It is overcome by the normal tone of the ciliary muscle. It is detected only when the ciliary muscle is paralysed by atropine.
2. **Manifest hypermetropia**—It is detected without paralysing the ciliary muscle.
     i. *Facultative*—It can be overcome by an effort of accommodation.
    ii. *Absolute*—It cannot be overcome by an effort of accommodation.

Symptoms

These are noticed specially in the evenings after close work.
1. There is blurring of vision for near work.
2. There may be frontal headache and eye strain.
3. Burning and dryness in the eyes are usually present.
4. In adults, presbyopia commences at an earlier age.

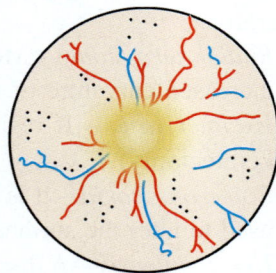

Pseudopapillitis

Signs

1. There is typical small eye as a whole. It is prone to cause closed angle glaucoma.
2. Accommodative convergent squint may be present.
3. Fundus examination
   • It may show no abnormality.
   • A bright reflex, i.e. watered silk appearance may be seen.
   • Pseudopapillitis, i.e. hyperaemic disc with blurred margin may be present which is similar to papillitis (inflammation of optic nerve head).

Treatment—It is treated by prescribing suitable correcting spherical convex lenses.

ASTIGMATISM

It is that condition of refraction in which a point of light cannot be made to produce a punctate image upon the retina by any spherical correcting lens (astigmatism = a point).

Etiology

1. There is unequal curvature of the cornea in different meridians.
2. There is decentring of the lens, e.g. as in subluxation of lens.

Types

1. *Regular*
    i. *Simple*
    ii. *Compound*
    iii. *Mixed*
2. *Irregular*

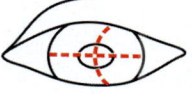 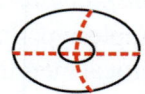

'With the rule' astigmatism

1. Regular Astigmatism

Normally cornea is flatter from side to side (horizontal meridian) perhaps because of the pressure of the eyelids. It is curved above downwards (vertical meridian).

Regular astigmatism is present when the two principal meridians are at right angles. It can be corrected by lenses.

i. *According to the rule*—The vertical meridian is more curved, e.g. as in normal cornea.
ii. *Against the rule*—The horizontal meridian is more curved, e.g. as after cataract surgery.

Sturm's Conoid

A regular astigmatic surface is said to have a *toric curvature*. Thus, the more curved meridian will have more convergent power than the less curved.

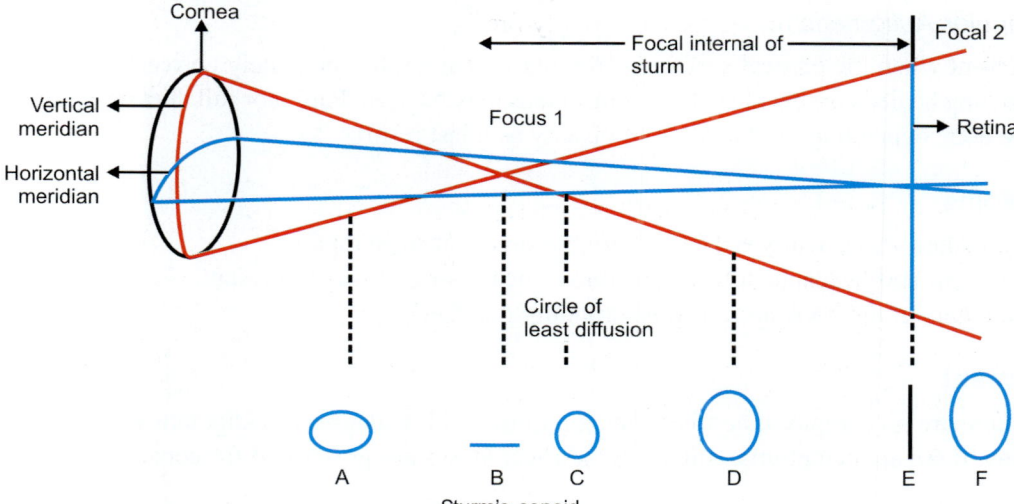

Sturm's conoid

- If parallel rays fall upon such a surface, the vertical rays will come to a focus sooner than the horizontal.
- Both the rays after refraction are perfectly symmetrical but they have two foci.
- The whole bundle of rays is called the *"Sturm's conoid"*.
- The distance between the two foci is called the *"Focal interval of sturm"*.
- If the retina is situated at A to E, the image will be blurred as rays never come to a focus in a single point.

Retinal plane at A
  Compound hypermetropic astigmatism
  Both the foci are behind the retina.

Retinal plane at B
  Simple hypermetropic astigmatism
  Vertical meridian—Emmetropic
  Horizontal meridian—Hypermetropic

Retinal plane at C and D
  Mixed astigmatism [circle of least diffusion]
  Vertical meridian—Myopic
  Horizontal meridian—Hypermetropic

Retinal plane at E
  Simple myopic astigmatism
  Vertical meridian—Myopic
  Horizontal meridian—Emmetropic

Retinal plane at F
  Compound myopic astigmatism
  Both the foci are in front of the retina

2. Irregular Astigmatism

It is present when the corneal surface is irregular. It cannot be adequately corrected by lenses, e.g. as following healed corneal ulcer. Soft contact lens may be used. Partial or full thickness keratoplasty may be done depending on the depth of opacity as a last resort.

Symptoms

1. Diminished visual acuity is the most troublesome clinical symptom.
2. Eye strain and headache after short-time of near work is usually present.
3. The letters in the book appear to be "running together".

Treatment

1. If there are no symptom, no treatment is required in low degree of astigmatism.
2. When there are symptoms, suitable cylindrical lenses are prescribed for constant use.

Prognosis

1. Regular astigmatism is the only form susceptible to treatment by lenses.
2. Mixed astigmatism has good prognosis as "circle of least diffusion" falls upon or near the retina.

APHAKIA

Aphakia is a condition of the eye where lens has been removed, i.e. absence of lens. It is a classical example of acquired high hypermetropia.

Optical Condition

1. The eye is hypermetropic. Parallel rays of light reach a focus about 31 mm behind the cornea.
2. There is loss of accommodation.
3. The retinal image is about 25% larger.
4. Astigmatism [against the rule]—The surgical scar at the corneoscleral junction in the upper part of the cornea flattens the vertical meridian of the cornea.

Aphakic eye   Correction with convex lens

Symptom

There is gross dimness of vision because of acquired high hypermetropia.

Signs

1. A linear semicircular corneo-scleral scar mark is seen in the upper half of cornea.
2. The iris shows peripheral buttonhole iridectomy at or near 12 o'clock position.
3. The anterior chamber is deep due to lack of support of the iris by the lens.
4. There is often iridodonesis or tremulousness of the iris due to lack of support.
5. The pupil is jet black.
6. Purkinje-Sanson 3rd and 4th images are absent.
7. In pseudophakia, i.e. where intraocular lens (IOL) has been placed in the posterior chamber, a peculiar shining reflex is seen through the pupil.

Treatment

1. Correction by Spectacles

Aphakia is treated by prescribing suitable spherical convex lens (+ 10 D approximately) and convex cylindrical lens (+1 to +2D at 180°) 6 weeks after the operation, i.e. when the scar has healed completely and the refraction has become stable.

Advantages
1. It is cheap and readily available.
2. It is easy to handle particularly by old persons.

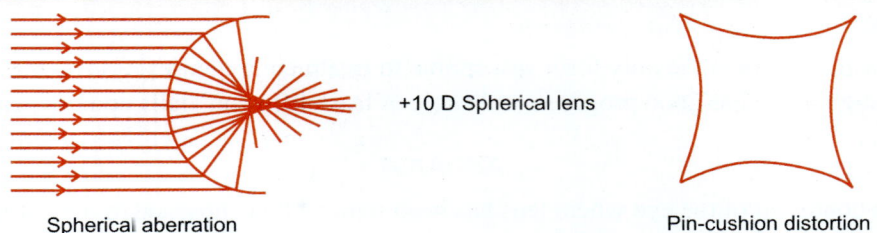

Spherical aberration   Pin-cushion distortion

Disadvantages
1. There is 25% retinal image magnification.
2. Spherical aberration causes 'pin cushion effect'. There is greater refraction at the periphery of spherical lens than near the centre. Thus, the incoming rays of light do not come to a point focus.
3. Chromatic aberration may be present.
4. "Jack in the box" ring scotoma is seen due to total internal reflection of light.
5. The peripheral visual fields are reduced.
6. There is difficulty in co-ordination and orientation.
7. Physical inconvenience and cosmetic deficiency is often present.

2. Contact Lens

Advantages
There is minimum retinal image magnification, therefore it is useful in unilateral aphakia. It looks good cosmetically.

Disadvantages
1. Corneal epithelium oedema may occur due to hypoxia.
2. Corneal erosion and ulcer may result from epithelial damage.
3. Corneal vascularization may occur due to constant irritation.
4. Papillary conjunctivitis may occur due to the growth of pathogens.
5. Intolerance and foreign body sensation are common complaints.
6. Loss, breakage and deterioration of lens leads to financial loss.

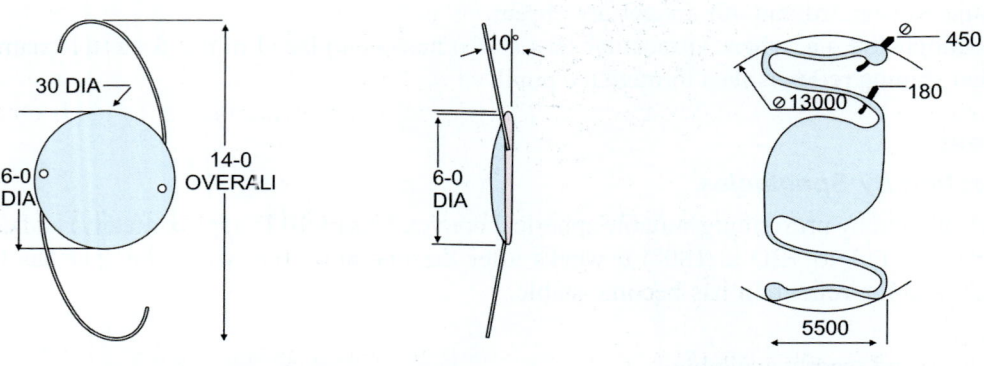

Single piece PMMA posterior chamber IOL   Anterior chamber IOL

3. Intraocular Lens [IOL] Implantation

This is also known as *pseudophakia*. Posterior chamber IOL implantation is best as they are placed in the normal physiological position of lens.
1. Intraocular lens is made up of hard material PMMA (polymethyl methacrylate) or soft material HEMA (hydroxyethyl methacrylate).
2. Lenses are biconvex or planoconvex measuring 4-6 mm in diameter.

Lens power is calculated by:
   i. Ultrasonography (A-scan) (axial length)
   ii. Keratometry
   iii. Standard calculation tables.
   The standard power of +19.5 D of posterior chamber IOL = +11 D spherical lens.

Advantages
1. There is minimum retinal image magnification
2. There is early return of binocular vision
3. The peripheral vision is normal
4. It has cosmetic advantage.

Complications
1. Corneal dystrophy may occur due to endothelial damage with anterior chamber lens.
2. Dislocation of IOL may occur in the vitreous or anterior chamber.
3. Pupillary block glaucoma results in raised tension postoperatively.
4. Cystoid maculopathy leads to impaired vision.
5. Postoperative iridocyclitis may occur occasionally.

ANISOMETROPIA

It is the optical condition the eyes in which the refraction of the two eyes differs in variety and degree.

Types

1. *Congenital*
   i. One eye is emmetropic and the other eye is ametropic.
   ii. Both eyes are ametropic (either myopic or hypermetropic) but differ in degree, e.g. one eye has refractive power of –2D and the other eye has –6D.
   iii. Both eyes are ametropic but differ in variety, e.g. one eye is hypermetropic and the other eye is myopic.
2. *Acquired*

It is seen after unilateral cataract extraction. One eye is emmetropic and the operated eye is hypermetropic.

Symptoms

1. There is eye strain due to aniseikonia, i.e. difference in the size of the retinal images.
2. Diplopia or seeing double objects may be present in severe cases and unilateral aphakia.

Signs

1. In low degree, binocular vision is usually present.
2. In high degree (more than 2-3 D), only uniocular vision is present. The other eye may become divergent and take the position of rest.
3. Alternating vision—The hypermetropic eye is used for distance and the myopic eye is used for near.

Treatment

1. It is treated by prescribing suitable correcting lenses for refractive difference of up to 2-3 D.
2. Contact lenses are useful in correcting aniseikonia, i.e. difference in size of retinal images.
3. Iseikonic or size lenses are indicated in complicated cases of anisometropia.

PRESBYOPIA

It is an insufficiency of accommodation due to advancing age (usually 40 years). It is not an error of refraction.

Etiology

There is physiological failure of accommodation due to:
- *Hardening of the lens with age*
- *Weakness of the ciliary muscle and suspensory ligament*
- *Excessive close work*
- *Prodromal stage of close angle glaucoma.*

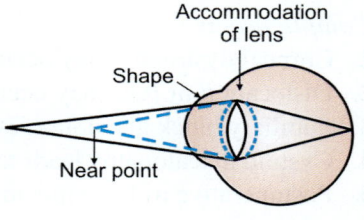

Presbyopia

Symptoms

1. There is blurring of vision for near work specially reading. The vision improves if the book is held further away from the ordinary reading distance, i.e. about 30 cm.
2. Symptoms appear early in persons doing too much close work, e.g. goldsmith, clerk.
3. Symptoms depend on existing error of refraction.
   In hypermetropia—There is early onset of presbyopia.
   In myopia—There is delayed onset of presbyopia.

Sign

Near vision is impaired. It can be tested by Snellen's near test types.

The average eye glass adds for various age group	
40 years	+ 0.5 D
45 years	+ 1.0 D
50 years	+ 1.5 D
55 years	+ 2.0 D
60 years	+ 2.5 D

Treatment

1. Presbyopia is treated by prescribing suitable convex spherical lenses for near work.
2. This correction for near work is added to the correcting lenses for the distant vision.

DETERMINATION OF REFRACTION

Determination of refraction is the term applied to the various testing procedures used to measure the refractive errors of the eye and to provide proper correction.

Determination of refraction is done by the following methods:

1. Objective Methods
  i. *Retinoscopy*—It is done after dilatation of the pupil.
  ii. *Auto-refractometer*—Refraction is tested automatically using electronic and computer technology.
  iii. *Keratometer*—It is useful for testing corneal astigmatism particularly.

2. Subjective Methods
Postmydriatic test (PMT).

RETINOSCOPY [Skiascopy or Shadow Test]

A retinoscope is an instrument that the examiner uses to shine light through the patient's pupil. He observes the reflex formed by the light rays reflected from the patient's retina.

Optical Principle

When light is reflected from a mirror into the observer's eye, the direction in which the light moves across the pupil varies with the refraction of the eye.

Mydriatics in Refraction

The pupil is dilated by a suitable mydriatic depending on the age of patient.

In children—Atropine ointment application three times a day for 3 days is preferred up to 8 years of age as it paralyses the ciliary muscle. Children have great power of accommodation.

In adults—Phenylephrine, homatropine cyclopentolate, tropicamide may be used.

COMMONLY USED TOPICAL MYDRIATICS AND CYCLOPLEGICS

Drugs	MYDRIASIS		CYCLOPLEGIA	
	Maximum effect (minutes)	Full recovery (days)	Maximum effect (hours)	Full recovery (days)
Atropine 1%	40	10	6	14
Homatropine 2%	60	3	1	3
Cyclopentolate	60	1	1	1
Tropicamide 0.5%	40	0.25	0.5	0.25
Phenylephrine 10%	20	0.25	Nil	Nil

Method

Retinoscopy is done in a dark room.
- The examiner sits at 1 m distance from the patient.

- The patient wears a trial frame and fixes a spot at the far end of the room so that the light rays entering the eye are parallel.
- A light is placed behind and above the patient's head.
- The examiner looks through a central hole in the plane mirror in the patient's eye.
- The mirror is moved slowly from one side to the other. The direction in which the shadow moves is noted.
- The horizontal meridian is observed first, and then the vertical.

Observations and Inferences

1. *In hypermetropia:* The shadow moves in the same direction as the mirror.
2. *In myopia (above –1 D):* The shadow moves in the opposite direction.
3. *In myopia of –1 D:* There is no shadow.
4. *In emmetropia and myopia of less than –1 D:* There is a very faint shadow moving in the same direction.
5. *In astigmatism:* The shadow appears to swirl around (scissor-shaped).

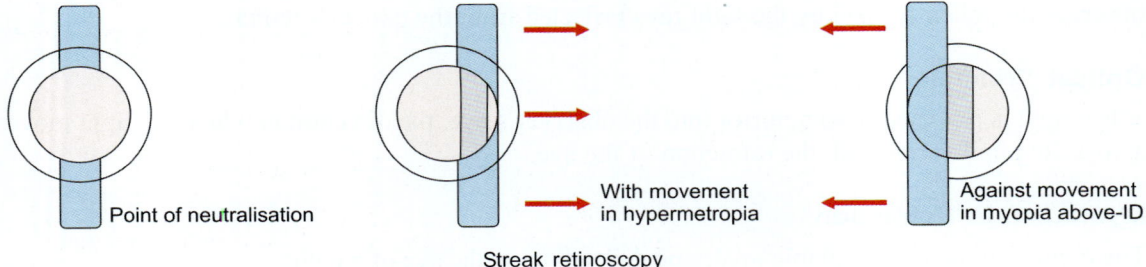

Streak retinoscopy

Neutralisation

When the shadow moves with the mirror, progressively stronger convex lenses are put in the trial frame until,
   i. No shadow is seen
   ii. The shadow moves in the opposite direction.

This is known as *'the point of reversal'*. Similarly, when the shadow moves against the mirror, progressively stronger concave lenses are put in the trial frame until *the point of reversal* is reached.

POSTMYDRIATIC TEST (PMT)

In postmydriatic test appropriate lenses as found by the retinoscopy are inserted in the trial frame. Each eye is tested separately. Then the two eyes are finally tested and corrected together for distant vision.

The correction for near vision by convex spherical lenses is made over 40 years of age usually. It is always undercorrected. It is added to the correction for distant vision.

CORRECTION OF AMETROPIA WITH LENSES

1. Spectacles

- In children spectacles with large round or oval lenses should be ordered as they may look over them.
- In adults and with astigmatism, rigid spectacles must be ordered.
- For distant vision, the lenses are centred properly so that the optical centres are opposite the pupil.
- For near vision, the lenses are decentered inwards and tilted at an angle of 15°.
- Bifocal, trifocal or multifocal lenses are used.
- Tinted glasses are used in high myopia, albinism or in tropical countries.
- Photochromatic lenses become dark automatically in bright light and remain white in dim light.

1. LENSES

Types

1. Spherical lens—Convex, concave
2. Cylindrical lens—Convex, concave

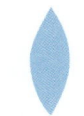
Convex spherical lens

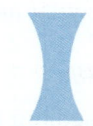
Concave spherical lens

1. Spherical Lens

It has equal curvature in all meridians.

1. *Convex lens*—It is a transparent medium bounded by two spherical surfaces.

   Identification
   i. When the lens is moved in front of the eye, the objects move in the opposite direction.
   ii. If an object is held close to the lens, it appears to be magnified.

   Uses
   It is used in the treatment of:
   - *Hypermetropia*
   - *Presbyopia*
   - *Aphakia*
   - *Magnifying lens.*

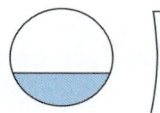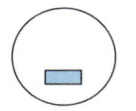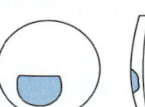
Type of bifocals

2. *Concave lens*—It is transparent medium bounded by concave surfaces.

   Identification
   i. When the lens is moved in front of the eye, the objects move in the same direction
   ii. An object seen through the lens appears to be diminished in size.

   Uses
   It is used in the treatment of:
   - Myopia
   - Hruby's lens (–58.6 D)

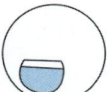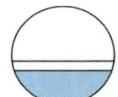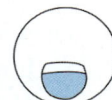
Types of trifocals

2. Cylindrical Lens

It is a segment of a cylinder of glass cut parallel to its axis. The axis of a cylindrical lens is parallel to that of the cylinder of which it is a part.

Identification
  i. Two marks are seen on the lens indicating the axis of the lens.
  ii. When the lens is moved in the direction of the axis, there is no movement of the objects.
  iii. When the lens is moved in a direction at right angles to the axis
    Convex cylinder—The objects move in the opposite direction.
    Concave cylinder—The objects move in the same direction.
Use Regular astigmatism can be treated by suitable cylindrical lenses.

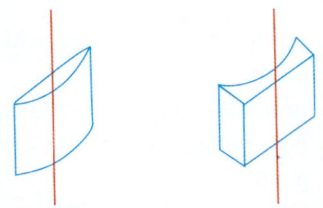

Convex cylinder   Concave cylinder

2. PRISM

It is a medium bounded by two plain refractive surfaces at an angle to each other. This angle is called, "the angle of the prism". The "base of the prism" is situated opposite this angle.

Uses

It is used in the treatment of:
- Heterophoria
- Convergence insufficiency
- It is used in various optical instruments.

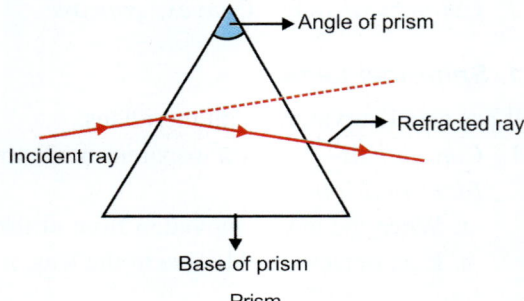

Prism

2. Contact Lenses

Principle

Contact lens alters the vergence power of the anterior surface of the eye.
- Contact lenses rest on the corneal surface.

Types

1. **Hard lens**—It consists of PMMA (Polymethyl methacrylate) a plastic, non-toxic material.
   Advantage—It is durable, firm and inert.
   Disadvantage—The corneal hypoxia leads to corneal oedema.
   - It may cause foreign body sensation.
2. **Soft lens**—It consists of HEMA (hydroxyethyl methacrylate) or related polymer and is hydrophilic in nature.

Advantage—It is comfortable and stable.

Disadvantage—It is delicate and has a short lifespan.

3. ***Gas permeable lens***—It consists of mixture of hard and soft material, e.g. CAB (cellulose acetate butyrate), silicone, silicone with PMMA.

   Advantage—It causes minimum corneal hypoxia.

   Disadvantage—It tends to scratch and break.

Method of Calculating the Power

It is done by keratometry and refraction.

Indications

They are mainly refractive, therapeutic, occupational and cosmetic.

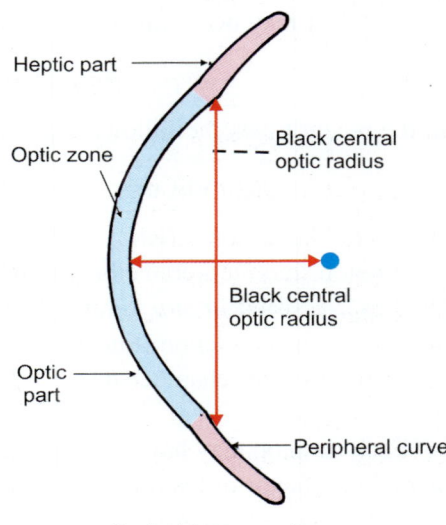

Contact lens curvatures

1. Refractive

   i. Unilateral aphakia—It prevents diplopia as there is no refinal image magnification.
   ii. Irregular astigmatism—Soft contact lenses are useful.
   iii. High myopia with macular degeneration.
   iv. Keratoconus or conical cornea—It provides regular corneal surface and mechanical support.

2. Therapeutic

   i. It has epithelial healing effect, e.g. as in corneal ulcers, filamentary keratitis.
   ii. It is used as a vehicle for drug delivery, e.g. soft hydrophilic lens.
   iii. It prevents symblepharon formation, e.g. as in chemical burn.
   iv. It encourages natural healing process, e.g. as in descemetocele and wound leaks.

3. Occupational

In athletes—There is less chances of serious injury, better optics and wider field.

4. Cosmetic

It improves the cosmetic appearance specially in young marriageable girls.

Disadvantages

1. Contact lenses are expensive, difficult to handle and manoeuvrable.
2. It is easily lost or destroyed by mucoproteins, fungus and calcium deposits.
3. Hard contact lenses are initially uncomfortable to wear. They cause corneal hypoxia resulting in corneal oedema, superficial punctate keratitis (SPK) and opacity.

Complications

1. *Conjunctiva*—Allergic or infective conjunctivitis may occur occasionally.
2. *Cornea*—Corneal epithelial oedema results due to corneal hypoxia.
   - Vascularization results due to hypoxia, infection and foreign body sensation.
   - Ulcer may occur due to improper hygiene and infection.

REFRACTIVE CORNEAL SURGERY

In the recent times the following procedures have been accepted by the refractive surgeons

CLINICAL PROCEDURES	CORRECTION OF MYOPIA
1. Radial keratotomy (RK)	–1.0 to –6.0 D
2. Photorefractive keratectomy (PRK)	–1.0 to –8.0 D
3. Laser-assisted *in situ* keratomileusis (LASIK)	–8.0 to –16.0 D
4. Clear lens extraction (Fucala's operation) with posterior chamber IOL.	–16 to –26 D

Each surgeon may have a preference for a particular procedure depending on economic reasons, availability factor or his own personal satisfaction with the end results.

1. RADIAL KERATOTOMY (RK)

It is still an excellent procedure for low myopias, i.e. from –1.0 to –6.0 D in young adults. Ideally 4 to 8 cut incisions are given with a calibrated diamond knife up to the level of Descemet's membrane.

Principle

It decreases myopia by flattening the corneal curvature.

Method

The central optical zone measuring 3-4 mm in diameter is marked out. With a specially calibrated diamond knife 4-8 deep radial incisions (depending on the degree of myopia) are made up to the Descemet's membrane in between the limbus and the optical zone.

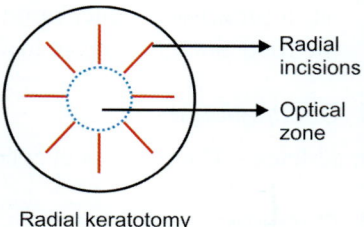

Radial keratotomy

Indication

It is suitable for young adults with stable myopia of –1 to –6 D with minimum astigmatism.

Advantages

1. The main advantage of RK is that the optical centre of 3 mm is spared unlike PRK where the optical zone of 6 to 7 mm is reshaped by laser with the fear of residual corneal haze.
2. Cost factor—It is comparatively cheap and almost 1/4 of the cost of PRK.

Disadvantages

1. Uneven healing may lead to irregular astigmatism which is difficult to correct. The person may feel that he is looking through the waves.
2. Weakening of eyeball may rarely lead to globe rupture on minimum trauma.
3. There may be glare at night.
4. Intrastromal inclusion cyst may occur due to radial incisions.

ASTIGMATIC KERATOTOMY

It is an extension of the principles of radial keratotomy. The aim of astigmatic keratotomy is to flatten the more curved meridian by asymmetrical incisional surgery. To achieve this various considerations are kept in mind such as the number and position of the transverse incisions. The main indication is in the management of postkeratoplasty patients. The results are often unpredictable.

2. PHOTOREFRACTIVE KERATECTOMY (PRK) BY EXCIMER LASER

PRK is the treatment of choice for myopia of –1.0 to –8.0 D. The central part of the cornea (optical zone) is reshaped by the laser after corneal epithelial debridement. PRK uses the computer-controlled accuracy and precision of the excimer laser to sculpt the surface of the cornea, correcting myopia, hypermetropia and astigmatism. As very thin layers of the cornea is removed, PRK does not weaken the eye.

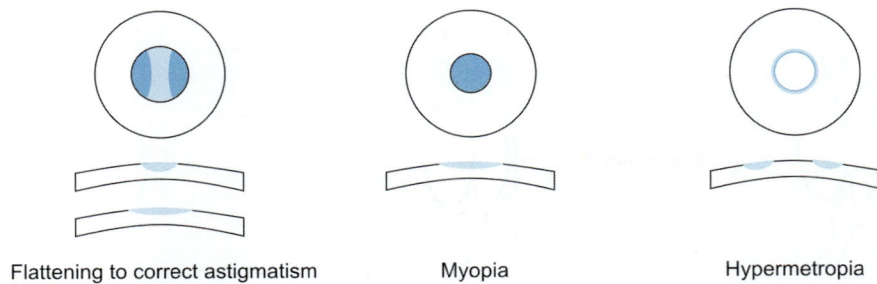

Flattening to correct astigmatism   Myopia   Hypermetropia

Excimer laser photorefractive keratectomy directly alters the central cornea

Method

Excimer lasers (excited dimer) act by tissue modelling (Photoablation). It is a source of far ultraviolet radiation which allows removal of corneal tissue with the accuracy of a fraction of a micron. It modifies and flattens the optical zone of cornea. Laser energy has been used to perform radial keratotomy as the laser incision is more accurate and predictable than a diamond knife incision.

Indications

1. Photorefractive keratectomy (PRK) for correction of refractive errors.
2. Phototherapeutic keratectomy (PTK) for corneal diseases such as band-shaped keratopathy may be done.

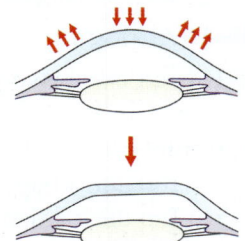

Advantages

1. The results are excellent with an accuracy of 95% in achieving a +/– 0.5D correction with nil to negligible corneal haze.
2. There are no cuts or weakening of the globe as may rarely occur with RK.

Disadvantages

There may be residual corneal haze in the centre affecting clear vision.

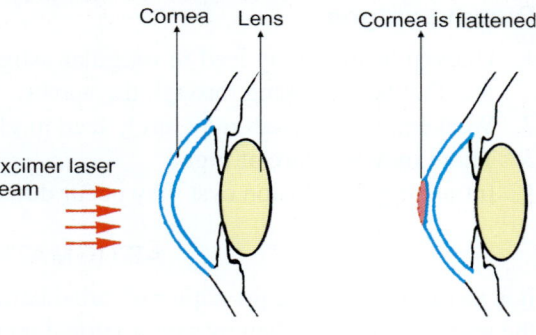

Photorefractive keratectomy (PRK)

3. LASER-ASSISTED *IN SITU* KERATOMILEUSIS (LASIK)

Method

LASIK is a modification of PRK. In this procedure a 160 micron hinged corneal flap is lifted from the central 8 to 9 mm of cornea with the help of a microkeratome. This flap is folded to the side and the excimer laser is then used to remove tissue from the exposed surface, correcting myopia and astigmatism. The corneal flap is replaced back.

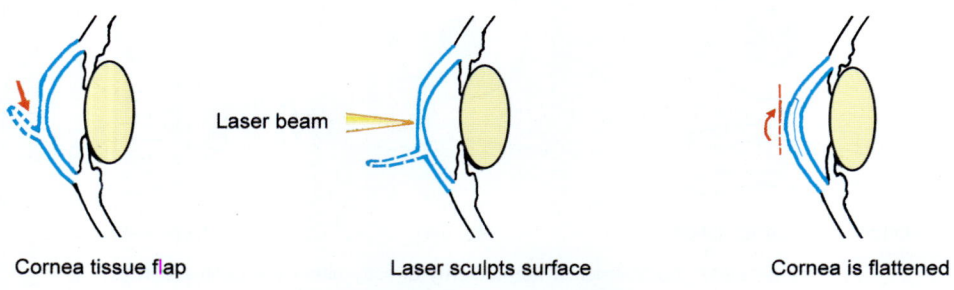

Laser-assisted *in situ* keratomileusis (LASIK)

Advantages

1. Patient has good vision at the end of the same day.
2. There is no pain, watering (RK) or corneal haze (PRK) as compared to RK and PRK respectively.

Disadvantages

1. It is an expensive procedure and requires greater surgical skill for correction of myopia from –8 to –16 D.
2. Complications of LASIK are related to the corneal flap
    - Too thin a flap can cause wrinkling of the flap on repositioning.
    - Too thick a flap will leave very little of the corneal stromal tissue to work on.

4. CLEAR LENS EXTRACTION (FUCALA'S OPERATION) AND PC IOL

This procedure can be done for correcting myopia of –16 to –26 D. It is now accepted that a zero power posterior chamber IOL is better than no IOL at all.
  i. It retards posterior capsular opacification.
  ii. It reinforces the posterior capsule to hold the vitreous phase thus minimising incidence of retinal detachment.

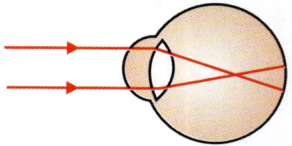

High myopia

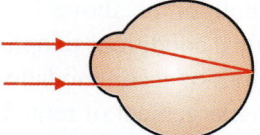

Clear lens extraction (Fucala's operation)

Advantage
There is a clear untouched cornea after surgery which is amendable to further treatment by PRK if need be at a later date.

EPIKERATOPHAKIA

Principle
It is a procedure in which a lenticule of donor tissue is used to alter the surface topography of the cornea.

Method
The donor lenticule of the desired power is sutured into the keratectomy with 10-0 nylon sutures. It is a surgical procedure whereby unilateral high myopia up to –18 D can be corrected.

Indications
In myopia—Minus lenticule is used.
In aphakia in children—Plus lenticule is used.
In keratoconus—Planolenticule is used.

Complications
1. Intolerable glare may be present
2. Chronic epithelial defects may occur.

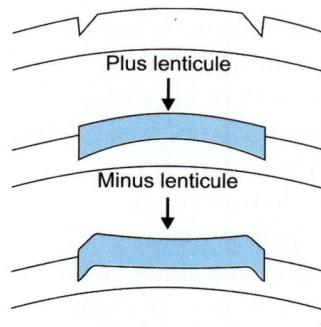

Epikeratophakia

KERATOMILEUSIS

It is a surgical procedure whereby unilateral high myopia up to –18 D can be corrected. A disc of 8 mm × 0.35 mm is removed from the patients cornea using a microtome. This disc is placed on a lathe machine equipped with freezing apparatus and keratomileusis (grinding) is performed. Thus, the surface of cornea is flattened.

Recently Coherent Schwind laser and fourth generation fractile mask spiral lasers are under trial which will further decrease the corneal ablation time.

MULTIPLE CHOICE QUESTIONS

1. Temporal crescent is seen typically in
   a. astigmatism
   b. hypermetropia
   c. myopia
   d. none of the above
2. Blurring of vision for near work occurs in
   a. hypermetropia
   b. presbyopia
   c. both of the above
   d. none of the above
3. Optical conditions of aphakia include all *EXCEPT*
   a. loss of accommodation
   b. astigmatism against rule
   c. enlargement of retinal image
   d. myopia
4. Unilateral aphakia can be treated by
   a. contact lens
   b. intraocular lens implant
   c. both
   d. none
5. Standard power of posterior chamber intraocular lens is
   a. + 20 D
   b. +10 D
   c. + 5 D
   d. + 15 D
6. Cylindrical lenses are prescribed in
   a. presbyopia
   b. astigmatism
   c. myopia
   d. squint
7. A newborn is invariably
   a. hypermetropic
   b. myopic
   c. astigmatic
   d. aphakic
8. Astigmatism is a type of
   a. axial ametropia
   b. index ametropia
   c. curvature ametropia
   d. spherical aberration
9. Hypermetropia causes
   a. divergent squint
   b. convergent squint
   c. both of the above
   d. none of the above
10. In retinoscopy using a plane mirror, when the mirror is tilted to the right the shadow in the pupil moves to the left in
    a. hypermetropia
    b. myopia more than –1 D
    c. emmetropia
    d. myopia less than –1 D
11. Optical condition of the eye in which the refraction of the two eyes differs is
    a. mixed astigmatism
    b. irregular astigmatism
    c. anisometropia
    d. compound astigmatism
12. Latent hypermetropia is detected when following mydriatic is used
    a. adrenaline
    b. phenylephrine
    c. cyclopentolate
    d. atropine
13. Radial keratotomy is useful in
    a. myopia
    b. hypermetropia
    c. presbyopia
    d. aphakia

14. Incident parallel rays come to a focus posterior to the light sensitive layer of retina in
    a. aphakia
    b. hypermetropia
    c. both of the above
    d. none of the above
15. The complications of myopia include all EXCEPT
    a. vitreous degeneration
    b. retinal detachment
    c. cataract
    d. closed angle glaucoma
16. Indistinct distant vision is seen in
    a. presbyopia
    b. myopia
    c. hypermetropia
    d. none of the above
17. The type of lens used for correction of regular astigmatism includes
    a. biconvex lens
    b. biconcave lens
    c. cylindrical lens
    d. none of the above
18. Pseudopapillitis is seen in
    a. hypermetropia
    b. myopia
    c. presbyopia
    d. none of the above
19. Contact lenses may be useful in treatment of all EXCEPT
    a. keratoconus
    b. refractive anisometropia
    c. Fuch's endothelial dystrophy
    d. severe keratoconjunctivitis sicca
20. Prisms are used in ophthalmology to measure and to treat
    a. heterophoria
    b. heterotropia
    c. both
    d. none
21. Hard contact lens is made up of
    a. HEMA
    b. PMMA
    c. PVP
    d. PVC
22. Biconvex lens is used in all EXCEPT
    a. aphakia
    b. presbyopia
    c. astigmatism
    d. hypermetropia
23. In compound hypermetropic astigmatism
    a. both the foci are in front of retina
    b. both the foci are behind the retina
    c. one focus is in front and one focus is behind the retina
    d. none of the above
24. Determination of the refraction is done by all EXCEPT
    a. retinoscopy
    b. refractometer
    c. keratometer
    d. perimeter
25. Retinoscopy is done in a dark room at a distance of
    a. 1 m
    b. 2 m
    c. 3 m
    d. 6 m
26. Drug of choice for pupillary dilatation in children is
    a. atropine
    b. homatropine
    c. scopolamine
    d. cyclopentolate

27. Out of the following which is the shortest acting mydriatic
    a. tropicamide
    b. homatropine
    c. cyclopentolate
    d. atropine
28. Frequent change of presbyopic glasses is an early symptom of
    a. closed angle glaucoma
    b. open angle glaucome
    c. senile cataract
    d. after cataract
29. Accommodation is maximum in
    a. childhood
    b. adulthood
    c. middle-age
    d. old age
30. Treatment of choice in aphakia is
    a. spectacles
    b. contact lens
    c. anterior chamber IOL
    d. posterior chamber IOL

ANSWERS

1—c	2—c	3—d	4—c	5—a
6—b	7—c	8—c	9—b	10—b
11—c	12—d	13—a	14—c	15—d
16—b	17—c	18—a	19—c	20—c
21—b	22—c	23—b	24—d	25—a
26—a	27—a	28—a	29—a	30—d

CHAPTER 6
The Conjunctiva

APPLIED ANATOMY

Conjunctiva is a thin, translucent, vascular mucous membrane which covers the under surface of the lids and is reflected over the anterior part of the eyeball upto the limbus. It is exposed to dust, wind, heat and radiation and therefore prone to get infected.

Parts

It consists of following parts namely,
1. *Palpebral*—It covers the under surface of both upper and lower lids. The palpebral conjunctiva is adherent to the tarsus and cannot be easily dissected. It is very thin.
2. *Bulbar*—It covers the anterior part of the eyeball. It is loosely attached to the underlying tissue but it is firmly adherent to the Tenon's capsule 3 mm around the limbus.
3. *Fornices*—These are folds of the conjunctiva formed by the reflection of the mucous membrane from the lids to the eyeball. It is a loose but thick membrane.
4. *Plica semilunaris*—It is a crescentic fold of the conjunctiva situated at the inner canthus.

Structure

It consists of two layers,
1. *The epithelium*—There are 2-5 layers of epithelial cells.
2. *The stroma*—It consists of blood vessels, connective tissue, glands such as glands of Krause, glands of Wolfring and goblet cells.

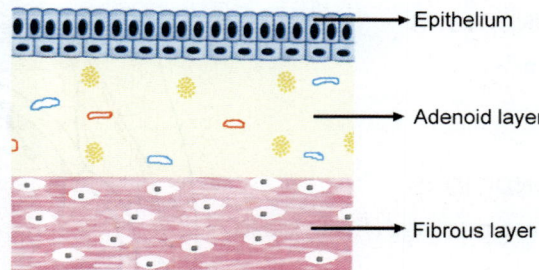

Structure of conjunctiva

Blood Supply

The anterior and posterior conjunctival arteries and veins.

Lymphatic Drainage

The preauricular and submandibular lymph nodes.

Nerve Supply

It is supplied by two different sets of nerves:
1. *Sensory nerves*—These are branches of ophthalmic and maxillary division of the 5th cranial nerve.
2. *Sympathetic nerves*—These are derived from the sympathetic plexus.

Bacteriology

Most of the organisms normally present are non-pathogenic but some are morphologically identical with pathogenic types.

Non-pathogenic bacteria—Diplococcus, Corynebacterium xerosis, Staphylococcus albus, etc.

Pathogenic bacteria—Staphylococcus, Streptococcus, Pneumococcus, Ps. Pyocyanea, E. coli, B. proteus, etc. are pathogenic but rare.

The bacterial growth is inhibited by:
  i. Mechanical washing away action of tears.
  ii. The tear contains lysozyme, IgA, IgG which are bacteriostatic.
  iii. Low temperature due to evaporation of tear, exposure and moderate blood supply.

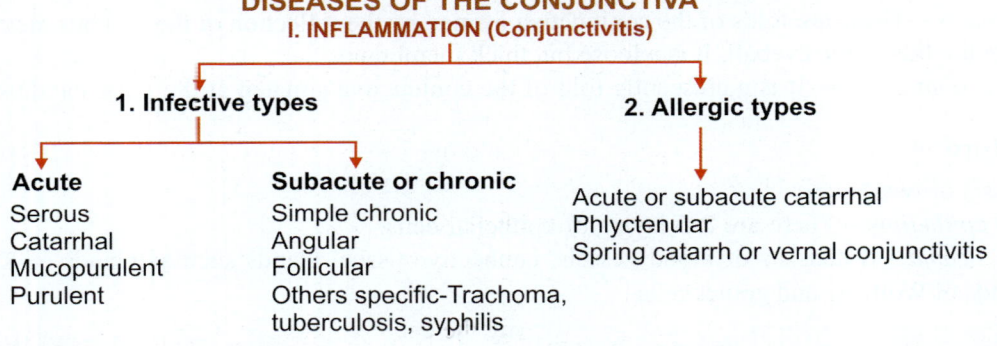

II. DEGENERATIVE CONDITIONS
1. Concretions (lithiasis)
2. Pinguecula
3. Pterygium

III. SYMPTOMATIC CONDITIONS
1. Subconjunctival haemorrhage (Ecchymosis)
2. Xerosis
3. Chemosis
4. Argyrosis

IV. CYSTS AND TUMOURS
1. Retention cyst, implantation cyst
2. Dermoid, dermolipoma, papilloma, epithelioma
3. Pigmented naevi and malignant melanoma

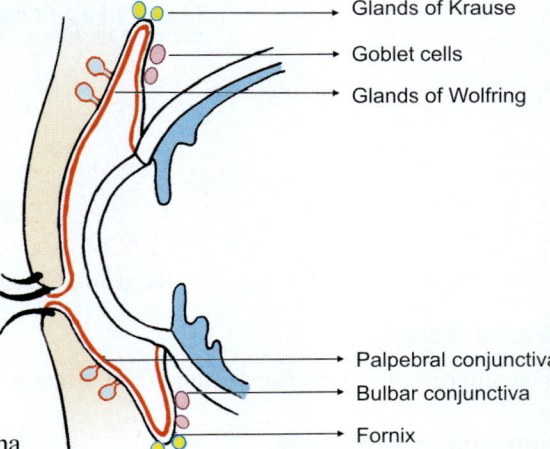

Parts of conjunctiva

I. INFLAMMATION (CONJUNCTIVITIS)

I. EVALUATION

Evaluation of conjunctival inflammation is done by:
1. The type of discharge.
2. The characteristics of conjunctival reactions.
3. The presence of lymphadenopathy.

1. Discharge

It consists of serous exudate, epithelial debris, mucus and tears.

Watery—It is present in acute allergic and viral conjunctivitis.

Mucin—It is seen in spring catarrh and keratoconjunctivitis sicca.

Mucopurulent—It is present in mild bacterial infection and chlamydial infection.

Purulent—It is seen in severe acute bacterial infection.

2. Conjunctival Reactions

Hyperaemia—It is seen maximum in the fornices and minimum at the limbus. It is due to congestion of the conjunctival vessels.

Oedema and chemosis—It is due to swelling of the conjunctiva as a result of exudation from capillaries. It is seen maximum in the fornices and the bulbar conjunctiva as they are lax.

Follicle—There is lymphoid hyperplasia with a germinal centre. They are usually multiple, discrete, slightly elevated, round, measuring 0.5-5 mm in size.

Papilla—It is a vascular structure invaded by the inflammatory cells.

Membrane

i. *True membrane*—It is a coagulum involving the entire epithelium. Its removal causes tearing of epithelium and bleeding, e.g. diphtherial, β-haemolytic streptococcal conjunctivitis.
ii. *Pseudomembrane*—It is a coagulum on the surface of the epithelium. It can be easily peeled off leaving the epithelium intact, e.g. pneumococcal, streptococcal, gonococcal, adenovirus and autoimmune conjunctivitis.

DIFFERENCES BETWEEN TRUE AND PSEUDOMEMBRANE

	TRUE MEMBRANE	PSEUDOMEMBRANE
1. Structure	Fibrinous exudate is situated over and within the conjunctival epithelium	Fibrinous exudate is situated over the surface of conjunctival epithelium.
2. On peeling	It cannot be peeled off easily.	It is separated easily.
3. Bleeding	Bleeding occurs when the membrane is removed.	There is no bleeding.

3. Lymphadenopathy

The preauricular nodes are enlarged in viral and chlamydial infections.

II. DIAGNOSIS

The diagnosis of conjunctivitis is confirmed by:
  i. Bacteriological examination for the presence of bacteria and inclusion bodies.
  ii. Histological examination of the secretion and scrapings of the epithelium taken by a platinum loop and stained with Giemsa stain and Gram stain.
  iii. Conjunctival culture—It is taken from lid margin and conjunctival sac with sterile cotton tipped applicators.

III. TREATMENT OF CONJUNCTIVITIS

1. *Antibiotic drops*—Antibiotic drops commonly used to treat conjunctivitis include the following:
    i. Norfloxacin is a quinolone antibiotic with broad spectrum activity and low toxicity.
    ii. Ciprofloxacin—It has similar properties as norfloxacin.
    iii. Other antibiotics include chloramphenicol, gentamicin, framycin, tobramycin, neomycin, polymyxin, etc. They are instilled 4-6 times daily.
2. *Antibiotic ointments*—Ointments provide higher concentration of antibiotic for longer period than drops. As they cause blurred vision during the day, ointments are used at night or during sleep.

    Antibiotics available in ointment form are : Chloromycetin, gentamicin, tetracycline, framycetin, neomycin, polymyxin and ciprofloxacin.

ACUTE CONJUNCTIVITIS
1. Acute Mucopurulent Conjunctivitis

Etiology

It is caused by several organisms such as *Staphylococcus, Streptococcus, Pneumococcus, Haemophilus aegyptius*, adenovirus, etc. It is often associated with measles and scarlet fever.

Incidence

1. It occurs in epidemics and is bilateral usually.
2. It is contagious and spreads by flies, fingers and fomites.
3. It is often self-limiting.

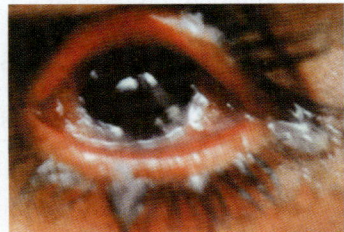

Acute mucopurulent conjunctivitis

Symptoms

1. There is redness and grittiness, i.e. feeling of foreign body sensation.
2. Mucopurulent discharge and crusting is present in the fornices and margins of lids.

3. There is sticking together of lids specially in the morning because of accumulation of mucous discharge during the night.
4. Coloured halos due to flakes of mucus passing across the cornea may be present.

Signs
1. Conjunctival congestion is always present. The conjunctiva is fiery red (pink eye or red eye).
2. Chemosis and subconjunctival haemorrhage may be present.

Complications
These are rare but superficial keratitis, marginal corneal ulcer, chronic conjunctivitis may occur.

Treatment
1. *Cleanliness*—Frequent washing of the eyes with warm saline or clean water.
2. *Control of infection*
    i. Frequent instillation of appropriate bacteriostatic antibiotic eye drops and application of eye ointment at bedtime after doing culture and sensitivity. Conjunctival swab is taken prior to starting treatment. Application of ointment prevents the lids from sticking together.
    ii. The eyes should not be bandaged as this prevents the free exit of secretion and encourage bacterial growth due to warmth and stasis.
    iii. In case of photophobia, dark glasses or an eye shade may be worn.

Prophylaxis
1. Isolation of the patient should be done when possible.
2. Avoid using the patients towel or other fomites.
3. Avoid contact with the infected eye as it is highly contagious.
4. Patient must keep his hands clean by washing them often.

2. Purulent Conjunctivitis (Acute Blenorrhoea)

Types
It is a much more serious condition occurring in two forms.
1. *In adults*—Acute purulent conjunctivitis.
2. *In babies*—Ophthalmia neonatorum. It is rare nowadays due to improved prophylactic measures before, during and after the birth of the child.

Acute Purulent Conjunctivitis
It is an acute inflammation of conjunctiva occurring in adults.

Etiology
Most cases are caused by gonococcus but same clinical picture may be seen with *Staphylococcus, Streptococcus diphtheriae, Chlamydia oculogenitalis* and in mixed infections.

Incidence
1. It occurs in males commonly affecting the right eye first.
2. There may be associated infection in the genital area and urethritis.
3. The incubation period is from a few hours to 3 days.

Symptoms
1. There is acute onset with much swelling of the lids and conjunctiva.
2. Purulent discharge is present at lid borders, canthi and fornices.
3. There may be constitutional disturbances including a rise of temperature and mental depression.

Signs
1. Marked conjunctival congestion is seen. Palpebral conjunctiva is red and velvety.
2. Severe chemosis and pus discharge are present.
3. Lids are swollen, red, tense and tender. The upper lid overhangs over the lower lid.
4. Pseudomembrane over palpebral conjunctiva may be seen rarely.
5. Preauricular lymphadenopathy may be present.

Complications
1. Subacute conjunctivitis with papillary thickening of the conjunctiva.
2. Corneal ulcers (marginal) are common. There is direct invasion of the bacteria.
3. Iritis and iridocyclitis lead to serious diminution of vision.
4. Perforation of cornea leads to blindness.
5. Arthritis, endocarditis, septicaemia may occur rarely.

Prognosis
It depends on the condition of the other eye. It is bad in untreated cases.

Treatment
1. Frequent washing of the conjunctival sac with warm saline.
2. Instillation of aqueous solution of benzyl penicillin drops (10,000 units per ml) every minute × half an hour. Later it can be continued 4 hourly × 3 days.
3. If allergic to penicillin, ciprofloxacin, tobramycin gentamicin, tetracycline or any other suitable antibiotics are instilled every few minutes initially. Later on they are applied four times daily.
4. Atropine is applied if there is corneal involvement and associated iritis.

Prophylaxis
1. Protect the other eye by protective covering and topical antibiotics.
2. Isolation of the patient should be done.

OPHTHALMIA NEONATORUM

It is a preventable disease occurring in newborn babies.

Etiology

Virulent gonococcus infection used to be responsible for 50% blindness in children but due to effective methods of prophylaxis and treatment, it is rare nowadays. *Chlamydia oculogenitalis, Streptococcus pneumoniae* or other organism cause mild infection.

Incidence

1. It is bilateral usually.
2. It commonly occurs in the newborns due to maternal infection.

Symptoms

1. Any discharge from a baby's eye during the 1st week of life is alarming as tears are secreted only 3-4 weeks after birth.
2. The conjunctiva is bright red and swollen with pouring out of thick yellow pus.
3. Thick pus accumulates at the lid borders, lashes and canthi.
4. Sticking together of the lids is a common feature.

Signs

1. Lids are swollen and tense due to dense infiltration of the bulbar conjunctiva.
2. Conjunctiva is markedly congested and chemosed. Lids are separated by lid retractors to see the cornea. Pseudomembrane may be present.
3. Later the conjunctiva becomes puckered and velvety with free discharge of pus, serum and blood.

Complications

These are common in untreated cases.
1. Corneal ulcer and opacity.
2. Perforated corneal ulcer with prolapse of iris.
3. Adherent leucoma and panophthalmitis.
4. Metastatic stomatitis and arthritis involving knee, wrist and ankle joints occur rarely.
5. In case of corneal opacity, there may be nystagmus as macular fixation occurs during the first 3-4 weeks of life.

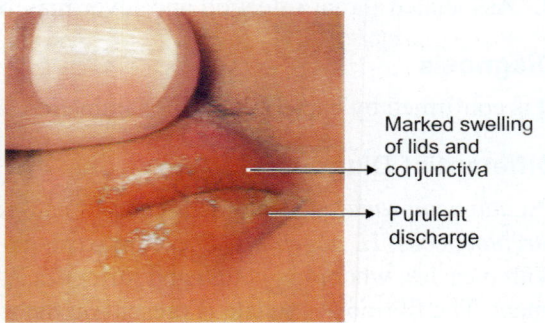

Ophthalmia neonatorum

Treatment

It is same as for adults. Topical therapy is supplemented by parenteral penicillin or newer cephalosporin (cefotaxime) for 3-5 days.

Prophylaxis

1. Aseptic delivery using gloves and sterile technique.
2. Proper antenatal care and treatment of any vaginal discharge prior to delivery.
3. Instil penicillin or broad spectrum antibiotic eyedrops immediately after birth.

3. Membraneous Conjunctivitis (Diphtheritic Conjunctivitis)

The conjunctival surface is covered by a fibrinous membrane.

Etiology

Corynebacterium diphtheriae is the most common pathogen. Other organisms such as gonococcus, pneumococcus, *Streptococcus* can also produce a membrane specially in sick, malnourished children.

Incidence

It is commonly seen in children who are not immunized previously. It often occurs in weak children after measles, scarlet fever or in cases of impetigo.

Symptoms

In mild cases there is swelling of the lids along with serous or mucopurulent discharge.

Signs

1. Lids are swollen, tense and tender with impaired mobility.
2. On everting the lids, a white membrane is seen covering the palpebral conjunctiva which peels off rapidly without much bleeding in mild cases.
3. In severe cases, the membrane does not peel off easily and underlying surface bleeds.
4. Preauricular nodes may be enlarged and tender. They may even suppurate.
5. Associated throat infection and fever may be present.

Membraneous conjunctivitis

Diagnosis

It is confirmed by bacteriological examination and culture of the conjunctival swab.

Differential Diagnosis

Pseudomembrane—Pseudomembrane is caused by gonococcus, *Staphylococcus*, pneumococcus, *Streptococcus, H. aegyptius, E. coli* in weak children who are not immunized. It is often associated with measles, whooping cough and influenza. It peels off readily leaving the underlying epithelium intact. The fibrinous exudate is present on the surface of the conjunctival epithelium.

Complications

1. Corneal ulcer due to secondary infection and iritis is often present.
2. Symblepharon may occur due to adhesions forming in between the palpebral and bulbar conjunctiva.
3. Postdiphtheritic paralysis even of accommodation may occur.

Treatment

1. Every case having membrane is treated as diphtherial unless conjunctival and throat swabs and culture are negative.
2. Intensive local and general administration of penicillin or other suitable antibiotic.
3. Prompt injection of antidiphtheritic serum (4-6-10000 units repeated in 12 hours) and topical application.
4. Protect the other eye from infection.

Prophylaxis

Isolation of the patient should be done.

CHRONIC CONJUNCTIVITIS
1. Simple Chronic Conjunctivitis

Simple chronic conjunctivitis often occurs as a continuation of acute conjunctivitis.

Etiology

1. Irritation by smoke, dust, heat, allergen, late hours is a common cause.
2. Concretions, misplaced eye lashes, dacryocystitis, chronic rhinitis aggravate it.
3. Retained foreign body in the fornix may cause unilateral conjunctivititis.
4. Seborrhoea, chronic intranasal infection and dandruff of scalp are common associated conditions.

Symptoms

1. There is burning discomfort and grittiness specially in the evening.
2. The edges of the lids feel hot and dry.
3. There is difficulty in keeping the lids open.
4. Mild serous discharge may be present.

Signs

1. The surface of the conjunctiva looks sticky.
2. Congestion of fornices and palpebral conjunctiva is seen.
3. Papillae may be present in palpebral conjunctiva (velvety appearance).

Treatment

1. Treat the underlying cause in the lacrimal sac, scalp and nose.
2. Protective glasses should be used to avoid irritants particularly in industries.
3. Bacteriological examination is done and a short course of suitable local antibiotic drops and ointment is given.
4. Conjunctivitis meibomiana, i.e. abnormal amount of secretion from the tarsal gland is treated by repeated massage of the lids. This results in squeezing out the contents of glands.

2. Angular Conjunctivitis (Diplobacillary Conjunctivitis)

The reddening of the conjunctiva is confined exclusively to the intermarginal strip of the bulbar conjunctiva.

Etiology

It is caused by Morax-Axenfield diplobacillus. It produces proteolytic ferment which macerates the conjunctival epithelium. It is often found in the nasal cavity and nasal discharge in case of angular conjunctivitis.

Symptoms

1. Red eye is the most common feature.
2. There is discomfort and frequent blinking.
3. Mild mucopurulent discharge may be present.

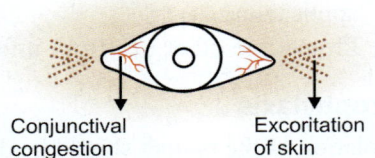

Angular conjunctivitis

Signs

1. Reddening of the bulbar conjunctiva is seen limited to the intermarginal strip specially at the inner and outer canthi.
2. There is excoriation of skin at the outer and inner canthi.

Complications

1. Blepharitis occurs in chronic untreated cases.
2. Marginal, central or hypopyon corneal ulcer may occur.
3. Recurrences are common.

Treatment

1. Oxytetracycline ointment is the drug of choice (bacteriostatic action).
2. Zinc sulphate lotion though less effective acts by inhibiting the proteolytic enzymes produced by Morax-Axenfield bacillus. It forms a coagulum in which the bacilli get enmeshed.
3. Zinc oxide ointment may be applied to the lids at night.

3. Follicular Conjunctivitis

In this condition, conjunctivitis is associated with the development of follicles. In infants, the follicles develop only after the age of 3 months.

Etiology

1. It may be due to exposure to certain chemicals and toxins, e.g. pilocarpine, eserine.
2. It is commonly caused by viruses, e.g. herpes and adenovirus
3. Any conjunctivitis of long duration may cause this condition.

Symptoms

1. There is slight irritation and discomfort.
2. Foreign body sensation is often present.

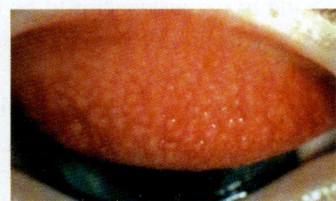

Follicular conjunctivitis

Signs
Multiple follicles are mainly present in the lower fornix. Follicle is a rounded swelling measuring 1-2 mm in size. There is no scarring which differentiates it from trachoma.

Types
Several types of acute follicular conjunctivitis may occur:
  i. *Inclusion conjunctivitis*—It is caused by chlamydial infection and produce inclusion bodies similar to those occurring in trachoma. The primary source of infection is from urethritis in male and cervicitis in female.
 ii. *Epidemic keratoconjunctivitis*—It is associated with several types (3, 7, 8, 19) of adenovirus. It is treated by adenine arabinoside (Ara—A).
iii. *Pharyngoconjunctival fever*—There is associated pharyngitis and fever. It is also caused by adenovirus.
iv. *Acute herpetic conjunctivitis*—It is common in young children. Corneal dendritic ulcers are often present.
 v. *New castle conjunctivitis*—It is caused by newcastle virus from infected fowls.

Complications
Follicles may persist for several years but always resolve without scarring.

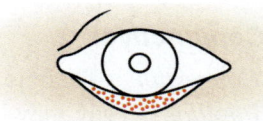

Follicular conjunctivitis

Treatment
1. Astringent eyedrops are applied frequently.
2. Improve general health and nutrition of the patient.
3. Treat associated adenoids, tonsils and upper respiratory tract infection promptly and adequately.

4. Trachoma (Egyptian Ophthalmia)
Trachoma in Greek means 'rough'. Though the disease is known for long, its etiology was not clear. Inclusion organisms were demonstrated in 1907 and the organism was isolated in 1957. The organisms isolated is known as Chlamydia trachomatis.

Etiology
Trachoma is caused by:
- *Chlamydia trachomatis*, a Bedsonian organism (serotypes A, B, Ba and C).
- It belongs to psittacosis lymphogranuloma group.
- It lies between bacteria and virus.
- They multiply by binary fission. They stay inside the cells, which makes them relative immune from effects of the drugs.
- It is seen in the conjunctival scrapings of the epithelial cells as the *Halberstaedter-Prowazek inclusion bodies*.

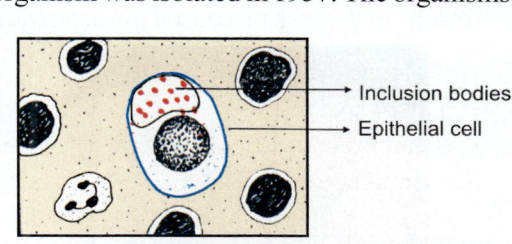

An epithelial cell with multiple inclusions

Incidence

1. It is estimated that 1/5 of world population is affected by trachoma.
2. It is prevalent in Europe, Asia (Iran, India, China, Japan, Middle East), Africa and South America, Australia.
3. In India it is common and endemic in north Gujarat, Rajasthan, Haryana and Punjab.
4. It is commonly seen in unhygienic, crowded, dusty and dirty environment.
5. It is contagious in the acute stage. It spreads by finger, flies, towels and fomites.
6. Maintenance of facial cleanliness is found to be the best measure to reduce the spread of trachoma.

Symptoms

1. Mild irritation and foreign body sensation is often present.
2. Frequent blinking may be present.
3. Mild itching is a common complaint.
4. In chronic stage, cornea is involved causing pain, lacrimation and photophobia.

Signs

The primary infection is epithelial and involves the epithelium of both the conjunctiva and the cornea.

1. Conjunctival

1. *Congestion*—There is red, velvety, jelly-like thickening of the palpebral conjunctiva.
2. *Papillae*—They may be present in the palpebral conjunctiva.
3. *Follicles*—Follicles are seen in the upper and lower fornix, palpebral conjunctiva, plica, bulbar conjunctiva (pathognomonic). They measure 1-5 mm in size.
4. *Typical star-shaped scarring* is seen at the centre of the follicles in late stages.
5. *Arlt's line*—A line of palpebral conjunctival scarring is seen 2 mm from the upper lid margin.

2. Corneal

1. *Superficial keratitis* may be present in the upper part.
2. *Herbert's pits*—There is follicle-like infiltration near the limbus in the upper part. This later results in depression caused by cicatrization of limbal follicles.

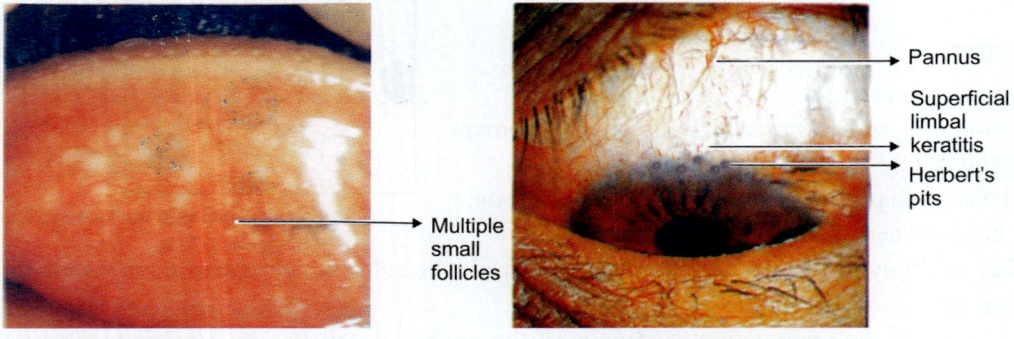

Early trachoma-follicles and papillae

Trachomatous scarring at limbus

3. *Pannus*—There is lymphoid infiltration with vascularization seen in the upper part of cornea. Pannus may resolve completely if Bowman's membrane is not destroyed.
    i. *Progressive pannus*—Superficial blood vessels are parallel and directed downwards. They extend to a horizontal level beyond which zone of infiltration and haze is present.
    ii. *Regressive pannus*—The area of infiltration stops short and the blood vessels extend beyond this haze. This is important in evaluating the result of treatment and progress of disease.

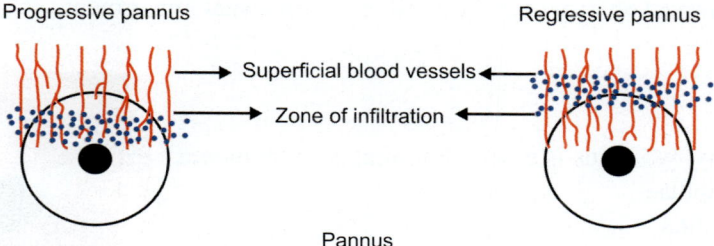

Pannus

I. Mac Callan Classification

There are four clinical stages according to Mac Callan classification.
Trachoma I (subclinical stage)
   It is the earliest stage before clinical diagnosis is possible.
Trachoma II (Stage of typical trachomatous lesions)
   It includes the period between the appearance of typical trachomatous lesions and development of scar tissue.
   i. Follicles or papillae
   ii. Epithelial keratitis
   iii. Pannus
Trachoma III (Stage of scarring)
   Typical star-shaped scarring is obvious.
Trachoma IV (Stage of sequelae and complications)
   The disease is quiet and cured but cicatrization gives rise to symptoms.

II. World Health Organization (WHO) Classification

WHO has suggested the following classifications in 1987.
1. TF *(Trachomatous inflammation—Follicular)*
    a. Atleast five or more follicles (each 0.5mm or more in diameter) should be present on the upper tarsal conjunctiva.
    b. The deep tarsal vessels should be visible through the follicles.
2. TI *(Trachomatous inflammation—Intense)*
    a. There is marked inflammatory thickening of the upper tarsal conjunctiva which appears red, rough, thickened with numerous follicles.
    b. This obscures 50% or more of the deep tarsal vessels.

3. **TS** *(Trachomatous scarring)*
   Presence of scarring is seen in the upper tarsal conjunctiva. Which is seen as white fibrous lines, bands or sheets.
4. **TT** *(Trachomatous trichiasis)*
   a. Atleast one or more misdirected eyelashes rub against the eyeball.
   b. Evidence of recent removal of inturned eyelashes should be regarded as trichiasis.
5. **CO** *(Corneal opacity)*
   Easily visible corneal opacity over the pupil results in visual impairment.

Diagnosis

1. Clinical

The presence of any two signs is essential to diagnose trachoma.
   i. Follicles or papillae
   ii. Epithelial keratitis
   iii. Pannus
   iv. Typical star-shaped scarring of the conjunctiva.

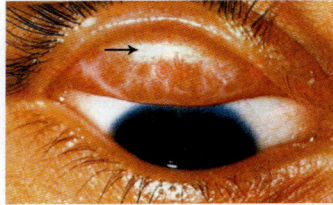

Arlt's line and star-shaped scarring

2. Laboratory

   i. Histological demonstration of the inclusion bodies
   ii. Culture in irradiated McCoy cells
   iii. Microimmunofluorescence test (micro-IF)
   iv. IgA-IPA light microscopy test
   v. Monoclonal antibody direct test.

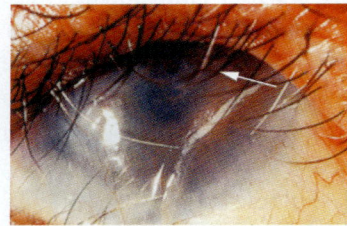

Trichiasis and corneal ulcer

Sequelae and Complications

The only complication of trachoma is corneal ulcer. All the rest are sequelae of trachoma.
1. *Trichiasis*—Misdirected eyelashes occur due to conjunctival scarring.
2. *Entropion*—In rolling of the lid margin results from scarring.
3. *Corneal ulcer*—It is often due to dry eye and misdirected eyelashes.
4. *Corneal opacity*—It results from corneal ulceration.

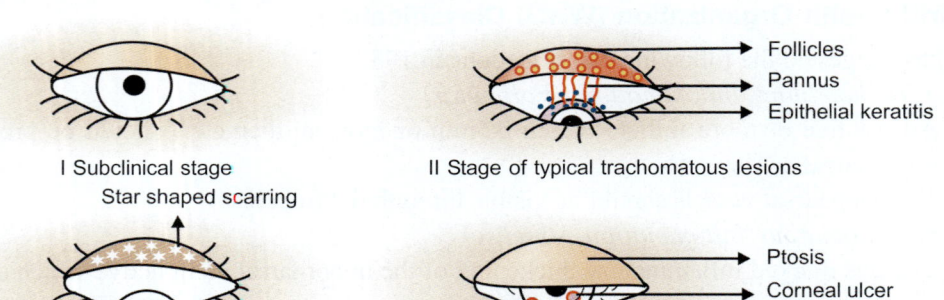

I Subclinical stage
Star shaped scarring

II Stage of typical trachomatous lesions
→ Follicles
→ Pannus
→ Epithelial keratitis

III Stage of scarring

IV Stage of sequelae and complications
→ Ptosis
→ Corneal ulcer
→ Trichiasis

5. *Xerosis*—Scarring of conjunctiva results in destruction of goblet cells which secrete mucus.
6. *Ptosis*—It occurs due to large follicles formation. It is rare nowadays.
7. *Blindness*—Perforation of corneal ulcer is a common cause of blindness.

Treatment

The ideal antimicrobial treatment has not been developed as yet.

1. Medical

Trachoma organisms are sensitive to tetracycline, sulphonamides, erythromycin, rifampicin, ciprofloxacin, azithromycine and sparfloxacine is also effective in trachoma. As the organisms live inside the cells, effect of antibiotic is slow. Therefore treatment should be continued for a longer period of time.

A. *Topical treatment*
   1. Sulphacetamide 20-30% eyedrops are instilled four times daily for 6 weeks. This treatment should be followed by an intermittent treatment in endemic areas.
   2. Elinimation of secondary infection of conjunctiva is done by antibiotic eyedrops, e.g. chloramphenicol, ciprofloxacin, etc.
   3. Addition of artificial tears is beneficial in treating associated xerosis.
   4. Topical treatment with 1% erythromycin, 1% tetracycline or rifampicin ointment is far more effective. It is applied twice daily for 3-6 weeks. It may be given for 5 consecutive days a month × 12 months in endemic areas.

B. *Systemic treatment*
   1. Systemic administration of tetracycline, erythromycin, rifampicin and sulphonamides is effective. Tetracycline or erythromycine 250 mg four time daily may be given for 3-4 weeks. Unfortunately each drug has some risk of side-reaction, e.g.
      i. Sulphonamides can cause allergic reaction like Stevens-Johnson syndrome, skin rash.
      ii. Tetracycline cannot be given to young children, pregnant women and nursing mothers as it adversely affects the enamel formation of the teeth.
   2. Initially oral doxycycline 100 mg is given twice daily for 3-4 weeks. Oral doxycycline 5 mg/kg body weight is given once per month × 12 months. It is a long acting tetracycline and is as effective as topical tetracycline.
   3. Nowadays treatment with a single dose of azithromycin 2 mg/kg body weight has been recommended.

C. *Combined topical and systemic treatment*
   It is preferred when the ocular infection is severe.
   1. 1% tetracycline or erythromycin ointment is applied 4 times a day for 6 weeks.
   2. Tetracycline and erythromycin 250 mg orally is given 4 times a day for 6 weeks.

2. Surgical Treatment

It is not necessary usually with the advent of antibiotics.
   i. Excision of fornix—If the follicles in the upper fornix are very large and closely packed, excision of the fornix can be done.

ii. **Tarsectomy**—If the tarsal plate is much diseased and distorted, tarsectomy may rarely be performed.
iii. Treatment of various sequelae such as trichiasis, entropion, dry eye should be done.

Prophylaxis

1. Personal hygiene and environmental sanitation is improved.
2. A good water supply improves washing habbits.
3. Blanket antibiotic treatment may be given in endemic area. WHO has recommended the following regime to be carried out in endemic areas to minimise the severity of disease. The regime is to apply 1% tetracycline eye ointment twice daily for 5 days per month. This is done for 6 months regularly.

ALLERGIC CONJUNCTIVITIS
1. Acute or Subacute Catarrhal Conjunctivitis

Etiology

It is an acute or subacute non-specific urticarial reaction to allergen.

1. Bacterial protein of endogenous nature, e.g. *Staphylococcus* in nose or upper respiratory tract can cause this condition commonly.
2. Exogenous protein as in hay fever, contact with animals (horse, cat), pollens or flowers.
3. Chemicals, cosmetics, drugs, e.g. atropine, hair dye, etc. can cause severe conjunctivitis and dermatitis.

Symptoms

1. Itching is the most prominent feature of allergic conjunctivitis.
2. There is associated watery secretion.
3. Marked redness of the conjunctiva is always present.

Signs

1. There is marked congestion of the conjunctiva with multiple follicles.
2. Watery mucoid discharge is present.
3. Skin of the lid is red and swollen.

Differential Diagnosis

It can be differentiated from acute bacterial infection by the following features:
   i. In allergic conjunctivitis there is presence of marked hyperaemia with itching.
  ii. Watery secretion contains large number of eosinophils.
 iii. There is chronic course with subacute remissions.

Treatment

1. Removal of the allergen is absolutely necessary. If this cannot be done, desensitization may be done by long course of injections.

2. Astringent lotions are applied frequently.
3. Vasoconstrictor, e.g. adrenaline solution (1 in 10000) reduces the congestion.
4. Antihistamine drugs (antistine privine 1%) are effective in controlling allergic reaction.
5. Disodium cromoglycate 2% is a mast cell stabilizer, thus, preventing the release of histamine. It is safe and can be used for long period.
6. Corticosteroid drops are effective in the treatment of severe cases.
7. In atropine irritation, the drug should be withdrawn. Phenylephrine (10%) or mydricaine injection (subconjunctival) may be substituted.

2. Phlyctenular Conjunctivitis (Eczematous Conjunctivitis)

It is an allergic reaction of the conjunctiva caused by endogenous protein characterised by formation of bleb or nodule near the limbus (phlycten = bleb).

Etiology

1. It is caused by allergic reaction to endogenous bacterial protein such as tuberculosis.
2. Chronic mild infections of tonsils and adenoids may also result in phlyctenular conjunctivitis. *Staphylococcus* protein is now thought to account for most of these cases.

Histopathology

The bleb is composed of compact mass of mononuclear cells, lymphocytes and polymorphs underneath the epithelium.

Incidence

1. Age—It is common in children between 4 and 14 years.
2. Unhygienic living conditions and malnutrition are important predisposing factors.

Symptoms

Discomfort, irritation, itching, reflex lacrimation are common complaints.

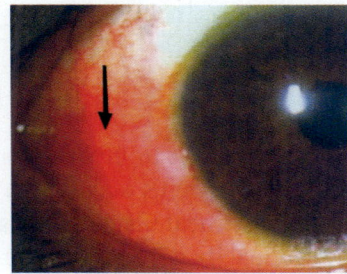
Phlyctenular conjunctivitis

Signs

1. One or more small, round, grey-yellow nodules measuring 1-3 mm in diameter, raised slightly above the surface is seen on the bulbar conjunctiva at or near the limbus.
2. Congestion is seen all around the nodule.

Clinical Types

1. *Phlyctenular conjunctivitis*—When the conjunctiva alone is involved.
2. *Phlyctenular kerato-conjunctivitis*—When phlycten is situated at the limbus, it involves both the conjunctiva and the cornea.
3. *Phlyctenular keratitis*—When cornea alone is involved (rare).
   It may present in two forms:
   a. Ulcerative phlyctenular keratitis
   b. Diffuse infiltrative keratitis

a. **Ulcerative phlyctenular keratitis**
   i. *Sacrofulous ulcer*—It is a shallow marginal ulcer formed due to breakdown of small limbal phlycten.
   ii. *Fascicular ulcer*—It has a prominent parallel leash of blood vessels. This ulcer usually remains superficial but leaves behind a band-shaped superficial opacity after healing.
   iii. *Miliary ulcer*—Multiple small ulcers are scattered over a portion of or whole of the cornea.
b. **Diffuse infiltrative phlyctenular keratitis**
   It may appear in the form of central infiltration of cornea with characteristic rich vascularization from the periphery all around the limbus.

DIFFERENTIAL DIAGNOSIS OF NODULE AT THE LIMBUS

1. Inflammations	• Episcleritis, scleritis
2. Allergic conditions	• Phlycten
	• Spring catarrh (bulbar form)
3. Degenerations	• Pterygium
	• Pinguecula
4. Cyst	• Dermoid, retention, implantation, parasitic
5. Tumours	• Squamous cell carcinoma
	• Papilloma, lymphoma, haemangioma
	• Naevus, malignant melanoma
	• Kaposis sarcoma (AIDS)
6. Granuloma	• Tuberculosis, syphilis
7. Filtering bleb	• Cystoid cicatrix following glaucoma surgery

Complications
These are mainly due to involvement of the cornea which is quite frequent.
1. Keratoconjunctivitis occurs as a result of involvement of cornea.
2. Fascicular corneal ulcer—A leash of blood vessel may follow the corneal ulcer at times.
3. Corneal opacity with base at the limbus is occasionally present.

Course
1. Vesicular stage—Initially phlycten resembles a bleb. This is a true vesicular stage.
2. Stage of ulceration—The surface epithelium becomes necrotic and ulcers are formed on the conjunctiva.
3. Healing stage—Ulcers heal rapidly without scar formation.

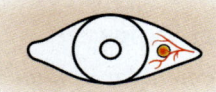
Phlyctenular conjunctivitis

Treatment
1. *Local*
   i. Corticosteroid drops and ointment are very effective.
   ii. Antibiotic drops and ointment are applied if there is associated conjunctivitis due to secondary infection.
   iii. Atropine eye ointment is applied if there is associated corneal ulcer.
   iv. Dark glasses or eyeshade are soothing.

2. **General**
    i. Improvement of general health and nutrition is necessary.
    ii. Treatment of the cause, e.g. tuberculosis, adenoids, tonsillitis is essential.

3. Spring Catarrh (Vernal Conjunctivitis)

It is a recurrent, bilateral/seasonal (conjunctivitis occurring with the onset of hot weather).

Etiology

It is caused by exogenous allergen. It occurs due to hypersensitivity reaction to exogenous allergen such as pollens and dust. It is mediated by IgE as shown by the accompanying eosinophilia.

Incidence

1. It affects young boys usually 5 to 10 years.
2. It is a bilateral and recurrent condition.
3. It usually occurs at the onset of hot weather (spring season) and subsides during winter.
4. It is sporadic and non-contagious in nature. It is seen in all classes of society.

Histopathology

   i. There are tuft of capillaries, dense fibrous tissue along with large number of eosinophils, plasma cells and histocytes.
   ii. The covering epithelium is hypertrophied and may show hyaline degeneration.

Symptoms

1. Itching is the most common complaint.
2. Thick, white, ropy mucous discharge is characteristic.
3. Burning and foreign body sensation may be present.
4. Photophobia is present in cases of corneal involvement.
5. Lacrimation or watering is a associated feature.

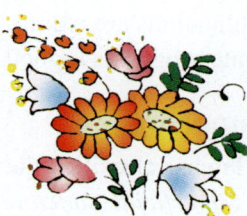
Exogenous allergen

Types

Two typical forms are seen. Both forms may occur together as mixed type.

1. Palpebral Form

   i. There is conjunctival hyperaemia and chemosis.
   ii. On everting the upper lid, palpebral conjunctiva shows multiple polygonal-shaped raised areas like cobblestones, due to diffuse papillary hypertrophy.
   iii. The colour is milky white due to thickened epithelium of the conjunctiva.
   iv. The nodules are hard and consist of dense fibrous tissue (hypertrophied papillae).
   v. Eosinophils are present in great number.

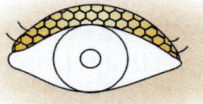
Palpebral form

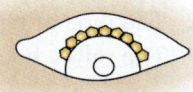
Bulbar form

Spring catarrh

2. Bulbar Form

   i. Multiple nodules or gelatinous thickening appears all around or in the upper part of the limbus. It is diagnostic of spring catarrh.
   ii. Discrete chalky white superficial spots (Horner-Tranta's dots) composed of eosinophils may be seen at the limbus.

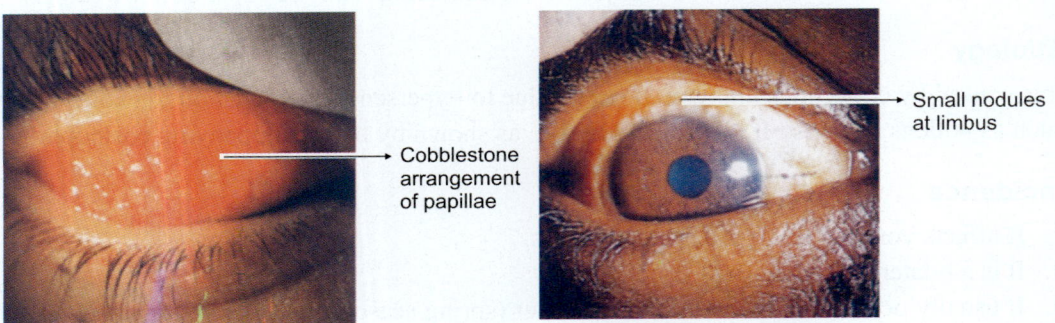

Spring catarrh - Palpebral form

Spring catarrh - Bulbar form

Course

It may persist for several years. Seasonal recurrences with exacerbations and remissions are common. In majority of cases, disease eventually subsides around puberty.

Complications

Complications are mainly due to corneal involvement. Serious complications are never seen and the ultimate prognosis is good.

Keratopathy

Buckley has classified the corneal involvement into 5 clinical stages:
   i. *Superficial punctate keratitis*—These are tiny microerosions in upper cornea.
   ii. *Epithelial macroerosion and ulceration* occurs due to epithelial loss.
   iii. *Plaque*—There is bare area caused by macroerosion of epithelium which becomes coated with mucus.
   iv. *Ring scar* is formed as a result of subepithelial corneal scarring.
   v. *Pseudogeron toxon*—It resembles arcus senilis with appearance of 'cupid's bow'.

Differential Diagnosis

Palpebral form may resemble trachoma. It is differentiated by,
   i. The type of patient, i.e. young boys
   ii. The milky hue of conjunctiva is present in spring catarrh.

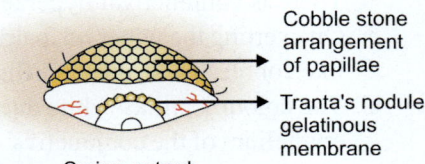

Spring catarrh

iii. There is freedom of the fornix from implication
iv. Characteristic recurrence in hot weather.

Treatment

It is purely symptomatic. Patient is encouraged to tolerate mild discomfort and use less harmful topical therapy.

1. Topical corticosteroids—Frequent application of steroid drops (0.1% dexamethasone or betamethasone) and ointment is very effective. A maintenance dose 3-4 times daily is given during the season. Prolonged use of steroids can cause steroid-induced glaucoma and cataract. Steroid drops are now available in low concentration, e.g. fluorometholone 0.1% which minimizes complications.
2. Acetylcysteine 10-20% drops controls excess mucus formation. It may be useful in the treatment of early plaque formation.
3. Disodium cromoglycate 2% drops is applied four times daily. It acts as an adjuvant to steroid therapy. It stabilizes mast cells thus preventing histamine release. It can be used for longer period.
4. Lodoxamide 0.1% drops is a new preparation that may be superior to cromoglycate.
5. Cryotherapy of the nodule may be effective at times but it causes scarring. Cold compresses are useful in milder cases.
6. Tinted glasses provide considerable comfort and relief.
7. Non-steroidal anti-inflammatory drugs (NSAIDs), e.g. flurbiprofen, indomethacin, diclofenac 0.1%, ketorolac tromethamine can be used safely for a longer period. They act by inhibiting arachidonic acid.
8. Supratarsal injection of steroid is very effective in patients with severe disease not responding to conventional topical steroid therapy.
9. Recently topical cyclosporine 1% has been found to be useful in steroid resistant cases.
10. Surgical management—It is useful for severe vernal keratopathy.
    - Debridement of large mucous plaques may speed up repair of persistent epithelial defects.
    - Lamellar keratectomy of densely adherent plaques may also be beneficial.

Prophylaxis

1. Beta-radiation is given in proliferative cases at monthly intervals during the months of February, March and April to prevent the onset of symptoms. This does not cure the disease.
2. Disodium cromoglycate 2% eyedrops are applied 3-4 times before the onset of the disease.
3. Desensitization has also been tried without much rewarding results.

DIFFERENTIAL DIAGNOSIS OF VARIOUS CONJUNCTIVITIS

CLINICAL FEATURES	BACTERIAL	VIRAL	TRACHOMA INCLUSION	SPRING CATARRH
1. *Injection*	Marked	Moderate	Mild	Mild to moderate
2. *Haemorrhage*	+	+	–	–
3. *Chemosis*	++	+ or –	+ or –	++
4. *Exudate*	Purulent or mucopurulent	Scanty watery	Scanty	Ropy white
5. *Pseudomembrane*	+ or –	+ or –	–	–
6. *Papillae*	+ or –	+ or –	+ or –	+
7. *Follicles*	–	+	+	–
8. *Pannus*	–	–	+	–
9. *Preauricular lymph nodes*	–	–	–	–

II. DEGENERATIONS

1. Concretions [Lithiasis]

Incidence
It is common in the elderly persons. There is accumulation of epithelial cells and inspissated mucus in Henle's glands. They never become calcified so the term 'lithiasis' or 'stone' is a misnomer.

Symptoms
Foreign body sensation and irritation are common complaints.

Signs
1. There are minute hard yellow spots seen in the palpebral conjunctiva.
2. They project from the surface rubbing against the lid or the cornea.

Treatment
Concretions are removed with a sharp needle.

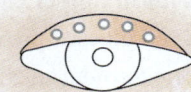

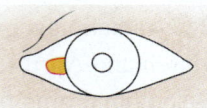

Concretions

2. Pinguecula [Pinguis = Fat]

It is a triangular yellow patch on conjunctiva near the limbus in the palpebral aperture.

Etiology
It commonly occurs in elderly persons exposed to strong sunlight, dust, wind, etc.

Pinguecula

Signs
There is a triangular yellow patch, seen first on the nasal side.
- It is situated near the limbus in the palpebral aperture. The base is always towards the limbus and the apex away from cornea.

Pathology

There is hyaline infiltration and elastotic degeneration of submucous tissue. It is considered to be precursor of pterygium.

Treatment

No treatment is required as it is a symptomless condition. Surgical excision is done for cosmatic reasons.

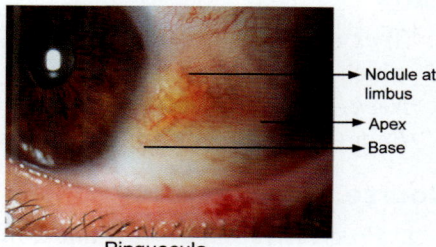
Pinguecula

3. Pterygium

Pterygium is a Greek word-meaning wing of a butterfly, like the butterfly it has got a head, neck and body. A pterygium is a triangular sheet of fibrovascular tissue which invades the cornea. It consists of three parts: a head or apex, i.e. the part which rests on the cornea, a neck and a body.

Etiology

- It frequently follows a pinguecula.
- It is common in dry sunny (ultraviolet rays) climate with sandy soil as in Australia, South Africa, Texas or the Middle East.

Incidence

The nasal side is affected first but it may be bilateral.

Symptoms

1. It is usually symptomless.
2. There is cosmetic disfigurement.
3. Vision is impaired due to astigmatism or if the pupillary area is covered by the progressive pterygium.
4. Rarely, diplopia (seeing double objects) may be present due to limitation of ocular movements specially in postoperative cases (due to injury to medial rectus muscle).

Signs

1. There is a triangular encroachment of the conjunctiva on the cornea from the inner canthus in the palpebral aperture. Pterygium is loosely adherent to the sclera in its whole length.
2. Numerous small opacities, i.e. deposits of iron (Stocker's line) may lie in front of the blunt apex of pterygium.
3. There may be limitation of inward ocular movements occasionally.

Pathology

1. It is a degenerative condition of the sub-conjunctival tissue which proliferates as vascularized granulation tissue.
2. It invades the cornea and destroys the superficial layers of stroma and Bowman's membrane.

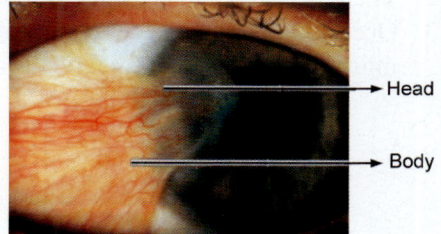
Progressive pterygium

Parts

1. *Apex or head*—It is the triangular foremost part which encroaches on cornea.
2. *Neck*—It is the narrow part near the limbus.
3. *Body*—It is the remaining fleshy part.

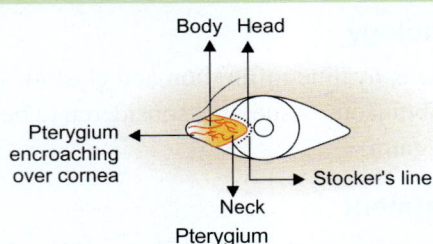

Course

i. *Progressive stage*—It is thick, fleshy and vascular in the early stage. It gradually increases in size and encroaches towards the centre of the cornea. At times it may cover the whole pupillary area.
ii. *Atrophic stage*—Later on it becomes thin and pale when it stops growing. However, it never disappears completely.

Differential Diagnosis

Pseudopterygium—It is formed due to adhesion of bulbar conjunctiva to a marginal corneal ulcer as in chemical burn. It is treated by simple excision.

Probe test—A probe can be passed easily beneath the neck of pseudopterygium as it is fixed to the cornea only at its apex.

DIFFERENCES BETWEEN PTERYGIUM AND PSEUDOPTERYGIUM

	PTERYGIUM	PSEUDOPTERYGIUM
1. *Age*	— Elderly	— Any age
2. *Etiology*	— Degeneration of subconjunctival tissue	— Inflammation (peripheral corneal ulcer)
3. *Site*	— Always situated at 3 or 9 o'clock	— Chemical burn — Situated at any meridian
4. *Probe test*	— A probe cannot be passed under the neck	— A probe can be passed
5. *Course*	— Progressive usually	— Stationary

Complications

1. Astigmatism is a common complication.
2. There is visual impairment if pupillary area is involved.
3. Occasionally there may be diplopia due to limitation of movement of the eyeball as a result of injury or fibrosis of medial rectus muscle.

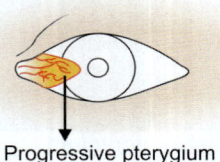
Progressive pterygium

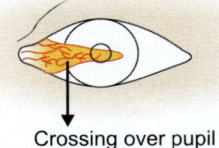
Crossing over pupil

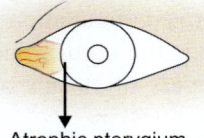
Atrophic pterygium

Treatment

I. Atrophic Pterygium

No treatment is required unless it is progressing towards the pupillary area or causing disfigurement. Atrophic pterygium is best left alone with periodic follow-up.

II. Progressive Pterygium

Indications for surgery include visual impairment, astigmatism, cosmetic reasons, limitation of ocular movement and diplopia.

1. SIMPLE EXCISION (OMBRAIN'S METHOD)
    i. Hold the neck of the pterygium with the fixation forceps and dissect the apex from the cornea. Care is taken not to cut the cornea too deeply. The surface of the cornea should be smooth and even.
    ii. The pterygium is then freed from the sclera along its length and from conjunctiva by doing subconjunctival dissection.
    iii. Make two parallel incisions on either side of the pterygium in the conjunctiva.

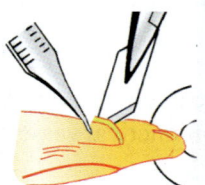
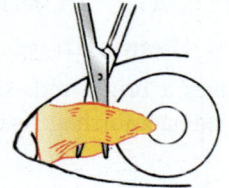
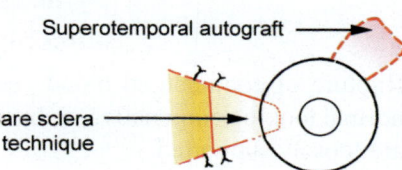

Simple excision (Ombrain's method)

    iv. The head, neck and body of the pterygium (3-4 mm) are excised leaving a bare area of the sclera at the edge of the cornea (bare sclera technique). A part of conjunctiva is also excised and the cut ends of the conjunctiva may be sutured to the episcleral tissue or together. Care is taken not to injure the medial rectus.
2. PTERYGIUM INVOLVING THE PUPILLARY AREA—Simple excision or resection of the pterygium with 'key-hole' lamellar keratoplasty is the treatment of choice. Earlier on pterygium was allowed to grow until it crosses pupillary area to prevent cornea haze.
3. RECURRENT PTERYGIUM
    i. *Mucous membrane autograft*—When the area of bare sclera is more than 5 mm, graft from the bulbar surface (preferably from superotemporal quadrant due to its large area) of the same or other eye or buccal mucosa should be applied.
    ii. *Transposition method* (McReynolds')—Simple excision is done. The cut end of pterygium is inserted below the conjunctiva at 6 O'clock position in the lower fornix. A mattress suture is passed to hold it in place. Thus, the direction of blood vessels is altered. This may result in thick and vascularised lower fornix
    iii. *Lamellar corneal graft* is applied after the apex is freed from the cornea. It is indicated specially when the pterygium is in the pupillary area or in cases of corneal thinning.

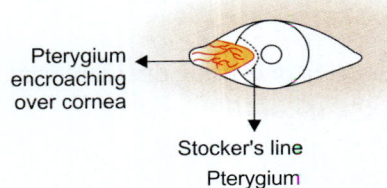
Pterygium encroaching over cornea

Stocker's line
Pterygium

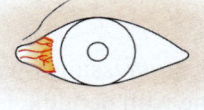
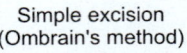
Simple excision (Ombrain's method)

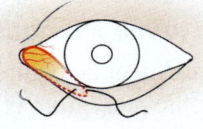
Transposition in lower fornix (McReynoids' method)

iv. *Beta-radiation* from the strontium-90 source is applied to the limbus postoperatively. 2500 rads are given in the first week following surgery.
v. *Thiotepa* 1:2000 solution is applied 4 times daily for 6 weeks. It prevents the growth of pterygium. It is given for at least 7 days postoperatively.
vi. *Alternatively, mitomycin C*, an anti-metabolite may also be effective in the prevention of recurrence. It is used as eye drops in the concentration of 2 mg powder dissolved in 5 ml of normal saline or 5% glucose starting from first postoperative day and continued for 7 days.
vii. *Argon laser* beam can be applied to obliterate the new blood vessels.

III. SYMPTOMATIC CONDITIONS
1. Subconjunctival Haemorrhage (Ecchymosis)

Rupture of conjunctival blood vessel causes a bright red, sharply delineated area surrounded by normal looking conjunctiva. Subconjunctival haemorrhage is common since the conjunctival vessels are loosely supported.

Etiology
There is rupture of small blood vessels in the conjunctiva due to :
- Minor injury to the eyeball and orbit
- Spontaneous/haemorrhage.
- Severe conjunctivitis due to, e.g. pneumococcus, adenovirus, etc.
- Mechanical straining, e.g. vomiting, whooping cough lifting heavy weight, etc.
- Bleeding disorder, e.g. purpura, scurvy, leukemia, etc.
- Head injury, e.g. fracture of the base of skull
- Prolonged pressure on thorax and abdomen leads to venous congestion.

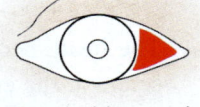
Subconjunctival haemorrhage

Symptom
Red eye is the most predominant feature.

Sign
Fresh bright red blood is visible under the conjunctiva.

Course
i. At first it is bright red in colour (oxyhaemoglobin).
ii. Subsequently, it looks blackish—red or orange-yellow. This is due to the breakdown of oxyhaemoglobin.
iii. Ultimately it gets absorbed within 2-3 weeks depending on the amount of haemorrhage.

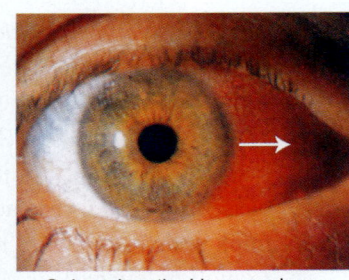
Subconjunctival haemorrhage

Treatment

1. Assurance is given to the patient that it is not a serious condition by itself.
2. No treatment is required as blood gets absorbed in 1-3 weeks.
3. Vitamin C may help in healing process.
4. Cold fomentation is given to stop further bleeding.

2. Xerosis [Dry eye]

It is a dry, lustreless condition of the conjunctiva due to the unstable tear film, exposing the conjunctival and corneal epithelium to evaporation.

The tear film consists of three layers:
i. *Outer lipid layer*—It is secreted by the meibomian and Zeis glands. It retards the evaporation of aqueous layer and lubricates the eyelids.
ii. *Middle aqueous layer*—It is secreted by the lacrimal and accessory lacrimal glands. It supplies atmospheric oxygen to cornea, has antibacterial function and washes away debris.
iii. *Inner mucin layer*—It is secreted by goblet cells, glands of Henle and Manz. It makes the corneal surface hydrophilic so that tear film sticks to cornea.

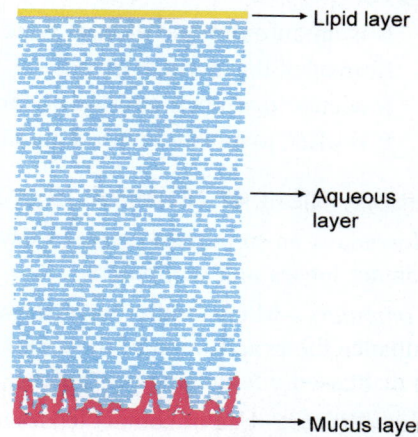
The tear film

Etiology

1. **Deficiency of tears**—It is the most common cause of dry eye.
    i. Sjögren's syndrome (keratoconjunctivitis sicca)
    ii. Senile or ideopathic atrophy of the lacrimal gland
2. **Deficiency of conjunctival mucus**—It occurs due to the scarring of the conjunctiva resulting in the destruction of goblet cells which secret mucus as in.
    i. Trachoma
    ii. Vitamin A deficiency
    iii. Burns—chemical, thermal, radiation
    iv. Stevens-Johnson syndrome
    v. Ocular pemphigoid
    vi. Erythema multiforme
    vii. Drug induced—Sulfonamides, epinephrine, etc.
3. **Irregular corneal surface**—It results in poor wetting of cornea as in healed corneal ulcer.
4. **Insufficient resurfacing of the cornea**—It occurs in lid paralysis (facial nerve palsy), proptosis and decreased blink rate in very sick and morbid patients.

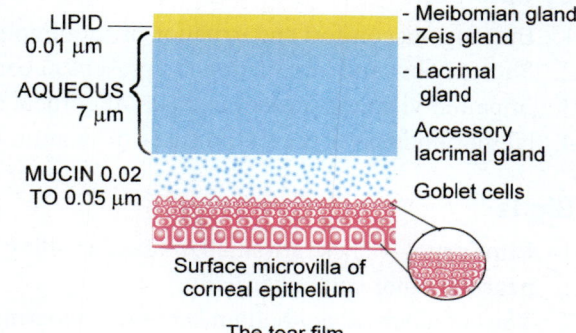
The tear film

5. *Lipid layer abnormality*
   i. Chronic blepharitis
   ii. Acne rosacea
6. *Visual display terminal syndrome (VDTS)* It is seen in contact lens and computer users.

Keratoconjunctivitis Sicca (Sjögren's Syndrome)

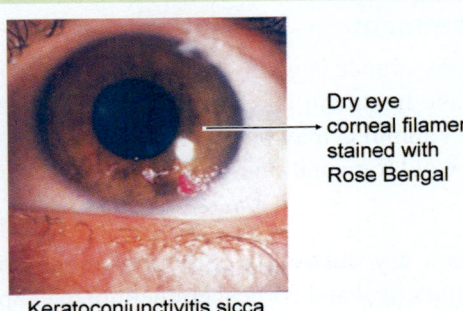

Keratoconjunctivitis sicca

- It is an autoimmune disease which results in the fibrosis of the lacrimal glands.
- It occurs in women after menopause usually female to male ratio of 9:1.
- It is often associated with rheumatoid arthritis and presence of antinuclear antibody.

VISUAL DISPLAY TERMINAL SYNDROME (VDTS)

Nowadays an important cause of dry eyes is use of contact lenses and computers.

Computers—Many studies have shown that computer screens kept at or above the level of the eyes enhance the evaporation of the tears. This is because the palpebral fissure is widened and blink rate is decreased while using computer.

Contact lens—Use of contact lenses also contribute to the development of dry eyes due to following reasons,
   i. Rigid lenses disrupt the lipid layer enhancing evaporation of the tear film.
   ii. Soft contact lenses actively deplete the mucus layer to maintain their hydration level.
   iii. Contact lenses also decrease the corneal sensation, a factor which may be necessary for the tear secretion.

Symptoms

1. Burning, discomfort and irritation are common complaints.
2. Photophobia and lacrimation are present in corneal involvement.
3. Impaired vision is present in cases of corneal opacity formation.
4. Night blindness is present in cases of vitamin A deficiency.

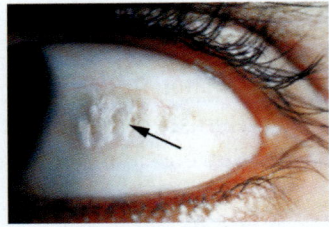

Bitot's spot

Signs

1. Bitot's spot—These are small, triangular, shiny, silver white patches seen on the bulbar conjunctiva near the outer canthus usually.
2. The conjunctival epithelium becomes epidermoid like that of skin.
3. There may be excessive mucus secretion (white coloured) due to deficiency of aqueous layer.

Complications

- Corneal stromal ulcers are common.
- Conjunctivitis and blepharitis occur due to loss of defence mechanism.

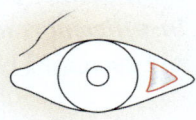

Bitot's spot

WHO CLASSIFICATION OF XEROPHTHALMIA (VITAMIN A DEFICIENCY)

Primary signs	
X1A	Conjunctival xerosis
X1B	Bitot's spots with conjunctiva xerosis < 1/3 corneal surface
X2	Corneal xerosis
X3A	Corneal ulceration with xerosis 1/3 corneal surface
X3B	Keratomalacia 1/3 corneal surface > 1/3 corneal surface
Secondary signs	
XN	Night blindness
XF	Xerophthalmia fundus (pale yellow spots)
XS	Xerophthalmia scars (in cornea)

- Band-shaped keratopathy may occur.
- There may be keratinization of cornea and conjunctival epithelium.

Investigations

1. *Slit-lamp examination* is most important in diagnosis of dry eye.
2. *Fluorescein staining*—It shows areas of denuded epithelium.
3. *Staining with alcian blue* shows the presence of particulate matter in the tear film due to excess mucus.
4. *Staining with Rose Bengal dye* 1%- It stains the devitalized cells red in colour.
5. *Tear lysozyme ratio* is between 0.9 and 0.6 usually. Tear lysozyme is also reduced.
6. *Schirmer test I*—It measures the rate of tear formation.

    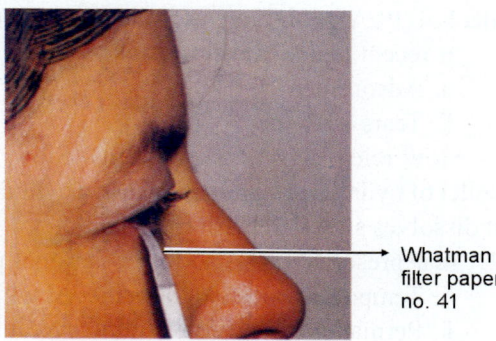
    Schirmer test

    Procedure—Take a 5 × 30 mm strip of no. 41 Whatman filter paper. A 5 mm tab is folded and gently inserted into the lower lid. If the wetting is less than 6 mm after 5 minutes, it is diagnostic of dry eye (normal range is 10-25 mm).

    Schirmer test II—It tests the reflex secretion of tears.
    The above procedure is repeated while stimulating the nasal mucosa with fumes of ammonia or a wisp of cotton.

    Normal Schirmer's test (more than 10 mm in 5 min) → Whatman filter paper no. 41

7. *Basic secretion test*—The purpose of this test is to measure the basal secretion of tears by eliminating reflex tearing.
    Procedure—Topical anesthetic is instilled into the conjunctival sac and a few minutes allowed to pass until reactive hyperaemia has subsided. The room is darkened and the procedure is the same as Schirmer test I and interpretation of the results is also similar. The difference between the two tests is measurement of reflex secretion. Less than 5 mm wetting of the filter paper confirms the diagnosis of hyposecretion of tears.

8. *Tear film break-up time (BUT)*—This is a test for the stability of the tear film. Deficiency of mucus layer is measured by the 'tear film break-up time'. The rapidity of appearance of dry spots on the cornea between blinks becomes an index of the adequacy of the mucin layer.
   Procedure—A few drops of fluorescein dye is instilled into the conjunctival sac. Ask the patient to close and open his eyes. Immediately scan the cornea with cobalt blue illumination of the slit-lamp for the first sign of dry (fluorescein free) areas. If the tear film breaks in less than 10 seconds, it is diagnostic of mucus deficiency (normal range is 15-35 seconds).
9. *Other tests*—There are several other sophisticated tests which can be done to confirm the diagnosis of dry eye such as,
   - Tear clearing test (TCT),
   - Tear function index (TFI),
   - Tear osmolarity test
   - Tear lactoferrin test
   - Ocular ferning test
   - Conjunctival biopsy

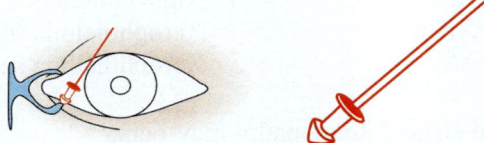
Freemans punctum silicon plug

Treatment

It is done by supplementation and preservation of tears.
1. Tear substitutes—Essentially three types of tear substitutes are available as,
   i. Eyedrops—It is instilled hourly in severe cases.
   ii. Eye ointment—It is applied at bedtime.
   iii. Insert—It is a slow release device inserted in the inferior fornix.
   Tear substitutes are inert substances and have high viscosity. These should form a stable tear film due to lubricant properties, e.g. hydroxy propyl methyl cellulose (HPMC), polymers cellulose, polyvinyl alcohol (PVA), polyvinyl pyrrolidene (PVP), hypromellose, parolein, etc.
   In recent years two newer drops are available.
   i. Adsorbotear
   ii. Tears naturale
   Slow releasing inserts (ocusert)- Slow releasing artificial tear (SR-AT) insert is a small 5 mg pellet of hydroxypropyl cellulose in a cylindrical form. It is placed in the lower fornix in the morning. It dissolves slowly releasing the polymer. Loss of insert and blurred vision are common problems.
2. Tear preservation—The lower lacrimal punctum can be blocked.
   i. Temporary occlusion is achieved with gelatin or silicon plugs.
   ii. Permanent occlusion is done by cautery or argon laser.
   This prolongs the action of artificial tears and preserves existing tears.
3. Treat the basic cause of dry eye, e.g. vitamin A deficiency, trachoma, etc.
4. Vitamin A is given in high doses in cases of vitamin A deficiency. Concentrated solution of vitamin A, i.e. 200,000 I.U. are given every six months prophylactically to children between 1-6 years of age. Topical vitamin A (Tretinoin) 0.1% applied 1-3 times daily is also useful in correcting squamous metaplasia. Deworming should be done periodically in children as intestinal worms can cause vitamin A deficiency.

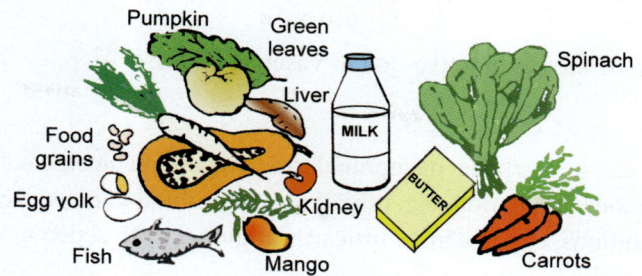

Foods rich in vitamin A

5. Supplement the diet with foods rich in vitamin A, e.g. fish, liver, egg, milk, carrot, spinach, (drumsticks) papaya and mango, etc.
6. Dark glasses or eye shields should be worn as they are soothing and comfortable.
7. Tarsorrhaphy (Lateral) is indicated in facial nerve palsy with exposure keratitis and corneal ulcer.
8. Other medical therapy—Recently following drugs are being tried.
    i. *Bromhexine hydrochloride*- It alters the mucus phase in keratoconjunctivitis sicca with improvement in BUT and Schirmer's test. It is given in three divided doses of 24-48 mg/day for 2-3 weeks. It is a tear stimulant.
    ii. *Topical cyclosporine* (0.05%)—Recent studies have shown that there is an immune based inflammation seen in dry eyes with local production of cytokines. Topical cyclosporine improves the signs and symptoms of dry eyes.
    iii. *Isobutyl—methyl—xanthine*—This has also been shown to increase tear secretion in some studies.
    iv. *Acetyl cysteine*—It may be used as a topical ocular solution 2-5% in artificial tears. It acts by lowering the viscosity of mucus.
9. Contact lenses—Bandage contact lenses provide prompt relief in cases of Filamentary keratitis. However there is increased deposits on the contact lens.
10. Topical vitamin A (0.01%-0.1%)—Tretinoin when applied topically is useful in reversing squamous metaplasia seen in various dry eye condition. It is applied once to three times a day.
11. Surgical measures—Various surgical methods are used in the treatment of dry eye. It includes mucous membrane grafting, conjunctival transplant, amniotic membrane transplant keratoprosthesis, correction of ectropion, entropion, trichiasis etc.

    In some cases autologuous nasal mucous membrane (stem cell) transplantation have been tried with good results.

Prophylaxis

- Avoid dry and hot atmosphere as it results in evaporation of tears.
- Prolonged computer use, i.e. without frequent breaks should be avoided.
- Discontinue any unnecessary prolonged topical medications which may cause toxic effects on the conjunctiva.

3. Chemosis

There is marked oedema of the conjunctiva due to vascular stasis.

Etiology

1. Acute inflammation, e.g. gonorrhoea, panophthalmitis, hypopyon ulcer, etc.
2. Obstruction to the venous circulation, e.g. orbital tumour, orbital varices, etc.
3. Abnormal blood conditions, e.g. anaemia, urticaria, angioneurotic oedema of face, etc.

4. Argyrosis

There is staining of the conjunctiva a deep brown colour due to prolonged application of silver salt (nitrate, proteinate, etc.) for the treatment of chronic conjunctivitis.

IV. CYSTS AND TUMOURS

1. Cysts

The common conjunctival cysts are due to:
- Dilatation of lymph spaces
- Epithelial implantation cyst
- Retention cysts of accessory lacrimal gland
- Cysticercus and hydatid cysts are rare.

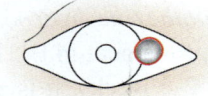

Dermoid cyst

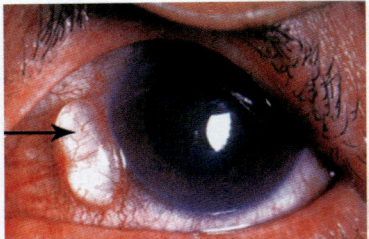

Retention cyst

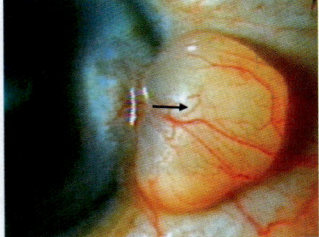

Implantation cyst

2. Tumours

1. Congenital

i. *Dermoid*—Dermoids are choristomas. It is yellow-grey in colour.
- They are smooth, solid round lesions
- It is situated astride the corneal margin on the outer side of limbus.
- Epibulbar dermoid may be associated with other congenital anomalies of the body.
- It consists of epidermoid, epithelium, sebaceous glands and hair.
- It is usually stationary in growth.
- Dermoids when large may cause corneal astigmatism.
- It is dissected off and replaced by lamellar corneal graft for cosmetic region.

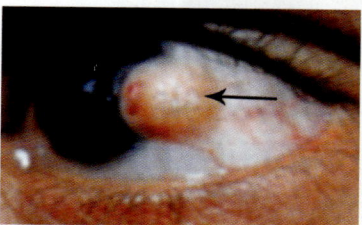
Dermoid

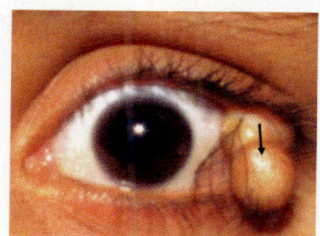
Dermolipoma

ii. *Dermolipoma* is situated at the outer canthus usually.
- It consists of fibrous tissue and fat.
- It should be removed surgically.

2. Papilloma
- It occurs at the inner canthus, fornices and the limbus.
- It should be removed as it may turn malignant.

3. Simple Granuloma
- It consists of exuberant granulation tissue.
- It is polypoid and is usually seen at the chalazion site when chalazion is insufficiently scraped.
- It should be completely removed by scissors.

4. Squamous Cell Carcinoma
- It occurs at the limbus or lid margin (transitional zone).
- It spreads over the surface and into the fornices.
- It may penetrate the eyeball.
- It is removed and the base is cauterized by diathermy.
- If it recurs, or in extensive lesions the eye is enucleated.

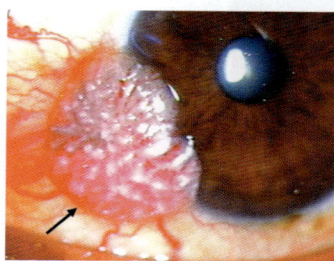
Squamous cell carcinoma

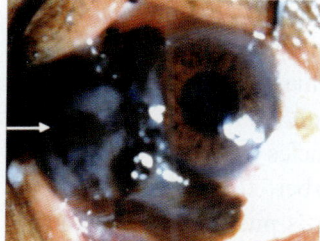
Malignant melanoma

5. Pigmented Tumours
i. Naevi or congenital mole is rarely malignant.
ii. Precancerous melanosis is a diffusely spreading pigmentation of the conjunctiva seen in elderly persons.
iii. Malignant melanoma occurs typically at the limbus in old people. It spreads over the surface of the eyeball. Recurrences and metastases occur elsewhere in the body commonly. It is treated by enucleation of the globe or exenteration of the orbit in cases of extraocular extension.

MULTIPLE CHOICE QUESTIONS

1. All the following are serous acinous glands *EXCEPT*
   a. Krause's glands
   b. meibomian gland
   c. lacrimal glands
   d. salivary gland
2. Natural protective mechanisms of conjunctiva include
   a. low temperature
   b. flushing due to tears
   c. blinking of eyelids
   d. all of the above
3. Follicles are not seen in which of the following
   a. spring catarrh
   b. trachoma
   c. adenovirus conjunctivitis
   d. streptococcal conjunctivitis
4. Angular conjunctivitis is caused by
   a. *Staphylococcus*
   b. pneumococcus
   c. virus
   d. Morax-Axenfeld bacillus
5. Eyes should not be bandaged in
   a. corneal ulcer
   b. purulent conjunctivitis
   c. glaucoma
   d. retinal detachment
6. Blood vessels in a trachomatous pannus lie
   a. beneath the Descemet's membrane
   b. in the stroma
   c. between Bowman's membrane and stroma
   d. between Bowman's membrane and epithelium
7. Cobblestone appearance of the conjunctiva is seen in
   a. spring catarrh
   b. angular conjunctivitis
   c. eczematous conjunctivitis
   d. trachoma
8. The HP inclusion bodies in trachoma are
   a. intranuclear
   b. intracytoplasmic
   c. both
   d. none
9. Sequelae of trachoma include
   a. pseudoptosis
   b. cicatricial entropion
   c. trichiasis
   d. all of the above
10. The pathognomonic features of trachoma are all *EXCEPT*
    a. follicles
    b. papillae
    c. Herbert's pits
    d. pannus
11. Herbert's pits are seen on the
    a. lid margin
    b. palpebral conjunctiva
    c. Arlt's line
    d. limbus
12. Promising treatment of epidemic keratoconjunctivitis is by
    a. oxytetracycline
    b. sulphacetamide 30%
    c. chloramphenicol
    d. adenine arabinoside
13. As a complication of acute mucopurulent conjunctivitis, the corneal ulcers that develop are
    a. marginal
    b. central
    c. anywhere on cornea
    d. no where

14. True membranous conjunctivitis is caused by
    a. trachoma
    b. Morax-Axenfeld bacillus
    c. virus
    d. diphtheria
15. Phlyctenular conjunctivitis is due to
    a. pneumococcus
    b. *Pseudomonas pyocyanea*
    c. allergy to endogenous protein
    d. allergy to exogenous protein
16. Concretions are due to accumulation of epithelial cells and mucus in
    a. Zeis's gland
    b. meibomian gland
    c. Moll's gland
    d. Henle's gland
17. Pinguecula is due to the infiltration of
    a. hyaline
    b. lipid
    c. calcium
    d. fatty acids
18. Bitot's spots are associated with
    a. vitamin A deficiency
    b. vitamin D deficiency
    c. vitamin E dificiency
    d. all of the above
19. Most common conjunctival cyst is due to
    a. dilatation of lymph spaces
    b. implantation cyst
    c. retention cyst
    d. hydatid cyst
20. The association of keratoconjunctivitis sicca with rheumatoid arthritis is
    a. Reiter's syndrome
    b. Sjögren's syndrome
    c. Stevens-Johnson syndrome
    d. Mikulicz's syndrome
21. The treatment of angular conjunctivitis is
    a. oxytetracycline ointment
    b. zinc oxide
    c. both
    d. none
22. Bilateral fat-like nodular area on nasal side is described as
    a. pinguecula
    b. pterygium
    c. phlycten
    d. pemphigoid
23. Dryness of eye is seen in all *EXCEPT*
    a. vitamin A deficiency
    b. trachoma stage IV
    c. keratoconjunctivitis sicca
    d. Horner's syndrome
24. The following are the features of conjunctival concretions *EXCEPT*
    a. calcification
    b. palpebral location
    c. age related
    d. corneal abrasions
25. Deficiency of vitamin A can cause all *EXCEPT*
    a. xerosis
    b. keratomalacia
    c. night blindness
    d. dermoid
26. Herbert's pits are seen in
    a. trachoma
    b. herpetic conjunctivitis
    c. ophthalmia neonatorum
    d. spring catarrh

27. Trantas nodules are seen in
    a. blepharoconjunctivitis
    b. vernal conjunctivitis
    c. phlyctenular conjunctivitis
    d. herpes keratitis
28. All is true about Sjögren's syndrome *EXCEPT*
    a. occurs in males
    b. polyarthritis
    c. dryness of eyes
    d. dryness of mouth
29. Most common cause of blindness in India is
    a. cataract
    b. glaucoma
    c. trachoma
    d. vitamin A deficency
30. Organism causing ophthalmia neonatorum is
    a. *Neisseria gonorrhoeae*
    b. staphylococci
    c. streptococci
    d. *Neisseria meningitidis*

ANSWERS

1—b	2—d	3—a	4—d	5—b
6—d	7—a	8—b	9—d	10—b
11—d	12—d	13—a	14—d	15—c
16—d	17—a	18—a	19—a	20—b
21—c	22—a	23—d	24—a	25—d
26—a	27—b	28—a	29—a	30—a

CHAPTER 7

The Cornea

APPLIED ANATOMY

Cornea is a clear transparent and elliptical structure with a smooth shining surface.
The average diameter is 11-12 mm (horizontal = 12 mm, vertical = 11 mm).
The thickness of the central part is 0.52 mm and the peripheral part is 0.67 mm.
The central one-third is known as the *optical zone*. Refractive index of cornea is 1.37.
The dioptric power of the cornea is approximately + 43 to + 45 D.

Structure

The cornea consists of five layers namely:

1. *The epithelium*—Stratified squamous type of epithelium consists of three cell types namely the basal columnar cells, two or three layers of wing cells and surface cells. It is normally replaced within 7 days when damaged.
2. *Bowman's membrane*—It is made up of collagen fibrils. It does not regenerate when damaged. This results in the formation of permanent corneal opacity.
3. *Substantia propria or stroma*—It forms 90% of corneal thickness. It consists of keratocytes, regularly arranged collagen fibrils and ground substance.
4. *Descemet's membrane*—It is a thin but strong homogeneous elastic membrane which can regenerate.
5. *The endothelium*—It is a single layer of flattened hexagonal cells. The cell density is about 3000 cells mm^2 at birth which decreases with advancing age. Corneal decompensation occurs only when more than 75% cells are damaged. It is measured by specular microscopy.

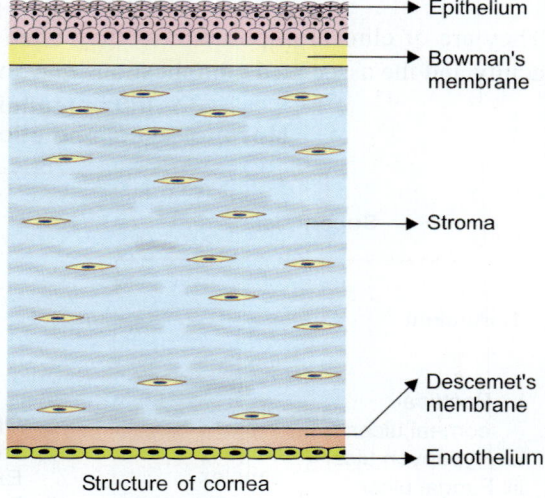

Structure of cornea

Nutrition of the Cornea

Cornea is an avascular structure. It derives nutrition from:
1. Perilimbal blood vessels—Anterior ciliary vessels invade the periphery of the cornea (limbus) for about 1 mm.
2. Aqueous humor—It supplies glucose and other nutrients by process of simple diffusion or active transport.
3. Oxygen from atmospheric air is derived directly through the tear film.

108 Basic Ophthalmology

Nerve Supply

The nerve supply is purely sensory. It is derived from the ophthalmic division of the 5th cranial nerve through the nasociliary branch.

Functions

There are two primary functions of the cornea.
1. It acts as a major refracting medium.
2. It protects the intraocular contents.

This is possible by maintaining corneal transparency and replacement of its tissues. Transparency is maintained by:
  i. Regular arrangement of corneal lamellae (lattice theory of cornea)
  ii. Avascularity
  iii. Relative state of dehydration.

DISEASES OF THE CORNEA

They are of clinical importance as they often leave permanent opacities which lowers the visual acuity and the associated complications may even lead to blindness.

1. Inflammations [Keratitis]
Morphological and etiological classification

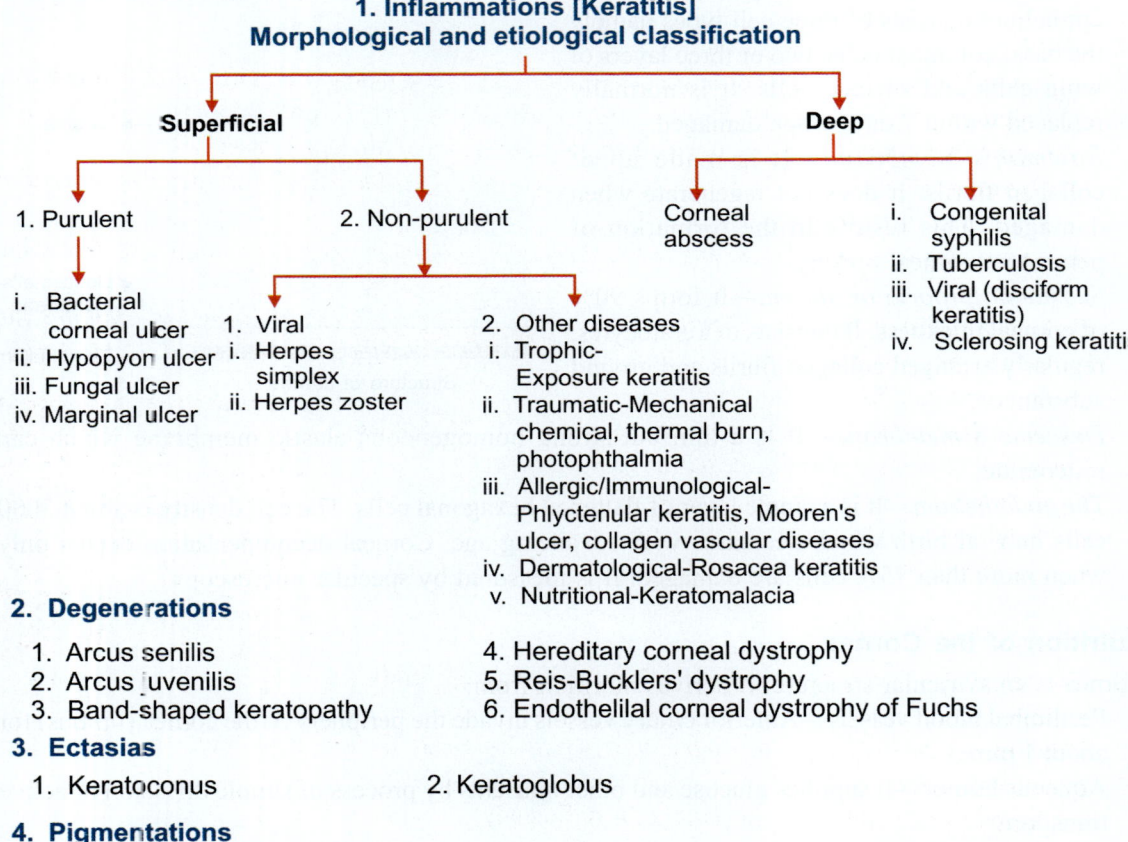

Superficial

1. Purulent
   i. Bacterial corneal ulcer
   ii. Hypopyon ulcer
   iii. Fungal ulcer
   iv. Marginal ulcer

2. Non-purulent
   1. Viral
      i. Herpes simplex
      ii. Herpes zoster
   2. Other diseases
      i. Trophic-Exposure keratitis
      ii. Traumatic-Mechanical chemical, thermal burn, photophthalmia
      iii. Allergic/Immunological-Phlyctenular keratitis, Mooren's ulcer, collagen vascular diseases
      iv. Dermatological-Rosacea keratitis
      v. Nutritional-Keratomalacia

Deep

Corneal abscess

  i. Congenital syphilis
  ii. Tuberculosis
  iii. Viral (disciform keratitis)
  iv. Sclerosing keratitis

4. Hereditary corneal dystrophy
5. Reis-Bucklers' dystrophy
6. Endothelilal corneal dystrophy of Fuchs

2. Degenerations
1. Arcus senilis
2. Arcus juvenilis
3. Band-shaped keratopathy

3. Ectasias
1. Keratoconus
2. Keratoglobus

4. Pigmentations
1. Blood staining
2. Argyrosis
3. Kayser-Fleisher's ring

INFLAMMATIONS OF THE CORNEA

Inflammation of the cornea (keratitis) is characterized by corneal oedema, cellular infiltration and associated conjunctival reaction.

1. *Exogenous infection,* e.g. *Staphylococcus, Streptococcus pneumoniae,* pneumococcus, *Pseudomonas pyocyanea, E.coli, Proteus, Klebsiella, H. influenzae,* etc. Usually organisms in the conjunctival sac, lacrimal sac (dacryocystitis), infected foreign body, etc. cause inflammation of the cornea.
2. *From the ocular tissue*
    i. Conjunctival diseases spread to the epithelium
    ii. Scleral diseases spread to the stroma
    iii. Uveal tract diseases spread to the endothelium
3. *Endogenous infection*—It is usually due to hypersensitivity reaction.

PURULENT KERATITIS
CORNEAL ULCER

There is a loss in the continuity of the corneal epithelium associated with tissue infiltration and necrosis.

Etiology

It is always exogenous infection commonly due to pyogenic organisms which invade the cornea from outside such as *Staphylococcus, Pneumococcus, Pseudomonas, E. coli,* etc.

The common causative bacterial organisms of corneal ulcer are as follows:

i. **Gram-positive cocci**—*Staphylococcus aureus, S. albus, Streptococcus hemolyticus, S. pneumoniae (Pneumococcus).*
ii. **Gram-negative cocci**—*Neisseria gonorrhoea (gonococcus), N. meningitidis (meningococcus).*
iii. **Gram-positive bacilli**—*Nocardia asteroides, Corynebacterium diphtheriae (diplobacilli).*
iv. **Gram-negative bacilli**—*Pseudomonas aeruginosa, Proteus, Klebsiella, Moraxella, Hemophilus, Escherichia coli,* etc.
v. **Mycobacteria**—*Mycobacterium tuberculosis, M. leprae.*

Three pathogens can invade normal intact epithelium:
- *Neisseria gonorrhoeae*
- *Neisseria meningitidis*
- *Corynebacterium diphtheriae*

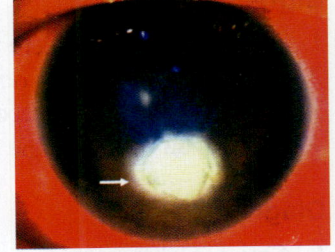

Corneal ulcer – Bacterial

Predisposing Factors

1. *Epithelial damage* due to trauma, e.g. minute foreign body, misdirected eyelash.
2. *Virulent organisms,* e.g. *Pneumococcus, Pseudomonas, Gonococcus,* etc.
3. *Poor resistance*
    - Xerosis and keratomalacia (vitamin A deficiency)
    - Protein calorie malnutrition

- Corneal oedema leads to desquamation of epithelium
- Neuroparalytic keratitis, e.g. herpes zoster, leprosy
- Exposure of the cornea due to proptosis, 7 nerve palsy

Stages of Corneal Ulcer

There are three stages namely;
1. *Progressive stage*
    - There is grey zone of infiltration by polymorphs.
    - Localised necrosis and sloughing of sequestrum is present.
    - Saucer-shaped ulcer with overhanging edges due to oedema is characteristic.
2. *Regressive stage*
    - The dead material is thrown off and the oedema subsides.
    - The floor and edges of the ulcer are smooth and transparent.
3. *Healing stage*
    - Minute superficial vessels grow in from the limbus near the ulcer.
    - There is formation of fibrous tissue which fills the gap. The irregular arrangement of fibrous tissue results in opacity, as the new fibres refract the light irregularly. As Bowman's membrane *never* regenerates, permanent opacity remains if it is damaged.

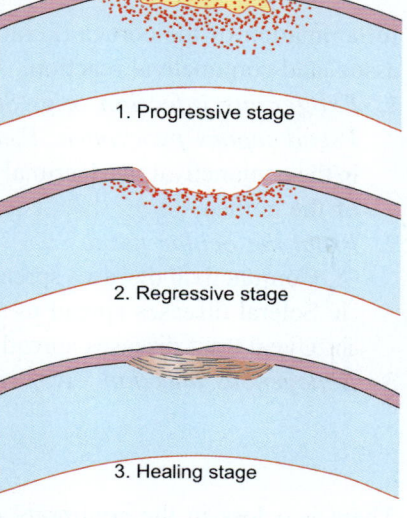

Stages of corneal ulcer

Symptoms

1. Pain—Cornea is richly supplied by ophthalmic division of the 5th nerve.
2. Photophobia—There is undue sensitivity to light.
3. Impairment of visual acuity occurs due to corneal opacity.
4. Lacrimation—There is excessive reflex tear production.

Signs

1. Blepharospasm—There is tight closure of the eyelids specially in children.
2. Corneal opacification occurs due to infiltration and oedema.
3. Ciliary congestion with conjunctival hyperaemia is present.
4. Hypopyon or pus in the anterior chamber may be present.

Diagnosis

1. Staining of the cornea by fluorescein stain:
    a. *Superficial staining*—It stains the margin of the ulcer bright brilliant green.
    Method—A drop of fluorescein is instilled in the conjunctival sac. Alternatively, disposable strip of fluorescein stain may be used.
    After few seconds, excess dye is washed off with normal saline.

b. *Deep staining*—It stains the stromal infiltration defect grass green and the endothelium yellow in colour respectively.

Method—After instillation of fluorescein dye in the conjunctival sac, the lids are kept closed for about 5 minutes. Excess dye is washed off with normal saline.

2. Slit-lamp examination shows irregular margins of the ulcer and details of anterior segment of the eye.

Complications
1. Corneal Opacity

1. *Nebula*—If the corneal scar involves Bowman's membrane and superficial layers of stroma, the resulting opacity is slight. It is so very faint that the finer details of iris are clearly visible through the opacity.

   A thin diffuse nebula covering the pupillary area interferes more with vision than localized dense leucoma not covering the whole pupillary area.

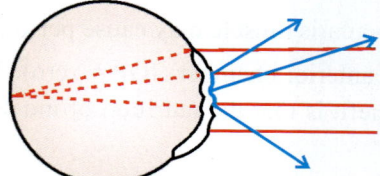
Optical effect of nebula
• irregular astigmatism

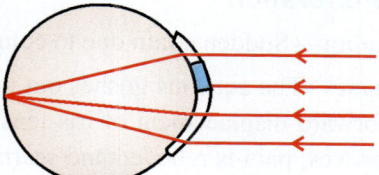
Optical effects of Leucoma
• stops all light which falls upon it
• loss of brightness but not definition

2. *Macula*—The corneal opacity is dense when it involves about half the thickness of the stroma. The fine details of the deeper structures are observed partially.
3. *Leucoma*—A thick white, dense and totally opaque scar results when almost full thickness of stroma is involved. Nothing can be seen through the leucoma.

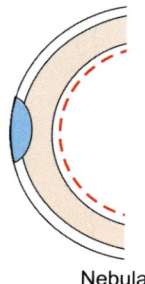
Nebula

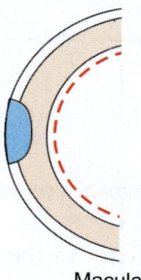
Macula

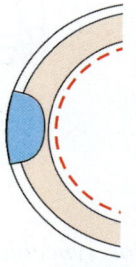
Leucoma

2. Ectatic Cicatrix [Keratectasia] (ectasia = bulge forwards, cicatrix = fibrous scar)

There is marked thinning at the site of ulcer. It bulges forwards even in the presence of normal intraocular pressure. There is no iris adhesion to the cornea. The cicatrix may become consolidated and flat later on.

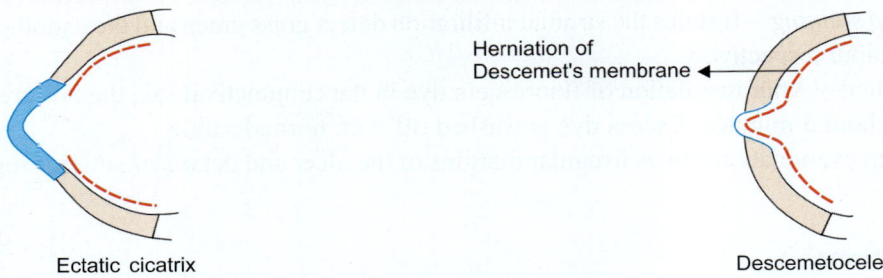

Ectatic cicatrix   Descemetocele

3. Descemetocele [Keratocele]

Few ulcers specially those due to pneumococcus and septic organisms extend rapidly. Descemet's membrane offers great resistance but eventually it may herniate as a transparent vesicle called the descemetocele. It may persist surrounded by white cicatricial ring or it may rupture.

4. Perforation

Etiology—Sudden strain due to cough, sneez or spasm of orbicularis muscle may cause perforation.

Course—The aqueous gushes out resulting in the collapse of anterior chamber (IOP = zero). There is forward displacement of iris-lens diaphragm. The only benefit is that the nutrition of the cornea improves, pain is relieved and scarring takes place.

Complications of Perforation

These are of extreme danger to the sight.
1. *Prolapse of iris*—When part of iris protrudes through the ulcer it is known as prolapse of iris.

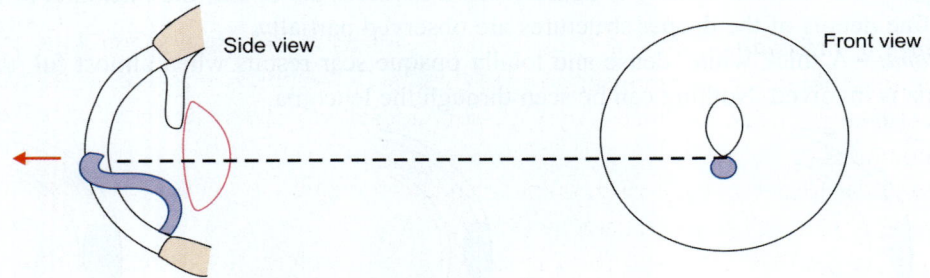

Perforated corneal ulcer with prolapse of iris

2. *Anterior synechia*—The adhesion of iris to the posterior surface of cornea is known as the anterior synechia. There is no incarceration of iris within the layers of the cornea.
3. *Adherent leucoma*—It is a leucomatous opacity in which the iris tissue is incarcerated within the layers of the cornea.

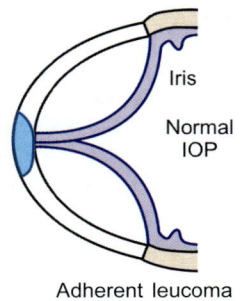
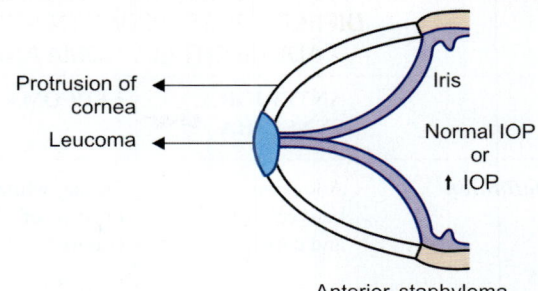

Adherent leucoma   Anterior staphyloma

4. *Anterior staphyloma*—The adherent leucoma becomes ectatic due to secondary glaucoma or weakness of corneal scar tissue. The ectatic cicatrix in which iris is incarcerated is called anterior staphyloma.
5. *Corneal fistula*—The ulcer ruptures repeatedly due to straining factors. The opening in the cornea is lined by the epithelium therefore it does not heal leading to fistula formation. The aqueous leaks continuously through the corneal fistula. It is usually situated in the centre.
6. *Anterior capsular cataract*—It is formed when the lens comes in contact with the ulcer.
7. *Dislocation or subluxation of lens* occurs due to stretching and rupture of zonule.
8. *Intraocular haemorrhage*—Sudden lowering of intraocular pressure results in dilatation and rupture of choroidal blood vessels leading to intraocular haemorrhage.
9. *Purulent iridocyclitis and panophthalmitis* usually occurs in gonococcal infection and hypopyon ulcers.

TREATMENT OF CORNEAL ULCER

Principles

1. **Control of infection** Infection is controlled by intensive local use of antibiotic drops. Broad-spectrum antibiotic drops, ointment, are given frequently 4-6 times a day. Subconjunctival injections may also be given once or twice daily. Culture and sensitivity should be done before the application of antibiotics.
2. **Cleanliness** Irrigation with warm saline or sodabicarb lotion is advised. It washes away necrotic material, toxin, secretion and pathogenic organisms.
3. **Heat** Heat prevents stasis and encourages repair of the ulcer. Hot fomentation may be given.
4. **Rest**
    i. 1% atropine either as drops or ointment is applied 2-3 times a day. It paralyses the ciliary muscles and provides comfort to the eye by preventing ciliary spasm. There is associated iritis always in cases of corneal ulcer due to penetration of endotoxin across the endothelium in the anterior chamber. It also prevents most of the dangerous complications of iritis.
    ii. Pad and bandage give rest to the eyeball by restricting its movements.
5. **Protection**
    i. Pad and bandage protect the eye from dust, wind and harmful external agencies.

DIFFERENCES BETWEEN ANTERIOR SYNECHIA, LEUCOMA, ADHERENT LEUCOMA AND ANTERIOR STAPHYLOMA

	ANTERIOR SYNECHIA	**LEUCOMA**	**ADHERENT LEUCOMA**	**ANTERIOR STAPHYLOMA**
Definition	Adhesion between iris and cornea	Dense, white opacity of cornea	Adhesion between iris and leucoma	• Adhesion between iris and leucoma. • There is ectasia due to secondary glaucoma usually. Same as adherent leucoma
Etiology	• Perforated corneal ulcer • Iridocyclitis • Closed angle glaucoma • Foreign body • Corneal dystrophy	• Healed corneal ulcer • Healed keratitis • Penetrating injury	• Perforated corneal ulcer • Penetrating injury • Operating wound	
	Anterior synechia	Leucoma	Adherent leucoma	Anterior staphyloma
Symptoms				
1. Visual acuity	Normal	Impaired if situated over pupillary area	Impaired if situated over pupillary area	Impaired
Signs				
1. Corneal surface	Flat	Flat	Flat	Ectatic
2. Pigments	Nil	Fine yellowish brown lines in the epithelium (Hudson Stahlis) haemosiderin, melanin	Brown pigment from iris are present	Brown pigment from iris are seen
3. Anterior chamber	Normal or shallow	Normal	Irregular or shallow where iris comes forwards	Usually absent or very shallow
4. Pupil	Normal	Normal	Drawn towards adhesion	Not seen
5. Corneal sensation	Normal	Impaired over opacity	Impaired over opacity	Impaired
6. Intraocular tension	Normal or raised when more than 3/4 circumference is involved (closed angle glaucoma)	Normal	Normal or raised (secondary glaucoma)	Raised usually

ii. A shield or dark glasses are used if there is associated conjunctival discharge to avoid retention of secretion, which in turn favours bacterial growth due to warmth and stasis.

Procedure

Bacterial corneal ulcer is a serious condition that requires immediate treatment by identification and eradication of causative organism.

Causative organism can be identified by smear preparation, culture and sensitivity test of the scrapings taken from the base of the ulcer. However, treatment cannot be delayed for the report to be available. It should be started immediately with broad spectrum antibiotics available.

a. Gram-positive bacteria usually responds to chloramphenicol, cephazoline, ciprofloxacin and penicillin, etc.
b. Gram-negative bacteria usually responds to gentamicin, tobramycin, norfloxacin, etc.

1. *Broad spectrum antibiotics*
    i. Topical antibiotic drops are instilled at half hourly interval in initial stages. Later on frequency can be reduced depending upon the response.
    Nowadays topical fortified preparations are preferred choice over commercially available antibiotic drops. It is the most effective way to maintain a high and sustained level of antibiotics at the site of infection.
    Fortified gentamicin drops can be prepared by adding 2 ml of parenteral gentamicin (80 mg) into 5 ml of commercially available gentamicin eyedrops. The resultant solution contains 15 mg/ml of gentamicin and is stable for 30 days.
    Similarly fortified cephazoline (50 mg/ml) drops can also be prepared by dissolving 500 mg of cephazoline powder into 10 ml distilled water, which should be used within 24 hours.
    ii. Antibiotic eye ointment should be applied at night as it has prolonged action.
    iii. Subconjunctival injection of gentamicin 40 mg and cephazoline 125 mg once a day for 5 days should also be given in moderate to severe cases.
    If the response is good, then there is no need to change the initial broad spectrum antibiotics but if it is not so, the subsequent therapy is decided depending upon the culture and sensitivity report.
    iv. Systemic antibiotics are usually not required except in fulminating cases with perforation.
2. *Atropine sulphate* (1%) drops or ointment should be used to reduce pain from ciliary spasm and to prevent formation of posterior synaechiae from secondary iridocyclitis.
    Atropine also increases blood supply to anterior uvea and brings more antibodies in the aqueous humour. It also reduces exudation by decreasing hyperaemia and vascular permeability.
    Other cycloplegics like homatropine (2%) or cyclopenlolate (1%) can be used in less severe cases.
3. *Analgesics and anti-inflammatory drugs* Systemic analgesics and anti-inflammatory drugs may be added to relieve pain and oedema.

4. *General measures* Rest, hot fomentation or dry heat, good diet and fresh air helps in faster healing.

IN GENERAL CORTICOSTEROIDS ARE CONTRAINDICATED IN THE TREATMENT OF CORNEAL ULCER.

Please note that *corticosteroids* are not given in routine cases of corneal ulcer as they inhibit healing by fibrosis and also retard epithelialisation. However, if the reaction is very severe, steroids can be administered with caution for a short period under cover of antibiotics. As soon as the inflammation is controlled steroids are discontinued as their prolong use may cause perforation.

TREATMENT OF NON-HEALING CORNEAL ULCER

In spite of all the above mentioned measures ulceration progresses and pain continues. A non-healing corneal ulcer does not respond to routine treatment for corneal ulcer due to following causes :

1. Local

1. Chronic dacryocystitis—It is a continuous source of pathogenic bacterial infection.
2. Increased intraocular pressure—It adversely affects the nutrition of the cornea.
3. Trichiasis—There is constant rubbing of the eyelashes against the cornea.
4. Retained foreign body—It is a source of constant irritation.
5. Neuroparalytic ulcers—There is complete loss of sensation in the cornea.

2. General

1. Diabetes mellitus—It reduces the resistance of the body against infections.
2. Vitamin A deficiency—It leads to xerosis and keratomalacia, thus, decreasing the resistance of the cornea.
3. Malnutrition—This results in delayed healing.
4. Immunosuppressive drugs and AIDS—There is decreased body resistance to infection.

Treatment

Non-healing corneal ulcer can be treated by:
1. *Cauterization*—The chemical cautery acts as an antiseptic.
    i. Pure carbolic acid—It acts both as an antiseptic and caustic.
    ii. Trichloracetic acid 10-20%
    iii. Silver nitrate 1%. It is a mild antiseptic.

Pure carbolic acid has the advantage of penetrating little more deeply than is actually applied. Therefore, it extends its antiseptic properties widely.

Method—Local anaesthetic agent is instilled in the eye frequently. Wait for 2-3 minutes for cornea to get anaesthetised. A drop of fluorescein dye may be applied to demarcate the ulcer (optional) . Apply carbolic acid soaked in a sterile wooden stick over the ulcer. The touched part becomes white immediately, but the normal epithelium recovers rapidly. The excess acid is washed off with normal saline. The acid should not touch the conjunctiva to prevent adhesions (symblepharon) between the lids and eyeball. Antibiotic eye ointment and pad and bandage is applied.

2. *Paracentesis*—Aqueous is released slowly by making an opening in the lower temporal quadrant of cornea. It improves the nutrition of the cornea by bringing in fresh aqueous. It prevents complications of spontaneous perforation which usually occurs in the centre of the cornea involving the visual axis.
3. *Conjunctival flap*—The non-healing ulcer may be covered with the conjunctival flap.
4. *Therapeutic keratoplasty*—Full thickness graft is applied to enhance healing and to prevent perforation.
5. *Tarsorrhaphy*—It is done in cases of neuroparalytic ulcers and exposure keratitis.
6. Treat the underlying cause which is responsible for non-healing ulcer.

TREATMENT OF IMPENDING PERFORATION (DESCEMETOCELE)

1. *Rest*—Preferably bed-rest is advised.
2. *Pressure pad and bandage*—By applying extra pad and tight bandage over the eye, support is given to the cornea.
3. *Intraocular pressure* is kept low by giving oral acetazolamide.
4. *Paracentesis* may be done to prevent central perforation.
5. *Straining factors are avoided*, e.g. coughing, sneezing or straining at passing stool.
6. *Therapeutic full thickness or penetrating keratoplasty* is done as the last resort.

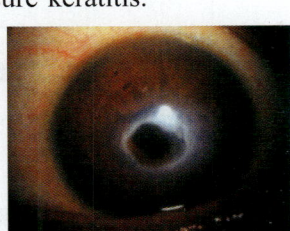
Descemetocele

TREATMENT OF CORNEAL ABSCESS

There is a localised collection of pus in the corneal stroma. The epithelium is usually intact and therefore the fluorescein staining is negative. The clinical features are similar to corneal ulcer.

Treatment

1. Evacuation of pus is done first by a sterile autoclaved fine needle or knife before starting the topical antibiotic treatment as for corneal ulcer.
2. Cauterization done by chemical (carbolic acid) cautery is also effective.

TREATMENT OF PERFORATED CORNEAL ULCER

1. **Immediate**—It depends on the site and size of perforation.
   1. If perforation is small in the pupillary area and there is no prolapse of iris:
      i. Rest in bed is advised.
      ii. Atropine and antibiotic ointment are applied.
      iii. Pressure pad and bandage helps in sealing perforation.
   2. Tissue adhesives, e.g. isobutyl cyanoacrylate may be used.
   3. Soft contact lens helps in the healing process.

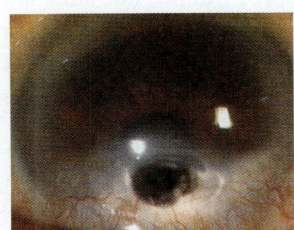
Perforated corneal ulcer

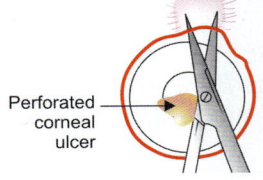
Perforated corneal ulcer

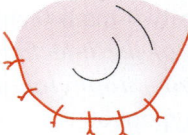

Conjunctival flap

118 Basic Ophthalmology

4. Conjunctival flap covers the perforation site and aids healing.
5. Therapeutic penetrating keratoplasty may be done as a final resort.

2. Late
1. *Leucoma*
   i. *Optical iridectomy* The pupil is extended to the periphery by a slit-like iridectomy. It is indicated when the vision is quite good and where facilities for keratoplasty are not available

Optical iridectomy

Site— 1. Temporal—When greater field of vision is required, e.g. farmers.
       2. Nasal—For near work, e.g., clerk, goldsmith.
   ii. Full thickness keratoplasty is preferred treatment when the ulcer has healed and the vision is markedly reduced.
   iii. Tattooing with gold (brown) or platinum (black) is advised for cosmetic purpose only in *firm blind eyes* usually.

   Method—The affected part is denuded of epithelium. A piece of blotting paper of the same size, soaked in fresh 2% platinum chloride solution is kept over the opacity. On removing this filter paper, few drops of fresh 2% hydrazine hydrate solution are applied over the area which in turn becomes black. Eye is washed with saline. A drop of parolein is instilled and a pad and bandage applied. The epithelium grows over the black coloured deposit of platinum.

2. *Adherent leucoma*—The treatment is same as for leucoma. In addition, synechiotomy is done, i.e. adhesion of the iris is separated by iris repositor to break the peripheral anterior synechiae. This prevents the occurrence of secondary glaucoma.
3. *Corneal fistula*—Full thickness keratoplasty is indicated as the fistulous tract is lined by the epithelium which prevents healing.

HYPOPYON ULCER

Hypopyon ulcer is a corneal ulcer associated with hypopyon, i.e., sterile pus in the anterior chamber, as a result of iridocyclitis. It is important to note that hypopyon is *sterile* as the leucocytosis is due to the toxins and not by actual invasion of the bacteria.

Etiology

It depends on two main factors
1. *Virulence of the infecting organism*—Pyogenic organisms, e.g. *Pneumococcus, Pseudomonas pyocyanea, Staphylococcus, Streptococcus, Gonococcus, Moraxella,* fungus, etc. may produce hypopyon.

2. *Resistance of the host*—It is commonly seen in old, debilitated, alcoholic, malnourished and immunologically deficient persons. It may occur during or after acute infectious diseases, e.g. measles, scarelet fever or chickenpox.

Predisposing Factors
1. Chronic dacryocystitis is a continuous source of infection particularly of *Pseudomonas pyocyanea* and pneumococcus bacteria.
2. Minor injury, e.g. scratches with the nail.
3. Retained minute foreign bodies such as stone, coal, etc.
4. Old, debilitated and alcoholic patients usually suffer from malnourishment.
5. Acute infections such as measles, scarlet fever, etc. occurring commonly in children.

Pathogenesis
1. In case of a corneal ulcer there is always associated iridocyclitis due to the liberation of toxins by the bacteria, which diffuses into the anterior chamber via the endothelium.
2. This results in dilatation of the blood vessels and outpouring of leucocytes which become enmeshed in the fibrin network. Such hypopyons are fluid and change their position with gravity when the patient's head is changed.
3. These gravitate to the bottom of anterior chamber. It may fill half of the anterior chamber, having straight upper margin. In severe cases, it may completely fill the anterior chamber thus obscuring the iris.
4. The hypopyon is *sterile* and it usually gets absorbed when hypopyon corneal ulcer is adequately treated with routine treatment for corneal ulcer.

Types
It varies in type according to the infective agent and age of the patient.
1. Ulcus serpens.
2. Mycotic hypopyon ulcer.

1. ULCUS SERPENS

It is the most common type of hypopyon ulcer. It occurs in adults due to pneumococcus bacteria usually.

It has a tendency to creep over the cornea in a serpiginous fashion.

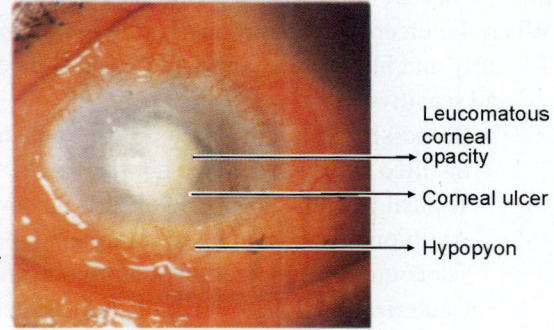

Hypopyon corneal ulcer

Symptoms
1. There is marked pain in the eye and lacrimation.
2. A variable amount of photophobia is present.

Signs
1. Cornea is lustreless and hazy. A greyish white or yellow disc is seen in the centre.

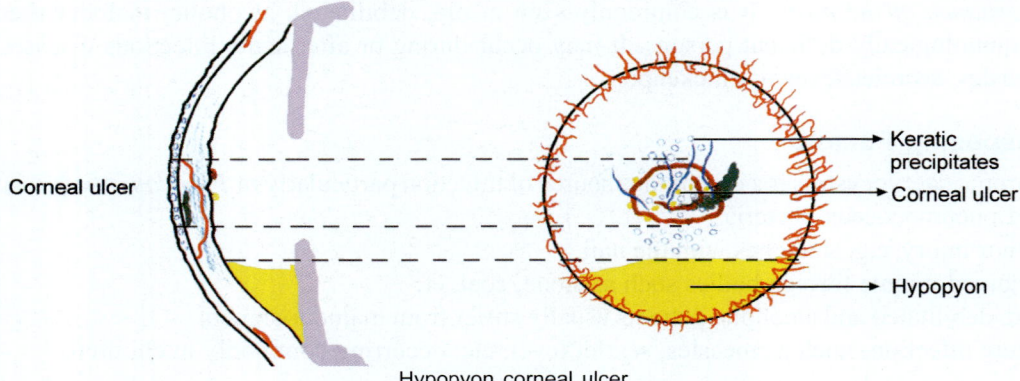

Hypopyon corneal ulcer

2. The opacity is greater at the advancing edge in one particular direction than centre.
3. The tissues breakdown on the side of the densest infiltration (yellow crescent) and ulcer spreads in size and depth.
4. Often there is infiltration anterior to Descemet's membrane at the floor of the ulcer while the intervening stroma is normal.
5. Marked iritis with cloudy aqueous (hypopyon), conjunctival and ciliary congestion is usually present. The lids are red and swollen.

Complications

1. Perforation with iris prolapse may occur due to thinning of cornea.
2. Panophthalmitis may occur due to rapid growth and spread of the virulent organisms.
3. Perforation may heal resulting in leucoma, adherent leucoma, anterior staphyloma or occlusio-pupillae causing marked visual impairment.
4. Secondary glaucoma usually follows perforation due to synechia formation.

Treatment

It is a well-known surgical rule that pus anywhere in the body has to be removed. However, this is not true in case of hypopyon ulcer. The fact that the hypopyon is *sterile* has great practical importance. When the ulcer is treated properly, the hypopyon gets absorbed automatically.

1. Early and intensive treatment of corneal ulcer as mentioned earlier is started at once after culture and sensitivity.
   - Broad-spectrum antibiotic drops are instilled every few minutes for the first hour. Later it is instilled hourly and then 2 hourly.
   - Topical atropine is applied even if the tension is raised.
   - Antibiotic and atropine eye ointment are applied at bedtime.
   - Subconjunctival injection of antibiotic and atropine may be given.
   - Cauterization if done skillfully may be helpful.
2. Secondary glaucoma is the most common cause of failure of treatment in elderly persons. It affects the nutrition and resistance of the cornea. It is treated by
   - Topical atropine 1%

- Oral acetazolamide (carbonic anhydrase inhibitor)
- Intravenous mannitol 20%, 200 ml (hyperosmotic agent)
- Paracentesis helps in lowering the tension and brings fresh aqueous and nutrient. It is done only in cases of markedly raised intraocular tension.

3. If there is associated chronic dacryocystitis, dacryocystorhinostomy (DCR) is performed.

2. MYCOTIC HYPOPYON ULCER
(KERATOMYCOSIS, FUNGAL CORNEAL ULCER)

This is a rare type of hypopyon corneal ulcer caused by injury by vegetable matter.

Etiology

It is commonly caused by *Candida albicans, Aspergillus fumigatus, Fusarium, Cephalosporium, Streptothrix actinomycosis,* etc.

Filamentous fungi—e.g. *Aspergillus* species (most common) *Fusarium*. They are most prevalent in agricultural areas.

Yeast—e.g. *Candida albicans*. It frequently affects the compromised host.

Incidence

It is common in rural agricultural areas. It usually occurs due to ocular trauma involving vegetable matter, e.g. thorn, sharp wooden stick, wheat and paddy husk, branches of tree, etc.

Predisposing Factors

1. They are same as for bacterial keratitis.
2. Indiscriminate use of topical or systemic steroids alters host defence mechanism.
3. It occurs commonly in immunocompromised subjects.

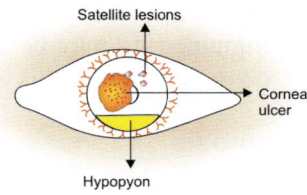

Fungal corneal ulcer

Symptoms

These are same as for the bacterial ulcer but they are less prominent than equal-sized bacterial ulcer. There is mild pain, irritation, watering and presence of yellow patch in the cornea.

Signs

1. A typical lesion is a yellow-white coloured ulcer with indistinct margin. There is minimum vascularization usually.
2. It is dry in appearance with small satellite lesions around the ulcer due to the stromal infiltration with delicate feathery, finger-like hyphate edges protruding into adjacent stroma.
3. Ulcer margin is often elevated above the surface.

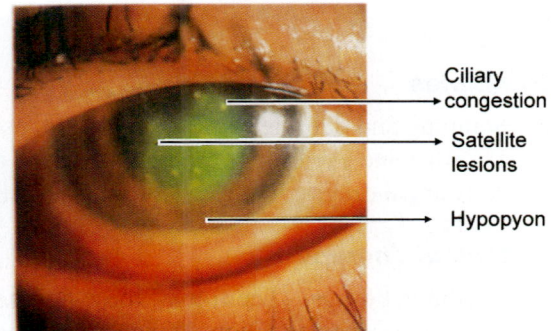

Fungal keratitis ulcer stained with fluorescein

DIFFERENCES BETWEEN BACTERIAL AND FUNGAL CORNEAL ULCERS

	BACTERIAL ULCERS	FUNGAL ULCERS
1. History of injury	Non-specific	With vegetable matter
2. Onset after injury	24-72 hours	One to two weeks
3. Predisposing factors	Non-specific	Systemic immunosuppressives, local or systemic steroids therapy
4. Course	Rapid	Usually slow but can be rapid if activated by steroids
5. Clinical features	Proportionate	Signs out of proportion to symptoms.
6. Description of ulcer	i. Moist look	• Dry necrotic look, yellowish-white in colour
	ii. Soft slough	• Thick solid slough
	iii. Marked infiltration with gross destruction of tissue	• Hyphate margins, satellite lesions, immune ring
	iv. Highly vascular	• Minimum vascularisation
	v. Perforation common	• Perforation less common
7. Hypopyon	Fluid and mobile	Dense and immobile

4. Massive hypopyon is present commonly which is dense and organized.
5. Slit-lamp examination—Endothelial plaque and immune ring may be seen around the ulcer. Some degree of iridocyclitis is usually present.

Diagnosis

Scraping of the ulcer at the margin and inoculation of media should be done promptly. As the organism is often situated deep within the stroma, corneal biopsy may be taken at times.
1. Staining with methamine silver, Gram and Giemsa stains.
2. Culture in Sabouraud's medium, blood-agar plate or brain-heart infusion broth is essential.

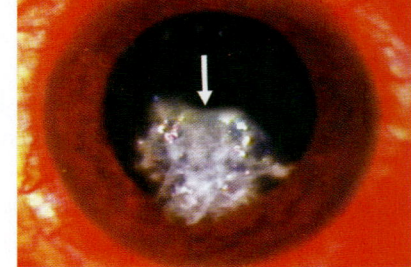

Fungal corneal ulcer

Treatment

Principles

1. Scraping and debridement of the ulcer is useful in drug penetration.
2. 1% Atropine eyedrop or ointment controls associated iritis and prevents synechiae formation.
3. Antifungal drugs—The available antifungal drugs are mainly fungistatic.

I. Medical Therapy

1. Antifungal drugs—The role of these drugs is limited due to the few approved antifungal drugs and their poor penetration. Topical antifungals are to be instilled for a long-time, as the response is often delayed.

ANTIFUNGAL THERAPEUTIC REGIMEN USED IN FUNGAL KERATITIS

1. Amphotericin B	Topical—0.3% every hour. Taper over several weeks Subconjunctival—100 -300 mg on alternate day × 1-2 doses Intravitreal—5-10 µg Systemic—By infusion, 5-10 mg total dose is given/day.
2. Ketoconazole	Oral 200- 400 mg /day for at least 14 days
3. Miconazole	Topical—10 mg /ml eyedrops every hour, taper gradually.
4. Clotrimazole	Topical 1% eyedrop every hour. Taper over several weeks
5. Natamycin	Topical 5% drops every hour. Taper over several weeks
6. Flucytosine	Topical 10 mg/ml drop every hour, then taper gradually.
7. Nystatin	Topical eye ointment is applied.

a. *Topical*
   i. Natamycin (5%) eyedrop is instilled 1 hourly. It is effective against the most common fungi.
   ii. Miconazole (1%) eye ointment is applied 5 times daily.
   iii. Nystatin eye ointment is applied 5 times daily. It is only effective against *Candida* and is less potent.
   iv. Topical amphoterecin B (0.25%) is instilled 1 hourly. It is effective against *Aspergillus* and *Candida*.
2. Systemic—Systemic antifungals are indicated if the infection spreads to the sclera and there is impending perforation, e.g. oral ketoconazole or fluconazole 200 mg daily may be given for 2-3 weeks.
3. Cycloplegics such as atropine is used to prevent posterior synechiae formation and to control iritis by paralysing the ciliary muscle. It also causes vasodilatation.
4. Corticosteroids are *contraindicated* as they enhance fungal growth.

II. Surgical Treatment

1. Debridement and superficial keratectomy help in drug penetration.
2. Cauterization of the ulcer may be done in non-responsive cases.
3. Conjunctival flap is useful in non-healing fungal ulcers.
4. Therapeutic full-thickness keratoplasty is much better solution in cases of non-healing fungal keratitis. Corneal graft is indicated for corneal opacity.

MARGINAL ULCER

Etiology

It is caused by Morax-Axenfeld bacillus, *Staphylococcus, H. aegyptius,* etc. It is often associated with chronic blepharo-conjunctivitis.

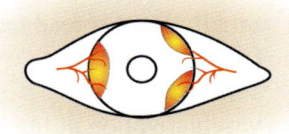

Marginal ulcer

Incidence

It is seen in old debilitated people usually. Deep marginal ulcer may occur rarely in cases of polyarteritis nodosa, systemic lupus erythematosus due to antigen-antibody complexes.

Symptoms

There is neuralgic pain in the face and head. Recurrence is common.

Signs

1. Shallow, slightly infiltrated, multiple ulcers are seen near the limbus.
2. The ulcers are often vascularised.

Complications

1. Deep marginal ulcers—These are seen in autoimmune diseases.
2. There may be formation of ring ulcer.
3. This may be followed by necrosis of the whole cornea.

Treatment

- Suitable antibiotic eyedrops and ointment are applied.
- Chemical cautery may be done with 1% silver nitrate in mild recurrent ulcers.
- Steroid drops and ointment may give temporary benefit.
- In severe cases, systemic steroids and cytotoxic drugs may be useful.

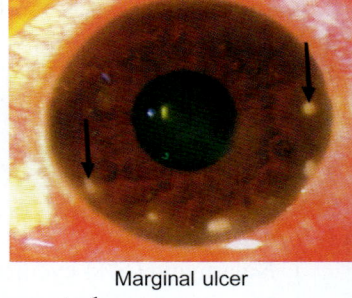

Marginal ulcer

CHRONIC SERPIGINOUS ULCER (RODENT OR MOOREN'S ULCER)

It is a rare superficial progressive marginal ulcer of a degenerative type.

Etiology

It occurs as a result of degenerative process due to ischaemia of cornea. It starts at the corneal margin and spreads over the whole of cornea. Erosion is due to autoimmune lysis of the epithelium. This is followed by the release of collagenolytic enzyme.

Incidence

It is common in elderly males.

Symptoms

There is severe persistent neuralgic pain with lacrimation.

Signs

1. It starts as one or more grey infiltrations which breakdown to form small ulcers.
2. Small ulcers spread centripetally and coalesce with each other.
3. Characteristic white overhanging edges are seen as the ulcer spreads below the epithelium and superficial layers of stroma. This resembles the ears of the rabbit (rodent ulcer). There is vascularization at the base of the ulcer.

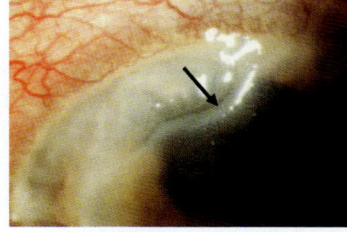

Mooren's ulcer

Complications

1. It rarely perforates but recurrences are common.
2. Thin nebular opacity may form over the whole cornea.

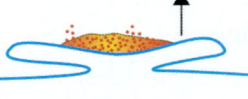

Over hanging edge

Rodent ulcer

Treatment

It is very difficult because of corneal ischaemia.
1. Excision of 4-6 mm strip of adjacent conjunctiva with or without cryotherapy is often effective. This removes conjunctival source of collagenase and proteoglycanase.
2. Immunosuppressive like cyclosporine A or cytotoxic agents may be quite useful.
3. Topical application of antibiotics and steroids are usually ineffective.
4. In case of perforation, cyanoacrylate adhesive and soft contact lens may be used.
5. Lamellar keratoplasty with intravenous methotrexate may be useful.

EXPOSURE KERATITIS

There is exposure of the cornea due to insufficient closure of the eye (Lagophthalmos).

Etiology

This condition is commonly seen,
- In eyes insufficiently covered by the lids due to paralysis of the orbicularis muscle.
- In extreme proptosis, e.g. exophthalmos, orbital tumour.
- There is absence of reflex blinking in extremely ill or comatose patients.

Sign

- There is corneal erosion with ulcer formation as the epithelium becomes desiccated.
- There is absence of reflex blinking and defective closure of lids during sleep.

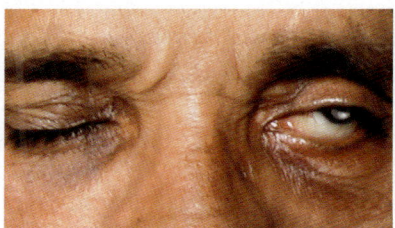
Exposure keratitis

Treatment

1. Keep the cornea well-covered by applying eye shade and bandage.
2. Artificial tears and ointment are applied frequently to lubricate the cornea.
3. Tarsorrhaphy may be done to protect the cornea.
4. Treat the underlying cause of proptosis.

NEUROPARALYTIC KERATITIS

There is loss of corneal sensation which results in the formation of corneal ulcer.

Etiology

There is 5th nerve (trigeminal nerve) paralysis. It occurs typically as a result of injecting alcohol in gasserian ganglion in cases of trigeminal neuralgia.

Symptom

It is a painless condition due to corneal anaesthesia.

Signs

The characteristic feature is desquamation of corneal epithelium.
1. Large corneal ulcers are seen due to peeling of the epithelium.

CLINICAL FEATURES OF DIFFERENT CORNEAL ULCERS

CLINICAL FEATURES	BACTERIAL	VIRAL	FUNGAL
Symptoms			
1. *Discharge*	Mucopurulent ++	Watery	May be present
2. *Pain*	Severe	Moderate	Mild
3. *Systemic-Fever headache, etc.*	—	++	—
4. *Recurrence*	—	++	—
5. *History of trauma*	Common with penetrating injury	—	Vegetative matter injury
Signs			
1. *Injection*	Marked	Moderate	Marked
2. *Follicles*	—	+	—
3. *Ulcer*	Central disc with necrotic material	Typical dendritic and geographical pattern	Dry yellow-grey with satellite lesions
4. *Depth*	May be deep	Usually superficial	Deep
5. *Corneal sensations*	Present	Absent	Present
6. *Preauricular*	+	+	—

2. The stroma is cloudy and yellow often associated with hypopyon.
3. Ciliary congestion is marked.
4. There is corneal anaesthesia.

Treatment

1. Treat the corneal ulcer on usual line of treatment. Special care is taken to protect the eye with an eye shield.
2. Artificial tears and eye ointment are applied to lubricate the cornea.
3. Closure of the lacrimal puncta may be done to conserve moisture.
4. Paramedian or lateral tarsorrhaphy is indicated in these cases.

NONPURULENT KERATITIS

HERPES SIMPLEX

Etiology

It is caused by herpes simplex virus type I (HSV I).

Incidence

It occurs in children or young adults usually.
- There is recurrence due to febrile cold, pneumonia, physical exhaustion or exposure to sunlight.

Types
1. **Primary ocular herpes**—There is acute follicular keratoconjunctivitis with regional lymphadenitis and skin involvement.
2. **Recurrent herpes**—It has following characteristic features:
   - Epithelial ulcers
   - Stromal interstitial keratitis
   - Disciform keratitis
   - Iridocyclitis.

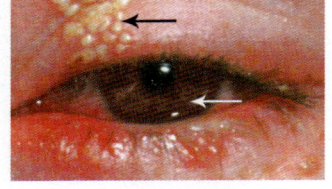

Herpes simplex

Symptoms
- Vesicles are seen on lips, nose, cornea (Herpes simplex virus type I / HSV I) and genitals (Herpes simplex virus type II / HSV II).
- Great irritation, lacrimation and blepharospasm is present.

Signs
1. **Skin lesion**—Initially vesicles with superficial crusts are formed. These vesicles heal without scar formation.
2. Severe follicular keratoconjunctivitis is present usually in children.
3. There may be regional lymphadenitis (preauricular lymph nodes).
4. Slit-lamp examination of the cornea shows:
   i. *Superficial punctate keratitis*
   - Numerous, white plaques of epithelial cells are present all over the corneal surface.
   - These are of minute pin—head size.
   - They are arranged in rows or groups.
   - There is absence of vascularization and corneal sensation.

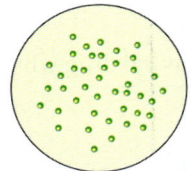 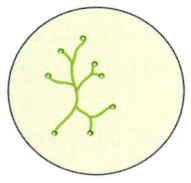 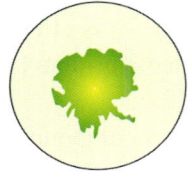 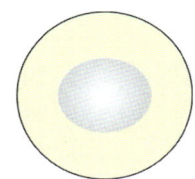

Superficial punctate keratitis   Dendritic ulcer   Confluent ulcer   Disciform keratitis

   ii. *Dendritic ulcer*—Erosions coalesce to form typical dendritic figure like liverwort. It is pathognomonic of herpes simplex.
   iii. *Confluent ulcer*—Large geographical pattern type of ulcers are seen.
   iv. *Disciform (deep) keratitis*—It involves the stroma forming disc-like opacity.

Complications
- Chronic epithelial ulcer with recurrence is a common complication.
- Corneal opacity is present in deep or stromal keratitis.
- Iritis and iridocyclitis is often associated with a severe herpetic keratitis.
- Hypopyon may be present in severe cases.

Diagnosis

1. Immunological tests—By immunofluorescence of epithelial scrapings.
2. Tissue biopsy and tissue culture—Elementary bodies are seen with suitable staining.

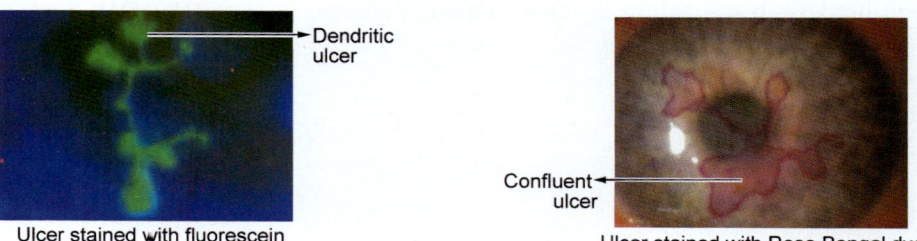

Ulcer stained with fluorescein — Dendritic ulcer

Ulcer stained with Rose Bengal dye — Confluent ulcer

Treatment

1. *Antiviral drugs*
   a. Systemic—Oral acyclovir 400 mg twice daily × 7 days. Ideally it should be started prior to the onset of symptoms. It is the method of choice in cases of recurrent herpes labialis. It has low toxicity.
   b. Topical
      i. 5-iodo-2-deoxyuridine (IDU)—0.1% eyedrops and 5% eye ointment. It is applied 5 times a day and at bedtime for 10-21 days. Treatment should not be prolonged beyond 3 weeks since this may lead to corneal toxicity.
      ii. Acyclovir—3% eye ointment is applied 5 times daily for 10-21 days.
      iii. Adenine arabinoside (Ara-A) and vidarabine (Vira-A) 3% ointment—It is not effective in stromal disease.
      iv. Trifluorothymidine (F_3T)—Trifluridine 1% eyedrops are applied 5-9 times daily for 14 days.
      v. Acycloguanosine—It is effective in cases of stromal disease and iritis
      vi. Bromovinyl—deoxyuridine 1% ointment and 0.1% drops is a new antiviral drug which is as potent as F_3T.
      vii. A very potent new compound 9-guanine (ganciclovir) is under trial.
2. *Debridement*—It may be used for dendritic but not for geographical ulcers. The corneal surface is wiped with sterile cellulose sponge 2 mm beyond the edge of the ulcer (as pathology extends beyond visible lesion)
   - This protects healthy epithelium from infection
   - It eliminates the antigenic stimulus to stromal inflammation.
3. *Atropine and warm compresses are useful in controlling iritis.*
4. *Topical corticosteroids* are only useful in deep or disciform keratitis. Steroids are contraindicated in epithelial lesions.
5. *Full thickness keratoplasty* is done in cases of permanent corneal opacity. The eye must be quiet for a year at least.

HERPES ZOSTER

Etiology
It is an acute infection of dorsal root ganglion by varicella—zoster virus. It is identical with chickenpox virus.

Incidence
It is associated with the chickenpox infection in youth or childhood. It often occurs in elderly with depressed cellular immunity, e.g. as in diabetics, alcoholics and in persons suffering from cancer or AIDS. It is unilateral always affecting the gasserian ganglion from where the virus travels down the branches of ophthalmic nerve.

Clinical Stages
It can be divided into three stages namely:
1. Acute phase—It occurs within the first 4 weeks which may totally resolve.
2. Chronic phase—It may persist for several years (10 yrs).
3. Relapsing phase—There is recurrence of the disease process even years later.

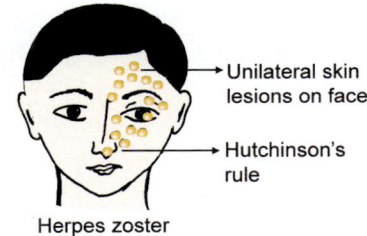

Herpes zoster

Symptoms
1. Rows of vesicular eruption take place along the branches of the ophthalmic division of the 5th cranial nerve. These suppurate, bleed and cause pitted scar.
   - Supraorbital nerve
   - Supratrochlear nerve
   - Infratrochlear nerve
   - Nasociliary nerve
   - Infraorbital nerve
2. Severe neuralgic pain along the course of the nerves is present due to neuritis.
3. Fever and malaise are present at the onset.
4. Skin of lid and face becomes red and oedematous.

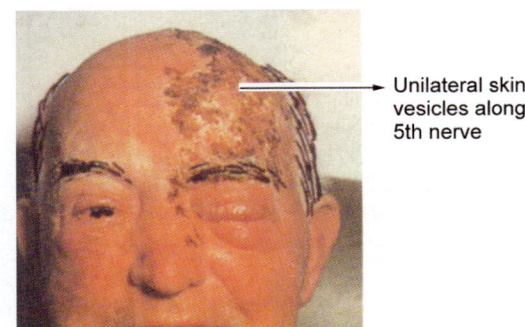

Herpes zoster

Signs
1. Hutchinson's rule—Ocular involvement is usually associated with eruption of vesicles on the skin of tip of the nose (nasociliary branch) during the acute stage.
2. Corneal and skin anaesthesias are characteristic and persist for a long-time.
3. Slit-lamp examination—
   - Superficial punctate keratitis is a most common feature. Numerous round white dots are seen in the epithelium which involve the stroma later.

DIFFERENCES BETWEEN HERPES SIMPLEX AND HERPES ZOSTER

	HERPES SIMPLEX	HERPES ZOSTER
1. Incidence	Children and young adult usually.	Elderly with depressed cellular immunity.
2. Etiology	Herpes simplex virus. There is recurrence in, • Febrile cold • Pneumonia, malaria • Exposure to sunlight • Physical exhaustion	Varicella zoster virus. It is identical with that causing chickenpox. Associated with chickenpox infection in youth.

3. Clinical features
  a. Systemic
 	
  b. Ocular
	• There are vesicles on lips, nose and genitals.
	• Bilateral usually.
	1. Follicular keratoconjunctivitis.
	2. Superficial punctate keratitis.
	3. Dendritic ulcer.
	4. Confluent ulcer.
	5. Disciform keratitis.
		Fever, malaise, severe pain along 5th nerve fibres.
		• Unilateral always.
		1. Eruption of rows of vesicles along ophthalmic division of 5th nerve.
		2. Vesicles suppurate and bleed forming small scars.
		3. Superficial punctate keratitis
		4. Subepithelial coarse punctate keratitis.
		5. Stroma may be involved in late stages.

4. Complications	• Iritis • Corneal opacity	• 3rd, 6th and 7th cranial nerve paralysis which usually passes off within 6 weeks • Exposure keratitis • Acute retinal necrosis • Optic neuritis • Corneal opacity

5. Treatment
  a. Systemic
 	
  b. Local
	• Oral acyclovir 400 mg twice daily × 7 days
	
	• Acyclovir eye ointment
	• IDU eyedrops and ointment
	• Vidarabine (Vira-A)
	• Adenine arabinoside (Ara-A)
	• Trifluorothymidine (F_3T)
	• Acycloguanosine
	• Corticosteroid drops
		• Oral acyclovir 800 mg 5 times daily × 10 days
		• Analgesic and anti-inflammatory
		• Acyclovir eye ointment
		• Artificial tears
		• Corticosteroid drops
		• Atropine

Similarity
1. Corneal anaesthesia—Both cause corneal anaesthesia.
2. Site of lesion—Both cause superficial corneal lesions therefore perforation is rare.

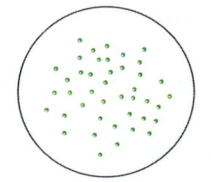 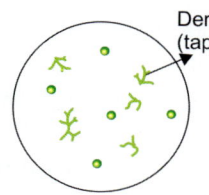 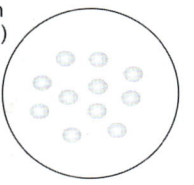 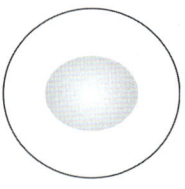

Superficial punctate keratitis | Coarse subepithelial punctate keratitis | Nummular keratits | Disciform keratitis

- Coarse subepithelial punctate keratitis occurs at a later stage.
- Micro dendritic epithelial ulcers—Unlike herpes simplex, these ulcers are small, peripheral, stellate and with tapered ends, i.e. without rounded bulbs.
- Nummular keratitis—Larger discoid lesions surrounded by stromal haze are seen.
- Disciform keratitis may be seen in few cases.
- Deep stromal involvement is often associated with iridocyclitis.

Complications

- Iridocyclitis and scleritis are associated with disciform keratitis.
- Secondary glaucoma may occur due to trabeculitis or peripheral anterior synechia, after the initial low tension.
- 3rd, 6th, 7th cranial nerve palsy and optic neuritis may occur in severe infection.
- Exposure keratitis results due to facial nerve paralysis.
- Postherpetic neuralgia may persist for several months and years.
- Acute retinal necrosis may develop after 5 days to 3 months after the skin infection.

Treatment

This is essentially symptomatic
1. Antiviral drugs
   a. *Systemic*—Oral acyclovir 800 mg is given five times daily × 10 days. It should be started within 3 days of appearance of skin rash. It shortens the duration of viral shedding and enhances epithelial healing.
   b. *Topical*
      i. Acyclovir 3% eye ointment is applied 5 times daily for 10-21 days.
      ii. Treatment of skin lesion consists of antiviral cream (acyclovir, IDU) and a steroid-antibiotic preparation. These are applied three times daily.
2. Analgesics and anti-inflammatory—In severe cases even pethidine may be given.
3. Topical atropine is applied in cases of keratitis, iridocyclitis, and scleritis.
4. Antibiotics are given if epithelium is ulcerated or when topical steroids are in use. Antibiotic skin ointment is applied over the skin lesion to prevent secondary infection.
5. Corticosteroids
   a. Topical steroids are useful particularly in disciform keratitis, scleritis and iridocyclitis.
   b. Systemic steroids are indicated in cranial nerve palsy, e.g. total 3 nerve palsy, optic neuritis, 7 nerve palsy.

6. Antidepressants such as amitriptylene 25-150 mg or imipramine may be given in acute phase for accompanying depression or in postherpetic neuralgia.
7. Artificial tears and lateral tarsorrhaphy are indicated in neuroparalytic ulcers and in cases of dry eye.
8. Full thickness keratoplasty is advised in neglected cases of disciform and scleral keratitis causing opacity. The eye must be quiet for a year at least.

ACANTHAMOEBA KERATITIS

Acanthamoeba keratitis has gained importance recently because of its increasing incidence, difficulty in diagnosis and unsatisfactory treatment.

Etiology
It is caused by *Acanthamoebae*, which are free living protozoans found in air, soil and fresh or brackish waters. They exist in both active (trophozoite) and dormant (cystic) forms.

Predisposing Factors
1. Keratitis may occur following a minor corneal abrasion.
2. Contact lens wearers who use distilled water and salt tablets instead of commercially prepared saline solutions for their lens care are at particular risk.

Symptoms
There is very severe pain (out of proportion to the degree of inflammation), watering, photophobia, blepharospasm and blurred vision.

Signs
Acanthamoeba keratitis evolves over several months as a gradual worsening keratitis with periods of temporary remissions.
1. Initial lesions of *Acanthamoeba* keratitis are in the form of coarse and opaque streaks. Fine epithelial and subepithelial opacities are also seen.
2. Advanced cases show a central or paracentral ring-shaped lesion with stromal infiltrates. There is an overlying epithelial defect.
3. Severe cases show associated *radial keratoneuritis*, in the form of perineural infiltrates along corneal nerves.

Diagnosis
1. *Clinical diagnosis*—It is difficult and is usually made by exclusion and with strong clinical suspicion in non-responsive patients being treated for herpetic, bacterial or fungal keratitis.
2. *Laboratory diagnosis*—Corneal scrapings may be helpful in some cases which can be stained.
   i. *Potassium hydroxide mount* is reliable in experienced hands for recognition of *Acanthamoeba* cysts.

ii. *Calcifluor white stain* is a chemifluorescent dye which stains the cysts of *Acanthamoeba* bright apple green.
iii. *Lactophenol cotton blue stained* film is also useful for demonstration of *Acanthamoeba* cysts in corneal scrapings.
iv. *Culture on non-nutrient agar* (*E. coli* enriched) may show trophozoites within 48 hours which gradually become cysts. *E. coli* prevents other organisms to grow whereas *Acanthamoeba* thrives on it.
3. *Confocal microscopy*—Acanthamoebae cysts can be demonstrated in optically cut parallel sections of cornea under confocal microscopy.

Treatment

It is usually unsatisfactory.
1. *Non-specific treatment* is on the general lines for corneal ulcer.
2. *Specific medical* treatment includes :
    A. Topical treatment
       - Propamidine isethionate (Brolene) 0.1% drops are used hourly
       - Neomycin drops
       - Polyhexamethylene biguanide (0.01-0.02%) drops are used hourly
       - Chlorhexidine drops
       - Paromomycin drops
       - Clotrimazole drops 1%
       - Polymyxin B drop
    B. Systemic treatment
    Oral ketoconazole 200 mg may be given four times a day for 2-3 weeks.
3. *Penetrating keratoplasty* is frequently required in non-responsive cases.

Acanthamoeba keratitis – Early

Acanthamoeba keratitis – Late

PHLYCTENULAR KERATITIS

Conjunctival phlycten may involve the corneal margin in later stages. It is an allergic reaction to an endogenous allergen, e.g. tuberculo-protein.

Symptoms

It causes much pain and photophobia.

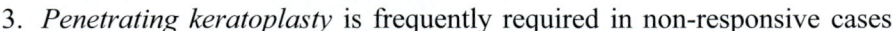

Phlyctenular keratitis → Fascicular ulcer

Signs

1. There is a grey nodule raised above the surface followed by formation of superficial yellow corneal ulcer.
2. Fascicular ulcer—A leash of blood vessel may follow the corneal ulcer at times.

Treatment

Intensive application of topical atropine and corticosteroids are very effective.

ACNE ROSACEA

Etiology

It is associated with pyogenic skin infection caused by *Staphylococcus*. It is seen in elderly women usually.

Signs

1. Mucopurulent conjunctivitis with phlycten-like lesions may be present.
2. There are multiple, small yellow-white intractable ulcers which keep recurring.
3. Heavy vascularization of the ulcers takes place eventually.
4. Iritis may be present in severe cases.

Treatment

- Topical atropine and corticosteroids are effective.
- A course of systemic broad-spectrum antibiotics is very useful in treating the underlying skin condition.

PHOTOPHTHALMIA

Etiology

It commonly occurs due to:
1. Exposure to ultraviolet rays by the bright flash of a short circuit or exposure to naked arc light in welding and cinema studio results in photophthalmia.
2. Snow blindness—The ultraviolet rays are reflected from snow surface.

Symptoms

There is extreme burning pain, photophobia, lacrimation and blepharospasm due to desquamation of corneal epithelium.

Signs

There are multiple epithelial erosions associated with blepharospasm and swelling of the palpebral conjunctiva and retrotarsal folds.

Treatment

- Cold compresses, astringent lotions and atropine ointment are effective.
- Bandage both eyes for 24 hours. This helps in regeneration of the epithelium.

Prophylaxis

Wearing of dark glasses (Crooke's glasses) made of such materials which cut off practically all the infrared and ultraviolet rays when such exposure is anticipated.

DEEP KERATITIS

The deep forms of keratitis affect the stroma of the cornea.

Etiology

1. *Congenital syphilis*—It is characterised by bilateral interstitial keratitis, vascularization (Salmon patches) and uveitis. It affects children between the age of 5-15 years.
2. *Tuberculosis*—There is presence of interstitial keratitis in this condition.
3. *Viral infections (disciform keratitis)*—A central grey disc is seen in the stroma. It is unilateral and seen in adults usually.
4. *Sclerosing keratitis*—It spreads from scleritis involving the corneal stroma.

Treatment

The basic cause of deep keratitis is treated along with routine treatment of corneal ulcer.

CONGENITAL ANOMALIES OF CORNEA

Megalocornea

It is a bilateral condition in which the corneal diameter is more than 14 mm. The cornea is usually clear with normal thickness and vision. It is often associated with Marfan's syndrome.
Differential diagnosis Megalocornea can be differentiated from buphthalmos and keratoglobus
   i. *Buphthalmos*—In this condition IOP is raised and eyeball is enlarged as a whole. Enlarged cornea is associated with Descemet's membrane tears.
  ii. *Keratoglobus*—There is congenital bilateral hemispherical protrusion of the whole cornea.

Keratoglobus

In this condition there is thinning and excessive protrusion of cornea which seems enlarged but its diameter is usually normal.

Microcornea

The corneal diameter is less than 10 mm with decreased radius of curvature. Hypermetropia and narrow angle glaucoma may be found in later years. The condition may occur as an isolated anomaly or in association with microphthalmos.

Cornea Plana

It is a rare anomaly in which cornea is comparatively flat since birth. It may be associated with microcornea.

Posterior Embryotoxon

There is an unusual prominence of Schwalbe's line which is peripheral termination of Descemet's membrane. It appears as a ring opacity in deeper layer of cornea.

CORNEAL DEGENERATIONS AND DYSTROPHIES

Corneal degenerations and dystrophies usually lead to a lot of confusion as far as their diagnosis is concerned. It is important to know how to differentiate between these two. In corneal degeneration tissue undergo some pathologic changes in circumstances such as ageing, inflammation, trauma or systemic diseases etc. whereas in dystrophies the lesions are not related to any particular systemic or local disease process and are often inherited.

Corneal Dystrophies

Corneal dystrophies are progressive, hereditary corneal disorders which are bilateral, symmetrical, non-vascularised, show no signs of inflammation and there is no associated systemic disease. They affect a particular layer of the cornea usually.

Classifications of Corneal Degenerations

1. **Central degenerations**
   - Cornea farinata
   - Salzman's Nodular degeneration
   - Hyaline degeneration
   - Lipid degeneration
   - Pigmentary degeneration

2. **Peripheral degenerations**
   - Arcus senilis
   - White limbal girdle of vogt
   - Terriens marginal degeneration
   - Pellucid marginal degeneration
   - Mooren's ulcer
   - Hepatolenticular degeneration

Corneal Degenerations

These are non hereditary and usually unilateral. They can be divided into three categories:
  i. Primary degeneration
  ii. Secondary degeneration
  iii. Infiltration associated with metabolic disturbance, e.g. fatty degeneration, hyaline degeneration, amyloid degeneration, calcific degeneration (Band shaped keratopathy) etc.
The basic difference between degenerations and dystrophies are as under:

Arcus Senilis

There is bilateral annular lipid infiltration of cornea in old persons with no symptoms. It does not require any treatment as it does not affect the vision or vitality of the cornea.

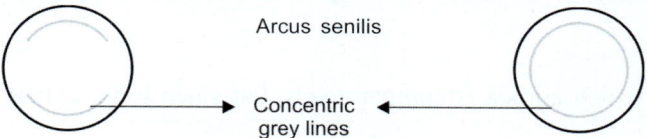

Arcus senilis
Concentric grey lines

- There are concentric grey lines in the upper and lower part of the cornea.
- The lines join to form a ring 1 mm broad which is separated from the margin by a rim of clear cornea about 1.5 mm. It is also known as lucid interval of Vogt. The outer border of the arcus is

sharp but the inner border appears faint. It is found in approximately 60% of population between the age of 40 to 60 years and almost in all persons above the age of 80 years. The arcus is formed by deposition of cholesterol, cholesterol esters, phospholipids and triglycerides in the substantial propria layer.

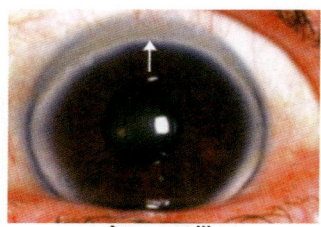
Arus senilis

Arcus Juvenilis

It usually occurs below 40 years of age. It is a rare condition. A serum lipid profile is indicated to rule out hereditary anomaly which has a serious prognosis.

White Limbal Girdle of Vogt

It is seen mostly in the age group of 40-60 years. It is seen as chalky line in the nasal and temporal periphery of inter-palpebral area of cornea. The opacity is at the level of Bowman's membrane. It is due to elastotic degeneration of tissues.

Amyloid Degeneration

Amyloid degeneration of cornea is characterized by deposition of amyloid material underneath its epithelium. It could be either primary or secondary due to some disease.

Pigmentary Degeneration

Pigment deposition in cornea could be iron, blood pigment, melanin and other metallic pigments like cooper, silver, gold etc.
a. Hudson-Stahli-line—It is a horizontal line at the lower half of the cornea due to deposition of hemosiderin pigment
b. Fleischer's ring is seen at the base of keratoconus
c. Stocker-Busaca line—It is seen in front of a Pterygium.

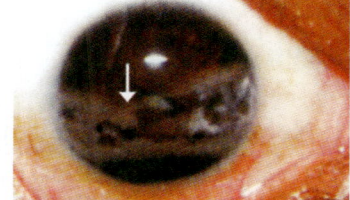
Band-shaped keratopathy

Band-shaped Keratopathy

- It is common in old, blind, shrunken eyes and in Still's disease of children.
- It is associated with hyperthyroidism, vitamin D poisoning or sarcoidosis.
- It could be either primary or secondary to hypercalcaemia, chronic uveitis, chronic glaucoma, interstitial keratitis etc.
- A continuous band lies in the interpalpebral area starting in the inner and outer side.
- It is due to hyaline infiltration in the superficial stroma followed by calcareous salt deposition.

DIFFERENTIALS BETWEEN CORNEAL DEGENERATIONS AND DYSTROPHIES

	DEGENERATION	DYSTROPHY
1. Incidence	Mostly unilateral	Most bilateral
2. Site	Peripheral	Mostly central
3. Onset	Usually occur in the middle of life or later	Occur early in life
4. Pattern	Asymmetrical lesion	Symmetric lesion
5. Vascularisation	Present	Absent
6. Inheritance	Non-hereditary	Always hereditary
7. Course	Often progressive	May remain stationary or progressive slowly
8. Cause	Mostly consequent to some local or systemic disease.	Primary lesions. Not related to any systemic or local disease.

DYSTROPHIES OF CORNEA
Classification of dystrophies

1. Anterior dystrophies
(Epithelium and Bowman's membrane)
- Cogan's microcystic
- Reis-Bucklers
- Recurrent corneal erosion syndrome

2. Stromal dystrophies
(Substantia propria or stroma)
- Granular
- Macular
- Lattice
- Central crystalline
- Congenital hereditary stromal

2. Posterior dystrophies
(Endothelium and Descemet's membtane)
- Fuchs' endothelial
- Cornea guttata
- Posterior polymorphous

ANTERIOR DYSTROPHIES

1. Reis-Buckler's Dystrophy

It is bilaterally symmetrical dystrophy, which starts in early childhood as recurrent corneal erosions. Later there is diffuse scarring of Bowman's membrane. Corneal surface becomes rough with diminished sensation. The opacities have typical ring like appearance. It is an autosomal dominant condition. It starts near the Bowman's membrane. There are subepithelial grey opacities arranged in a fish net pattern.

2. Cogan's Microcystic Dystrophy

It is the commonest epithelial dystrophy with dot, map or fingerprint opacities characterized by recurrent attacks of severe pain, watering, photophobia and blepharospasm. There is increased hydration of cornea and formation of microcysts under the epithelium.

3. Messman's Juvenile Epithelial Dystrophy (Recurrent Corneal Erosion Syndrome)

Characterized by appearance of small vesicles between epithelium and Bowman's membrane. It is an autosomal dominant inherited bilateral symmetrical condition. There are minimum symptoms and visual loss is very less, hence it does not require any treatment.

STROMAL DYSTROPHIES

1. Granular Dystrophy

- It is autosomal dominant dystrophy.
- There is milky granular hyaline deposits in anterior stroma.
- There is clear cornea between opacities.
- It develops in first decade of life and vision remains good until 40 years of life.

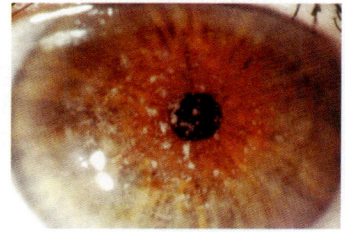

Granular dystrophy

2. Macular Dystrophy

- It is autosomal recessive dystrophy.
- There is dense opacity in central cornea.
- There is deposition of mycopolysaccharides.
- It starts in first decade and vision lost early in life.
- It requires penetrating keratoplasty.

3. Lattice Dystrophy

- There is autosomal dominant inheritance.
- There are amyloid deposits in corneal stroma.
- Spider like opacities are seen in cornea.
- It starts early in life.
- Cornea becomes hazy by the age of 20 years.
- It requires penetrating keratoplasty.

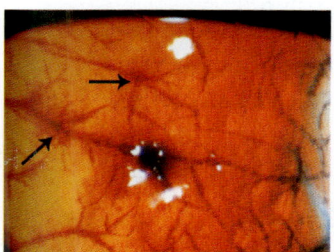

Lattice dystrophy

ENDOTHELIAL DYSTROPHIES

1. Fuch's Endothelial Dystrophy

- It was described by Fuch's in 1910.
- It usually occurs after 50 years of age.
- The female to male ratio is 4:1.
- There is atrophy of the endothelial cells along with oedema and formation of vesicles. Grey punctate opacities are seen in the stroma.
- The clinical features are divided into four stages
  a. Stage of cornea guttata

b. Oedematous stage
c. Stage of bullous keratopathy
d. Stage of scarring
- Treatment
    a. 5% sodium chloride ointment or solution (hypertonic saline) is useful.
    b. Hydrated soft contact lenses may be useful.
    c. Penetrating keratoplasty can be done.

2. Cornea Guttata

- It manifests are middle age.
- Females are most affected.
- It has autosomal dominant inheritance.
- There are bilateral symmetric lesions, which appear as golden hue on the posterior surface of cornea.
- It rarely affects vision.

ECTATIC CONDITIONS OF CORNEA

The ectatic conditions of the cornea may result from:
1. *Inflammation*
    i. Ectatic cicatrix
    ii. Anterior staphyloma
2. *Congenital*
    i. Keratoconus
    ii. Keratoglobus
    iii. Megalocornea.

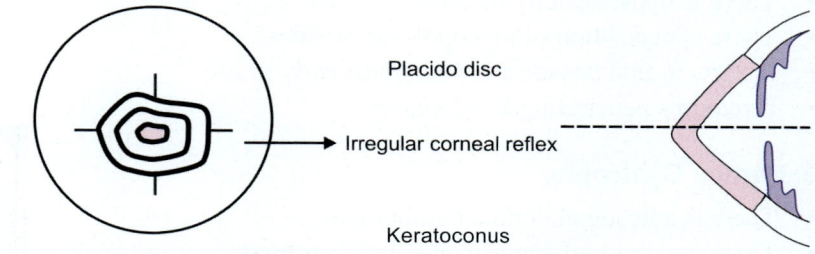

KERATOCONUS [CONICAL CORNEA]

Etiology

It is often due to congenital weakness of the central part of the cornea. It may occur in association with other ocular anomalies such as blue sclera, ectopia lentis, retinitis pigmentosa, Down's, Marfan's and Ehlers-Danlos syndrome.

Incidence

It is a bilateral condition occurring at puberty in girls usually.

Classification

1. **Keratoconus** can be classified by doing keratometry as follows:
    i. Mild < 48 D
    ii. Moderate 48-54 D
    iii. Severe > 54 D

2. **Morphological classification** is dependent on the shape.
    i. *Nipple cones*—These are characterised by their small size (5 mm) and steep curvature. The apical centre is often either central or paracentral and displaced inferonasally.
    ii. *Oval cones*—These are longer (5-6 mm), ellipsoid and commonly displaced inferotemporally.
    iii. *Globus cones*—These are largest (> 6 mm) and may involve 75% of the cornea.

Symptoms

There is impaired vision due to progressive myopia. This cannot be corrected by ordinary glasses due to parabolic nature of the corneal curvature.

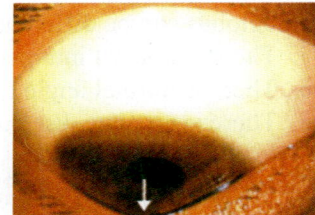

Munson's sign

Signs

1. *Early signs*
    i. Ophthalmoscopy shows an 'oil droplet' reflex.
    ii. Retinoscopy shows an irregular 'scissor reflex'.
    iii. Keratometry initially shows irregular astigmatism where the principal meridians are no longer 90° apart and the mires cannot be superimposed.
2. *Late signs*
    i. Conical shape of the cornea is characteristic. The apex of the cone is always situated below the centre of the cornea.
    ii. Placido disc shows distortion of corneal reflex.
    iii. Munson's sign—There is indentation or acute bulge of the lower lid, when the patient looks down.
    iv. Slit-lamp examination
        a. Vogt's lines—Fine, parallel lines are seen at the apex. These are vertical folds at the level of deep stroma and Descemet's membrane.
        b. Fleischer ring—A brownish ring is seen at the base due to haemosiderin pigment.
        c. There is oedema and opacity of the stroma due to rupture in Descemet's membrane.

Munson's sign

Treatment

1. Spectacles and soft contact lens are helpful in the early stage.
2. If vision does not improve than combination of hard over soft contact lenses known as "Piggy back" contact lenses may be tried.
3. Intrastromal insertion of stromal ring of 0.25 to 0.45 mm thickness may be inserted in the stroma in corneal periphery.
4. Keratoplasty, penetrating or deep lamellar, is indicated in advanced progressive disease.

KERATOGLOBUS

Etiology

There is a congenital, bilateral hemispherical protrusion of the whole cornea. It is a familial and hereditary condition. It is seen in Marchesane syndrome.

Differential Diagnosis

Keratoglobus can be differentiated from buphthalmos by the following features:
  i. There is normal intraocular pressure in keratoglobus.
 ii. There is normal angle of anterior chamber in keratoglobus.
iii. There is no optic disc cupping in keratoglobus.

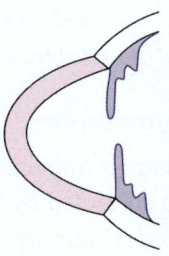

Keratoglobus

PIGMENTATIONS OF THE CORNEA

1. *Argyrosis*—Black coloured pigments are deposited in the elastic fibres of Descemet's membrane due to prolonged use of silver nitrate salt.
2. *Blood staining*—Rust coloured stain (haemosiderin) is seen in the corneal stroma due to traumatic hyphaema with raised intraocular tension. Raised tension damages the endothelium thus allowing the passage of haemosiderin pigment in the stroma.
3. *Kayser-Fleischer ring*—There is a green-golden brown coloured pigment ring seen around the periphery of cornea in the deeper layers of stroma and Descemet's membrane in Wilson's disease and retained copper foreign body (chalcosis).

PIGMENT DEPOSITION IN THE CORNEA

TYPE OF PIGMENT	DISORDERS	CORNEAL LOCATION
IRON	• Keratoconus (Fleischer's ring)	Epithelium
	• Pterygium (Stocker's line)	Epithelium
	• Filtering bleb (Ferry's line)	Epithelium
	• Old opacity (Hudson-Stähli line)	Epithelium
	• Siderosis	Mainly stroma
	• Blood staining of the cornea	Mainly stroma
COPPER	• Wilson's disease	Descemet's membrane
	• Chalcosis	
	• (Kayser-Fleischer ring)	
MELANIN	• Pigment dispersion syndrome	Endothelium
	• (Krukenberg's spindle)	

OPERATIONS ON THE CORNEA

Paracentesis

Aqueous is slowly released from the anterior chamber. This improves the nutrition of the cornea.

Indications
- Hypopyon ulcer or hyphaema with raised tension.
- Impending perforation of corneal ulcer (descemetocele).

Method
- A small incision is made in the lower temporal quadrant, 2 mm within the limbus by a paracentesis needle, pointed blade or a broad needle.
- Aqueous is evacuated slowly to avoid intraocular haemorrhage or prolapse of iris.

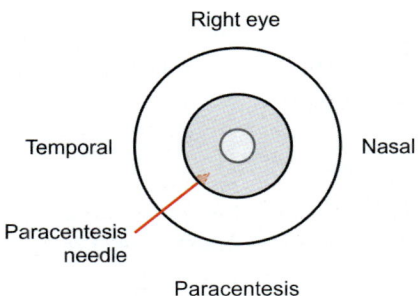

TARSORRHAPHY

The aim is to achieve lid closure so that palpebral aperture is narrowed. It is not strictly a corneal operation, but it is performed for corneal conditions.

Indications
- Neuroparalytic keratitis as a result of 5th nerve paralysis.
- Exposure keratitis due to inadequate closure of palpebral aperture as a result of 7th nerve paralysis or proptosis.

Method
Palpebral aperture is narrowed by placement of mattress sutures through the small raw areas in the lid margins and skin. The sutures are tied over rubber sheet in the skin.

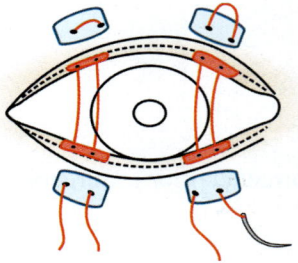

Paramedian tarsorrhaphy

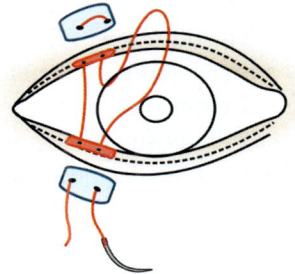

Lateral tarsorrhaphy

Types
1. *Lateral tarsorrhaphy*—The suture is placed at the junction of middle and lateral third of lid margin.
2. *Paramedian tarsorrhaphy*—Two sutures are placed on either side of the middle line as shown in the diagram.

KERATOPLASTY (Corneal Transplant or Graft)

Keratoplasty is an operation by which the patient's opaque corneal tissue is replaced by the donor's clear cornea. Keratoplasty aims at attaining normal visual acuity and protecting intraocular structures of recipient.

Types
1. *Full thickness (penetrating)*—Full thickness of cornea is replaced.
2. *Partial thickness (lamellar)*—Superficial layers of stroma are replaced.

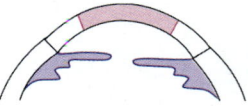
Penetrating keratoplasty

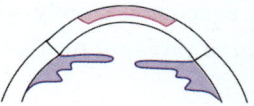
Partial thickness lamellar keratoplasty

Indications
1. *Optical*—Central corneal opacity (leucoma, macula, nebula) results in marked diminution of vision. Other causes include pseudophakic or aphakic bullous keratopathy, regraft due to graft failure, Fuch's and other corneal dystrophies.
2. *Therapeutic*—Bacterial, fungal and viral infection not responding to standard treatment.
3. *Structural*—To restore corneal anatomy, e.g. Descemetocele, fistula, after pterygium and dermoid excision, keratoconus.
4. *Cosmetic*—It is a relatively rare indication.

Contraindications
The following factors (recipient eye) may result in graft failure,
1. Dry eye—The nutrition of the epithelial cells is disturbed.
2. Marked corneal stromal vascularization.
3. Absence of corneal sensation.
4. Diseases of the posterior segment of the eye.
5. Abnormality of lids, e.g. ectropion, entropion, trichiasis are corrected prior to surgery.

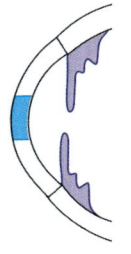
Corneal opacity

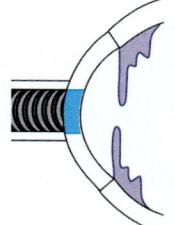
Trephine application

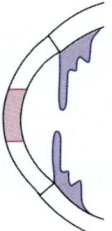
Donor's clear cornea

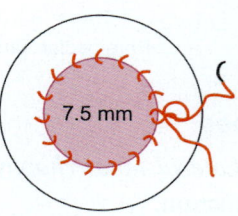
Continuous suture

Technique of penetrating keratoplasty

Method

1. *Excision of the donor eye*—It must be done as early as possible, i.e. within 6 hours after death. Cornea receives nutrition from oxygen present in the aqueous humor even after death. It is stored in sterile containers having McCarey-Kaufman (MK) or chondroitin sulphate (CDS) corneal preservation medium at 4°C.
2. *Excision of the donor's cornea*—An ideal size of the donor is 7.5 mm. Great care is taken not to damage the endothelium during trephining and during suturing the graft.
3. *Excision of diseased host cornea*—It is done by a trephine. Care is taken not to damage the iris and lens while trephining. Viscoelastic substances such as methylcellulose may be injected in the anterior chamber to prevent endothelium damage.
4. *Fixation of donor's clear graft*—It is done by continuous 10.0 nylon sutures. The anterior chamber is reformed. Corticosteroids and antibiotic drops are instilled postoperatively. Short acting mydriatic may be used to prevent synechiae formation.

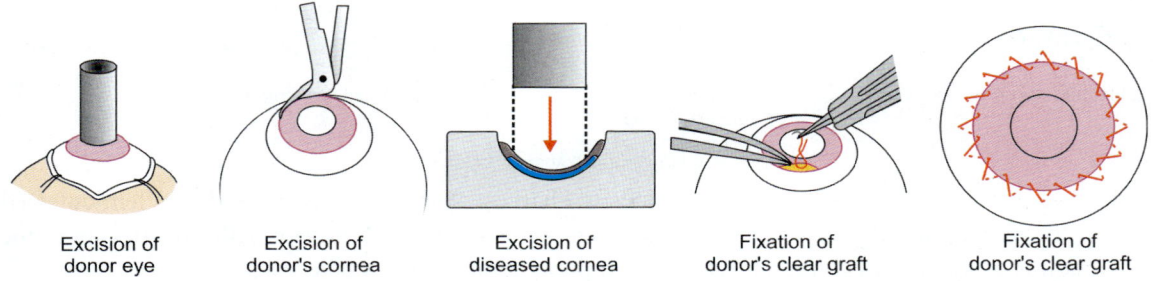

Schematic diagram of technique of penetrating keratoplasty

Complications

The complications can arise early or late.
1. *Early*
    i. Flat anterior chamber occurs due to improper suturing and leakage.
    ii. Iris prolapse may take place due to raised tension postoperatively.
    iii. Infection can occur in cases of bacterial corneal ulcer.
2. *Late*
    i. Graft failure results in haziness of cornea.
    ii. Secondary glaucoma can occur due to anterior peripheral synechiae.
    iii. Astigmatism is common due to irregular healing.

STEM CELL TRANSPLANT

Indications

This is indicated in a large number of cases with corneal damage which includes postchemical burns, postradiation, Stevens-Johnson syndrome, ocular cicatricial pemphigoid, extensive symblepharon of any etiology, chronic contact lens use, multiple limbal surgeries like pterygium, dermoid, benign and malignant limbal tumours.

Procedure

i. After recessing conjunctiva from the limbus and sclera, the undermined tissue is scraped with blunt dissector.
ii. Two trephines 9 mm and 11 mm in size, are used to make 2 marks 0.1 mm deep on the cornea and limbus respectively. The encompassed tissue is removed. Similar limbal lenticules are removed from the other eye (Antograft) or from the eye of near relative (homograft) or from freshly enucleated eyeballs.

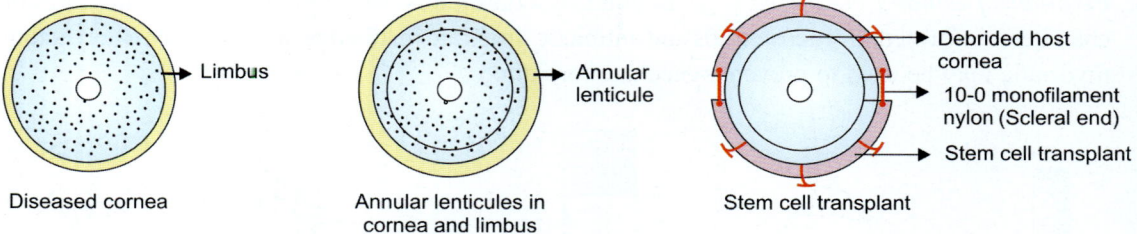

Onlay limbal transplantation

iii. The annular lenticules are bisected into two halves. While removing the donor lenticules (if removed in piecemeal) care is taken to retain both superior and inferior pallisade of Vogt of the donor as these sites contain the maximum population of stem cells.
iv. Two circumferential sutures with 10-0 monofilament nylon are applied separately at the extreme ends of each lenticule and the knots are burried. One to three extra sutures are applied at the scleral end of each lenticule depending upon the length of the lenticule. No sutures are applied on the corneal side as it results in much irritation and foreign body sensation.
v. Pad and bandage is applied after instillation of antibiotic drops.

EYE BANK

The primary function of an eye bank is to collect, store good quality donor's cornea and make it available for cornea transplantation for therapeutic use and research.

Objective of Eye Bank

The main objectives of an eye bank can be summarized as follows,
1. Collection of donor eyes.
2. Preservation of donor cornea.
3. Distribution of highest quality of donor tissue for cornea transplantation.
4. Promotion, awareness about eye donation from potential donors.

A person makes a pledge to donate his eyes after death. No living individual can donate his eye because the law does not permit it and moreover it is not practical. The eye cannot be sold or purchased. Eye bank personnel collect the eyes after getting information about death and proper written consent from close relative. It is important to know the age of the donor, cause of death and time of death. Eyes should be removed as early as possible or atleast within 5-6 hours after death.

Equipments for an Eye Bank

The equipments required for any eye bank are listed below,

COMPULSORY	DESIRABLE
• Refrigerator with temperature recording device • Operation theatre • Slit-lamp • Sterilization facilities • Enucleation and corneal excision instruments	• Incubator • Specular microscope • Ice machine • Microbiology facilities • Centrifuge

Enucleation

Eyes should be enucleated soon after death. A relatively longer interval of 4-6 hours may be allowed in winter months but in summer, not more than 2-3 hours should elapse between death and enucleation.

The eyes should carry the following information about the donor:
1. Age and sex.
2. Cause of death.
3. Time and date of death.
4. Time and date of enucleation.

Enucleation should be done aseptically and the eyeballs should be transported to the eye bank in a wide mouth sterile glass bottle in an ice box or thermos flask. The eyeballs are washed with normal saline, antibiotic drops instilled and the cornea is examined with good illumination and magnification, preferably with slit-lamp. Clinical viability is graded depending upon the degree of stromal oedema and folds. Usable eyeballs are then transferred to autoclaved wide mouth bottles containing sterile cotton gauze pad. Adequate antibiotic solution is instilled to moisten the pad. The eyeball rests on the pad with cornea straight up and without touching any part of the bottle. It is better to have a mouldable clamp in the bottle to hold the eyeball erect to protect the cornea. This is particularly important when these eyes are to be transported to distant corneal surgeons. The bottles should have tight screw caps so that even if ice has melted off in the container, fluid does not enter the bottle. The Eye Bank Association has designed a thermocol container which has provision for carrying one or two pairs of eyeballs with adequate amount of ice for 18 to 24 hours transport. If Descemet's membrane folds and stromal oedema exceed acceptable limits, the cornea is designated unusable for therapeutic purpose but can be used for surgical training and experimental purposes.

One may conclude that when media preservation facilities are not available, eyeballs enucleated from a relatively younger person who dies after an acute episode such as accident, suicide, homicide, etc. and preserved in moist chamber at 4° C provide the best donor cornea.

Contraindications for Collection of Donor Eyes

There are certain conditions when the donor's eye are not suitable for corneal transplant.
1. **Systemic causes**—These include death due to:
   - AIDS (HIV positive)
   - Hepatitis B
   - Rabies
   - Poison
   - Severe burn
   - Malignancy, leukaemia, lymphoma
   - Death from unknown cause.
2. **Ocular causes**
   - Corneal opacities and dystrophy
   - Retinoblastoma, malignant melanoma
   - Active inflammatory diseases, e.g. conjunctivitis, iridocyclitis, endophthalmitis
   - Congenital abnormalities, e.g. keratoconus, keratoglobus
   - Prior refractive procedures, e.g. radial keratotomy, laser photoablation
   - Anterior segment surgical procedures, e.g. cataract, glaucoma.

Evaluation of Donor Tissue

1. Gross examination with torch and loupe.
2. Slit-lamp examination.
3. Specular microscopy (for endothelial cell count and morphology).

A careful slit-lamp examination provides an overall status of the endothelium. The normal endothelium shows a pattern of cells of similar size and shape with no abnormal structures. The normal cell density is usually between 2000 to 3500 cells per sq. mm.

CORNEA WITH SPECULAR ENDOTHELIUM PATTERNS—UNFIT FOR TRANSPLANT

1. Endothelial cell density less than 1500 cells/mm^2
2. Marked pleomorphism of the endothelial cells
3. Abnormally shaped cells such as fused cells (these are seen in stressed endothelium)
4. Presence of central cornea guttata
5. Severe oedema of endothelium
6. Presence of inflammatory cells or bacteria on endothelium.

Preservation of the Donor Eye

Traditionally corneal preservation is described under short-term, intermediate-term and long-term preservations.

1. *Short-term Preservation (up to 96 hours)*

   i. *Moist chamber method*—Whole globe is preserved in a moist chamber at 4°C in a refrigerator for 24 hours.

ii. *M.K. (McCarey-Kaufman) medium*—It consists of tissue culture (TC)-199, 5% Dextran-40, HEPES buffer to adjust pH at 7.4, Gentamicin 0.1 mg/ml, colour-pink.

Corneoscleral button can also be preserved in M-K medium at 4° C for upto 96 hours. It is superior than conventional moist-chamber method and practised widely.

2. Intermediate-term Preservation (upto 2 weeks)

K-SOL medium, *dexol* medium, *optisol* medium, etc. are used for preservation.

3. Long-term Preservation (months to years)

i. *Viable*—Organ culture method, cryopreservation.
ii. *Non-viable*—Glycerine preservation.

Promotion and Awareness about Eye Donation

There is an acute shortage of donor eyes in most of the developing countries. In India, the estimated corneal blindness is 1.5 lakhs unilateral blind and 5.9 lakhs bilateral blind (NPCB-WHO 1986-89). Against this huge demand for donor eyes in India, eye collection numbered 12,000 in 1995 out of which only 50% eyes were of usable grade.

Grief Counseling

In general, there is great reluctance about eye donation at the time of family member's death resulting in less voluntary eye donations. Family member need assistance to overcome the moments of grief. A tactful reminder that a timely eye donation is possible for the good of mankind is very helpful. However, prior publicity is of utmost importance in voluntary eye donation.

Publicity

Public awareness plays a very important role in eye donation. Several publicity methods such as print media, audio-visual aids and lectures have been used to give useful informations about eye donation. Distributing and collecting pledge cards from the public for potential eye donations is necessary for popularizing the concept of eye donation. Publicity should also take care of informing the community about the operational steps of actual donation of eyes.

MULTIPLE CHOICE QUESTIONS

1. Which of the following is not a source of nutrients to cornea
   a. air
   b. aqueous humour
   c. perilimbal capillaries
   d. vitreous
2. Following pathogens can invade normal intact corneal epithelium EXCEPT
   a. *Pneumococcus*
   b. *N. gonorrhoeae*
   c. *N. meningitidis*
   d. *C. diphtheriae*
3. Treatment of impending perforation of corneal ulcer includes all EXCEPT
   a. contact lens
   b. acetazolamide (diamox)
   c. therapeutic corneal graft
   d. cautery
4. Ulcus serpens is caused in adults by
   a. *Mycobacterium tuberculosis*
   b. *Pneumococcus*
   c. *Corynebacterium*
   d. all of the above
5. The ectatic cicatrix in which iris is incarcerated is called
   a. adherent leucoma
   b. anterior synechia
   c. prolapse of iris
   d. anterior staphyloma
6. Central corneal ulceration may be associated with
   a. herpes virus
   b. bacteria
   c. fungus
   d. all of the above
7. Hypopyon corneal ulcer results in following complications EXCEPT
   a. perforation
   b. panophthalmitis
   c. secondary glaucoma
   d. corneal anaesthesia
8. The most common organism responsible for hypopyon corneal ulcer is
   a. *Staphylococcus*
   b. *Pneumococcus*
   c. *Pseudomonas*
   d. *Candida albicans*
9. Symptoms of corneal ulcer are following, EXCEPT
   a. mucopurulent discharge
   b. pain in the eye
   c. redness of the eye
   d. watering
10. Steroids are contraindicated in
    a. iritis
    b. corneal ulcer
    c. optic neuritis
    d. phlyctenular conjunctivitis
11. The dendritic corneal ulcer is typical of
    a. varicella zoster
    b. herpes simplex
    c. *Pseudomonas*
    d. *Aspergillus*
12. Satellite nodules in the cornea are caused by
    a. bacteria
    b. virus
    c. fungus
    d. rickettsia
13. The following is not used for cautery of corneal ulcer
    a. trichloracetic acid
    b. iodine
    c. carbolic acid
    d. mercurochrome

14. Atheromatous corneal ulcer is
    a. purulent
    b. degenerative
    c. allergic
    d. none of the above
15. Hudson-Stahli lines in cornea are
    a. red
    b. yellowish red
    c. yellowish brown
    d. yellow
16. Hutchinson's triad comprise all EXCEPT
    a. flat nose bridge
    b. interstitial keratitis
    c. Hutchinson's teeth
    d. 8th nerve deafness
17. 'Salmon patches' are seen in
    a. haemorrhage into the cornea
    b. interstitial keratitis
    c. retinitis pigmentosa
    d. phlyctenular keratitis
18. Cornea is thinned in
    a. keratoconus
    b. Fuchs' dystrophy
    c. keratoglobus
    d. all of the above
19. The deposits seen in arcus senilis is
    a. lipid
    b. calcium
    c. hyaline
    d. none of the above
20. Which of the following chemicals is not used for tattooing of corneal opacity
    a. gold chloride
    b. silver chloride
    c. platinum chloride
    d. hydrazine hydrate
21. The pigment deposited in Kayser-Fleischer ring is
    a. melanin
    b. haemosiderin
    c. copper
    d. none of the above
22. Band-shaped keratopathy is due to
    a. calcareous degeneration
    b. hyaline degeneration
    c. fatty degeneration
    d. elastotic degeneration
23. Munson's sign is seen in
    a. episcleritis
    b. chalcosis
    c. keratoconus
    d. retinal detachment
24. Common cause of non-healing corneal ulcer
    a. chronic dacryocystitis
    b. raised intraocular pressure
    c. diabetes mellitus
    d. all of the above
25. Antiviral drugs include the following EXCEPT
    a. acyclovir
    b. ketoconazole
    c. iodo-deoxyuridine
    d. trifluorothymidine
26. The earliest symptom to occur in corneal ulcer is
    a. pain
    b. photophobia
    c. loss of sensation
    d. diminished vision

27. Fascicular ulcer is present in
    a. Mooren's ulcer
    b. neuroparalytic keratitis
    c. herpes zoster
    d. marginal ulcer
28. Rupture of Descemet's membrane is seen in
    a. keratoconus
    b. rubella
    c. glaucoma
    d. retinoblastoma
29. Bullous keratopathy involves
    a. Descemet's membrane
    b. epithelium
    c. endothelium
    d. Bowman's membrane
30. In case of central dense leucoma (5 mm) treatment of choice
    a. penetrating keratoplasty
    b. lamellar keratoplasty
    c. tattooing
    d. enucleation

ANSWERS

1—d	2—a	3—d	4—b	5—d
6—d	7—d	8—b	9—a	10—b
11—b	12—c	13—d	14—c	15—c
16—a	17—b	18—a	19—a	20—b
21—c	22—b	23—c	24—d	25—b
26—b	27—a	28—a	29—b	30—a

CHAPTER 8
The Sclera

APPLIED ANATOMY

It is a strong, opaque, white fibrous layer which forms 5/6 of the external tunic of the eye. It is relatively avascular therefore infections rarely affect it. If they do occur, they are chronic and sluggish. It is blue (thin) in childhood and in pathological conditions where uvea shines through it. It may be yellow in old age due to fat deposition. It is about 1 mm thick. Sclera is thinnest at the attachment of extraocular muscles.

Apertures

There are three sets of apertures namely,
1. *Anterior*
   - *Anterior ciliary vessels*
   - *Perivascular lymphatics*
   - *Nerves*
2. *Middle*
   - *Four vena vorticosa exit 4 mm behind the equator*
3. *Posterior*
   - *Optic nerve exit 3 mm to the medial side and just above the posterior pole*
   - *Long and short ciliary vessels and nerves*

Functions

1. Stress and strain are overcome by the disposition of fibrous bands of the sclera.
2. Retina and choroid are maintained in the correct optical shape by the sclera.
3. It provides rigid insertion for the extraocular muscles.

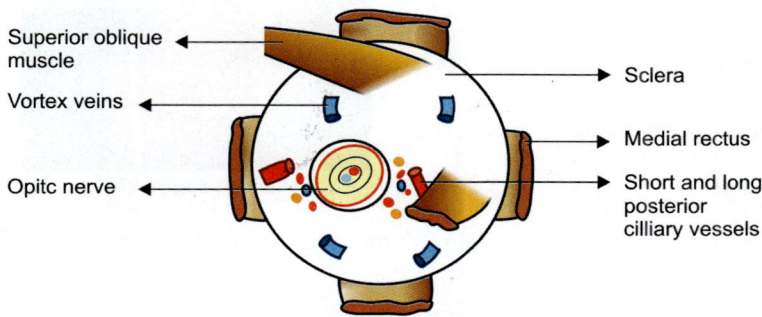

Posterior aspect of right eye

INFLAMMATION OF THE SCLERA

Types

Inflammations of the sclera are of two main types:
1. *Episcleritis (superficial)*
2. *Scleritis (deep)*.

EPISCLERITIS

An inflammation of the subconjunctival and episcleral tissue is known as episcleritis. It is usually benign in nature.

Etiology

1. It is an allergic reaction to endogenous protein or toxin.
2. It may be a collagen disease as history of rheumatoid arthritis is often associated.
3. It can be associated with prior episodes of herpes zoster and gout.

Incidence

- It occurs commonly in women.
- There is usually bilateral involvement.
- The peak age incidence is in the 4th decade.

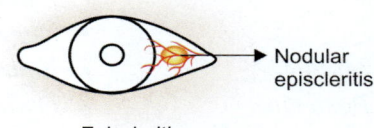

Episcleritis

Pathology

There is lymphocytic infiltration of subconjunctival and episcleral tissue.

Types

1. Simple diffuse episcleritis
2. Nodular episcleritis.

Symptoms

1. A localized redness is seen over sclera in nodular episcleritis.
2. Discomfort or mild to moderate pain is present.

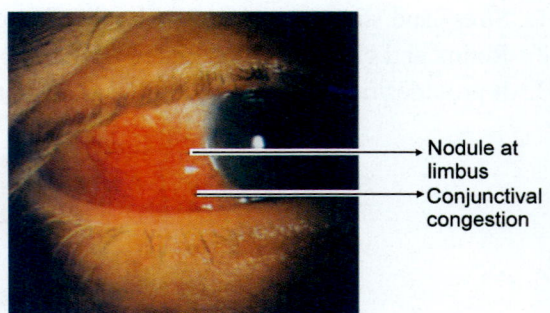

Nodular episcleritis

Signs

1. Circumscribed nodule-like lentil is situated 2-3 mm away from the limbus.
2. It is hard, immovable and tender.
3. The conjunctiva moves freely over the nodule.
4. The conjunctiva looks purple in colour as deep episcleral vessels traverse it.

Course

It is usually transient lasting for several days or weeks.
- Recurrence is common.
- In *episcleritis periodica fugax*—The attacks are fleeting but frequently repeated.
- It may be chronic but never ulcerates.

Complications

1. Severe neuralgia may occur due to nerve involvement.
2. Scleritis results from deeper infiltration of inflammation.
3. There may be associated uveitis.

Treatment

It is often difficult and unrewarding.
   i. *Local*
   - Corticosteroid eyedrops and ointment are applied.
   - Warm compresses are very soothing.
   ii. *General*
   - Anti-inflammatory and analgesics relieve pain and control inflammation.

SCLERITIS

An inflammation of the deep scleral tissue is known as scleritis. It can occur as anterior (95%) and posterior (5%) scleritis.

Etiology

1. In 50% cases, associated connective tissue diseases are present such as :
   - *Rheumatoid arthritis*
   - *Polyarteritis nodosa*
   - *Systemic lupus erythematosus*
   - *Non-specific arteritis*
   - *Wagener's granulomatosis*
   - *Dermatomyositis*
   - *Polychondritis*
2. It may be associated with prior episodes of herpes zoster and gout.

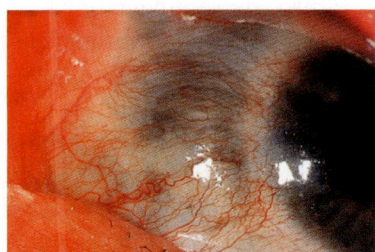

Necrotizing scleritis

Incidence

- Women are commonly affected in 4th-5th decade.
- There is bilateral involvement usually.

Pathology

There is dense lymphocytic infiltration of the sclera.

Types
1. Diffuse scleritis.
2. Nodular scleritis
3. Necrotizing scleritis.

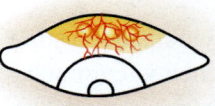
Necrotizing scleritis

Symptoms
1. A localized redness is seen in the deep scleral tissue in nodular scleritis.
2. Discomfort and mild to moderate pain is often present.

Signs
1. *Diffuse scleritis*
   - Multiple hard, whitish nodules, about the size of pin-head develop in the inflamed area of the sclera.
   - They disappear without disintegrating.
2. *Nodular scleritis*
   - One or more nodules are present.
   - It is less circumscribed than episcleritis.
   - The swelling is dark red or bluish at first but later it becomes purple and porcelain like, i.e. semitransparent.
3. *Necrotizing scleritis*
   - There are large areas of avascular sclera leading to necrosis.
   - Sclera may appear as a sequestrum or dead tissue.
   - There is exposure of the uveal pigment through a markedly thin sclera.
   - Anterior uveitis is usually present.
   - It is a serious condition.

Investigations
- Complete blood picture and total and differential white blood cell count.
- Erythrocyte sedimentation rate.
- Rheumatoid factor, antinuclear factor, plasma protein and immunoglobulin level.
- Uric acid estimation for gout
- Serologic tests for syphilis
- X-ray chest, hand, feet and lumbosacral spine
- Fluorescein angiography of anterior or posterior segment for evidence of vasculitis.

DIFFERENCES BETWEEN EPISCLERITIS AND SCLERITIS

CLINICAL FEATURES	EPISCLERITIS	SCLERITIS
1. *Corneal and uveal tract involvement*	Absent	Iritis, cyclitis and anterior choroiditis may be present.
2. *Secondary glaucoma*	Absent	Common Associated with ciliary staphyloma
3. *Ulceration*	Absent	There is no ulceration but much absorption is present. Sclera becomes thin.

Complications

1. Iritis, cyclitis, anterior choroiditis occur commonly.
2. Annular scleritis—There is ring-shaped involvement of the sclera.
3. Changes in the cornea—There are four characteristic patterns of corneal involvement.
    i. *Diffuse stromal keratitis*—Opacities occur with immune ring pattern and keratic precipitate in the corneal stroma.
    ii. *Sclerosing stromal keratitis*—Oedema and infiltration of the stroma occur with vascularization and scarring.
    iii. *Deep keratitis*—White opaque sheets of infiltration occur at the level of the Descemet's membrane.
    iv. *Limbal guttering and keratolysis*—Limbal gutter can progress to ectasia. There may be melting of the stroma.
4. Secondary glaucoma occurs as a result of uveitis or associated trabeculitis.
5. Ciliary staphyloma may result due to scleral thinning.
6. Scleromalacia perforans is a necrotizing scleritis without inflammation. There is exposure of the uvea but no pain.
7. Massive granuloma of the sclera
    - There is proliferation of chronic inflammatory cells.
    - The 'Brawny scleritis' is seen in the anterior segment of eye.
    - The sclera thickens and resembles tumour mass when posterior segment is involved.

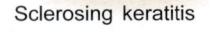

Sclerosing keratitis

Treatment

I. Medical therapy
It is the first line of defence.
1. *Local*—Corticosteroids are effective usually.
2. *General*
    i. Systemic corticosteroids are given starting with high doses and gradually reducing to maintenance dose.
    ii. Analgesics and anti-inflammatory drugs relieve pain and suppress inflammation.
    iii. Cytotoxic immunosuppressive drugs may be useful, e.g. cyclophosphamide.

II. Surgical treatment
1. Extreme scleral thinning or perforation requires reinforcement. Donor sclera or cornea may be used but they usually swell with oedema and soften. Fascia lata or periosteum is more resistant to the melting process. All grafts must be covered with conjunctiva to maintain their integrity.
2. Extreme corneal marginal ulceration or keratolysis may require corneal grafting usually as lamellar graft.

BLUE SCLEROTICS

The sclera and cornea are so thin that the uveal pigment shines through them. It is a hereditary condition. It occurs in babies and in both sex equally. It is associated with fragilitas ossium and deafness.

STAPHYLOMA

It is an ectatic condition of the sclera in which uveal tissue is incarcerated.

Etiology
Staphylomas are formed due to thinning of the sclera often associated with raised intraocular tension.

Clinical Types
1. *Anterior staphyloma*—It is associated with ectasia of the cornea and iris. The most common cause is perforating corneal ulcer or injury.
2. *Intercalary staphyloma*—It lies between the iris and the ciliary body. There is ectasia of sclera and root of iris. The most common cause is absolute glaucoma.
3. *Ciliary staphyloma*—There is ectasia of sclera and the ciliary body. The common causes are absolute glaucoma and scleritis.
4. *Equatorial staphyloma*—It is situated at the exit of vortex veins where the sclera is unsupported by the muscles. There is ectasia of sclera and the choroid due to absolute glaucoma.
5. *Posterior staphyloma*—There is ectasia of sclera and the choroid commonly in chorioretinal degeneration due to high myopia.

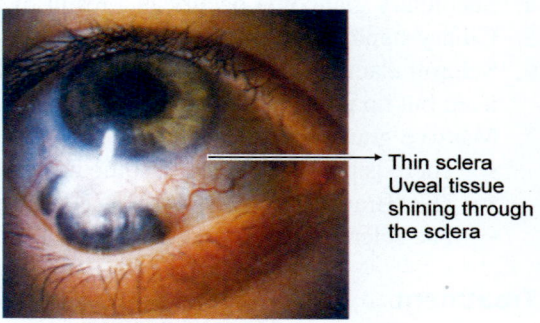

Ciliary staphyloma

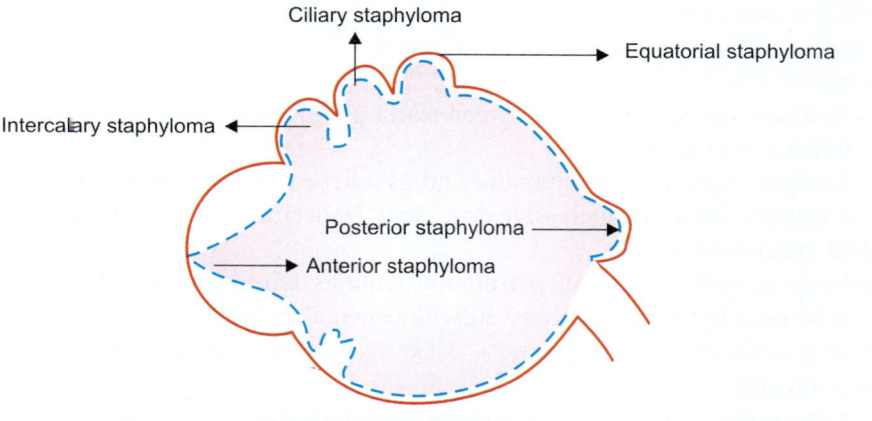

Different types of staphylomas

Treatment
1. No treatment is effective. The eye may be enucleated in cases of extreme disfigurement.
2. Posterior staphyloma can be treated by reinforcement surgery by fascia lata or silicon band in cases of high myopia.
3. Evisceration is indicated in cases of bleeding anterior staphylomas.

MULTIPLE CHOICE QUESTIONS

1. The thickness of sclera is
   a. 0.5 mm
   b. 0.1 mm
   c. 1 mm
   d. 2 mm
2. The vena vorticosa exit from sclera
   a. at the equator
   b. 4 mm behind the equator
   c. 4 mm in front of equator
   d. at posterior pole
3. In which of the following there is intense itching
   a. mucopurulent conjunctivitis
   b. episcleritis
   c. scleritis
   d. spring catarrh
4. Symptom differentiating scleritis from episcleritis is presence of
   a. cornea and uveal involvement
   b. ulceration
   c. secondary glaucoma
   d. all of the above
5. The optic nerve pierces the sclera
   a. anteriorly
   b. posteriorly
   c. at the equator
   d. 4 mm behind the equator
6. The classical features of episcleritis include all *EXCEPT*
   a. circumscribed nodule, 2-3 mm from limbus
   b. conjunctiva moves freely over it
   c. hard, movable and tender
   d. cornea and uveal tract involvement
7. Episcleritis and scleritis are common in
   a. women
   b. allergic reaction to endogenous toxin
   c. associated with collagen disease
   d. all of the above
8. The complications of scleritis include all *EXCEPT*
   a. annular scleritis
   b. ciliary staphyloma
   c. posterior staphyloma
   d. sclerosing keratitis
9. The following conditions are associated with blue sclerotics
   a. deafness
   b. fragilitas ossium
   c. both
   d. none
10. Common causes of staphyloma include
    a. increased IOP
    b. scleritis
    c. injury
    d. all of the above
11. Intercalary staphyloma is a type of
    a. equatorial staphyloma
    b. posterior staphyloma
    c. ciliary staphyloma
    d. anterior staphyloma
12. Anterior staphyloma occurs due to
    a. perforating corneal ulcer
    b. penetrating corneal injury
    c. secondary glaucoma
    d. all of the above
13. Scleritis is often associated with
    a. polyarteritis nodosa
    b. SLE
    c. dermatomyositis
    d. all of the above

14. Treatment of episcleritis includes *EXCEPT*
    a. corticosteroids
    b. anti-inflammatory
    c. analgesics
    d. atropine
15. Features of scleritis include
    a. pain
    b. thining of sclera
    c. associated with connective tissue disease
    d. all of the above

ANSWERS

1—c	2—b	3—d	4—b	5—b
6—d	7—c	8—c	9—c	10—d
11—a	12—d	13—d	14—d	15—d

CHAPTER 9

The Uveal Tract

APPLIED ANATOMY

The uveal tract consists of iris, ciliary body and choroid. Anatomically, they are continuous and so disease of one part may spread to the other. The uveal tract is the vascular layer of the eye.

I. IRIS

It is a coloured, free, circular diaphragm with a central aperture—*the pupil*, measuring about 4 mm. It regulates the amount of light rays reaching the retina. The pupillary margin slides to and fro upon the lens capsule. When pupil is constricted, more of the posterior surface of the iris is in contact with the lens capsule. When pupil is fully dilated, the iris may not touch the lens. It divides the space between the cornea and lens into the anterior and posterior chambers of eye. At the periphery, the iris is attached to the middle of anterior surface of the ciliary body.

Parts

Anterior surface of the iris can be divided into two zones by a zigzag line called the *collarette*.
1. *Ciliary zone*—There are series of radial streaks (due to underlying radial blood vessels) and crypts. Crypts are depressions where the endothelium layer is missing.
2. *Pupillary zone*—It is situated in between the collarette and the pigmented pupillary frill. It is relatively smooth and flat.

Structure

It consists of three layers.
1. *Endothelium*—It contains crypts or tissue spaces which communicate freely with the anterior chamber.

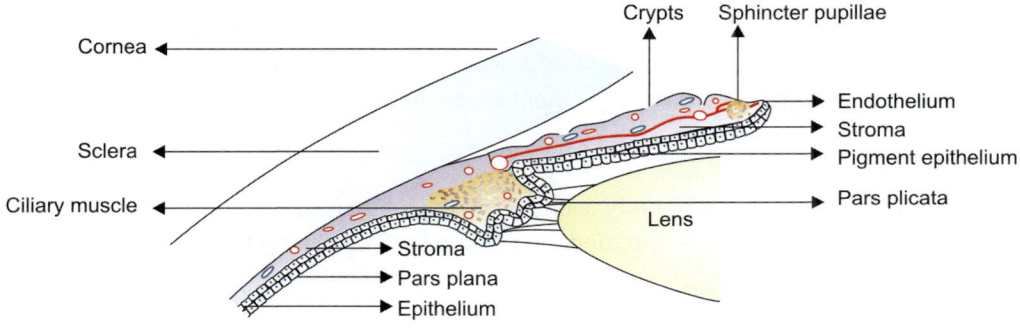

Structure of iris and ciliary body

2. *Stroma*—It consists of loosely arranged connective tissue, blood vessels, nerves and unstripped muscles namely,
    i. *Sphincter pupillae*—It is 1 mm, narrow circular band surrounding the pupil. It is supplied by the cervical parasympathetic nerves via third cranial nerve and causes constriction of the pupil.
    ii. *Dilator pupillae*—These are radial fibres extending from ciliary body to the pupillary margin. It is supplied by cervical sympathetic nerves and causes dilatation of the pupil.
3. *Pigment epithelium*—Two layers of pigment epithelium are situated on the posterior surface of iris.

II. CILIARY BODY

The shape of the ciliary body is like a isosceles triangle with base forwards. Iris is attached to about the middle of the base of the ciliary body. The outer side of the triangle lies against the sclera with the suprachoroidal space in between.

Parts

Ciliary body has two parts namely,
   i. *Pars plicata*—The anterior one-third of ciliary body (about 2 mm) is known as pars plicata.
   ii. *Pars plana*—The posterior two-third of ciliary body (about 4 mm) is known as pars plana. It is relatively avascular therefore posterior segment of the eye is entered through the pars plana incision 3-5 mm behind the limbus.

Structure

The ciliary body consists of four layers namely,
1. *Ciliary muscles*—These are flat bundles of non-striated muscle fibres which are helpful in accommodation of the lens.
2. *Stroma*—It consists of loose connective tissue of collagen and fibroblasts, nerves, pigments and blood vessels.
3. *Ciliary processes*—There are about 70 ciliary processes seen macroscopically. Suspensory ligament or zonule of Zinn is attached to them and the equator of the lens. Each finger-like process is lined by two layers of epithelial cells. The core of the ciliary process contains blood vessels and loose connective tissue. These processes are the main site of aqueous production.
4. *Epithelium*—There are two layers of pigmented and non-pigmented epithelial cells.

Functions

   i. Pars plicata part of the ciliary body secretes aqueous humour.
   ii. The ciliary muscle helps in accommodation of the lens for seeing near objects.

III. CHOROID

It is a dark brown, highly vascular layer situated in between the sclera and retina. It extends from the ora serrata upto the optic nerve aperture. The outer layers of retina are dependent for their nutrition

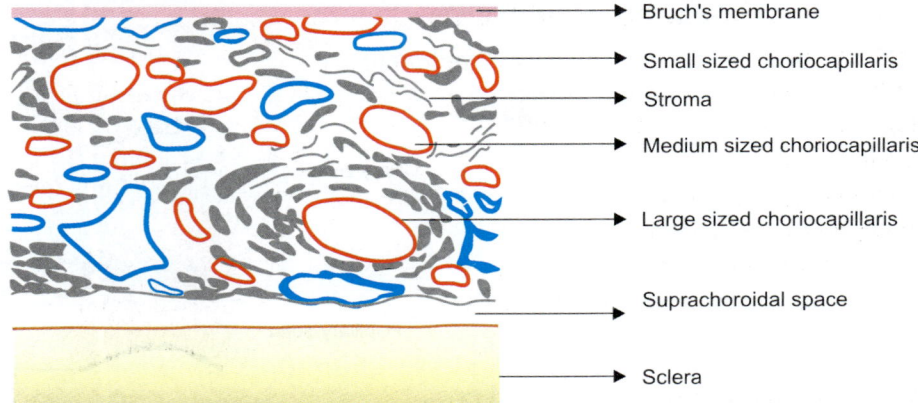
Structure of choroid

upon the choroid. The inflammation of choroid always involves the retina. It consists of suprachoroidal lamina, vascular layer and Bruch's membrane.

Structure

1. *Suprachoroidal lamina*—It is a thin membrane of collagen fibres, melanocytes and fibroblasts. The potential space between this membrane and sclera is known as suprachoroidal space.
2. *Vascular layer or stroma*—This layer contains loose collagenous tissue, pigment cells, macrophages, mast cells and plasma cells. Its main bulk is formed by blood vessels which are arranged in three layers.
   i. Layer of large vessels (Haller's layer)
   ii. Layer of medium vessels (Sattler's layer)
   iii. Layer of choriocapillaris—It nourishes the outer layers of the retina. The inner side of the choroid is covered by at thin elastic membrane lamina vitrea or membrane of Bruch.
3. *Bruch's membrane*—It lies in approximation with the pigment epithelium of the retina.

The Blood Supply

The blood supply of the uveal tract is almost entirely derived from the posterior ciliary and anterior ciliary arteries.

DISEASES OF THE UVEAL TRACT
I. INFLAMMATION

Uveitis
1. Anterior (iritis, iridocyclitis)
2. Intermediate uveitis (Pars planitis)
3. Posterior (choroiditis)
4. Panuveitis
5. Endophthalmitis
6. Panophthalmitis

Specific uveitis
1. Syphilis
2. Gonorrhoea
3. Tuberculosis
4. Leprosy
5. Toxoplasmosis
6. Sarcoidosis

II. SYNDROMES ASSOCIATED WITH UVEITIS
1. AIDS (Acquired immune deficiency syndrome)
2. Uveoparotitis (Heerfordt's disease)
3. Behcet's syndrome
4. Reiter's disease
5. Ankylosing spondylitis
6. Vogt-Koyanagi syndrome
7. Stevens-Johnson syndrome
8. Heterochromic iridocyclitis of Fuchs
9. Ocular histoplasma syndrome

III. VASCULAR DISTURBANCES
Rubeosis iridis

IV. DEGENERATIONS
1. **Iris**
   i. Senile atrophy
   ii. Essential atrophy
2. **Choroid**
   i. Primary degeneration
   ii. Secondary degeneration
3. **Detachment of choroid**

V. CONGENITAL ANOMALIES
1. Heterochromia iridum
2. Heterochromia iridis
3. Polycoria
4. Corectopia
5. Aniridia
6. Persistent pupillary membrane
7. Colobomata
8. Albinism
9. Cyst

VI. TUMOURS
Malignant melanoma.

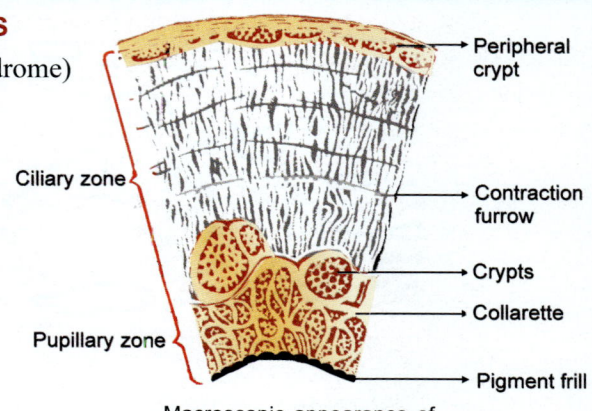

Macroscopic appearance of anterior surface of the iris

CLASSIFICATION OF UVEITIS
1. Anatomical
   i. Anterior uveitis
   ii. Intermediate uveitis
   iii. Posterior uveitis
   iv. Panuveitis
2. Clinical
   i. Acute uveitis
   ii. Chronic uveitis
   iii. Recurrent
3. Pathological
   i. Granulomatous uveitis
   ii. Exudative uveitis

I. INFLAMMATION OF THE UVEAL TRACT (UVEITIS)

The term uveitis strictly means inflammation of the uveal tissue only. However, there is always associated inflammation of the adjacent structures such as retina, vitreous, scleral and cornea.

Uveitis—The inflammation of the uveal tract.
Anterior uveitis—The inflammation of the iris (iritis) and pars plicata of the ciliary body (cyclitis), i.e. iridocyclitis.
Intermediate uveitis—The inflammation of the pars plana part of the ciliary body.
Posterior uveitis—The inflammation of the choroid (choroiditis).
Endophthalmitis—The inflammation of the internal structures of the eye.
Panophthalmitis—Purulent inflammation of all the structures of the eye.

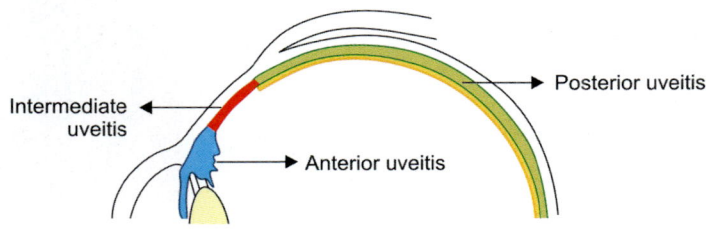

Classfication of uveitis

Classification

1. Anatomical classification—The International Uveitis Study Group has recommended the classification based on anatomical location of uveal tract.
    i. Anterior uveitis—It can be divided as follows:
        - *Iritis*—The inflammation mainly affects the iris.
        - *Iridocyclitis*—Iris and pars plicata part of the ciliary body are involved equally.
        - *Cyclitis*—Pars plicata part of the ciliary body is affected predominantly.
    ii. Intermediate uveitis—There is inflammation of pars plana part of the ciliary body and peripheral retina and underlying choroid. It is also called "pars planitis".
    iii. Posterior uveitis—There is inflammation of the choroid (choroiditis). There is associated inflammation of adjacent retina and hence the term "chorioretinitis" is used.
    iv. Panuveitis—There is inflammation of the whole uveal tract. It is commonest among chronic type of inflammation.

ANTERIOR UVEITIS	INTERMEDIATE UVEITIS	POSTERIOR UVEITIS	PANUVEITIS
Iritis	Posterior cyclitis	Choroiditis	
Anterior cyclitis	Pars planitis	Chorioretinitis	
Iridocyclitis	Hyalitis	Retinochoroiditis	
	Basal retinochoroiditis	Neuro-uveitis	

2. Clinical classification—Uveitis can also be categorized by the clinical courses as:
    i. *Acute uveitis*—The onset is sudden and it usually lasts for less than 3 weeks.
    ii. *Chronic uveitis*—The onset is insidious and the duration is more than 3 weeks.
    iii. *Recurrent uveitis*—The uveitis keeps recurring periodically.

3. *Pathological classification*—Uveitis can be further divided according to the pathological lesions which can be of two types:
   i. *Granulomatous uveitis*—It is infective in nature. Inflammation is insidious in onset, chronic in nature with minimum clinical features.
   ii. *Non-granulomatous uveitis*—It is usually due to allergic or immune related reaction. It is of acute onset and of short duration.
4. Etiological classification (Duke Elder's):
   i. Infective uveitis
   ii. Allergic or immune related uveitis
   iii. Toxic uveitis
   iv. Traumatic uveitis
   v. Uveitis associated with non-infective systemic diseases
   vi. Idiopathic uveitis.

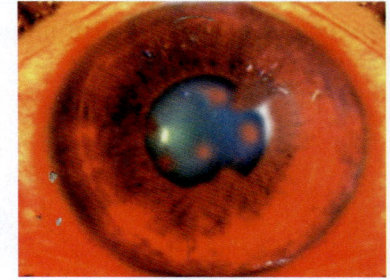

Iridocyclitis

Etiology

In most cases, uveitis is not due to direct infection. It is usually due to allergy or hypersensitivity reaction to an infectious agent.
1. *Exogenous infection*—It occurs due to a perforating wound or corneal ulcer. It causes acute purulent iridocyclitis and panophthalmitis.
2. *Secondary infection*—The inflammation spreads from cornea, sclera or retina.
3. *Endogenous infection*—Organisms lodged in some other organ of the body reach the eye through the bloodstream.
   i. *Bacterial*
      - Septicaemia due to *Streptococcus, Staphylococcus, Meningococcus, Pneumococcus*, etc.
      - Tuberculosis, syphilis, gonorrhoea, etc.
   ii. *Viral*—Mumps, measles, influenza, herpes, etc.
   iii. *Protoza*—Toxoplasma, toxocara, cysticercosis.
4. *Allergic inflammation*—It occurs in a sensitized ocular tissue which comes in contact again with the same organism or its protein (antigen-antibody reaction), e.g. tubercular lesion in lymph nodes, streptococcal and other infections in teeth, tonsils, paranasal sinuses, urinary and genital tract.
5. *Hypersensitivity reaction*—It occurs due to hypersensitivity reaction to autologous tissue components (autoimmune reaction). Therefore uveitis occurs commonly in association with: rheumatoid arthritis, systemic lupus erythematosus, sarcoidosis, ankylosing spondylitis, Reiter's disease, Behcet's syndrome.

BASIC MECHANISM OF OCULAR INFLAMMATION AND SIGNS OF UVEITIS

BASIC MECHANISM		OCULAR SIGNS
i. Vessel dilatation	→	Circumcorneal ciliary injection
ii. Vascular permeability	→	Aqueous flare
iii. Migration of cells	→	Keratic precipitate, hypopyon, hyphaema

ANTERIOR UVEITIS

Inflammation of the iris and the ciliary body is known as anterior uveitis.

Clinical Forms

Anterior uveitis occurs in two forms namely,
1. *Infective (granulomatous)*—It is due to direct organismal infection. Inflammation is insidious in onset, chronic in nature with minimum clinical features. There is dense nodular infiltration of tissues by lymphocytes and plasma cells. It is characterized by presence of large greasy "mutton fat" keratic precipitates which are deposits of white blood cells (mainly lymphocytes), cluster of inflammatory cells on the pupillary border (Koeppe's nodules) or on the peripheral part of the anterior surface of iris (Busacca's nodules).
2. *Allergic (exudative or non-granulomatous)*—It is of acute onset and short duration. It is diffuse in an extension, i.e. without focal lesion in the iris. It is characterized by the presence of fine keratic precipitates which are composed of lymphoid cells and polymorphs.

DIFFERENCES BETWEEN GRANULOMATOUS AND EXUDATIVE ANTERIOR UVEITIS

CLINICAL FEATURES	GRANULOMATOUS UVEITIS	EXUDATIVE UVEITIS
1. *Onset*	Slow and insidious	Acute
2. *Course*	Chronic course with remissions and exacerbations	Short course
3. *Clinical features*	Features of low grade inflammation	Features of acute inflammation
i. *Keratic precipitate*	Mutton fat kp	Small kp
ii. *Aqueous flare*	Mild with few cells	Marked with numerous cells
iii. *Iris nodule*	Common	Absent
iv. *Posterior synechiae*	Marked and organised	Few in recurrent cases
v. *Posterior segment*	Commonly involved	Rarely involved

1. ACUTE IRIDOCYCLITIS

It is an acute inflammation of the iris (iritis) and the ciliary body (cyclitis).

Symptoms

1. Redness—It is due to circumciliary congestion.
2. Pain—It is worse at night. There is severe neuralgic pain referred to forehead, scalp, cheek, malar bone, nose and teeth (as the iris is richly supplied by sensory nerves from the ophthalmic division of 5th nerve).
3. Lacrimation and photophobia may be present (without any mucopurulent discharge) due to associated keratitis.

4. **Impaired vision**—It is mainly due to hazy plasmoid aqueous and opacity in the media.
5. **Photophobia** is due to pain induced by pupillary constriction and ciliary spasm because of inflammation.

Signs

1. **Circumciliary congestion**—There is hyperaemia around the limbus which is dull purple-red in colour. It is due to the dilation of anterior ciliary vessels.
2. **Anterior chamber**
   1. There is plasmoid aqueous containing leucocytes, minute flakes of coagulated proteins and fibrinous network.
      The slit-lamp examination shows the presence of :
      a. *Milky 'flare' or 'aqueous flare'*—Dust-like particles are seen moving in the beam of slit-lamp similar to Tyndall effect.

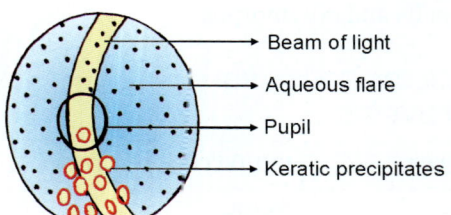
Slit-lamp examination in acute iridocyclitis

Aqueous flare grading
+1 Faint — Just detectable
+2 Moderate — Iris details clear
+3 Marked — Iris details hazy
+4 Intense — With severe fibrinous exudate

   b. *Keratic precipitates (kp)*—The exudate tends to stick to the damaged endothelium in the lower part of cornea in a triangular pattern due to the convection currents in anterior chamber and effect of gravity.
      There are three main types of kps:
      i. *Fresh kp*—These are multiple, circular and grey-white coloured. They consist of lymphocytes predominantly. They are seen in active anterior uveitis and cyclitis typically.
      ii. *Old kp*—These are pigmented, small with crenated edges. They consist of plasma cells mainly. They are evidence of past uveitis.

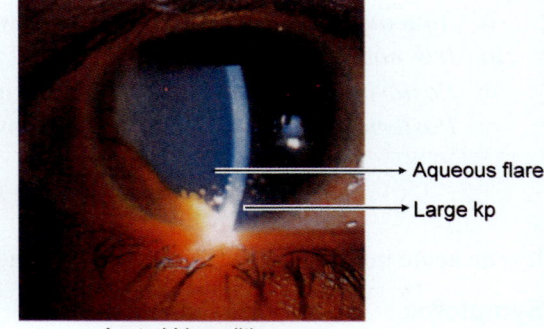
Acute iridocyclitis

      iii. *Mutton fat kp*—These are few, large, yellow, greasy waxy kps. They are characteristic of granulomatous uveitis with predominance of macrophages.
   2. **Hypopyon**—In severe cases of iritis polymorphonuclear leucocytes are poured out which sink to the bottom of the anterior chamber forming hypopyon.
   3. **Hyphaema**—Blood in the anterior chamber rarely occurs due to spontaneous haemorrhage.

3. **Pupil**—It is constricted due to water logging and vasodilatation. It reacts sluggishly to light due to irritation of the third nerve endings in iris.
4. **Iris**
   1. There is loss of normal pattern of the iris.
   2. Iris appears muddy due to the collection of exudates.

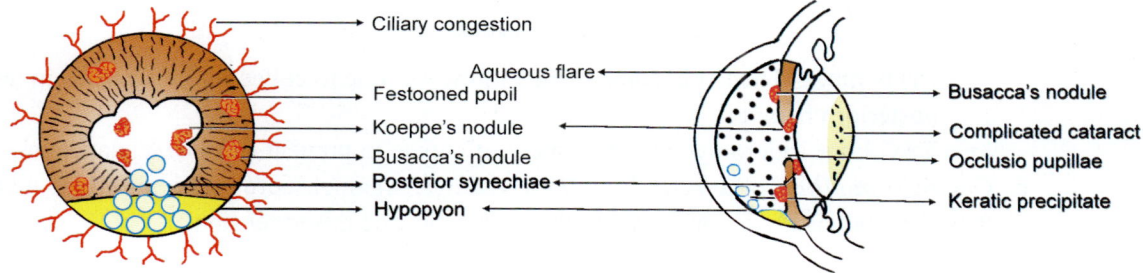

Signs of anterior uveitis

   3. Ectropion of uveal pigment is due to the contraction of exudates upon the iris so that the posterior surface of iris folds anteriorly.
   4. White coloured atrophic patches may appear later.
   5. Iris nodules are seen in granulomatous uveitis,
      i. Koeppe's nodules are small and situated at the pupillary border
      ii. Busacca's nodules are larger and located away from the pupil.
5. **Synechiae**—It is an adhesion or attachment of iris to the adjacent structures.
   1. *Anterior peripheral synechiae*—The iris gets attached to the periphery of the cornea. Intraocular pressure may rise when 3/4 circumference or more of the angle of anterior chamber is blocked.

Anterior peripheral synechiae

   2. *Posterior synechiae*
      i. Annular or ring synechiae (seclusio-pupillae)
         - Whole pupillary margin is tied to the lens capsule by exudates therefore anterior chamber becomes funnel-shaped.
         - Festooned pupil is seen on dilatation, i.e. the pupil dilated irregularly and looks like festive paper decoration.

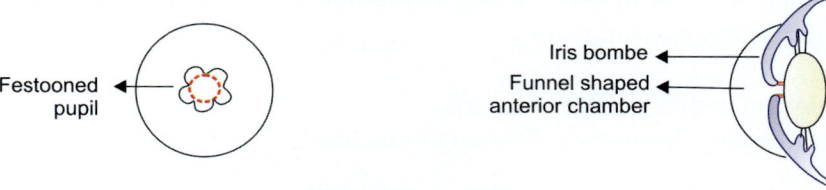

Annular or ring synechiae

- Iris bombe—The iris become bowed forewards due to collection of aqueous in the posterior chamber.
- YAG laser iridotomy is the treatment of choice to prevent secondary glaucoma.

ii. *Occlusio-pupillae or blocked pupil*—Exudates organize across the pupillary area therefore the vision is impaired and there is associated raised tension.

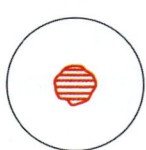
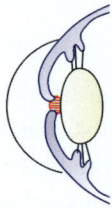

Occlusio-pupillae

iii. *Total posterior synechiae*—In severe cyclitis, the posterior chamber is filled with exudates which may organize tying down the iris to the lens capsule.

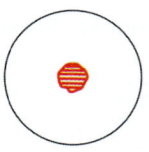
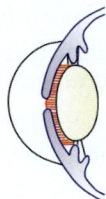

Total posterior synechiae

iv. *Cyclitic membrane*—In worst cases of plastic iridocyclitis, a cyclitic membrane may form behind the lens.

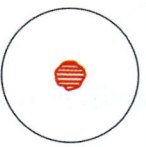
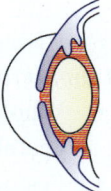

Cyclitic membrane

6. **Lens**
   1. *Complicated cataract*—There is typical posterior cortical cataract with bread crumb appearance and polychromatic lustre.
   2. *Pseudoglioma*—It is seen in young children.
7. **Vitreous**—Vitreous opacities due to leucocytes, coagulated fibrin and exudates may be present in severe cases.
8. **Intraocular tension**
   1. *In active stage*
      i. Hypertensive iridocyclitis may be present due to increase pressure in dilated capillaries and outpouring of leucocytes.
      ii. The sticky albuminous aqueous drains with difficulty thus raising the tension.
   2. *In later stage*
      i. Secondary glaucoma may be present due to pupillary block.
      ii. Phthisis bulbi (hypotony) may be present due to atrophy of the ciliary body.

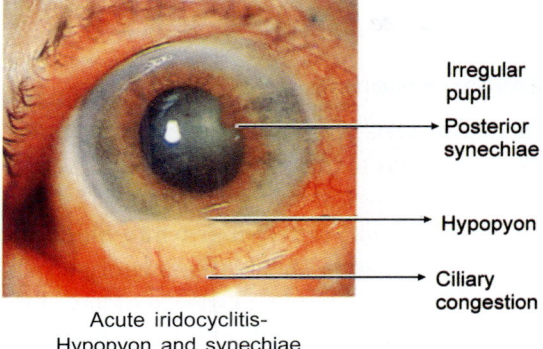

Acute iridocyclitis-
Hypopyon and synechiae

Complications and Sequelae

1. *Complicated cataract*—It is a common complication of iridocyclitis. It progress rapidly in the presence of posterior synechiae.
2. *Secondary glaucoma*—It may occur as an early or late complication of iridocyclitis.
    i. Early glaucoma (Inflammatory glaucoma)—In active phase of the disease, presence of exudates and inflammatory cells in the anterior chamber may block the trabedular meshwork resulting in decreased aqueous drainage and thus a rise in intraocular pressure (hypertensive uveitis).
    ii. Late glaucoma (postinflammatory glaucoma) is the results of pupil block (seclusio-pupillae due to ring synechiae formation or occlusio-pupillae due to organised exudates) not allowing the aqueous to flow from anterior to posterior chamber. There may or may not be associated peripheral anterior synechiae formation.
3. *Cyclitic membrane*—It results due to fibrosis of exudates present behind the lens. It is a late complication of acute plastic type of iridocyclitis.
4. *Choroiditis*—It may develop in prolonged cases of iridocyclitis owing to their anatomical continuity.
5. *Retinal complications*—These include cystoid macular oedema, macular degeneration, exudative retinal detachment and secondary periphlebitis retinae.
6. *Band-shaped keratopathy*—It occurs as a complication of long-standing chronic uveitis, especially in children having Still's disease.
7. *Phthisis bulbi*—It is the final stage end result of any form of chronic uveitis. In this condition, ciliary body is disorganised and atrophied. This leads to decrease production of aqueous. As a result the eye becomes soft and shrinks due to hypotony.

Diagnosis

Iritis should be differentiated from conjunctivitis and acute glaucoma as the treatment of these conditions differ drastically.
  i. *In iritis*—Atropine is *always* used.
  ii. *In acute glaucoma*—Atropine is *never* used.

Investigations

Series of tests should be done because of varied etiology of uveitis. However, a few common investigations required are listed below :
1. Haematological investigations
   - Total and differential white blood cell count (TLC and DLC) is done to have a general information about inflammatory response of the body.
   - ESR to ascertain existence of any chronic inflammatory condition.
   - Blood sugar levels to rule out diabetes mellitus.
   - Blood uric acid in patients suspected of having gout.
   - Serological tests for syphilis, toxoplasmosis, and histoplasmosis.
   - Tests for antinuclear antibodies, rheumatoid factor, LE cells, C-reactive proteins, etc.
2. Urine examination is done for WBC, pus cells, RBC and culture to rule out urinary tract infections.
3. Stool examination is done for cyst and ova to rule out parasitic infestations.
4. Radiological investigations include X-rays of chest, paranasal sinuses, sacroiliac joints and lumbar spine.
5. Skin test—These include tuberculin test, Kveim's test (sarcoidosis) and toxoplasmin test.

TREATMENT OF ANTERIOR UVEITIS

The aims of treating uveitis are:
1. To prevent vision-threatening complications.
2. To relieve the patient's discomfort and pain.
3. To treat the underlying cause of uveitis.

Principles

There are five main principles of treatment:
1. Rest to the eye is given by dilatation of the pupil with atropine.
2. Heat application improves blood circulation and relieves pain.
3. Control of acute phase of the inflammation with corticosteroids.
4. Analgesics and anti-inflammatory relieve pain and discomfort.
5. Modern broad-spectrum antibiotics which cross the blood-aqueous barrier are given in cases of infections.

1. *Atropine*

It is the most powerful, longest acting (2 weeks) and commonly used mydriatic and cycloplegic. Atropine acts in three ways:

DIFFERENCES BETWEEN CONJUNCTIVITIS, IRITIS AND ACUTE GLAUCOMA

CLINICAL FEATURES	CONJUNCTIVITIS	IRITIS	ACUTE GLAUCOMA
1. **Symptoms**			
1. *Onset*	Gradual	Usually gradual	Sudden
2. *Pain*	Mild discomfort	Moderate	Severe
3. *Discharge*	Mucopurulent	Watery	Watery
4. *Coloured halos*	May be present	Absent	Present
5. *Systemic complications*	Absent	Mild	Prostration and vomiting
2. **Signs**			
1. *Congestion*	Superficial conjunctival	Deep ciliary	Deep ciliary
2. *Tenderness*	Absent	Marked	Marked
3. *Media*	Clear	Opacities may be seen	Corneal oedema
4. *Anterior chamber*	Normal	May be deep	Shallow
5. *Pupil*	Normal	Small, irregular	Large, oval
3. **Investigations**			
1. *Vision*	Good	Fair	Poor
2. *Tension*	Normal	Normal or low	Raised
3. *Slit-lamp examination*	Normal	Aqueous flare and kp	Corneal oedema and anterior synechiae

i. It keeps iris and ciliary body at rest by paralysing the ciliary muscle. Thus, it also relaxes the ciliary muscle spasm which is always associated with iritis.

ii. It diminishes hyperaemia by causing vasodilation. It increases the blood supply to anterior uvea. As a result more antibodies reach the target tissue and more toxin are absorbed.

iii. It prevents formation of posterior synechiae and breaks down recently formed synechiae which are not firmly attached by dilating the pupil.

1% atropine eyedrop or ointment is applied twice daily. Subconjunctival injection of 'cocktail' of 0.3 ml mydricaine (atropine, procaine, adrenaline) may be given along with garamycin 20 mg (0.5 ml) and betamethasone 4 mg (0.1ml). In case of atropine allergy, other mydriatics like phenylephrine, cyclopentolate or tropicamide may be used.

In milder cases weaker, short-acting agents such as cyclopentolate 1% or homatropine 2% thrice daily may be used.

Dark glasses or an eyeshade may also be used to avoid glare, discomfort and lacrimation specially in sunlight.

2. Heat Application

Heat application in the form of hot fomentation or local dry heat is very soothing. It reduces pain, prevents stasis and increases blood circulation.

3. Corticosteroids

These are anti-inflammatory in action. They are very useful in controlling inflammation in the acute phase. Due to their anti-allergic and anti-fibrotic activity they reduce fibrosis and thus prevent disorganisation and destruction of tissues.

i. Topical—Eyedrops and eye ointment, e.g. 0.1% betamethasone or dexamethasone. Locally steroids are used as,
   a. Eyedrops 4-5 times a day.
   b. Eye ointment at bedtime.
ii. Subconjunctival injection, e.g. betamethasone 4 mg. It is given once or twice a day depending on the severity of disease.
iii. Periocular injection of depot steroids (e.g. 40-80 mg methylprednisolone or triamcinolone) in the sub-Tenon space. It is better to use full strength topical steroids for 6 weeks to make sure that patient is not having side effects such as raised intraocular pressure.
   It is indicated for
   - Severe acute anterior uveitis
   - As an adjunct to topical or systemic therapy in resistant chronic anterior uveitis
   - In cases of poor patient compliance with topical or systemic medication.
iv. Systemic steroids full course with maintenance tapering doses, e.g., prednisolone 1-1.5 mg/kg or equivalent quantity of other steroids (dexamethasone or betamethasone) is given four time daily for 1-2 weeks and then gradually reduced by a weekly interval over a period of 5-6 weeks.
   It is indicated in cases of
   - Severe uveitis
   - When there is no improvement on maximal topical and periocular steroids
v. Rimexolone (Vexol 1%)—A new drug is being used in United States of America for anterior uveitis. It has strong anti-inflammatory action with minimum side effects of steroids such as increased IOP and cataract formation.

4. Analgesics and Anti-inflammatory

These are useful in relieving pain and discomfort, e.g. aspirin, ibuprofen, etc.

5. Antibiotics

The modern broad-spectrum third generation antibiotics are of immense value particularly in fulminant cases of purulent uveitis. Although these are of not much use in allergic iridocyclitis, they provide an umbrella cover.

6. Non-steroidal Anti-inflammatory (NSAIDs) and Cytotoxic Drugs

Recently cyclosporin, a powerful anti-T cell immunosuppressive agent and cytotoxic drugs have been tried in steroid-resistant cases. Non-steroidal anti-inflammatory drugs act by inhibiting arachidonic acid, e.g. flurbiprofen, indomethacin, diclofenac. These are safer as prolonged use of steroids may produce open angle glaucoma by reducing outflow facility, cataract and secondary infection with bacteria or fungi.

Antimetabolites and systemic immunosuppresive like methotrexate, cyclophosphamide and cyclosporin are indicated for
- Sight-threatening uveitis which is bilateral, non-infectious reversible has failed to respond to adequate steroids
- Steroids-sparing therapy in patients with intolerable side effects from systemic steroids
- These drugs are specially useful in severe cases of Behcet's syndrome, sympathetic ophthalmitis, pars planitis and VKH (Vogt-Koyanagi-Harada) syndrome.

These agents should be administered with great caution under the supervision of haematologist or an oncologist as they have adverse side effects or kidney, liver and cause bone marrow depression.

Recently azathioprine, mycophenolate, mofetil, tacrolimus are used in unresponsive or intolerant patients.

7. Specific Treatment

Specific treatment of the underlying disease should be added if the etiology is identified e.g. Reiter's syndrome, Behcet's syndrome, syphilis, tuberculosis etc.

Treatment of Complications

1. *Secondary glaucoma (hypertensive uveitis)*—Drugs to lower intraocular pressure such as 0.5% timolol maleate eyedrops twice a day and tablet acetazolamide (250 mg thrice a day), should be added over and above the usual treatment of iridocyclitis.
2. *Post-inflammatory glaucoma* due to ring synechiae and iris bombe demand an iridectomy in all cases so that communication can be restored between anterior and posterior chambers. Surgical iridectomy should not be done during the acute phase of iritis (presence of 'kp'). Laser iridotomy is a preferred procedure.
3. *Complicated cataract* requires lens extraction with guarded prognosis in a quiet eye under cover of steroids. The presence of fresh kp is considered a contraindication for intraocular surgery.
4. *Retinal detachment* of exudative type usually settles itself if uveitis is treated aggressively. A tractional detachment requires vitrectomy.
5. *Phthisis bulbi* especially when painful requires removal by enucleation operation.

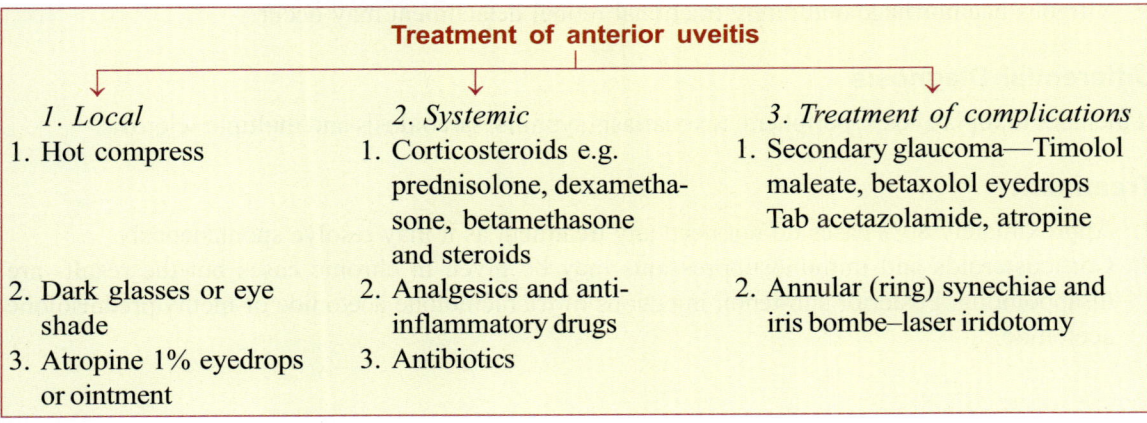

Treatment of anterior uveitis		
1. Local	2. Systemic	3. Treatment of complications
1. Hot compress	1. Corticosteroids e.g. prednisolone, dexamethasone, betamethasone and steroids	1. Secondary glaucoma—Timolol maleate, betaxolol eyedrops Tab acetazolamide, atropine
2. Dark glasses or eye shade	2. Analgesics and anti-inflammatory drugs	2. Annular (ring) synechiae and iris bombe–laser iridotomy
3. Atropine 1% eyedrops or ointment	3. Antibiotics	

2. INTERMEDIATE UVEITIS
(CHRONIC POSTERIOR CYCLITIS OR PARS PLANITIS)

It affects the pars plana of the ciliary body and the peripheral retina and underlying choroid.

Etiology

It is unknown. It is an idiopathic, insidious relapsing inflammatory disease.

Incidence

- It is common in children and young adults.
- Both eyes are affected in about 80% of cases.
- Females are more commonly affected than males.

Symptoms

1. Patient initially complains of seeing floaters.
2. There is diminished vision due to opacities in the anteior aqueous.
3. Later impairment of visual acuity results due to cystoid macular oedema.

Signs

1. Anterior vitiritis–There is mild aqueous flare with occasional keratic precipitates. It can be termed 'spill over' anterior vitiritis.
2. Peripheral retinal periphlebitis–It appears as isolated foci of inflammation or multifocal. It may also be diffuse.
3. Snowbanking, i.e. grey-white plaques involving the inferior pars plana are seen near ora serrata which may coalesce together giving the appearance of a snow bank.

Complications

1. Retrolenticular cyclitic membrane may form
2. Macular oedema, papilloedema or papillitis may be present.
3. Vitreous haemorrhage and rarely tractional retinal detachment may occur.

Differential Diagnosis

It includes toxoplasmosis, peripheral toxocariasis syphilis, sarcoidosis and multiple sclerosis.

Treatment

1. Approximately 80% cases do not need any treatment as it may resolve spontaneously.
2. Corticosteroids and immunosuppressants may be given in chronic cases but the results are disappointing. Posterior sub-tenon injections of triamcinolone acetonide or methylprednisolone acetonide.

3. POSTERIOR UVEITIS (CHOROIDITIS)

There is inflammation of the posterior uveal tract (choroid). It may be focal, multifocal and diffuse in location. As the outer layers of retina depend upon the choroid for nutrition, there is always associated inflammation of retina (chorio-retinitis).

Clinical Forms
It occurs in two forms which is similar to anterior uveitis.
1. Granulomatous choroiditis is due to direct pathogenic infection.
2. Non granulomatous choroiditis or exudative choroiditis is due to allergic reaction.

Symptoms
1. *There is diminution of vision* due to retinal lesions and opacities in the vitreous (floaters).
2. *Photopsia*—Flashes of light are seen due to irritation of the retina.
3. *Metamorphopsia*—Straight line appears wavy due to oedema of the retina.
4. *Micropsia*—The objects appear smaller than they actually are due to separation of rods and cones.
5. *Macropsia*—The objects appear larger than they actually are due to overcrowding of rods and cones.

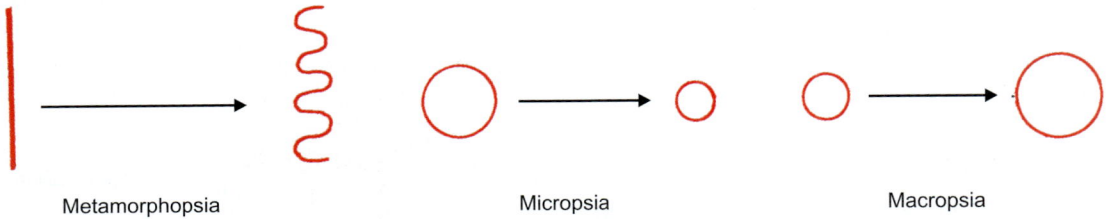

Metamorphopsia   Micropsia   Macropsia

6. *Positive scotoma*—Patient complains of seeing a black spot in front of the eye corresponding to the retinal lesion.
7. *Negative scotoma*—A black spot is present in the field of vision similar to the blind spot, corresponding to the retinal lesion.

Signs
Fundus Examination
1. In early stage one or more yellowish areas with ill-defined edges are seen deep to retinal vessels. This appearance is due to infiltration of the choroid and presence of exudates which hide the choroidal vessels. There may be sheathing of retinal vessels.
2. Black spots are seen floating in the vitreous (vitritis).
3. 'Spill over' uveitis—Anterior segment inflammation such as posterior synechia, kp, aqueous flare may be present.
4. In the healing stage—Yellow lesions become white due to fibrosis and the lesions are surrounded by black pigments.

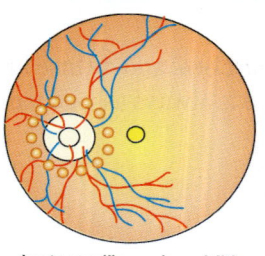
Juxtapapillary choroiditis

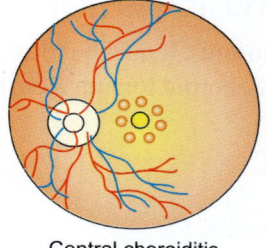
Central choroiditis

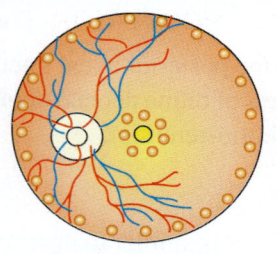
Anterior choroiditis

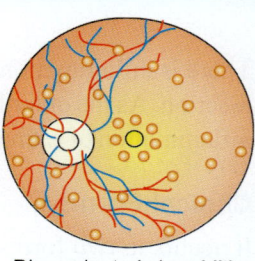
Disseminated choroiditis

Differential Diagnosis

It includes toxoplasmosis, peripheral toxocariasis syphilis, multiple sclerosis and sarcoidosis.

Clinical Types

Choroiditis is usually classified according to number and site of lesions.
1. *Disseminated (diffuse) choroiditis*—The lesions are seen scattered all over the fundus, e.g. as in syphilis and tuberculosis.
2. *Anterior choroiditis*—The lesions are seen in the peripheral parts (near equator) of the fundus, e.g. as in syphilis.
3. *Central choroiditis*—It involves the macular area or posterior pole, e.g. as in toxoplasmosis, histoplasmosis.
4. *Juxtapapillary choroiditis (of Jensen)*—The lesions are present around the optic disc. It occurs in young persons.

Complications

In late stages following complications are seen:
- Complicated cataract
- Secondary glaucoma
- Choroidal neovascularisation
- Retinal detachment.

Treatment

It is usually unsatisfactory as great damage is usually done to the retina before the condition can be controlled,
1. Atropine provides rest to the eye by paralysing the ciliary muscles.
2. Heat application by diathermy or an electric pad may be useful.
3. Corticosteroids—Systemic administration of corticosteroids or ACTH cuts short an attack and hastens healing.
4. Specific treatment is required for causative organism such as toxoplamosis, toxocariasis, tuberculosis, syphilis, etc.

Disseminated choroiditis

CHRONIC IRIDOCYCLITIS (Simple Cyclitis)

Chronic iridocyclitis deserves special mention as it is a extremely chronic disease with insidious onset. It is difficult to diagnose it as there are very few signs and symptoms.

Symptoms
There is gradual diminution of vision with mild pain.

Signs
1. Mild ciliary congestion is usually present.
2. There is tenderness on pressure over the ciliary region.
3. Anterior chamber may be deep or funnel-shaped due to the formation of occlusio-pupillae or ring synechiae.
4. The colour of iris changes. It looks muddy and there may be white atrophic patches.
5. Total posterior synechiae and cyclitic membrane may be present.

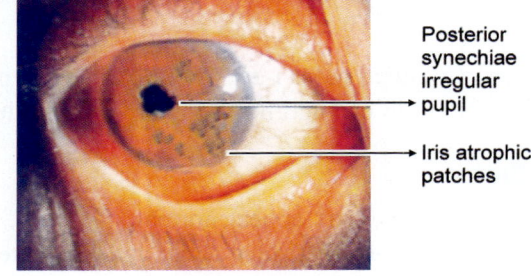

Posterior synechiae irregular pupil

Iris atrophic patches

Slit-lamp Examination
1. Keratic precipitates are scattered over a triangular area in the lower part of cornea.
2. Mutton fat kp—Small kp coalesce together forming small plaques which gradually become translucent.
3. Vitreous shows dust-like opacities.
4. Vitreous gel becomes liquefied or fluid like.

Complications
1. Recurrence is a common feature.
2. Tractional retinal detachment—It may occur due to contraction of strands of fibrous tissue in the vitreous.
3. Phthisis bulbi—The ciliary epithelium is destroyed by the inflammatory process. The eyeball becomes shrunken due to marked hypotony.
4. Hypertensive iridocyclitic crisis of Posner and Schlossman may occur occasionally.

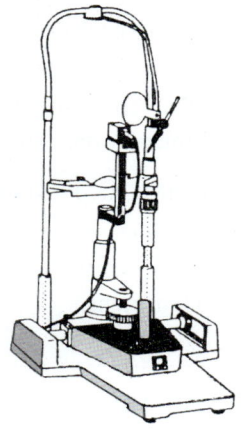

Slit-lamp

HYPERTENSIVE UVEITIS
(Hypertensive Iridocyclitic Crisis of Posner and Schlossman)

There are episodes of raised intraocular tension in association with chronic iridocyclitis.

Symptoms
  i. There is mild to moderate dimness of vision.

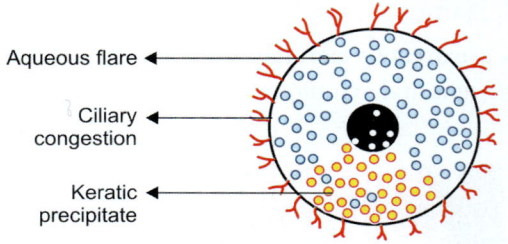 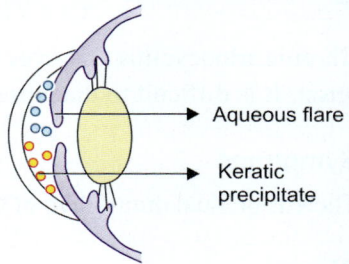

ii. Coloured halos may be seen around light due to corneal oedema.
iii. Pain in eye and headache are present due to raised tension.

Signs

i. The eye may appear normal.
ii. There are periodical acute and subacute attacks of raised tension.
iii. Slit-lamp examination shows presence of aqueous flare and keratic precipitates.

Differential Diagnosis

Hypertensive iridocyclitis should be differentiated from angle closure glaucoma.

Primary angle closure glaucoma—As the treatment of angle closure glaucoma is exactly opposite of iridocyclitis, this condition should be diagnosed carefully. There is absence of keratic precipitate and aqueous flare in angle closure glaucoma. Presence of open angle confirms the diagnosis.

CLINICAL FEATURES	HYPERTENSIVE UVEITIS	ANGLE CLOSURE GLAUCOMA
1. Slit-lamp examination	Presence of aqueous flare and kp	Absent
2. Gonioscopy	Presence of open angle	Narrow or closed angle
3. Treatment	Atropine and corticosteroids (No pilocarpine)	Pilocarpine (No atropine)

Treatment

It includes treatment of iridocyclitis and medical therapy to lower the IOP by use of β-blockers (timolol maleate, betaxolol) acetazolamide and hyperosmotic agents.

i. Atropine helps in controlling the iridocyclitis (no pilocarpine).
ii. Topical corticosteroids are effective anti-inflammatory agent.
iii. Oral acetazolamide, β-blockers and hyperosmotic agents should be given to control the raised tension.
iv. Treat the underlying cause of iridocyclitis in cases of recurrences.

ENDOPHTHALMITIS

Endophthalmitis is the inflammation of the internal structures of the eye, i.e. choroid, retina and vitreous.

Etiology

1. It occurs most commonly as an acute process 1-7 days following intraocular surgery such as cataract extraction and filtering operation. In India the incidence rate varies from 1 to 3%. Chances of infection are much greater if there is associated vitreous loss as vitreous is a very good culture medium for organisms. It is commonly caused by :
    i. *Bacteria*—*Staphylococcus, Pseudomonas, Pneumococcus, Streptococcus, E. coli,* etc.
    ii. *Fungus*—*Aspergillus fumigatus, Candida albicans, Nocardia asteroides, Fusarium,* etc.
    It occurs after injury with vegetable matter such as thorn or wooden stick.
    Sources
    - Bacterial flora of the eyelids, conjunctiva and lacrimal passage.
    - Contaminated instruments, solutions, environmental flora including that of surgeon and operating room personnel.
2. It may follow a penetrating injury with an infected object, e.g. wooden splinter, iron particle.
3. Perforation of suppurative corneal ulcer of *Pseudomonas pyocyanea* or fungal origin.
4. Systemic infection may cause metastatic infection (septic emboli), e.g. AIDS, viral fever, septicemia. It may occur in immunodeficient host and uncontrolled diabetic patients.

Clinical Features

Bacterial Endophthalmitis

1. There is sudden onset with severe pain and redness in the eye in acute cases.
2. Marked visual loss with defective projection of rays is an important feature.
3. Lid oedema, chemosis and corneal haze are present.
4. There is low intraocular tension (hypotony) due to cyclitis.
5. Fibrinous exudate or hypopyon is seen in the anterior chamber.
6. There is associated vitritis and haze in the vitreous.
7. There is yellowish reflex seen behind the lens. There is absence of red fundus reflex and inability to visualize the fundus even with indirect ophthalmoscope.

Fungal Endophthalmitis

1. It has an incubation period of several weeks.
2. There is mild pain and redness with transient hypopyon.
3. It affects the anterior vitreous and anterior uvea causing thick, organized hypopyon.
4. The whole vitreous turns into a granulomatous mass.

Differential Diagnosis

1. Retained cortical lens material following lens extraction may be associated with severe anterior uveitis.
2. Toxic reaction to the irrigating fluid, chemicals or foreign material.

3. **Panophthalmitis**—There is associated inflammation of extraocular tissues resulting in lid oedema, chemosis and painful limitation of movements of eyeball.

Complications

1. Panophthalmitis
2. Papillitis
3. Phthisis bulbi.

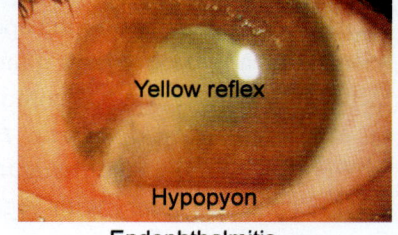

Endophthalmitis

Investigation

Identification and culture and sensitivity of the causative organism from the aqueous and vitreous taps confirms the diagnosis.

Treatment

1. Broad-spectrum antibiotics which cover gram-positive and gram-negative organisms are given.
   i. Intravitreal—An aminoglycoside (gentamicin or amikacin) and vancomycin should be injected slowly into the midvitreous cavity using a 25-gauge needle.
   ii. Periocular injections or subconjunctival injections of:
      - Vancomycin 25 mg and ceftazidine 100 mg daily for 5-7 days.
      - Gentamicin 20 mg and cefuroxime 125 mg daily for 5-7 days.
   iii. Topical therapy every 30-60 minutes.
   iv. Systemic—Intravenous ceftazidine (2 gm every 72 hours), cefotaxime (1 gm twice daily)
      - Oral ciprofloxacin (750 mg every 8 hours)

INTRAVITRIAL DRUGS FOR BACTERIAL ENDOPHTHALMITIS

ANTIBIOTIC	INITIAL CONCENTRATION	VOLUME OF DILUENT ADDED	FINAL CONCENTRATION	DOSE ORDERED
Amikacin	50 mg/ml	0.9 ml	5 mg/ml	0.4 mg/0.08 ml
Cefazolin	225 mg/ml	0.9 ml	22.5 mg/ml	2.25 mg/0.1ml
Dexamethasone	4 mg/ml			0.36 mg/0.09 ml
Gentamicin	40 mg/ml	0.5 ml	2 mg/ml	0.2 mg/0.1 ml
Tobramycin	40 mg/ml	0.5 ml	2 mg/ml	0.2 mg/0.1 ml
Vancomycin	50 mg/ml	0.8 ml	10 mg/ml	1 mg/0.1 ml

2. Corticosteroids are given topically, systemically and by periocular subconjunctival injections.
3. Atropine and analgesics are useful in giving rest to the eye and relieving pain.
4. Vitrectomy if done early may be useful in severe and resistant cases only. It is indicated particularly in fungal endophthalmitis along with intravitreal and systemic amphotericin B.

Prevention

1. Treatment of pre-existing infections before surgery, e.g. staphylococcal blepharitis, conjunctivitis and dacryocystitis should be done. Systemic antibiotics should be started preoperatively.
2. Preoperative prophylactic topical broad-spectrum antibiotics are instilled to decrease patients conjunctival bacterial flora. Eye is irrigated with normal saline or povidone iodine solution before surgery.
3. Postoperative subconjunctival injection of antibiotics and steroids is a must.
4. Meticulous attention to aseptic surgical technique is given.

PANOPHTHALMITIS

Panophthalmitis is the purulent inflammation of all the structures of the eye. There is inflammation of all the three coats of the eye and Tenon's capsule as well.

Etiology

1. *Exogenous*—It is usually due to infected wound which may be accidental, operative or after corneal ulcer perforation. The common pathogens are *Pneumococcus, Staphylococcus, Streptococcus, E. coli, Pseudomonas pyocyanea, Bacillus subtilis, C. welchii*, etc.
2. *Endogenous*—It is due to metastasis of the infected embolus in the retinal artery and choroidal vessels.

Clinical Features

1. There is severe pain and limitation of the movements of eye.
2. There is rise in temperature, headache, vomiting and rapid failure of vision.
3. The lids are red and swollen with marked conjunctival chemosis.
4. Purulent conjunctival discharge, marked conjunctival and ciliary congestion.
5. Corneal wound appears to be necrotic and hypopyon may be present.
6. Yellow reflex is seen through the pupil (vitreous abscess).
7. Fundus examination—Media is hazy so the yellow oedematous retina is faintly visible or often invisible.

Complications

1. Cyclitic membrane is present due to organized exudates.
2. Papillitis—Inflammation of optic disc and surrounding retina may occur.
3. Pus may burst through the globe just behind the limbus.
4. Phthisis bulbi occurs eventually.

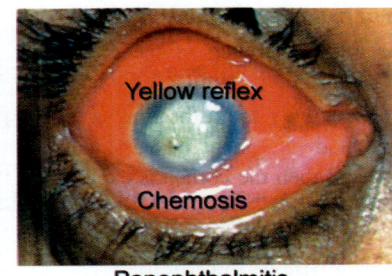

Panophthalmitis

Treatment

Medical

1. *Control the infection by administration of modern broad-spectrum antibiotics* by all possible routes:
   i. Topical frequent instillation of eyedrops and eye ointment at bedtime.

ii. Subconjunctival or periocular injection.
iii. Systemic administration by oral or parenteral routes.
High intraocular concentration of antibiotics is maintained. Multiple antibiotics are given to cover all pathogens. Third generation cephalosporins are given intravenously or intramuscularly.
2. *Corticosteroids*—Topical, subconjunctival injection and systemic administration of corticosteroids is essential. They are anti-inflammatory in action and preserve the ocular structure.
3. *Atropine*—Topical administration by drops or ointment and subconjunctival injection are given. It provides rest to the eye by paralysing the ciliary muscle.

Surgical
1. *Vitrectomy* may be done early to save useful vision.
2. *Evisceration* is done when eye cannot be saved and the patient is completely blind with no perception of light. It saves the patient from severe agonising pain.

PHTHISIS BULBI

There is shrinkage of the eyeball due to marked hypotony or low tension.

Etiology
1. It occurs as a result of destruction of ciliary body due to severe inflammation as in chronic iridocyclitis.
2. It commonly follows perforated corneal ulcer and penetrating corneal injury.

Clinical Features
1. There is no perception of light.
2. There is marked hypotony or low tension.
3. There may be ptosis due to lack of support.
4. Eyeball is shrunken and quadrilateral in shape due to the pressure by four recti muscles.
5. Different structures such as cornea, iris can not be seen clearly.

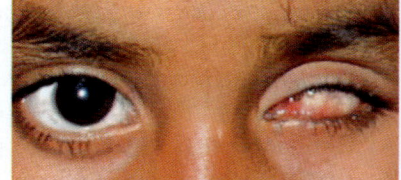

Phthisis bulbi – Left eye

Differential Diagnosis
Atrophic bulbi—It can be differentiated from phthisis bulbi by the following clinical features.

CLINICAL FEATURES	PHTHISIS BULBI	ATROPHIC BULBI
1. Size and shape of eyeball	Small, shrunken, quadrate	Normal usually
2. Intraocular pressure	Marked hypotony	Normal or raised as in absolute glaucoma
3. Identification of ocular structures	Cannot be differentiated	Can be clearly differentiated
4. Light perception	Nil	Nil

Treatment
Enucleation and application of artificial eye.

SPECIFIC TYPES OF UVEITIS

1. Syphilis

Incidence
It is bilateral usually.

Clinical Features
1. *Iritis*—Plastic and gummatous variety is seen in congenital syphilis and secondary stage. Herxheimer reaction—This occurs 24-48 hours after the first therapeutic dose of penicillin due to release of treponemal toxin in the blood.
2. *Cyclitis*—It is often associated with iritis.
3. *Choroiditis*—Disseminated, anterior and diffuse varieties are commonly seen.

Treatment
Systemic course of long acting penicillin is effective.

2. Gonorrhoea

Incidence
It is common in males and is bilateral usually.

Clinical Features
1. *Iritis*—Acute plastic form is often present.
2. *Cyclitis*—Fine vitreous opacities are seen commonly.
3. *Choroiditis*—Inflammation of choroid is rare.

Treatment
1. Local—Penicillin or other suitable antibiotics are given.
2. Systemic—Sulphonamides or other suitable antibiotics are administered.
3. Iritis is treated by atropine and corticosteroids.

3. Tuberculosis
Tuberculosis is a chronic granulomatous infection caused by bovine or human tubercle bacilli.

Incidence
It accounts for 1% of uveitis case in developed countries. The incidence is more in India and other underdeveloped countries.

Clinical Features
It may cause both anterior and posterior uveitis and also Eales disease.

1. *Iritis*—The metastatic granulomatous type occurs in following forms:
    i. *Miliary*—Multiple yellowish-white nodules are seen near pupillary and ciliary margin particularly in debilitated patients.
    ii. *Conglomerate tubercle*—Yellowish-white tumour containing giant cell system is present.

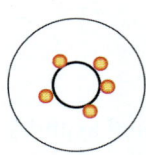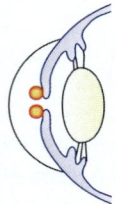

Koeppe's nodules seen in tuberculosis

   iii. *Exudative type*
    - It is allergic in nature.
    - It is usually recurrent and has a chronic course.
    - Large 'mutton fat' keratic precipitates are present.
    - Koeppe's nodules—Minute translucent nodules are seen on the surface of iris at the pupillary margin.
2. *Choroiditis*—It occurs in following two forms:
    i. Acute miliary form
    ii. Chronic disseminated form.

Treatment

Rifampicin with isoniazid or ethambutol is effective when given for 6 months to 1 year.

Miliary tuberculosis

Multiple yellowish white nodules

4. Leprosy

Incidence

Approximately one-third of leprosy patients have eye complications.

Types

1. *Lepromatous (cutaneous)*—Eye involvement often occurs in late stage.
    - There is conjunctivitis, keratitis, episcleritis and iritis.
2. *Tuberculoid (neural)*—Tuberculoid type results in neuroparalytic keratitis usually.

Treatment

Dapsone 50-100 mg daily is administered for several years.
   A course of rifampicin is also very effective.

5. Toxoplasmosis

Etiology
It is a protozoan infection acquired from cats and rodents.

Clinical Features
The signs and symptoms of choroiditis and retinitis are present.

Treatment
1. Medical—Corticosteroids, sulphatriad, pyrimethamine or clindamycin are given.
2. Photocoagulation may protect macular involvement.

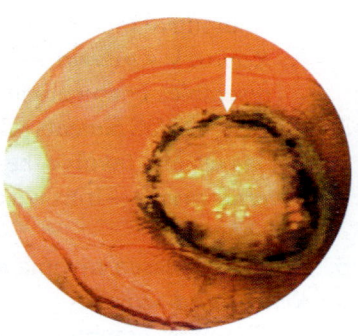

Toxoplasmosis – choroiditis

6. Sarcoidosis

It causes acute and chronic iridocyclitis and posterior uveitis. Uveal parotid fever (Heerfordt's disease) is characteristic.

II. SYNDROMES ASSOCIATED WITH UVEITIS
1. Acquired Immunodeficiency Syndrome (AIDS)

Etiology
It is caused by the HIV (Human immunodeficiency virus). The immune complex deposition leads to small vessel disease. This results in cotton wool spots and cytomegalovirus retinitis.

Incidence
It commonly occurs in homosexual men, haemophiliacs, female sexual partners and infants of women suffering with AIDS.

Clinical Features
About 50-75% of adult AIDS patients suffer from ocular lesions and complications.
1. *Eyelids*—Eyelids may show following clinical features:
    i. *Herpes zoster ophthalmicus* (HZO)—Any individual under the age of 50 years who presents with herpes zoster ophthalmicus (HZO) should be suspected of having HIV infection.
    ii. *Kaposi's sarcoma*—This may present as flat or very slightly raised purple papules on the eyelid. These lesions may be part of a multifocal presentation including conjunctiva or orbit.
    iii. *Molluscum contagiosum*—Molluscum contagiosum is a DNA pox virus that causes raised lesions with umbilicated centres, present along the eyelid. This growth may be associated with a follicular conjunctivitis.
2. *Conjunctival lesions*—Conjunctival involvement is a common feature.
    i. *Non-specific conjunctivitis*—Approximately 10% of AIDS patients develop non-specific conjunctivitis.
    ii. *Dry eye*—About 10% of AIDS patients experience dry eye syndrome. The cause is not clear but it may result due to malabsorption of nutrients essential for maintenance of healthy tear film.

iii. *Microvasculopathy*—There are dilated capillary segments, microaneurysmal formation and sludging of blood flow in the conjunctiva.
iv. *Kaposi's sarcoma*—Conjunctival Kaposi's sarcoma presents as a reddish plaque which resembles conjunctival haemorrhage or chalazion in about 1% or less of AIDS patients.
3. **Cornea**—AIDS patients seldom develop bacterial or fungal corneal ulcers. Herpes simplex keratitis lesions usually involve the periphery of cornea.
4. **Anterior uveitis**—Iritis is a common presentation in patients of AIDS which is sometimes associated with hypopyon.
5. **Lens**—Increased myopia and premature presbyopia have been reported.
6. **Retina and vitreous**
   i. The most common ocular manifestation is presence of cotton wool spots (CWS) in retina which occurs in 50% of cases. It results due to microvascular abnormalities, i.e. endothelial damage caused by circulating immune complex.
   ii. Intraretinal haemorrhages resembling Roths spots (intraretinal haemorrhages with white centres) are commonly seen. They are usually due to non-infectious microvascular retinopathy.

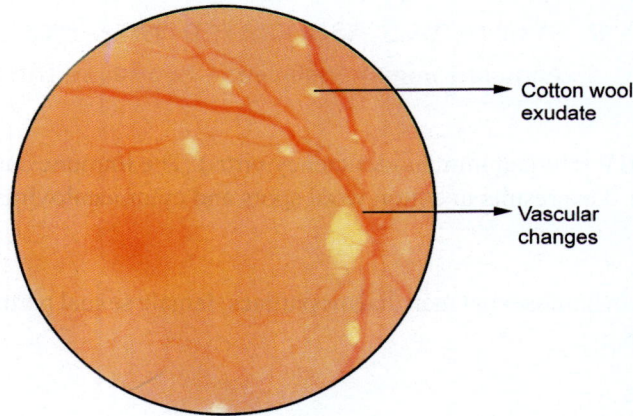

Fundus examination in AIDS

   iii. Retinal infections—These include retinitis caused by cytomegalovirus (CMV), syphilis, toxoplasmosis, candida, varicella, tuberculosis and herpes simplex. CMV retinitis is the most common intraocular infection in AIDS affecting about 25% of patients.
7. **Choroid**—Choroidal infiltrates are present as deep yellow or white lesions. These may result due to infections such as tuberculosis syphilis, *Pneumocystis carinii*, *Candida*, *Cryptococcus* and lymphoma.
8. **Orbit**—AIDS patients may present with unilateral painless and progressive proptosis with or without diplopia and periorbital lymphoedema.

Paediatric AIDS

The incidence of ocular manifestations in paediatric AIDS patients, especially non-infectious microvasculopathy, CMV retinitis and Kaposi's sarcoma seem to be significantly less than in adults. The reason for these differences is unclear.

Diagnosis of HIV infection

The diagnosis of HIV infection depends upon the demonstration of antibodies to HIV and/or the direct detection of HIV or one of its components. The antibodies to HIV generally appear in the circulation 2-12 weeks following infection.

1. **ELISA test**—It is also referred to as an enzyme immunoassay (EIA). This is the standard screening test for HIV infection. This solid phase assay is an extremely good screening test with a senstivity of > 99.5%.
2. **Western blot test**—It is the most commonly used confirmatory test for HIV infection.

WHO CASE DEFINITION OF AIDS

- Two major signs
- At least one minor sign
- Absence of other causes of immunodeficiency

MAJOR SIGNS	MINOR SIGNS
1. Loss of 10% body weight within a short period	1. Persistent cough for more than a month
2. Chronic diarrhoea for more than a month	2. Generalised dermatitis
3. Chronic fever for more than a month	3. Recurrent herpes zoster
	4. Oral candidiasis
	5. Chronic herpes simplex
	6. Generalised lymphadenopathy

Treatment

1. Ganciclovir and Forscarnet are used intravenously in treatment of CMV retinitis.
2. Zidovudine (Azeidothymidine AZT) is seen to be effective in HIV retinitis.
3. Kaposi's sarcoma is sensitive to radiotherapy.

2. Uveoparotitis (Heerfordt's Disease)

It is seen in sarcoidosis. There is bilateral involvement of the entire uveal tract, the parotid glands and 3rd, 7th cranial nerves.

3. Behcet's Syndrome (Recurrent Iridocyclitis with Hypopyon)

It is due to obliterative vasculitis with immunological basis. It is seen in young adults.

Clinical Features

i. Severe iridocyclitis with hypopyon is present.
ii. Ulcerative lesion in the conjunctiva, oral and genital mucosa are seen (Erythema multiforme).
iii. Neurological and articular involvement may also be associated.

Treatment
- No specific treatment is available.
- Systemic steroid may be given. It may be useful initially but ultimate response is poor.
- Oral chlorambucil 6-8 mg daily is administered for 1 year.

4. Reiter's Disease and Uveitis

It is characterized by a triad of urethritis, arthritis and conjunctivitis with or without iridocyclitis. It affects young males. It is associated with high incidence of HLA—B27 antigen.

Clinical Features
i. Uveitis
ii. Rheumatic manifestations
iii. Genitourinary infection
iv. Mucocutaneous lesions.

Treatment
Oral tetracycline 250 mg four times daily for 10 days is recommended.

5. Ankylosing Spondylitis

In young males acute recurrent iridocyclitis is associated with chronic progressive involvement of sacroiliac and posterior intervertebral joints.

6. Vogt-Koyanagi Syndrome

In young adults the chronic exudative iridocyclitis is associated with: vitiligo (white coloured patches of skin), poliosis (white coloured eyelashes) and deafness.

7. Stevens-Johnson Syndrome (Erythema Multiforme)

It is an acute inflammatory polymorphic skin disease with rash, vesicles and bullae of skin, mucous membrane and conjunctiva.

Etiology
In young—Herpes simplex or other virus diseases.
In adults—Reaction to sulpha group of drugs is the most common cause.

Complication
Corneal ulcer, dry eye (xerosis) and uveitis may occur.

Treatment
Immediate withdrawal of the drug should be done along with administration of anti-allergic treatment.

8. Heterochromic Iridocyclitis of Fuchs

It is a low grade chronic cyclitis. There is light coloured iris associated with presence of few keratic precipitates.

Complications

Iris atrophy, cataract, secondary glaucoma may occur.

9. Ocular Histoplasma Syndrome

It affects young person. There are bilateral disci form lesions at the macula.

Treatment

Argon laser application is the treatment of choice.

III. VASCULAR DISTURBANCES

The pathological vascular conditions involving the major arterial circle of iris affects both iris and ciliary body. The blood supply to choroid is segmental therefore isolated areas, are involved.

RUBEOSIS IRIDIS

It is a condition of neovascularisation of iris near its root and angle of anterior chamber.

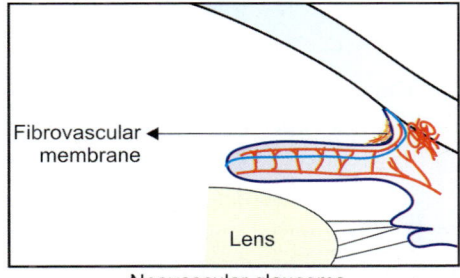

Neovascular glaucoma

Etiology

It occurs due to hypoxia of retina in the following conditions commonly:
1. Diabetes mellitus of long-standing causing proliferative retinopathy.
2. Central retinal vein occlusion (as the glaucoma usually develops after 3 months, it is called 90 days glaucoma)
3. Central retinal artery occlusion
4. Carotid artery diseases—Atherosclerotic obstruction, carotid cavernous fistula
5. Other causes—Eales' disease, Coats' disease, intraocular tumour, sickle cell retinopathy, angiomatosis retinae, retinopathy of prematurity, etc.

Clinical Features

1. Neovascularisation—There is development of new and enlarged blood vessels in the iris towards its root and angle of the anterior chamber.
2. Mild iritis may be present.
3. Neovascular glaucoma, i.e. rise in intraocular tension is a dangerous complication.

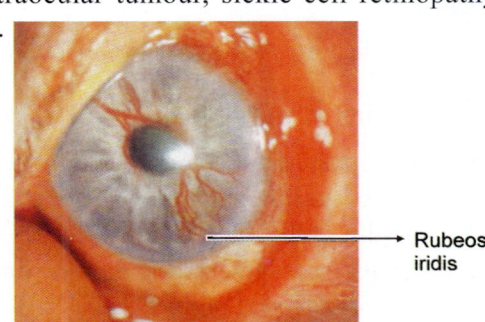

Neovascular glaucoma

Treatment

It is very difficult with poor visual prognosis. Destruction of the neovascular tissue by cyclocryopexy, trans-scleral laser or high intensity ultrasound application may be useful.

Prophylaxis

Panretinal photocoagulation (PRP) of the ischaemic retina is effective.

IV. DEGENERATIONS

1. SENILE IRIS ATROPHY

Depigmentation of the iris with atrophy of the stroma is seen in old people.

2. ESSENTIAL (PROGRESSIVE) ATROPHY OF IRIS

It is usually unilateral and is common in young adults. The etiology is unknown. It is slowly progressive with atrophic changes in iris tissue. Vision is eventually lost with the onset of glaucoma. Prognosis is poor.

3. PRIMARY CHOROIDAL DEGENERATIONS

The causes of primary choroidal degeneration include :
a. *Local degeneration*—Central choroidal atrophy occurs commonly in
  i. Myopia
  ii. Senile macular degeneration—drusen or colloid bodies are formed.
  iii. Obstructive vasosclerosis
b. *Generalized degeneration*
  i. Geographical choroidopathy
  ii. Serpiginous choroiditis
  iii. Essential (gyrate) atrophy of choroid—It is due to an inborn error of ornithine amino acid metabolism.

Treatment

It is unsatisfactory. Argon laser application may be useful.

4. SECONDARY CHOROIDAL DEGENERATIONS

It is usually postinflammatory resulting in localized spots of complete atrophy as in syphilis. This causes loss of nutrition to the retina which in turn results in
  i. Atrophy of the outer layers of retina.
  ii. Migration of pigment from pigment epithelium to perivascular spaces of veins. Thus, the retinal veins are mapped out.

DETACHMENT OF CHOROID

The choroid is apparently detached or separated from the sclera due to fluid accumulation.

Etiology

It is commonly seen in the following conditions :
1. First few days following intraocular surgery. There is sudden lowering of IOP, which leads to vasodilatation of choroid vessels and exudation in the outer layer of choroid. Thus, choroid is separated from sclera.
2. Plastic iridocyclitis and choroiditis.
3. Absolute glaucoma
4. Severe choroidal haemorrhage
5. Tumour mass in the choroid, e.g. malignant melanoma

Sudden lowering of IOP
↓
Vasodilatation of choroid vessels
↓
Exudation in the outer layer of choroid
↓
Choroid is separated from sclera

Signs
1. Anterior chamber is shallow.
2. Fundus examination—The detached choroid appears as a dark mass.
3. Examination by oblique illumination—The detached choroid appears as a dark brown mass.

Prognosis

The choroid becomes replaced and anterior chamber forms again usually by itself therefore the prognosis is good.

Complication

There may be formation of anterior peripheral synechiae causing obstructive glaucoma.

Treatment
1. No treatment is required usually.
2. In recalcitrant cases, drainage of subchoroidal fluid through the sclera with formation of anterior chamber with air may be done.

V. CONGENITAL ANOMALIES

1. Heterochromia Iridum

One iris may have a different colour from the other.

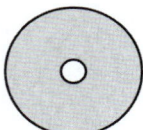 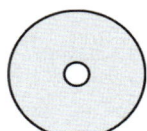

Heterochromia iridum

2. Heterochromia Iridis

Parts of one iris may have different colour.

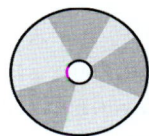 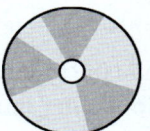

Heterochromia iridis

3. Polycoria

There are more than one pupil.

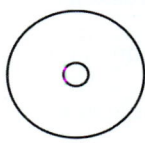 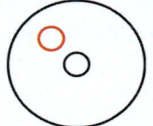

Normal Polycoria

4. Corectopia

The pupil is not central but displaced to the nasal side usually.

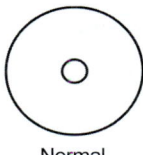 

Normal Corectopia

5. Aniridia

It is a bilateral condition. The iris is absent except for a narrow rim at the ciliary border. It often leads to secondary glaucoma.

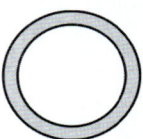 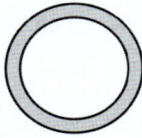

Bilateral aniridia

6. Persistent Pupillary Membrane

Incidence

It is commonly seen in babies.

Etiology

There is persistence of part of anterior vascular sheath of the lens which normally disappears before birth.

Clinical Features

- Fine threads stretch across the pupil.
- It may be attached to lens capsule.
- Pigments are seen on the lens surface as fine brown dots.
- It does not interfere with vision usually.

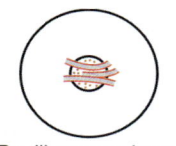
Pupillary membrane

Differential Diagnosis

It is differentiated from the posterior synechiae
  i. In persistent pupillary membrane, fine threads are attached to the anterior surface of iris just outside the pupillary margin.
  ii. There are no keratic precipitates or other signs of iritis.

7. Colobomata

Etiology

Coloboma is due to deficient closure of the embryonic cleft resulting in abnormal shape of the iris.

Clinical Features

1. *Iris*
   i. *Typical*—Pear-shaped coloboma is seen in the lower part and slightly inwards.
   ii. *Atypical*—Defect in iris is seen in any other direction.
2. *Choroid and retina*
   i. Fundus examination shows oval or comet-shaped defect with rounded apex towards the disc. The disc may be included in the defect. Few vessels are seen over the surface and edge.
   ii. The central vision is defective.
   iii. Field of vision—Scotoma is present corresponding to the defect.

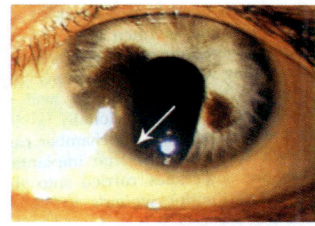

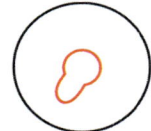
Pear-shaped coloboma

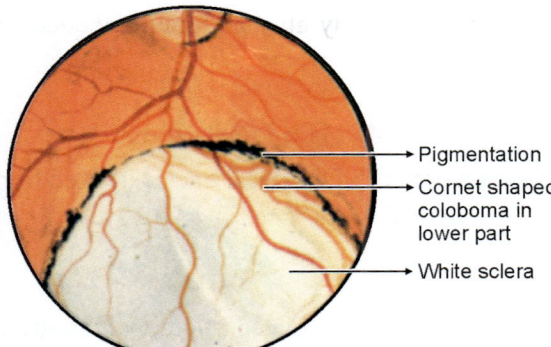
Retinal and choroidal coloboma

- Pigmentation
- Cornet shaped coloboma in lower part
- White sclera

8. Albinism

It is a hereditary condition of defective development of pigment throughout the body.

Type
There are three main clinical types of albinism namely,
1. *Ocular*
2. *Oculocutaneous*
3. *Cutaneous.*

Symptoms
1. There is defective vision.
2. Photophobia and dazzling may be present.
3. Nystagmus is usually associated if macula is involved.
4. Strabismus may be present.

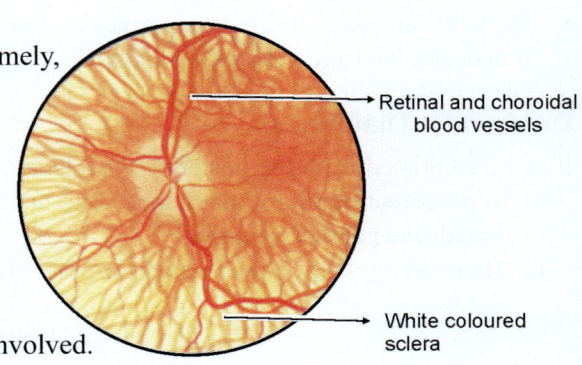

Albinism

Signs
1. Iris is pink in colour
2. Fundus examination—Retinal and choroidal vessels are seen with great clarity with glistening white sclera behind them.
3. Partial albinism is more common. The iris is blue and the pigments are absent from choroid and retina. The macula may be pigmented and may therefore look normal.

Treatment
Use of tinted glasses as a protection from glare is recommended.

9. Cysts
1. *Serous cyst*—It is due to closure of the iris crypts.
2. *Cyst of posterior epithelium*—It must be differentiated from iris bombe.
3. *Implantation cyst*—It occurs commonly after perforating wounds or operations.

VI. TUMOURS

Malignant Melanoma

The common primary malignant tumour of the uveal tract is derived from the sheaths of Schwann of sensory nerves and is thus ectodermal.

1. Iris
Malignant melanoma of iris occurs as an isolated nodule which grows rapidly. It may penetrate through the limbus.

It consists of pigmented or unpigmented spindle-shaped cells or round cells.

Treatment
- Wide iridectomy is performed which should include the tumour mass.
- Excise the eye if there is recurrence.

2. Ciliary Body
Clinical features and treatment are same as that for malignant melanoma of choroid.

3. Choroid
Incidence
It is commonly seen in 40-60 years age group unilateral and single usually.

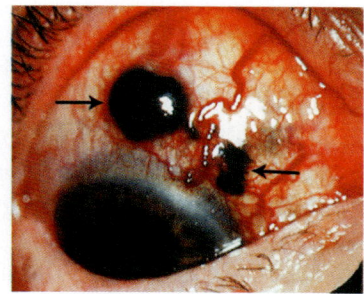

Malignant melanoma

Types
There are two main clinical types namely,
  i. *Pedunculated melanoma*
  ii. *Flat melanoma.*

Stages
  i. *Quiescent stage*—It is symptomless usually.
  ii. *Glaucomatous stage*—The clinical features of raised tension are present.
  iii. *Extraocular extension*—There is local spread into the orbital tissue.
  iv. *Metastasis*—Blood-borne metastasis to central nervous system and liver occur commonly.

Diagnosis
1. Defective vision—There is no perception of light probably.
2. Retinal detachment—The retinal detachment site is rounded and fixed at the summit of the tumour with patches of black uveal pigment over it.
3. A peculiar pattern of dilated blood vessels is seen over the tumour mass.
4. Transillumination indicates the tumour mass.

Investigations
1. *Ultrasonography (B-scan)*—It clearly denotes the tumour mass.
2. *Fluorescein angiography*—It outlines the abnormal blood vessels.
3. *Radioactive tracer*—Neoplastic tissue has an increased rate of phosphate (P32) uptake.

Treatment
1. Small tumours (less than 10 mm in diameter) may be treated by plaque brachytherapy external beam radiation, cryotherapy, laser ablation or transpupillary thermotherapy.
   Medium-sized tumours (10-15 mm in diameter) can be treated by plaque or external beam radiation.
2. *Enucleation*—Large tumours require enucleation. Excise the eye and cut the optic nerve as far back as possible.
3. *Orbital exenteration*—It is advised in cases of orbital spread and extraocular extension.

Prognosis
- If untreated, it is fatal within 5 years.
- The prognosis is fair if the tumour is small (less than 10 mm in size) and intraocular.

OPERATION UPON THE IRIS

IRIDECTOMY

Iridectomy consists of the abscission or cutting of a portion of the iris.

Indications
1. *Prolapsed iris*—A peripheral iridectomy including the prolapsed iris is usually effective.
2. *Closed angle glaucoma*—Usually a small peripheral (buttonhole) iridectomy is done.
3. *As part of cataract extraction*—A small peripheral iridectomy is done.
4. *Threatening ring synechia in iritis*—Sector iridectomy is done in the upper part of the iris to prevent the formation of ring synechia.
5. *Foreign body in the iris*—It is removed by abscissing the iris.
6. *Small cysts or tumours of the iris*—These can be excised totally along with wide iridectomy.
7. *Optical iridectomy*—In central leucomatous corneal opacity, temporal (for distant vision, e.g. farmers) or nasal (for near work, e.g. clerk, goldsmith) iridectomy is done according to the requirement and job of the patient.

Technique
- An easy and safe procedure is by the ab-externo incision of the cornea near the limbus at 12 O' clock position.
- A small incision is made by a few strokes of the blade to open the anterior chamber.
- Iris presents in the wound which is abscised near its base leaving the pupillary sphincter intact.

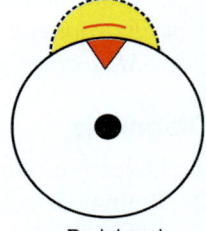

Peripheral iridectomy

IRIDOTOMY

This consists of section of the iris without the abscission of any portion of iris. It can be done surgically or by Argon Diode or Nd:YAG laser.

LASER PERIPHERAL IRIDOTOMY
Indications
i. Pupillary block with angle closure glaucoma
ii. Chronic angle closure glaucoma
iii. Fellow eye in patients of acute angle closure glaucoma
iv. Suspected malignant glaucoma to rule out pupillary block
v. Pupillary block after cataract surgery
vi. Updrawn pupil.

Contraindications

  i. Inability of the patient to sit at the slit-lamp.
  ii. A dense corneal opacity.

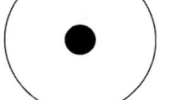

Iridotomy (after YAG laser treatment)

Pretreatment Regimen

a. Topical miotics, e.g. pilocarpine 1-4%, three applications every five minutes to tighten the iris and pull it away from the periphery.
b. Topical beta-blockers, if not contraindicated or carbonic anhydrase inhibitors to reduce the intraocular pressure.

Choice of Laser for Iridotomy

Among argon, diode and Nd: YAG lasers, Nd : YAG laser is the best as it can be used in all type of irides. In unusual instances such as a very thick brown iris or a vascular iris, argon or diode laser need to be used. Iridotomy should be minimum 150-200 microns size, the lens capsules should be easily seen on retro-illumination and good fundal glow should be seen through the iridotomy opening.

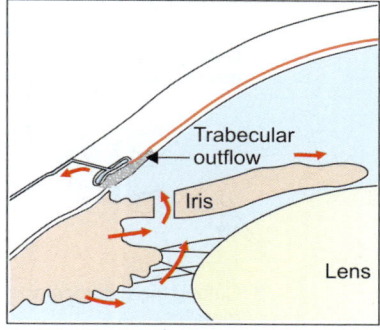

Laser iridotomy or peripheral iridectomy

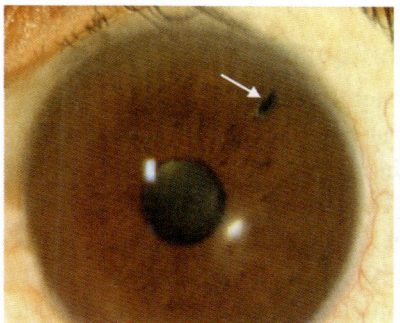

Nd: YAG Laser iridotomy

Post Laser

The patient is put on topical steroids, topical b-blockers or carbonic anhydrase inhibitors. Patients are reviewed after 1 hour, 1 day, 1 week and 4 weeks and intraocular pressure recorded.

Complications

1. Haemorrhage may occur specially with Nd: YAG laser. This can be managed by increasing the pressure over the eye using the lens.
2. Corneal burns
3. Lens opacities
4. Uveitis
5. Retinal burn
6. Diplopia—If iridotomy is performed in the horizontal meridian.

EXCISION OF THE EYEBALL

ENUCLEATION

In enucleation the eyeball is excised or cut off as a whole by cutting the optic nerve. Thus the meninges are opened.

Indications

1. *Absolute*
   i. *Malignant tumours of the eyeball*, e.g. retinoblastoma, malignant melanoma. This prevents dissemination or spread of malignant cells.
   ii. *Severely injured eye with no perception of light.* (This prevents sympathetic ophthalmitis in the good eye.
2. *Relative—Painful blind eye (without infection)*
   i. *Absolute glaucoma.* It prevents severe pain and agony.
   ii. *Anterior and ciliary staphyloma.* It is done for cosmetic purpose.

Technique

A general anaesthesia is always preferred.
- The conjunctiva is cut all around the cornea just outside the limbus.
- The rectus muscles are taken up one by one with the help of muscle hook and divided close to the globe.
- The optic nerve is cut as far back as possible by the enucleation scissors (in order to prevent spread of malignant cells to the brain).
- The eyeball is freely drawn forwards and removed.
- The conjunctiva is sutured, antibiotic ointment is applied and firm pad and bandage is tied.

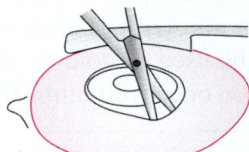
1. Cutting the conjunctiva around limbus

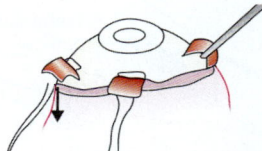
2. Cutting the extraocular muscles

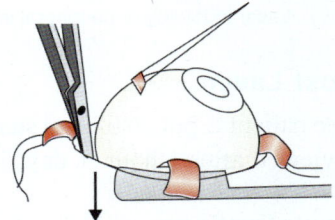
2. Cutting the optic nerve

Enculeation

EVISCERATION

In evisceration, the intraocular contents are removed or scooped out without cutting the optic nerve and without opening the meninges. It is useful in cases of infection.

Indications

1. *Panophthalmitis with no perception of light (PL)*—It prevents extension of infection up to the optic nerve sheath to brain.
2. *Bleeding anterior staphyloma*—To control the excessive bleeding from the uveal tract.

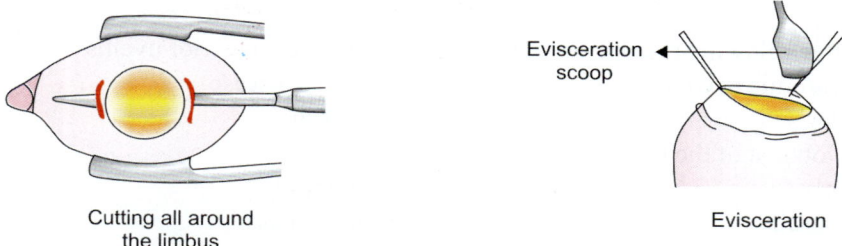

Cutting all around the limbus

Evisceration

Technique

- An opening is made into the cornea near the limbus which is cut and removed with the help of scissors.
- All the intraocular contents are scooped out and the inner surface of sclera is thoroughly cleaned with an evisceration scoop.

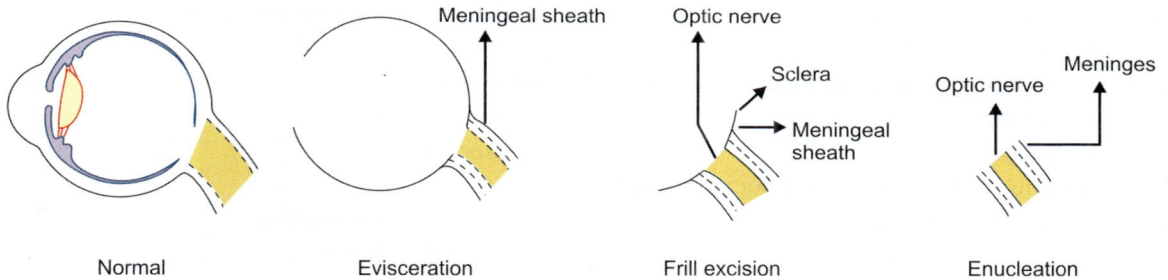

Normal   Evisceration   Frill excision   Enucleation

FRILL EXCISION

Frill excision is a variant of evisceration. It can be done in cases of panophthalmitis with associated scleral necrosis. If the entire sclera is left, there is considerable reaction and delayed healing. Therefore, only a small frill of sclera is left around the optic nerve so as to avoid opening of meninges.

Technique

- The insertions of extraocular muscles and greater part of the sclera is cut off leaving only a small collar of sclera around the optic nerve.
- Thus, the nerve sheaths remain unopened. There are no chances of spread of the infection to the meninges and brain involvement.

IMPLANT AND ARTIFICIAL EYE

Implant—It provides support for the artificial eye. Plastic implant is buried in Tenon's capsule and extraocular muscles are sutured to it.

Artificial eye—Plastic artificial eye is worn after 2-4 weeks of excision. It may be taken out and washed once daily.

Basic Ophthalmology

MULTIPLE CHOICE QUESTIONS

1. Which of the following is not a possible etiology for chronic anterior uveitis
   a. heterochromic uveitis
   b. Still's disease
   c. sarcoidosis
   d. syphilis
2. Typical coloboma of the iris is situated
   a. superiorly
   b. inferiorly
   c. superonasally
   d. inferonasally
3. Iridocyclitis is characterised by
   a. dilated pupil
   b. normal tension
   c. keratic precipitate
   d. all of the above
4. The earliest feature of anterior uveitis includes
   a. keratic precipitate
   b. hypopyon
   c. posterior synechiae
   d. aqueous flare
5. Rubeosis iridis is seen in
   a. diabetes
   b. central retinal vein occlusion
   c. both
   d. none
6. In subacute uveitis with glaucoma, which drug should *not* be given
   a. pilocarpine
   b. timolol maleate
   c. atropine
   d. eserine
7. Anterior uveitis is seen in association with
   a. rheumatoid arthritis
   b. ankylosing spondylitis
   c. Reiter's syndrome
   d. all of the above
8. Black spots floating in front of eyes is a symptom of
   a. panophthalmitis
   b. endophthalmitis
   c. iritis
   d. choroiditis
9. Complete loss of vision is seen at the onset
   a. panophthalmitis
   b. orbital cellulitis
   c. cavernous sinus thrombosis
   d. all of the above
10. In complete albinism the colour of iris is
    a. white
    b. blue
    c. pink
    d. black
11. Essential atrophy of choroid is due to inborn error of metabolism of amino acid
    a. cystine
    b. lysine
    c. arginine
    d. ornithine
12. "Mutton fat" keratic precipitates are typically seen in
    a. acute iritis
    b. chronic cyclitis
    c. central choroiditis
    d. juxtapapillary choroiditis
13. Koeppe's nodules are characteristic of
    a. granulomatous uveitis
    b. exudative uveitis
    c. posterior uveitis
    d. none of the above

14. The characteristic features of AIDS include
    a. cotton wool spots
    b. cytomegalovirus retinitis
    c. conjunctival Kaposi's sarcoma
    d. all of the above
15. Vogt-Koyanagi syndrome includes all EXCEPT
    a. vitiligo
    b. deafness
    c. poliosis
    d. genitourinary infection
16. The common causes of choroid detachment include all EXCEPT
    a. leaking section postoperatively
    b. plastic iridocyclitis
    c. new growth
    d. central choroidal atrophy
17. Aniridia is a congenital defect whereby there is
    a. absence of iris
    b. more than one pupil
    c. pupil is displaced from central position
    d. pear-shaped coloboma of iris
18. The treatment of intraocular malignant melanoma of the uveal tract includes
    a. enucleation
    b. evisceration
    c. exenteration
    d. chemotherapy
19. The common indications for peripheral iridectomy include all EXCEPT
    a. open angle glaucoma
    b. closed angle glaucoma
    c. prolapsed iris
    d. a part of cataract extraction
20. Hypertensive iridocyclitis occurs commonly due to all EXCEPT
    a. increased pressure in dilated capillaries of iris
    b. sticky albuminous aqueous humour
    c. outpouring of leucocytes into the anterior chamber
    d. acute congestive glaucoma
21. Behcet's syndrome includes
    a. recurrent iridocyclitis
    b. ulcerative lesions in conjunctiva, oral and genital mucosa
    c. hypopyon
    d. all of the above
22. Heerfordt's disease is seen in
    a. toxoplasmosis
    b. sarcoidosis
    c. tuberculosis
    d. histoplasmosis
23. In juxtapapillary choroiditis, the lesions are seen in
    a. macular area
    b. peripheral part
    c. around the disc
    d. all over the fundus
24. The symptoms of choroiditis include all EXCEPT
    a. metamorphopsia
    b. photopsia
    c. photophobia
    d. macropsia
25. The term endophthalmitis means inflammation of
    a. internal structures of the eye
    b. all the structures of the eye
    c. choroid
    d. retina

26. Drug of choice for acute iridocyclitis is
    a. acetazolamide
    b. atropine
    c. antibiotic
    d. aspirin
27. All the following are seen in albinism *EXCEPT*
    a. glaucoma
    b. refractive error
    c. nystagmus
    d. photophobia
28. Uveitis is characterized by all *EXCEPT*
    a. mucopurulent discharge
    b. small pupil
    c. moderate pain
    d. keratic precipitate
29. Chronic use of steroids may lead to
    a. iris atrophy
    b. glaucoma
    c. corneal opacity
    d. retinopathy
30. Uveitis occurs commonly in association with
    a. rheumatoid arthritis
    b. SLE
    c. Reiter's disease
    d. all of the above

ANSWERS

1—d	2—d	3—c	4—d	5—c
6—a	7—d	8—d	9—a	10—c
11—d	12—b	13—a	14—d	15—d
16—d	17—a	18—a	19—a	20—d
21—d	22—b	23—c	24—c	25—a
26—b	27—a	28—a	29—b	30—d

CHAPTER 10

The Lens

APPLIED ANATOMY

The lens is a transparent, biconvex structure of crystalline appearance placed between the iris and the vitreous. It is suspended by the suspensory ligament of the lens or zonule of Zinn which is attached to the ciliary body and equator of the lens. The accommodative power varies with age, being 14 to 16 D (at birth), 7 to 8 D (at 25 years of age) and 1 to 2 D (at 50 years).

The lens is composed of 64% water, 35% protein and 1% lipid, carbohydrate and trace elements. The metabolism of the lens is anaerobic. Glycolysis is responsible for 85% glucose utilization resulting in lactate formation.

Refractive index = 1.39
The dioptric power = 15 to 18 D
Diameter = 9-10 mm
Thickness = 4 mm
Radius of curvature
   i. *Anterior surface* = 10 mm (less convex or flat)
  ii. *Posterior surface* = 6 mm (more convex)
Weight = 250 mg (approximately). The lens grows in size continuously throughout life. At birth it weighs about 65 mg and by 80 years of age it weighs approximately 258 mg.

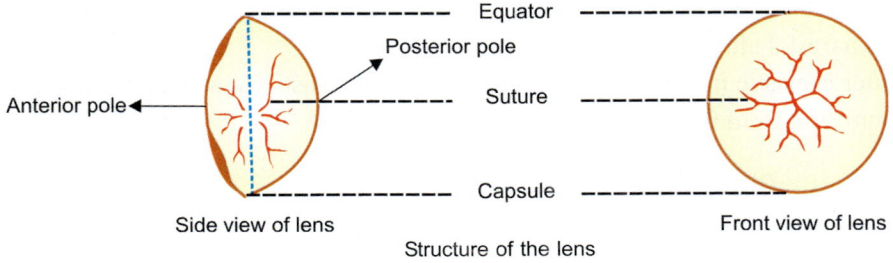

Structure of the lens

Structure

i. *Lenticular capsule*—It is a smooth, homogeneous, acellular envelope. The hyaline lens capsule is secreted by the underlying epithelial cells.
ii. *Lenticular epithelium*—It is a single layer of cuboidal cells just deep to the anterior capsule. There is no corresponding posterior epithelium.
iii. *Lenticular fibres*—The anterior cuboidal cells gradually become columnar and elongated (lens fibres) towards the equator. Anterior and posterior Y-shaped suture lines are formed at the junction of lens fibres.
iv. *Suspensory ligament or zonule of Zinn*—This consists of transparent, straight and inextensible fibres.

Parts

i. *Lens capsule*—It is a thin, transparent membrane which is thicker anteriorly. It is thinnest at the posterior pole measuring 4 m (pre-equator region = 14 m).
ii. *Cortex*—It lies in between the lens capsule and the nucleus. It consists of lens fibres.
iii. *Nucleus*—The lens has four nucleus which are formed at different stages of life upto late adolescence namely embryonic nucleus (1-3 months of gestation), fetal nucleus (from 3 months of gestation till at birth), infantile nucleus (from birth to puberty) and adult nucleus (early adult life).

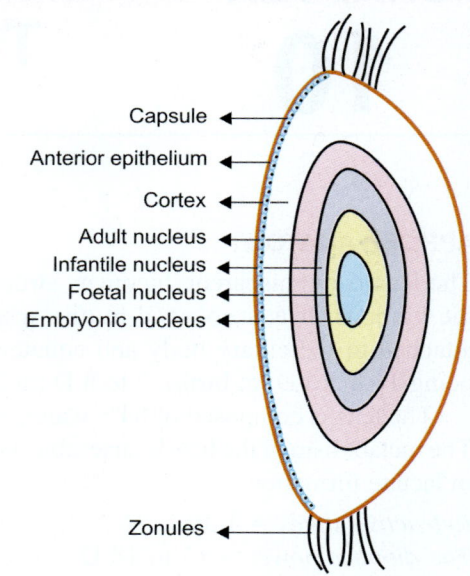

Major components of adult lens

Functions

The main functions of the lens are:
1. To maintain its own clarity and transparency. The lens (like the cornea) transmits 80% of light between 400 nm and 1400 nm.
2. To provide refractive power to the optical system of the eye. It is responsible for 35% of the refracting power of the eye.
3. To provide accommodation for near vision.
4. Absorption of harmful ultraviolet light.

The lens matter is elastic in nature but it gradually loses its elasticity with age. Lens is avascular and derives its nutrition from the aqueous humour.

DISEASES OF THE LENS
I. Cataract

Congenital or development cataract
1. Punctate cataract
2. Zonular cataract
3. Coronary cataract
4. Anterior capsular cataract
5. Posterior capsular cataract
6. Others—coralliform, discoid, axial, sutural cataract.

Acquired cataract
1. Senile—cortical and unclear cataract
2. Cataract associated with ocular diseases
3. Cataract associated with systemic diseases—diabetes, parathyroid tetany, galactosaemia, myotonic dystrophy, etc.
4. Cataract due to radiant heat of other energy
5. Traumatic cataract
6. After cataract

II. DISLOCATION AND SUBLUXATION
III. CONGENITAL ABNORMALITIES

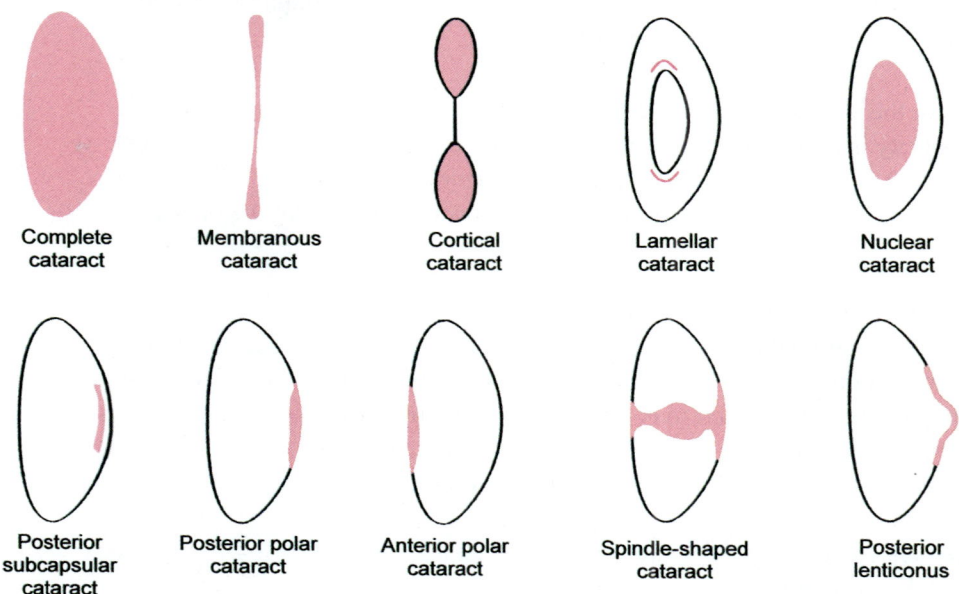

The various presentations of congenital cataract

CATARACT

Any opacity in the lens or its capsule whether developmental or acquired is called cataract.

CONGENITAL (DEVELOPMENTAL) CATARACT

Developmental cataract may be present at birth or it may occur in early childhood. It has a tendency to affect a particular zone. It is usually stationary but may be progressive.

Incidence

Congenital cataract occurs in about 3:10,000 live births. Two third of cases are bilateral.

Etiology

1. *Heredity*—It accounts for approximately 25% of all congenital cataracts. The most common cause is genetic mutation, usually autosomal dominant.
2. *Maternal causes*
   i. *Maternal malnutrition,* e.g. as in zonular cataract.
   ii. *Maternal infection by virus,* e.g. rubella in the first trimester.
3. *Foetal causes*
   i. *Deficient oxygenation* due to severe placental haemorrhage, e.g. placenta praevia.

ii. *Metabolic disorders* of the foetus or infant like galactosaemia, galactokinase deficiency
iii. *Chromosomal abnormalities*, e.g. as in Down syndrome (trisomy 21)
4. *Idiopathic*—Unilateral cataracts are usually sporadic and of unknown etiology.

Symptoms

It depends on the size and position of the opacity.
1. If the opacity is large and central in position, there is marked visual impairment.
2. White reflex is seen in the pupillary area (leucocoria).
3. Abnormal movements of the eye due to squint or nystagmus may be present.

Signs

1. White reflex is present in the pupillary area.
2. Plane mirror examination—There is black opacity against a red background.
3. Ophthalmoscopic examination—There is black opacity against a red background.
4. Congenital anomalies which may occur in association with developmental cataract:
    - Congenital heart disease (patent ductus arteriosus)
    - Microphthalmos
    - Microencephaly
    - Mental retardation
    - Deafness
    - Dental anomalies.

Clinical Types

1. *Punctate or blue-dot cataract*   It is the most common variety. Multiple small, opaque, scattered dots are seen. It does not interfere with vision usually.
2. *Zonular cataract*
    - It is bilateral with strong dominant hereditary tendency.
    - Malnutrition and lack of vitamin D may cause zonular cataract along with erosion of permanent incisors and canines. It is the most common congenital cataract.
    - An area around embryonic nucleus becomes opacified and two rings of opacity are seen. The opacity is sharply demarked and the area of the lens within and around the opacity is clear. Linear opacities or riders may run towards the equator.

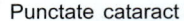
Punctate cataract

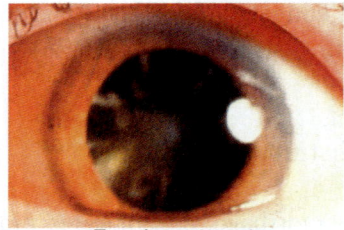
Zonular cataract

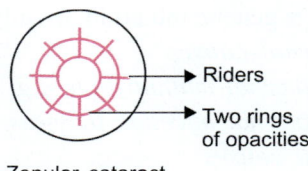
Zonular cataract

3. *Coronary cataract* It commonly occurs at puberty. It is situated in the deep layers of cortex and superficial layers of nucleus. There are multiple club-shaped opacities near the periphery of the lens usually hidden by the iris.

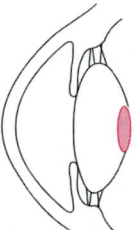

Coronary cataract

4. *Anterior capsular cataract* It is due to the delayed formation of the anterior chamber. It may occur following perforation of a corneal ulcer in ophthalmia neonatorum cases. It may project forwards into the anterior chamber like a pyramid (anterior pyramidal cataract). The underlying cortex may become opaque (anterior cortical cataract) occasionally.
5. *Posterior capsular cataract* It is often due to persistence of posterior part of vascular sheath. Persistence of hyaloid artery may eventually result in total cataract.

Anterior capsular cataract   Posterior capsular cataract

Investigations

1. Ocular examination
   - Density and morphology of cataract is noted based on childs vision and visibility of fundus on ophthalmoscopy.
   - Refraction by retinoscopy under atropine is done in partial cataract.
   - Associated ocular pathology, e.g. microphthalmos, congenital heart disease etc.
   - Intraocular pressure is noted.
   - B-scan ultrasonography is useful in assessing posterior segment of the eye in total cataract to rule out associated retinal detachment or retinoblastoma.
   - A-scan ultrasonography is done to record and compare the axial lenghts of two eyes.
2. Systemic investigations
   For bilateral non hereditary cataracts
   - Serum biochemistry is done to find out levels of fasting blood glucose, calcium and phosphorus, galactokinase and red blood cell transferase etc.
   - Urine analysis for the presence of reducing substances after milk feeding (galactosaemia), screening for aminoacids in urine (Lowe's syndrome)
   - Serological tests for estimating the titres of antibody for infections such as toxoplasmosis, rubella, cytomegalovirus, herpes simplex (TORCH) and hepatitis B virus.

Treatment

1. **No treatment**—No treatment is required if the vision is good.
2. **Mydriasis with atropine**—It is advocated atleast until puberty if the cataract is small, central and the vision is good. Atropine drop is instilled once a week.

3. **Optical iridectomy**—It may be done if the opacity is small, central and stationary.
4. **Lens aspiration**—Aspiration of lens matter can be done as the lens material is soft in children. This is followed by IOL implantation.
5. **Lensectomy**—In this operation, the lens including anterior and posterior capsule along with anterior vitreous are removed.

Lens Aspiration

The child should be operated earlier as the fixation reflex develops between 2-4 months of age. This is followed by intraocular lens (IOL) implant to establish binocular vision.

Indications

- It is done in young patients upto the age of 30 years as the nucleus is not hard.
- It is commonly indicated for congenital and traumatic cataracts when,
    i. Lens is completely opaque.
    ii. Pupil does not dilate.
    iii. There is development of squint.
    iv. There is development of nystagmus.

Contraindications

i. *It is difficult to perform anterior capsulotomy in totally shrunken cataract*
ii. *Presence of persistent hyaloid artery may lead to severe haemorrhage.*

Technique

Aspiration of lens matter can be done by limbal route, (either single incision or two-port bimanual technique) or corneo scleral tunnel technique.
- General anaesthesia is required in young patients.
- Pupil must be fully dilated with suitable mydriatic such as phenylephrine, tropicamide.
- The globe is fixed by superior rectus muscle suture.
- A small corneo-scleral incision 1-1.5 mm is made.
- A small peripheral buttonhole iridectomy is performed at 12 O'clock.
- Anterior capsulorrhexis is performed measuring about 5 mm size. In children the anterior capsule is more elastic therefore it may be difficult.
- Soft lens matter is aspirated and irrigation with BSS (balanced salt solution), Ringer's lactate or normal saline is done with a manual or automated irrigation-aspiration device.
- Posterior capsulorrhexis measuring 3-4 mm with limited anterior vitrectomy should be performed, specially in young children to prevent posterior capsule opacification.
- Suitable intraocular lens may be inserted in the posterior chamber (in the ciliary sulcus or preferably in the capsular bag). Generally IOL are favoured in children (over 2 years of age) whose ocular growth is almost complete and in unilateral cataract. The intraocular lens material recommended is heparin coated polymethyl-methacrylate (PMMA). Newer foldable hydrophobic acrylic polymer lenses are becoming popular.

- Wound is closed with monofilament silk or nylon sutures. A subconjunctival injection of gentamicin and dexamethasone is given postoperatively.
- The pupil is kept dilated with short acting mydriatic and topical steroid–antibiotic drops are applied several times each day for 2-3 weeks.

Postoperative Complications

1. Posterior capsular opacification—This is almost universal if the posterior capsule is retained. The incidence is reduced when posterior capsulorhexis is combined with vitrectomy.
2. Secondary membranes may form across the pupil. Thin membrane may be opened with an Nd: YAG laser while thick membranes may require surgery.
3. Proliferation of lens epithelium is common but may not be visually significant if visual axis is not involved.
4. Glaucoma may develop eventually in about 20% of eyes.

Lensectomy

In this operation, the lens including anterior and posterior capsule along with anterior vitreous are removed with the help of vitreous cutter, infusion and suction device.

Indication

- All cataracts occuring in childhood both congenital or acquired are easily treated by this procedure. It is specially useful in very young children (less than 2 years of age) in which primary IOL is not planned.
- Lensectomy is preferred in cataracts secondary to chronic anterior uveitis (Stills' disease) and in special cases of congenital cataracts, e.g. total rubella cataract, ectopia lentis, subluxated lens.

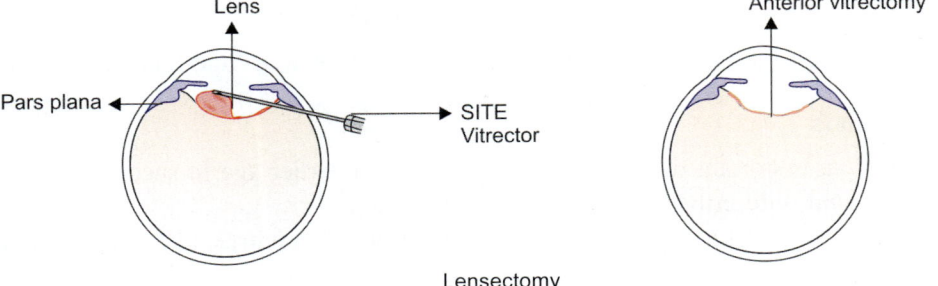

Lensectomy

Technique

Lensectomy is done preferably through a pars plana. Lens and the anterior phase of vitreous are removed by vitreous cutter.
- Anterior chamber is entered with keratome and filled with viscoelastic substance.
- A small limbal or pars plana incision is made about 3 mm behind the limbus.
- The anterior capsule and lens material is cut and aspirated through a fine bore needle or vitrectomy instruments such as:
    i. SITE (suction infusion time extractor) vitrector.
    ii. Vitreous stripper.
    iii. VISC (Vitreous infusion suction cutter).

- Finally the posterior capsule is removed and a shallow anterior vitrectomy performed.
- Viscoelastic substance is aspirated with the help of two way cannula.
- A well constructed sclera tunnel may not require suturing, but placement of one horizontal suture (with 10-0 nylon) ensures wound stability and reduces postoperative astigmatism.
- A peripheral rim of capsule can be left as an alternative to complete lensectomy for secondary IOL implantation at a later date by some surgeons.

Visual Rehabilitation

i. Spectales—They are useful for older children with bilateral aphakia but not for unilateral aphakia.
ii. Contact lenses—These are superior optical solution for both bilateral and unilateral aphakia
iii. IOL implantation—These are increasingly being performed in young children and even infants, specially in unilateral cataract. The IOL should be of a single piece type, i.e. optic and haptic in one piece with diameter not more than 12 mm. It is fitted in the capsular bag in the posterior chamber. Implantation of anterior chamber IOL is discontinued in the mid-1980s due to major complications such as corneal decompensation and secondary glaucoma.
- Rigid IOL—One piece rigid IOL is made of polymethyl methacrylate (PMMA)
- Foldable IOL—It is hydrophobic, foldable, acrylic polymer lens
- Rollable IOL—It is ultrathin and implanted through microincision (1 mm) after phaconit technique. It is made up of hydrogel.

Power of IOL—In children below 2 years, an undercorrection by 20% is recommended. In children between 2-8 years of age 10% undercorrection from the calculated biometric power is recommended to counter the 'myopic shift'.

iv. Occlusion—Occlusion of better eye is done to treat or prevent amblyopia.

SENILE CATARACT

This is the commonest type of acquired cataract. It is also known as 'age related cataract'.

Etiopathogenesis

- Heredity play an important role and it may appear at an earlier age in successive generations. This phenomenon is described as a history of 'anticipation'.
- The average age of onset is about 10 years earlier in tropical countries like India as compared to temperate climates. This may be due to exposure to sunlight (UV-A, UV-B radiation).
- Risk factors for cataract include increasing age, diabetes, atopic dermatitis, myotonic dystrophy, trauma, etc.

Cataract is caused by:
i. Degeneration and opacification of the lens fibres already formed.
ii. Formation of aberrant lens fibres—These are produced when the germinal epithelium of lens loses its ability to form normal fibres as happens in posterior subcapsular cataract.
iii. Fibrous metaplasia of the lens fibres may occur in complicated cataract.
iv. Abnormal product of metabolism, drugs or metals can be deposited in storage diseases (Fabry), metabolic diseases (Wilson) and toxic reactions (siderosis).

Classification

Morphologically, the senile cataract occurs in two forms:
1. Senile cortical cataract (soft cataract)
    i. Cuneiform cataract
    ii. Cupuliform cataract
2. Senile nuclear cataract (hard cataract).

It is common to find cortical and nuclear senile cataracts co-existing together in one eye. In general, the relative frequency of cunieform cataract is 70%, nuclear 25% and cupuliform cataract is 5% approximately.

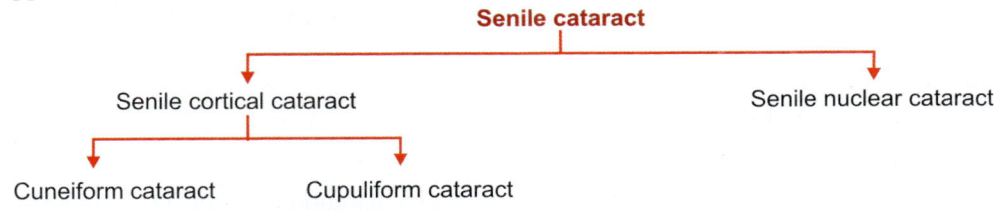

SENILE CORTICAL CATARACT (Soft Cataract)

It is the most common type of senile cataract.

Etiology

It occurs due to the degeneration of lens fibres already formed. Any physical or chemical factor which disturbs the intra and extracellular equilibrium of water and electrolytes causes opacification of lens.

Biochemical changes responsible for cataract formation are:
1. *Hydration*—It occurs due to osmotic changes and changes in the semipermeability of lens capsule. The entire lens swells up and becomes opaque.
2. *Denaturation and coagulation of proteins*—It leads to the formation of dense, irreversible lenticular opacity.

Incidence

Age—It is common after 50 years of age usually.
Sex—Both sexes are affected equally.

It is usually *bilateral* but develops in one eye earlier.

Symptoms

1. Frequent changes of glasses occur due to rapid change in the refractive index of lens.
2. Diminished visual acuity—It is gradual, painless and progressive. This is mainly due to reduction in transparency of the lens.
3. Monocular diplopia or polyopia—It is common in cortical spoke - like (cuneiform) opacities along with clear water clefts.
4. Glare—There is increased scattering of light.
5. Coloured halos around light are seen due to presence of irregular refractive index in different parts of the lens.

Morphological Types

i. Cuneiform cataract
ii. Cupuliform cataract

Clinical Stages

In senile cortical cataract presenile changes are the rule.

STAGES OF SENILE CORTICAL CATARACT

1. Immature cataract	i. Lamellar separation
	ii. Incipient
	iii. Intumescent
2. Mature cataract	
3. Hypermature or Morgangnian cataract	

1. ***Stage of lamellar separation***
   1. There is demarcation of cortical fibres due to their separation by fluid. This can be seen only by the slit-lamp or ophthalmoscopic examination.
   2. Grey appearance of pupil—It is due to increase in the refractive index of the cortex and due to increased reflection and scattering of light.

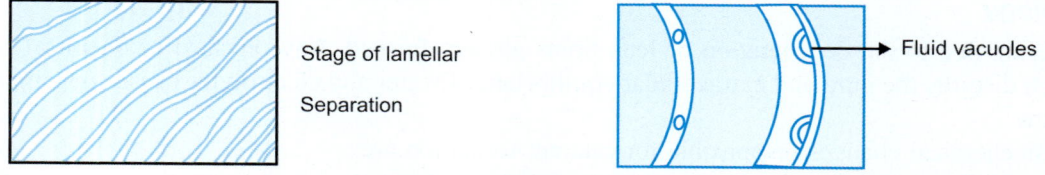

Stage of lamellar Separation

Stage of lamellar separation

2. ***Incipient cataract***
   1. Lens striae—The wedge-shaped or spokes-like opacities (Cuneiform opacities) appear in the periphery of the lens with clear areas in between. They are most common in the lower nasal quadrant. Later their apices appear within pupillary margin.
   2. Polyopia may be present due to irregular refraction.
   3. The vision is impaired as the visual axis is involved in the later stage.
   4. Coloured halos are seen which make and break while doing Fincham's test.

Incipient cataract

3. ***Intumescent cataract***
   1. Deeper layers of the cortex become cloudy and opaque.
   2. Progressive hydration causes swelling of the lens, making the anterior chamber shallow. It may lead to phacomorphic type of secondary glaucoma.
   3. Coloured halos may be seen due to hydration of the lens.

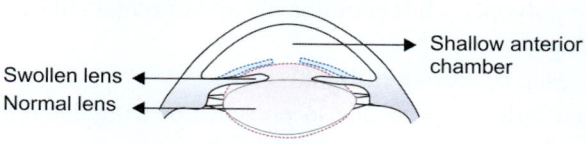

Intumescent cataract

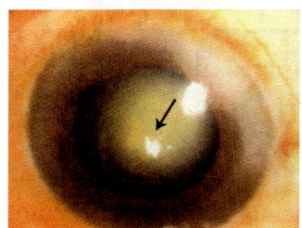
Immature cataract

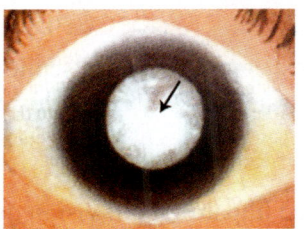
Mature cataract

4. **Mature cataract**
   1. Entire cortex is opaque and the swelling subsides.
   2. Nucleus suffers little change except there is progressive sclerosis.
   3. Iris shadow test—The iris shadow is absent.
      i. Immature cataract—When there is clear lens substance between the pupillary margin and the opacity, the iris throws a semilunar shadow on the deeper lens opacity.

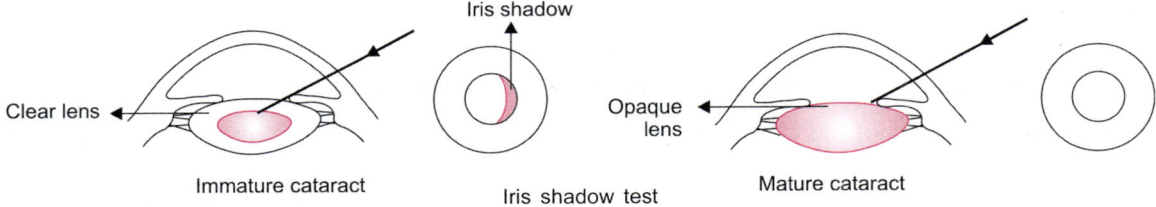

   ii. In mature cataract the cortex is completely opaque. The iris shadow is absent as iris is separated by only lens capsule from the opaque lens.

5. **Hypermature (Morgagnian) cataract**
   1. Cortex—It becomes fluid and appears milky.
   2. Nucleus—It is small, brownish and sinks by gravity in the bag of liquefied cortex (*Morgagnian cataract*). The edge of the nucleus is seen as brown semicircular line. The nucleus alters its position with the position of head.
   3. Anterior capsule—It is thickened with deposition of calcium salt on the surface. Later on fluid cortex may get absorbed due to leakage resulting in the formation of membranous cataract with a very small nucleus.

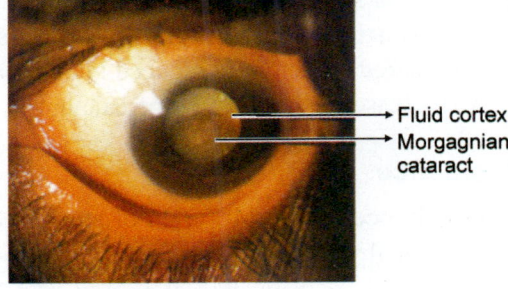
Hypermature morgagnian cataract

   4. Iridodonesis—There is tremulousness of iris as its support is lost due to shrinkage of lens.
   5. Anterior chamber is deep due to lack of support of the lens.
   6. Subluxation of lens may occur due to degeneration of suspensory ligament.
   7. Phacolytic glaucoma may occur due to leakage of lens protein which is ingested by the phagocytes. These large phagocytes obstruct the angle of anterior chamber.

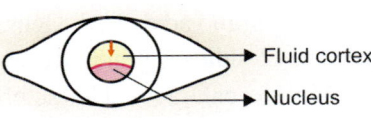
Hypermature cataract

   8. Phacoanaphylactic uveities—Lens protein may leak into the anterior chamber which act as antigens causing antigen antibody reaction leading to uveitis.

CUPULIFORM CATARACT

It is the second most common type of senile cortical cataract. There is dense aggregation of opacities just beneath the capsule usually in the posterior cortex.

Symptom
1. There is marked impairment of vision due to the opacity being near the nodal point of the eye.
2. Glare—There is increased scattering of light.
3. There is loss of ability to see objects in bright sunlight or being blinded by light when driving at night. This is due to loss of contrast sensitivity.

Signs
1. Slit-lamp examination—A yellow layer is seen in the posterior cortex.
2. Ophthalmoscopic examination—It is difficult to see the opacity clearly. A vaguely defined opacity is seen in the posterior cortex. It can be detected as a dark shadow on distant direct ophthalmoscopy.

SENILE NUCLEAR CATARACT

There is slow sclerosis of the central nuclear fibres but the cortical fibres remain transparent and clear.

Etiology
There is slow sclerosis of the nucleus due to long-term effect of the ultraviolet irradiation. There is photo-oxidation of aromatic amino acids. This results in the following biochemical changes in the lens
  i. Formation of brown pigment and deposition of abnormal lipoproteins.
 ii. Marked reduction in reduced glutathion.
iii. Increased concentration of calcium.

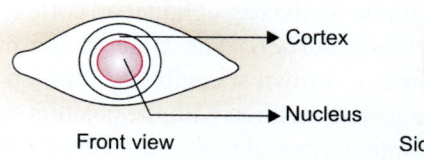

Senile nuclear cataract

Incidence
It usually occurs after 40 years of age, i.e. earlier than cortical variety.

Clinical Stages
1. Black cataract (Cataracta brunescens)—The nucleus becomes diffusely cloudy and dark. It may become brown, dusky red or black occasionally due to deposition of melanin pigment derived from amino acids in the lens.
2. The cloudiness gradually spreads towards the cortex.
3. Mature cataract—The sclerosis extends upto the capsule and the entire lens functions as a nucleus. There is progressive myopia.
4. Hypermaturity does not occur as the process is very slow.

Symptoms
1. There is visual impairment due to progressive myopia and central opacity.
2. There may be 'second sight' or 'myopic shift'. There is change in refractive index of the nucleus which causes index myopia, resulting in improvement of near vision.
3. Colour shift—The blue end of the spectrum is absorbed more by the cataractous lens. It becomes more obvious after cataract surgery.

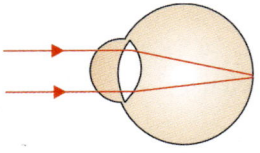

Normal eye

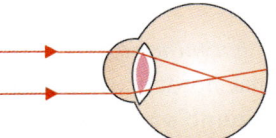

Nuclear cataract-Progressive myopia

Signs
1. Blackened pupillary reflex is seen due to nuclear sclerosis.
2. Ophthalmoscopic examination—The details of the fundus cannot be seen due to hazy media.

COMPLICATED CATARACT

Complicated cataract occurs as a result of any disease or pathology in the eye.

Etiology
There is disturbance to the nutrition of the lens due to the inflammatory or degenerative diseases of the other parts of the eye.

1. Inflammatory diseases
  i. Iridocyclitis
  ii. Choroiditis

2. Degenerative diseases
  i. High myopia
  ii. Pigmentary retinal dystrophy
  iii. Retinal detachment

Symptom
There is markedly impaired vision due to presence of opacity near the nodal point in the posterior cortex.

Signs
1. *Inflammation of the anterior segment*
    - It causes opacification of the cortex.
    - It usually progresses and matures rapidly.
2. *Posterior segment diseases*
    - It causes characteristic posterior cortical cataract.
3. *Ophthalmoscopic examination*—Vaguely defined, dark area is seen in the posterior cortex against red background.

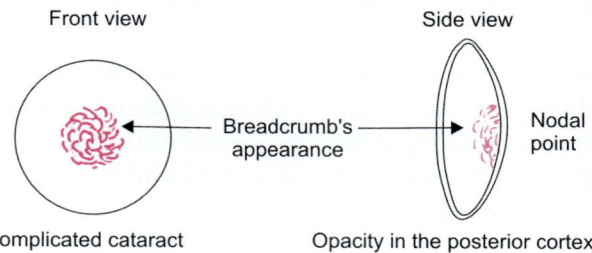

Complicated cataract — Opacity in the posterior cortex

4. *Slit-lamp examination*
    i. Irregular borders of opacity extend towards the equator and the nucleus.
    ii. Breadcrumb's appearance is seen.
    iii. Polychromatic lustre, i.e. rainbow display of different colours is present.

Course

1. It may remain stationary indefinitely.
2. Eventually whole of the posterior cortex is affected.
3. Total soft and uniform cataract is formed eventually.

DIABETIC CATARACT

In diabetes mellitus senile cataract develops early and progresses rapidly. True diabetic cataract is a rare condition occurring typically in young persons due to acute diabetes.

When blood sugar levels are elevated beyond 200 mg per ml, excess glucose is converted to sorbitol. This accumulates in the lens fibres and causes osmotic imbalance.

Slit-lamp Examination

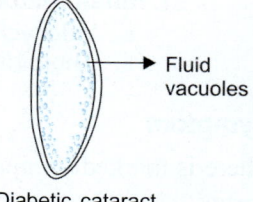

Diabetic cataract

i. Immense number of fluid vacuoles appear under the anterior and posterior capsule. It is a reversible process.
ii. Numerous snow flakes are seen all over the cortex causing milky white appearance.

PARATHYROID TETANY

There is deficiency of parathyroid hormone due to atrophic parathyroid gland or removal of parathyroid glands accidentally during thyroidectomy.

Slit-lamp Examination

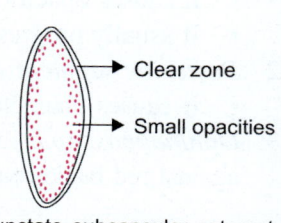

Punctate subcapsular cataract

i. Clouds of small discrete opacities appear in the cortex, separated from the capsule by a clear zone.
ii. They coalesce to form large crystalline flakes.
iii. Lens is opaque usually within 6 months. Operative prognosis is good.

MYOTONIC DYSTROPHY
Clinical features are same as above, i.e. punctate subcapsular cataract is formed.

MONGOLIAN IDIOCY (DOWN SYNDROME) AND CRETINISM
Clinical features are similar to punctate subcapsular cataract.

GALACTOSAEMIA
It is a rare congenital disease occurring in infants. It causes bilateral cataract typical (oil drop cataract) due to inborn inability to metabolize galactose. Therefore, milk and milk products are eliminated from the diet.

Drug Induced
Steroids, both systemic and topical are cataractogenic. Chlorpromazine, Busulphan, Amiodarone, Gold and Allopurinol are the other drugs associated with cataract.

CATARACT DUE TO RADIANT OR HEAT ENERGY
1. *Heat (infrared)*—It is common in glass and iron industry workers. It results in posterior cortical cataract.
2. *Irradiation*—Irradiation by X-ray, γ-rays and neutrons results in formation of posterior cortical cataract near posterior pole.
3. *Electric*—It occurs due to passage of a powerful current in the body. There is formation of punctate, subcapsular opacities which mature rapidly.
4. *Ultrasonic radiation*—Lens opacities are formed due to heat and concussion produced by ultrasonic radiation.

TRAUMATIC CATARACT
Concussion and perforating corneal injuries cause traumatic cataract. Early or late Rosette-shaped' cataract is formed usually in the posterior cortex or at times in the anterior cortex or both.

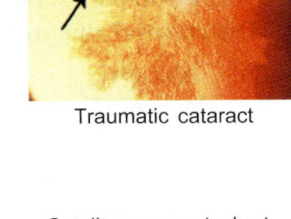

Traumatic cataract

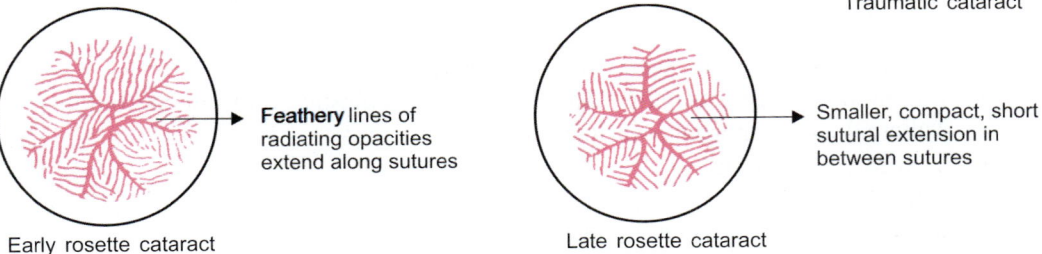

Early rosette cataract → **Feathery** lines of radiating opacities extend along sutures

Late rosette cataract → Smaller, compact, short sutural extension in between sutures

SYMPTOMS OF ACQUIRED CATARACT
These are entirely visual. There is gradual loss of vision.

Early
1. *Glare* is one of the earliest visual disturbances with cataract. It is the excessive awareness of light, such as direct sunlight or headlights of an oncoming motor vehicle. Commonly occurs with posterior subcapsular cataract due to excessive irregular scattering of light.

2. Frequent changes of glasses.
3. *Black spots* are seen before the eyes. These are stationary and retain their relative position in the field of vision. They can be easily differentiated from muscae volitantes in the vitreous which are mobile.
4. *Uniocular diplopia or polyopia*, i.e. seeing double or triple objects occur due to irregular refraction of lens particularly in the incipient stage.
5. *Coloured halos* are seen due to hydration of the lens which results in irregularity in the refractive index of different parts of the lens.
6. *Colour value changes* due to absorption of the shorter wavelength. Thus, red colour is accentuated (nuclear cataract).

Late

Central vision is impaired depending on position and density of opacity.
1. *Peripheral opacity*—Vision is not affected usually. Vision improves in bright light due to miosis or constriction of the pupil.
2. *Central opacity*—Early visual loss is present. Vision improves in dim light due to mydriasis or dilatation of pupil.
3. *Posterior cortical cataract*—Visual loss is out of proportion to the size of opacity as it is close to the nodal point.
4. *Nuclear sclerosis*—There is progressive myopia so the presbyopic person gets "second sight" or "improvement" in vision without the glasses.
5. *Mature cataract*—The vision is grossly reduced to counting fingers at few cm or hand movement or perception of light with good projection of rays.

SIGNS OF CATARACT

1. White pupillary reflex (leucocoria) is seen in mature cataract.
   Differential diagnosis of white pupillary reflex [Leucocoria]
   In Children
   i. Congenital cataract
   ii. Retinoblastoma.
   iii. Pseudogliomas—They are seen in children usually.
   - Inflammatory deposits in the vitreous following a plastic cyclitis or choroiditis.
   - Tuberculosis of choroid (confluent type).
   - Toxocara infestation.
   - Congenital defects due to persistent hyperplastic vitreous at the back of the lens.
   - Retrolental fibroplasia (Retinopathy of prematurity).
   iv. Other causes— i. Coats' disease, ii. Choroidal coloboma, iii. Retinal dysplasia.
   In Adults
   i. Senile mature and hypermature cataract
   ii. Occlusio-pupillae
   iii. Cyclitic membrane.
   iv. Total retinal detachment.
   v. After or secondary cataract.

2. Plane mirror examination—(at a distance of 1 M). This is done after dilatation of the pupil. Black coloured opacity is seen against a red background.
3. Plane mirror examination at a distance of 22 cm (distant direct ophthalmoscopy)—The exact position of the opacity is determined by parallactic displacement.
4. Direct ophthalmoscopy—The surgeon looks through a self-luminous ophthalmoscope and directs the light upon the pupil. Black coloured opacity is seen against a uniform red background.

COMMON CAUSES OF GRADUAL LOSS OF VISION

1. Cataract—Acquired, congenital, after cataract
2. Glaucoma—Open angle glaucoma, chronic congestive glaucoma
3. Refractive errors—Myopia, hypermetropia, astigmatism
4. Uveitis and its complications—Chronic iridocyclitis, secondary glaucoma, complicated cataract, choroiditis, etc.
5. Macular degeneration, dystrophy and diabetic maculopathy.
6. Retinal causes—Diabetic and hypertensive retinopathy, retinitis pigmentosa.
7. Keratitis, keratoconus and corneal dystrophies.
8. Vitreous degenerations and vitreous opacities.
9. Tobacco amblyopia

Complications

1. Phacoanaphylactic uveitis—In hypermature cataract lens proteins may leak into anterior chamber. These may act as antigens and induce antigen-antibody reaction leading to uveitis.
2. Lens-induced glaucoma—It may occur due to an intumescent lens (phacomorphic glaucoma) or due to leakage of proteins into the anterior chamber from an hypermature cataract (phacolytic glaucoma).
3. Subluxation and dislocation of lens may occur due to degeneration of zonules in hypermature stage.

DIFFERENCES BETWEEN IMMATURE AND MATURE CATARACT

SIGNS	IMMATURE CATARACT	MATURE CATARACT
1. Visual acuity	• Impaired	• Markedly impaired (HM, PL)
2. Pupillary reflex	• Grey	• White
3. Iris shadow	• Present	• Absent
4. Purkinje's image	• All 4 images are present	• Absence of 4th Purkinje's image
5. Plane mirror examination at 1 m	• Black opacity against a red background	• No red glow seen
6. Distant direct ophthalmoscopy at 22 cm	• Same as above	• Same as above
7. Ophthalmoscopic examination	• Same as above	• Same as above

PREOPERATIVE INVESTIGATIONS

Prior to planning cataract operation, including intraocular lens (IOL) implantation, it is important to know about the general health of the patient as well as the ocular condition.

1. *Examination of the eye* is done carefully specially in cases of complicated cataract.
    i. *Pupillary reactions*—The normal functions of optic nerve and retina are assessed.
    ii. *Visual acuity* and projection of rays indicate retinal function.
    iii. *Intraocular pressure* is recorded to rule out glaucoma.
    iv. *Patency of lacrimal apparatus* is tested to exclude chronic dacryocystitis.
2. *Systemic examination* is done for diabetes, hypertension, ischaemic heart disease and gross focal sepsis.
3. *Fundus examination* is done in both eyes to detect any retinal diseases.
4. *When fundus cannot be seen*, the following tests are done to find out the condition of posterior segment,
    I. *Projection of light*—This test is of utmost importance. The test is done in a dark room with one eye covered. Patient is asked to look straight ahead. Light is thrown from various directions and the patient points the correct direction.

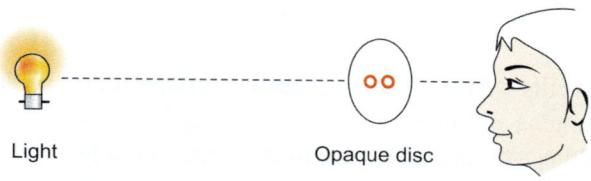

Two point discrimination test

II. *Macular function test*
   i. *Two point discrimination test*—Patient looks through an opaque disc perforated in the centre with two pinholes close together. If the central area of retina is good, the patient appreciates the two lights.
   ii. *Maddox rod test*—Patient looks at a distant light through the Maddox rod. The macular function is good if the red line is straight and unbroken.

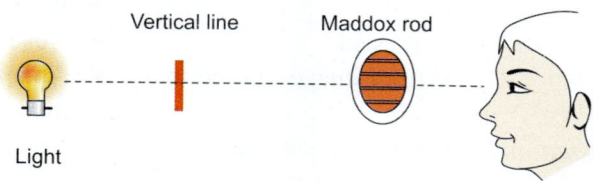

Maddox rod test

   iii. *Entoptic view of the retina*—The eyes are closed and globe is firmly massaged through the lower lid with a bare lighted bulb of a torch. The patient sees the vascular tree of the retina on an orange background. Any blanks or scotomas are noted.

iv. *Foveal electroretinogram (ERG)*—It indicates the condition of fovea and macula.
   v. *Ultrasonic investigation by B-scan*—Retinal detachment and vitreous pathology may be detected.
   vi. *Laser interference fringes*—Postoperative visual acuity is assessed by focusing light beams from two sources (helium—neon) which overlap equally posterior to the plane of the lens.
   vii. *Photo stress test*—The eye is exposed to bright light for 15 seconds and recovery time is noted. In macular disease, recovery time is prolonged.

INDICATIONS FOR CATARACT EXTRACTION

1. **Visual improvement**—Interference with the routine of a patient's life is the most important indication. A visual acuity of 6/12 or 6/18 with accommodation is considered better than 6/6 without accommodation. However, it depends on the individual's requirement and type of work.
2. **Medical causes**—Presence of cataract may adversely affect the eye as in,
   i. Phacolytic glaucoma—It results due to leakage of lens protein (hypermature cataract).
   ii. Phacomorphic glaucoma—The swollen lens pushes the iris forwards (intumescent stage).
   iii. Retinal diseases like diabetic retinopathy or retinal detachment, treatment of which cannot be done in presence of cataract.

TREATMENT OF SENILE CATARACT

Medical Treatment

No medical treatment is effective once opacities have developed.

Surgical Treatment

The technique of cataract extraction has changed drastically in recent years due to the introduction of operating microscope and intraocular lens implant. However, the modern trend is in favour of extracapsular lens extraction along with intraocular lens implantation. This reduces the incidence of vitreous loss to the minimum with superior visual results.

The type of operation depends on the individual case.

In elderly persons the nucleus is hard and it can be removed by the following methods:
1. *Intracapsular cataract extraction (ICCE)*—It has become obsolete nowadays.
2. *Extracapsular cataract extraction (ECCE)*
3. *Phacoemulsification*
4. *Phacolysis.*

Choice of Surgical Technique

In the modern age ECCE is considered as the procedure of choice. Intracapsular cataract extraction (ICCE) has become obsolete nowadays. The choice of a particular surgical technique depends upon the following factors:

1. *Age of patient*—ICCE is contraindicated (due to presence of strong zonules) below 40 years of age. Therefore ECCE technique is employed in young patients.
2. *Availability of surgical facilities*—If facilities for microsurgery are available then ECCE is performed for cataracts after the age of 40 years.
3. *Surgical skill of the surgeon*—If surgeon is trained in microsurgery then ECCE should be performed.
4. *Eye camps*—Nowadays in eye camps ECCE is performed.
5. *Posterior chamber intraocular lens (PCIOL) implantation*—ECCE is the choice of operation as PCIOL implantation is possible only after ECCE.
6. *In high myopia*—ECCE should be preferred due to presence of fluid vitreous.
7. *In subluxated and dislocated lens*—ICCE should be done as the lens is surrounded by vitreous.

I. PREOPERATIVE PREPARATIONS

1. *Prophylactic antibiotics*—Local and systemic broad-spectrum antibiotics should be started at least one day prior to surgery.
2. *The pupil is dilated* with a combination of medications which include topical cycloplegics which paralyze the sphincter pupillae (cyclopentolate, tropicamide or homatropine drops), mydriatics which stimulate the dilator pupillae (phenylephrine) and nonsteroidal anti-inflammatory agents (diclofenac or ketorolac). The latter inhibit prostaglandin release from the iris on mechanical stimulation during surgery and prevent intraoperative miosis.
3. *Anaesthesia and akinesia*—Most of the cataract surgery is done under local anaesthesia except in children and uncooperative patients.
    I. Topical—4% xylocaine, 0.5% proparacaine, etc. Topical anaesthesia with paracaine or 2% lignocaine jelly supplemented with intracameral injection of preservative free lignocaine, if required, provides only anaesthesia and is being increasingly used for phacoemulsification surgery.
    II. Block—2% xylocaine with adrenaline (epinephrine), 0.5% bupivacaine and hyaluronidase. In hypertensive patients, adrenaline should not be used.
        i. **Facial nerve block**
            a. *O' Briens' method*—5 cc of anaesthetic is injected on the neck of the mandible just below the condyle. The facial nerve is paralysed so that the patient is unable to squeeze the eyelids during operation due to orbicularis oculi muscle paralysis.
            b. *Van Lints method*—Local anaesthetic is injected near the outer canthus of the eye.
        ii. **Ciliary block by retrobulbar injection**
            1-2 cc of anaesthetic is injected into the neighbourhood of ciliary ganglion behind the eyeball. It causes anaesthesia of deeper structures like iris and lowers the intraocular pressure. It also results in mydriasis and akinesia of extraocular muscles. It is associated with risk of causing retrobulbar haemorrhage and bulbar penetration.
        iii. **Peribulbar anaesthesia**—It is a much safer alternative method. The patient looks up straight at the ceiling and 5 ml of local anaesthetic is injected from the lateral part of the lower lid. A 23 G needle measuring 2.5 cm is directed almost straight into the deeper

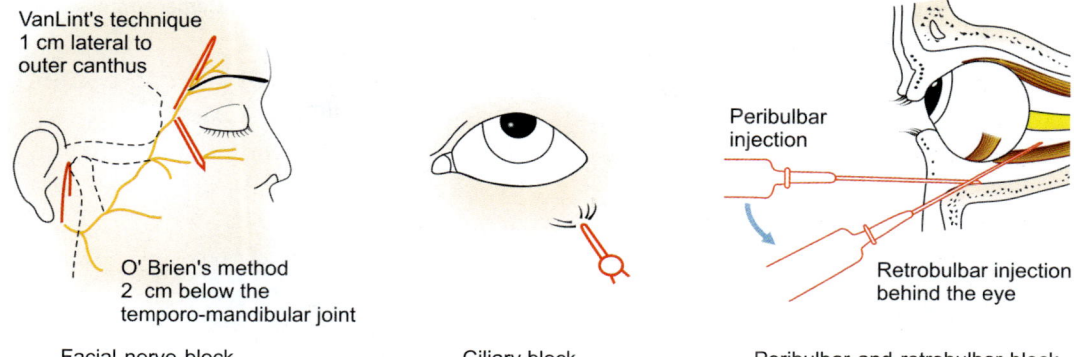

Facial nerve block • Ciliary block • Peribulbar and retrobulbar block

tissues and not in the muscle cone. The anaesthetic infiltrates into the retrobulbar space by the application of superpinkie ball (30 mm Hg pressure) for 15-20 minutes. Facial block is not required/necessary.

Complications of anaesthesia include:
- Retrobulbar or peribulbar haemorrhage
- Accidental globe perforation
- Accidental injection into optic nerve sheath with intracranial spread
- Anaphylactic shock
- Vasovagal reflex resulting in collapse and death.

4. *Ocular hypotony*—In most cases hypotony is achieved by the application of superpinkie ball or manual pressure. Single oral dose of 500 mg of acetazolamide or intravenous 200 ml mannitol (20%) given preoperatively is also effective.

II. OPERATIVE TECHNIQUES

A. Corneoscleral Section

i. **Ab-interno incision**—It has become obsolete nowadays.
It was made in the classical way by the von Graefe knife. It is introduced in the right eye at 9 O'clock position and is brought out at 3 O'clock and vice versa for the left eye. By slow zigzag movement of the knife, the corneoscleral section is completed. This was used for intracapsular lens extraction specially in eye camps.

ii. **Ab-externo incision**
A conjunctival flap is made 3 mm away from limbus around the upper half of cornea.
- While the eye is studied by a fixation forceps, a Bard-Parker knife with a D blade incises the sclera at the limbus.
- The anterior chamber is entered and the curved corneal scissors completes the incision.

Advantages of ab-externo Incision
i. There is great accuracy in the selection of site of corneoscleral section.
ii. Protection is offered to the corneoscleral section by the conjunctival flap.
iii. Gradual release of intraocular pressure prevents chances of expulsive haemorrhage.

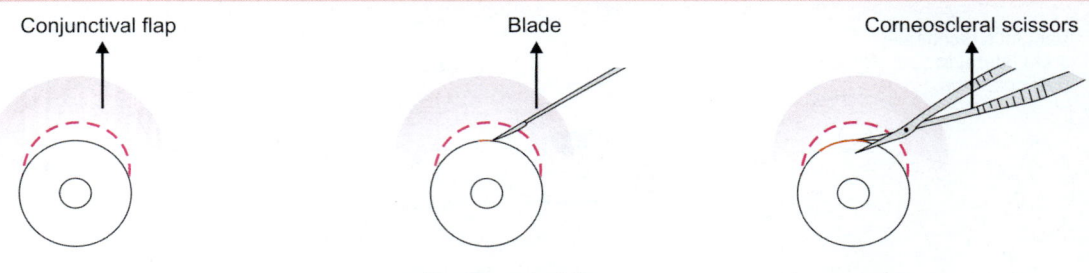

Ab-externo incision

B. Lens Extraction

1. INTRACAPSULAR CATARACT EXTRACTION (ICCE)

At present it has become obsolete. The entire lens along with the capsule is removed by intracapsular forceps or cryoprobe by rupturing the zonules.

ICCE has stood the test of time and has been widely used for about 50 years all over the world. However for the last 25 years it has been replaced by planned extracapsular technique.

Indications

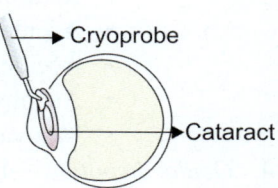

i. Subluxated lens—The lens is tilted due to partial rupture of zonule.
ii. Dislocated lens—The zonules are broken completely.

Technique

1. *Intracapsular forceps cataract extraction*
   - After the corneoscleral section is made, a small peripheral buttonhole iridectomy is performed at 12 O' clock position to prevent pupillary block.
   - Intracapsular forceps are introduced and the lens capsule is grasped just in front of the equator either above or below (capsule is thick at these sites).
2. *Cryoprobe cataract extraction*
   - Alternatively, the cornea is lifted by an assistant, anterior chamber is dried by spontex or cotton swab and cryoprobe is applied to the upper part of lens to form an iceball.
   - The lens is lifted, rotated and removed through the wound by sliding method.

Intracapsular Lens Extraction with Cryoprobe

- Sterile air is injected to reform the anterior chamber.
- Preplaced corneoscleral sutures (5-6) are tied and the conjunctival flap is sutured.
- A subconjunctival injection of gentamicin and dexamethasone is given postoperatively.

Advantages of cryoprobe application—It is the preferred technique for intracapsular lens extraction as there are less chances of capsular rupture and vitreous loss.

Complications

1. *Immediate Complications*

a. *Prolapse of vitreous* (vitreous loss) is a serious complication.

Prophylaxis: Vitreous loss can be prevented by lowering the tension:
  i. Preoperative administration of acetazolamide 500 mg oral or IV.
  ii. Mannitol (20%) 200 ml IV drip may be given preoperatively.
  iii. Flieringa ring used to be sewn on to the globe to avoid its collapse.
  iv. Preoperative digital pressure is applied intermittently.
  v. Use of relaxants by the anaesthetist during general anaesthesia.
  vi. Pressure by pinkie or super pinkie ball is applied for 15-20 minutes with intermittent release of pressure every few minutes.
  Treatment—Open sky vitrectomy should be performed.

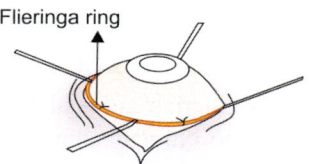
Position of Flieringa ring before the eye is opened

b. *Rupture of capsule*—The incidence of capsule rupture is minimum with cryoprobe.

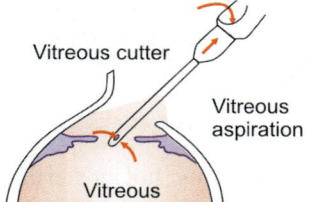
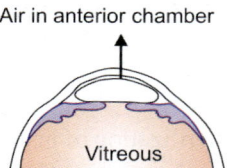

Management of vitreous loss by vitreous cutter

c. *Expulsive haemorrhage*—In hypertensive and arteriosclerotic patients and in cases of raised IOP, sudden lowering of intraocular pressure causes rupture of choroidal vessel. The lens, vitreous, retina and choroid are expelled out along with severe haemorrhage and the eye is lost.

2. Late Complications

a. *Striate keratitis* due to folds in Descemet's membrane and corneal oedema usually disappears in a few days postoperatively.
b. *Iris prolapse* may occur due to inadequate wound closure and raised tension.
c. *Hyphaema* may occur spontaneously or due to trauma.
d. *Delayed formation of anterior chamber* is seen due to leaking section, pupillary block or choroidal detachment.
e. *Cystoid macular oedema*—It is a common complication. Typically visual acuity is good initially and then declines few days after lens extraction.
f. *Infection* leading to iridocyclitis, endophthalmitis or panophthalmitis may occur following vitreous loss as vitreous is a good culture medium.

3. Delayed Complications

a. *Aphakic glaucoma* may occur due to pupillary block or presence of vitreous in the anterior chamber. This blocks the angle of anterior chamber.
b. *Detachment of retina* may result specially in cases of vitreous loss followed by formation of fibrous bands.

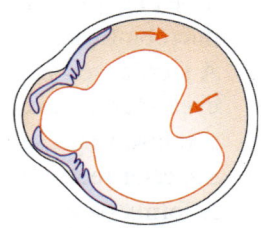
Aphakic glaucoma

c. *Epitheliazation of the anterior chamber* may occur due to the growth of the conjunctival epithelium in the anterior chamber specially over the angle.

2. EXTRACAPSULAR CATARACT EXTRACTION (ECCE)

The modern trend is in favour of ECCE with posterior chamber IOL implantation. This technique has replaced intracapsular cataract extraction. The posterior capsule and part of the anterior capsule are left behind after extracapsular lens extraction. The nucleus is removed along with aspiration and irrigation of cortex. The most essential requirements for extracapsular cataract extraction with IOL are:

i. Perfect coaxial illumination
ii. Adjustable magnification with zoom system
iii. Instrumentation for extracapsular surgery vary from simple to complex ones such as various cannulae, SITE (suction infusion time extractor) or Cavitron.

Sterilization

Various methods of sterilization of instruments include autoclaving, hot air sterilization, ethylene oxide gas, acetone and formalin vapour sterilization.

Indications

i. Posterior chamber intraocular lens implant in patients of all ages whether young or old. In young patients upto the age of 30 years lens aspiration or lensectomy is usually effective. In older patients the nucleus is hard and must be extracted.
ii. High myopia with degenerated fluid vitreous.

Technique

1. Conventional ECCE
2. Manual small incision cataract surgery
3. Phacoemulsification
4. Phakonit
5. Laser phacolysis.

1. CONVENTIONAL ECCE

1. Eye is cleaned with 5% betadine lotion applied to the skin of the eyelids and allowed to dry. One drop of 5% betadine lotion is instilled into the conjunctival sac to eliminate local saprophylactic microbiological flora.
2. A sterile, self adhesive plastic drape is applied to the skin on and around the eyelids and the eyelashes are excluded from the operative field by folding the edges of the drape around them and inserting a self-retaining speculum to hold the lids open.
3. Superior rectus bridle suture is passed to fix the eye in down gaze.
4. A fornix based conjunctival flap is raised and limbus exposed.
5. Haemostasis is achieved by applying gentle cautery.

6. A circumferential vertical partial thickness groove or gutter is made at the limbus through about two-thirds depth from 10 to 2 O' clock and the anterior chamber entered. Alternatively, a small 2-3 mm corneoscleral section is made and a small buttonhole peripheral iridectomy is done at 12 O'clock.
7. Viscoelastic substances (ocular viscosurgical device OVD) such as methylcellulose, healon is injected in the anterior chamber specially to protect the endothelium and deeper tissues and to maintain the anterior chamber. They are of two main categories:
   i. Dispersive such as hydroxypropyl methylcellulose (HPMC) 2% and chondroitin sulphate
   ii. Viscoadhesive such as sodium hyaluronate 1%, 1.4% and 5%.
8. A cystitome or bent 26 G needle makes a series of small radial cuts in the anterior capsule (can opener). This is known as "can-opener" technique. Anterior capsulotomy can also be done by making a superior linear or curved opening (envelope technique) or by tearing off a flap in a continuous curvilinear fashion (continuous curvilinear capsulorrhexis) for 360° in shape of a ring.

Envelope

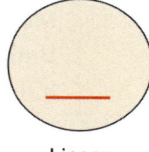
Linear

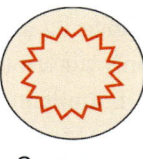
Canopener

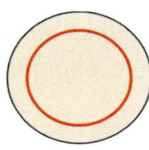
Continous circular capsulotomy (CCC)

Types of Anterior Capsulotomy

9. Hydrodissection—Balanced salt solution (BSS) is injected under the lens capsule to separate the cortex from the capsule.
10. Corneoscleral section is then enlarged (8-10 mm) using the corneoscleral section enlarging scissors.
11. Nucleus is delivered by pressing the scleral lip of the wound with an irrigating vectis and applying counter pressure at the opposite pole by gently pushing with a lens hook at the 6 O' clock position. (Pressure and counter pressure technique).
12. Residual cortical matter is aspirated using a two-way irrigation aspiration cannula. Cortical clean up is done with either a manual or automated infusion-aspiration device, e.g. Cavitron–Extraction–Irrigation system. Simcoe aspiration irrigation cannula, using balanced salt solution (BSS), Ringer's lactate or normal saline.
13. The capsular bag is inflated with viscoelastic substance.
14. Posterior chamber intraocular lens implant is gently inserted behind the iris with angled forceps (of Kelman and McPherson) under the lens capsule at 6 O' clock.
15. IOL is gently dialed with dialling hook (Sinskys) so that the haptics are placed at 180°.

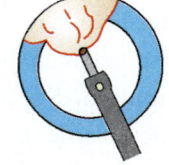
Aspiration of cortex

16. Viscoelastic substance is aspirated and incision is sutured by 3 to 5 interrupted or continuous 10.0 nylon sutures.
17. Conjunctival flap is reposited back and subconjunctival injection of dexamethasone and gentamicin is given.
18. Patching of the eye is done with a pad and a bandage may be applied.

COMPARATIVE STUDY OF INTRA- AND EXTRACAPSULAR CATARACT EXTRACTION

	INTRACAPSULAR	EXTRACAPSULAR
1. Vitreous loss	Risk of vitreous loss is present	No risk as the posterior capsule protects the vitreous
2. After cataract	Absent	May be present
3. Aphakic glaucoma	Usually in cases of vitreous loss or due to pupillary block	Rarely seen
4. Retinal detachment	Higher incidence	Minimum incidence
5. IOL implant	Only anterior chamber IOL implantation is possible	Both posterior and anterior IOL implantations are possible

Advantages of ECCE Over ICCE

1. The modern trend is in favour of ECCE with posterior chamber IOL implantation. ECCE can be performed at all ages except when zonules are not intact (subluxated, dislocated lens). Whereas ICCE cannot be performed below 40 years of age as the zonules are tight and there are greater chances of vitreous loss.
2. Posterior chamber IOL can be implanted only after ECCE. It cannot be implanted after ICCE.
3. Postoperative vitreous related problems (herniation in anterior chamber, pupillary block and vitreous touch syndrome) associated with ICCE are not seen after ECCE.
4. Incidence of postoperative complications such as endophthalimitis, cystoid macular oedema and retinal detachment are much less after ECCE as compared to that after ICCE.
5. Postoperative astigmatism is less as the incision is smaller in size.

Sutures

Sutures help in proper wound healing by keeping the cut edges of the cornea or limbus well apposed. Interrupted or continuous 10.0 monofilament nylon, perlon or absorbable vicryl (polyglactin) sutures are applied. Sutureless cataract surgery can be done with 2-3 mm incisions as in cases of phacoemulsification with scleral tunnel incision.

2. MANUAL SMALL INCISION CATARACT SURGERY

It is becoming very popular due to its merits over conventional ECCE. In this technique IOL implantation is done through a sutureless self-sealing valvular sclero-corneal tunnel incision.

1. Sclero-corneal tunnel incision—It consists of three components:
   - *Extenral scleral incision:* A 1/3 or 1/2 thickness external groove is made 1.5 - 2 mm behind the limbus. It varies from 5.5 - 7 mm in length depending on the size of the nucleus. It may be straight or semi-circular in shape.
   - *Sclero-corneal tunnel:* It is made with a crescent knife. It usually extends 1 - 1.5 mm into the clear cornea.
   - *Internal corneal incision:* It is made with a sharp 3.2 mm angled keratome.
2. Side-port entry is made at 9 O' clock position with a Stiletto or MVR (micro vitreal retinal) blade. A valvular self sealing incision about 1 mm wide is made at the limbus. This helps in aspiration of the sub-incisional cortex and increasing the depth of anterior chamber.
3. Anterior capsulotomy—It can be either a 'can-opener', envelop shaped or continuous circular capsulotomy (CCC). However, a large sized CCC is preferred.
4. Hydrodissection is essential to separate cortico-nuclear mass from the posterior capsule.
5. Removal of nucleus
   i. Prolapse of nucleus from the capsular bag into the anterior chamber is done during hydrodissection and completed by rotating the nucleus with Sinskey's hook.
   ii. Delivery of nucleus through the corneo-scleral tunnel is done by
      - Irrigating wire vectis method. It is used most commonly
      - Phacofracture technique
      - Phaco-sandwich technique
      - Blumenthals technique
      - Fish hook
      - Visco expression.

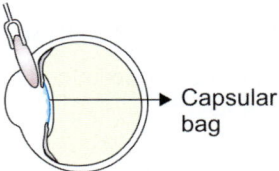
Capsular bag

6. Aspiration of the cortex is done by a two way irrigation and aspiration cannula from the main incision and side port entry.
7. A posterior chamber IOL is implanted in the capsular bag after filling it with viscoelastic substance (OVD).
8. Viscoelastic substance is then removed thoroughly from the anterior chamber and capsular bag with the help of a two way irrigation aspiration cannula.
9. Wound closure—The anterior chamber is deepened with balanced salt solution or Ringer's lactate (through side port entry). This results in self sealing the valvular incision. The conjunctival flap is reposited back.

3. PHACOEMULSIFICATION

Phacoemulsification is a sophisticated technique of extracapsular cataract extraction invented by Charles Kelman in 1967. It is the most popular method worldwide and has virtually replaced all other techniques in some well developed countries. This technique consists of breaking down of cataractous lens by application of ultrasonic vibrations. The machine is known as phacoemulsifier which has three functions:
   i. *Irrigation*—It is done by a gravity flow system. Balanced salt solution (BSS) is allowed to flow to the handpiece, which is controlled by foot switch.
   ii. *Aspiration*—The emulsified material is aspirated through peristaltic or venturi pump as irrigation maintains normal depth of the anterior chamber.

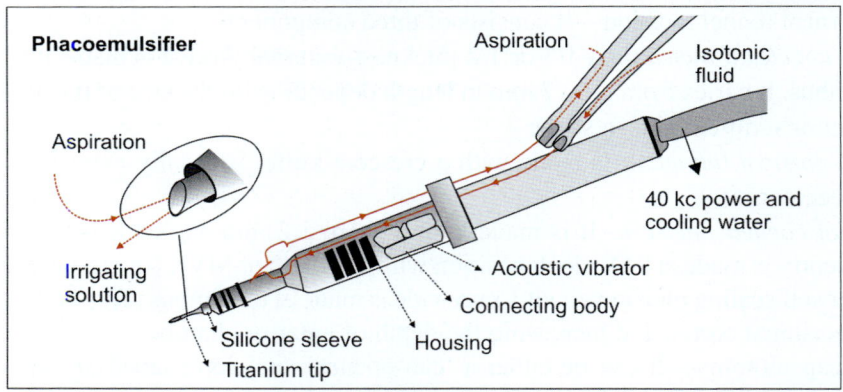

Phacoemulsifier

iii. *Fragmentation*—It is performed through a piezo-electric ultrasonic mechanism which activates a hollow 1 mm titanium needle, vibrating at the frequency of 40,000/sec (40 kilo-hertz ultrasonic energy). The amplitude of vibration is 0.038 mm from the resting point of the tip and the total to and fro motion is 0.076 mm (stroke length).

Technique of Phacoemulsification

The technique is constantly changing and has many variations. The basic steps are described as follows:

1. Phaco Incision

i. Scleral tunnel incision
ii. Clear corneal incision

At present scleral tunnel approach is most popular. Initially, incision is placed through half the scleral thickness, 1.5 to 2.0 mm away from the clear cornea. The length of the incision is about 3 mm. Dissection is carried out in the sclera and upto atleast 1 mm inside the cornea. The incision heals quickly, ambulation is quick and there is no induced astigmatism.

2. Anterior Capsulotomy [Continuous Curvilinear Capsulorrhexis (CCC)]

Continuous curvilinear capsulorrhexis of 4-6 mm is performed with bent needle cystitome or capsulorrhexis forceps after filling the anterior chamber with viscoelastic substance. Capsulorrhexis

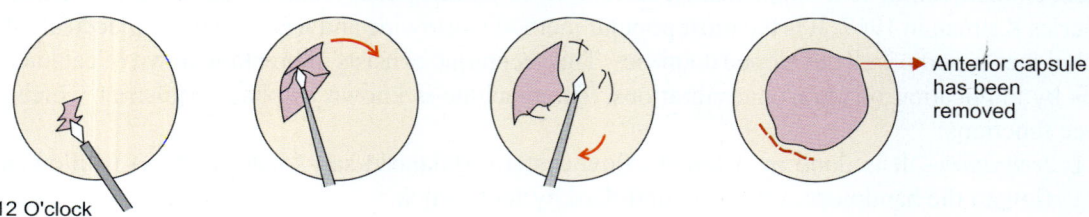

Continuous curvilinear capsulorrhexis

is started by making a small cut at the centre of the lens, pulling directly towards the 12 O'clock position and curving towards the left. This creates a central flap that tears in a circular pattern to the right. The flap is folded over and pulled by forceps in a circular motion and capsulorrhexis is complete.

3. *Hydroprocedures*

These procedures facilitate nucleus rotation and manipulation during phacoemulsification.
  i. *Hydrodissection*—It is the seperation of the capsule from the cortex by slowly injecting balanced saline solution between the two.
  ii. *Hydrodelineation*—A 26 gauze needle is inserted between the hard central nucleus and epinucleus and slowly balanced saline solution is injected. Thus cleavage is done between nucleus and epinucleus.

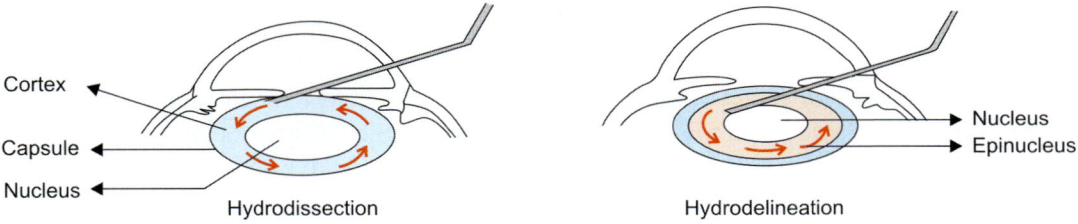

4. *Nucleus Emulsification*

The different densities of cataracts have created different methods of sculpting or breaking the nucleus in small fragments.
  i. In soft to moderately hard nucleus—A vertical 'trench' is sculpted and the procedure is called 'trench divide and conquer' (TDC).
  ii. In moderately hard to very hard nucleus—A deep central crater is sculpted and the procedure is called 'crater divide and conquer (CDC).

The other common methods are 'chip and flip technique' and 'phaco chop technique'. The nucleus is finally emulsified and aspirated.

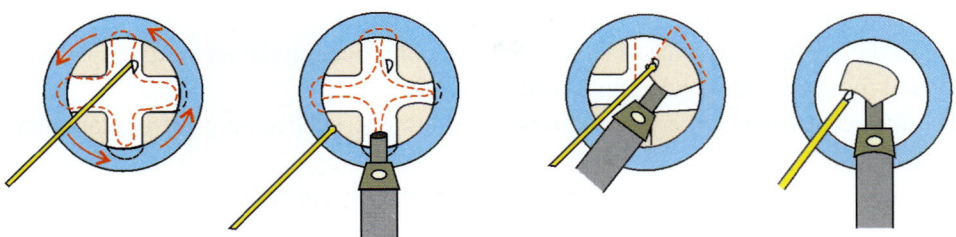

Nucleus emulsification by Divide and Conquer Technique (Four quadrant cracking)

5. *Aspiration of the Residual Cortex*

It is performed using the irrigation aspiration handpiece with a 0.3 mm aspiration port. The posterior capsule is polished with the same handpiece using very low aspiration pressure. The incision is then enlarged to a width sufficient to introduce the lens implant into the capsular bag.

6. Intraocular Lens Implantation

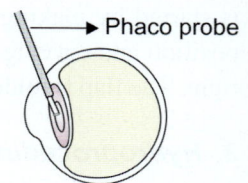

The intraocular lenses which may be used after phacoemulsification are,
  i. Single piece PMMA IOL—The rigid IOL used in phacosurgery should have an optic diameter of 5.5 mm or less.
  ii. Foldable IOL is made of soft acrylic, hydrogels or silicone materials. The design can be either 3 piece lenses or single piece plate haptic design. Presently, the 3 piece lenses are used and plate haptic design is used for toric IOLs to correct astigmatism of < 3 D.

Complications

1. Immediate Complications

  i. *Excessive bleeding* from conjunctiva during preparation of conjunctival flap. It is managed by gentle cautery.
  ii. *Damage to superior rectus* muscle while passing bridle suture may occur.
  iii. *Incision related complications* depend on type of cataract surgery being performed
     a. In conventional ECCE, irregular incision leading to defective coaptation of wound
     b. In phacoemulsification
        - Button holing of the anterior wall of the tunnel due to superficial dissection of the sclera flap. Re-entry at a deeper plane from the other side may be done
        - Premature entry into the anterior chamber due to deep dissection may occur. New dissection can be started at a lesser depth at the other end of the tunnel
        - Scleral disinsertion due to very deep groove incision may occur. There is complete separation of inferior sclera from the sclera superior to the incision. It is managed by radial sutures.
  iv. Complications related to anterior capsulorhexis. The capsulorhexis may sometimes escape, become very small or very large or may sometimes become eccentric.
  v. Injury to cornea, iris and lens may occur.
  vi. Iridodialysis may occur during intraoperative manipulations
  vii. Rupture of the posterior capsule—This is dreaded complications of any extracapsular cataract surgery and more so with phacoemulsification.
  viii. Zonular dehiscence may give rise to sunset and sunrise syndrome after implantation of an intraocular lens.
  ix. Vitreous loss—This is a serious complication which may occur following accidental rupture of posterior capsule during any technique of ECCE.
  x. Nucleus drop into vitreous cavity—This occurs more frequently with phacoemulsification. It is a dreaded complication which occurs due to sudden and large posterior capsular rupture. The case must be referred to a vitreoretinal surgeon without making any attempts to fish out the nucleus.
  xi. Posterior loss of lens fragments—This may occur after zonular dehiscence or posterior capsule rupture. It is a potentially serious complication because it may result in galucoma, chronic

uveitis, retinal detachment and chronic cystoid macular oedema. This complication is more commonly associated with phacoemulsification than conventional ECCE. The patient should be referred to a vitreoretinal surgeon after controlling any uveitis or raised intraocular pressure.

xii. Posterior dislocation of IOL—This is a rare but serious complication and has to be managed by pars plana vitrectomy, with repositioning or exchange of IOL.

xiii. Expulsive choroidal haemorrhage—This is one of the most dramatic and serious complications of open chamber surgery. There is bleeding into suprachoroidal space which may result in extrusion of intraocular contents (expulsive haemorrhage). Although the exact cause is not known, contributing factors include advanced age, glaucoma, systemic cardiovascular disease and vitreous loss.

2. Postoperative Complications

I. *Early postoperative (within first few days to 4 weeks)*

   i. Hyphaema—Collection of blood in the anterior chamber may occur from conjunctival or scleral vessels. It usually resolves spontanously.
   ii. Iris prolapse—This may occur after conventional ECCE due to inappropriate suturing.
   iii. Striate keratopathy—This occurs due to endothelial cell damage during surgery. It is characterized by mild corneal oedema with Descemet's membrane folds.
   iv. Flat or shallow anterior chamber—The incidence has decreased due to improved wound closure. It may be due to
      a. Wound leak—This is associated with hypotony. It is diagnosed by Seidel's test. In this test, a drop of fluorescein is instilled in the lower fornix and the patient is asked to blink. The incision is examined with slit lamp using cobalt-blue filter. Fluorescein will appear to be diluted by aqueous at the site of leak.
      b. Cilio-choroidal detachment may or may not be associated with wound leak.
   v. Postoperative anterior uveitis—It may be induced by instrumental trauma, handling of uveal tissue, reaction to residual cortex or chemical reaction.
   vi. Endophthalmitis—Acute postoperative endophthalmitis is a devastating complication which occurs in 1:1000 surgeries approximately. Causative organisms include staphylococci, pseudomonas and proteus sp. Source of infection is often thought to be patient's own external bacterial flora of the eyelids, conjunctiva and lacrimal drainage passages.
   Prevention—The following measures may be beneficial
      a. Preoperative treatment of pre-existing infection such as blepharitis, conjunctivitis, dacryocystitis etc.
      b. Povidone-iodine is instilled preoperatively as follows:
         Two drops of 5% betadine solution are instilled into the conjunctival sac several minutes prior to surgery. The solution is also used to paint the skin of the eyelids prior to draping. The eye is irrigated with saline solution prior to commencing surgery.
      c. Meticulous draping technique that ensures that the lashes and lid margins are isolated
      d. Prophylactic antibiotics should be given
      e. Postoperative injection of anterior sub-tenon antibiotics is commonly performed
      f. Intraoperative irrigation of anterior chamber by adding antibiotics such as vancomycin into the infusion fluid may be efficacious

TECHNIQUE	INTRACAPSULAR CATARACT EXTRACTION (ICCE)	EXTRACAPSULAR CATARACT EXTRACTION (ECCE)	PHACOEMULSIFICATION
1. General principles	Whole lens removed with intact capsule	Lens, nucleus and cortex are removed leaving the capsular bag behind	Same as ECCE
2. Dilatation of pupil	Required	Required	Required
3. Magnification	Binocular loupe or Microscope	Microscope	Microscope
4. Incision	Large, 180°, 10-12 mm Large incision	Medium, 120°, 7-8 mm Smaller incision	Small, 30°, 3.2–3.5 mm Smallest incision
5. Lens removal • Capsulotomy • Nucleus delivery • Cortex removal	 Nil Intact lens delivered Nil Cryoprobe → Cataract	 'Can-opener' or rhexis Manual sliding Irrigation aspiration, Manual or automated → Capsular bag	 Rhexis Phacoemulsification Irrigation aspiration, automated → Phaco probe
6. Intraocular lens	Anterior chamber or none	Posterior chamber 'in the bag'	Posterior chamber 'in the bag'
7. Sutures	Required, continuous or interrupted (5-7)	Required, continuous or interrupted (3-5)	Not required

II. *Late postoperative (after one month to years)*
   i. *Cystoid macular oedema*—It commonly occurs after complicated surgery involving rupture of posterior capsule and vitreous prolapse. There is collection of fluid in the form of cystic loculi in the Henle's layer of macula.
   ii. *Delayed chronic postoperative endophthalmitis.* It may occur when an organism of low virulence becomes trapped within the capsular bag.
   iii. *Retinal detachment*—Though uncommon following uneventful ECCE or phacoemulsification, it may sometime occur, specially in the presence of vitreous loss and high myopia.
   iv. *Pseudophakic bullous keratopathy*—It is usually a continuation of postoperative corneal oedema. It is a common indication of penetrating keratoplasty.

v. *Posterior capsular opacification (after or secondary cataract)*—It is the most common late complication of uncomplicated cataract surgery. It is the opacity which follows extracapsular extraction of the lens.

Advantages of Phacoemulsification

1. Intraoperatively, phacoemulsification allows excellent control of each phase of the operation for cataract removal.
2. The small incision technique involving a self-sealing 'no stitch' or 'sutureless' incision produces very secure and stable wound. There is rapid wound healing and shorter convalescence.
3. Removal of the nucleus occurs through a continuous circular capsulotomy (CCC) with the closed chamber. Aspiration of the cortex also occurs within a closed anterior chamber, with low risks of damaging the endothelium, iris and posterior chamber.
4. Phacoemulsification and small incision surgery are compatible with small size implants, i.e. foldable lenses. There is minimum or no astigmatism with early return of binocular vision.

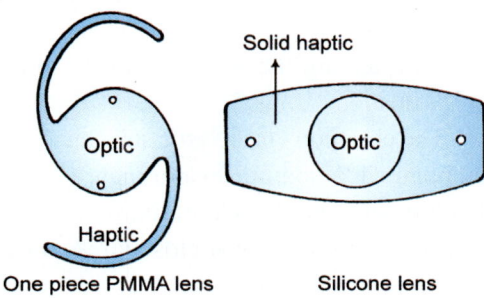

Disadvantages of Phacoemulsification

1. It is a difficult technique to master.
2. It requires expensive instrumentation.

4. PHAKONIT

It is a technique of phacoemulsification performed with a needle opening via an incision using the tip of a phacoprobe. The size of the incision is only 0.9 mm and after surgery an ultrathin rollable IOL is inserted into the capsular bag. The main advantage of this technique is that it is an astigmatism free cataract surgery.

5. LASER PHACOLYSIS

In recent times laser phacolysis is under trial whereby it is possible to lyse the lens matter through the intact anterior capsule by excimer, ruby or other newer lasers.

OCULAR VISCOSURGICAL DEVICE (OVD) (Viscoelastic substance)

Viscoelastic substance or OVD have been recently introduced in ophthalmology. They are useful in various diagnostic procedures as well as during surgery. These agents have high viscosity and elasticity.

1. Diagnostic Procedures
   i. Gonioscopy
  ii. Three mirror examination
 iii. Laser procedures

In diagnostic procedures these agents create a required working space, lubricate the instruments as in gonioscopy, three-mirror examination or even in performing laser procedures for glaucoma, after cataract and on the retina.

2. In Surgery

i. They are helpful in dissecting the tissues in the most atraumatic manner.
ii. For creating and maintaining surgical space as during insertion of intraocular lens during catract surgery.
iii. Protecting the endothelium from damage due to handling in keratoplasty and phacoemulsification.

The common viscoelastic substances are 1%, 2% hydroxy propyl methyl cellulose, 1% chondroitin sulphate, 1% sodium hyaluronate (Healon) and combinations of these like Viscoat (3% Sodium hyaluronate and 4% chondroitin sulphate). Sodium hyaluronate (1%, 1.4%, 5%) is obtained from rooster combs and most closely resembles the natural vitreous gel.

TREATMENT OF APHAKIA

1. Correction by Spectacles

Aphakia is treated by prescribing suitable spherical convex lens (+ 10 D approximately) and convex cylindrical lens (+1 to +2D at 180°) 6 weeks after the operation, i.e. when the corneo-scleral scar has healed completely and the refraction has become stable.

Advantages

It is cheap, easy to handle and readily available.

Disadvantages

- They are heavy and give a cosmetically poor appearance.
- There is 25% retinal image magnification hence it causes diplopia in unilateral aphakia.
- Spherical aberration can cause 'pin-cushion' effect. There may be chromatic aberration. This leads to visual distortion.
- There is 'jack in the box' ring scotoma and reduction in peripheral visual field.
- Physical invonvenience and cosmetic deficiency are usually present.

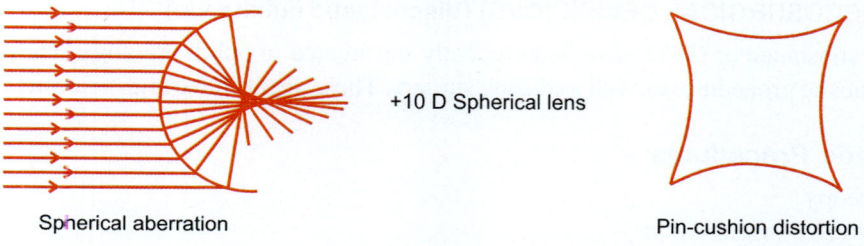

Spherical aberration   Pin-cushion distortion

2. Contact Lens

Advantage
There is minimum retinal image magnification therefore it is specially useful in case of unilateral aphakia. It also looks good cosmetically.

Disadvantages
- Daily cleaning and maintenance is essential.
- Their insertion and removal is cumbersome.
- Corneal epithelial oedema, erosion and vascularization may occur due to hypoxia
- Conjunctivitis, intolerance and foreign body sensation are common complaints.
- Loss, breakage and deterioration of the contact lens leads to financial loss.

3. Intraocular Lens (IOL) Implant

This is also known as 'pseudophakia'. The modern trend is in favour of posterior chamber IOL implantation as it offers best optical rehabilitation following removal of a cataractous lens.

Biometry
Removal of the crystalline lens substracts approximately 20D from the refracting system of the eye. Modern cataract surgery therefore involves the implantation of an intraocular lens (IOL). Biometry offers calculation of the lens power likely to result in emmetropia or a desired postoperative refraction.

Two ocular parameters are involved in biometry
 i. *Keratometry*—The curvature of anterior corneal surface (steepest and flattest meridians)
 ii. *Axial length*—The anteroposterior dimension of the eye measured using A-scan ultrasonography.

SRK formula—It is the most commonly used mathematical formula to calculate the IOL power. It was developed by Sanders, Retzlaff and Kraff and states that
$P = A - 2.5L - 0.9K$, where;
- P is the power of IOL
- A is a constant, which is specific for each lens type
- L is the axial length of eyeball in mm (A-scan ultrasonography)
- K is the average corneal curvature (Keratometry)

The ultrasound machine equipped with A-scan and IOL power calculation software is called *Biometer*.

The intraocular lens optic may be monofocal, toric or multifocal, but monofocal lenses with a separate pair of glasses for close work are most widely used.

Advantages
There is minimum retinal image magnification and early return of binocular vision. It also has cosmetic advantage.

Complications
- Pupillary block glaucoma may result in raised tension.

- Dislocation of IOL may occur in the vitreous or anterior chamber. Sunset phenomenon occurs when posterior chamber IOL dislocates inferiorly.
- Cystoid macular oedema, maculopathy and iridocyclitis.
- Corneal endothelial dystrophy may occur with anterior chamber lens.

TREATMENT OF UNILATERAL CATARACT

Unilateral cataract occurs commonly in cases of traumatic cataract and senile cataract. Treatment of unilateral cataract is often difficult and unsatisfactory when the vision is good in the fellow eye. It is best treated by extracapsular lens extraction with intraocular lens implantation (ECCE with IOL). Postoperative correction with spectacles causes intolerable diplopia due to difference in the size of retinal image (eyes can tolerate dioptric difference of 2 to 3 D). Binocular vision is only possible with:
  i. Contact lens
  ii. Intraocular lens implant.

TREATMENT OF ASSOCIATED RAISED TENSION

Increased intraocular tension may be present in association with cataract in:
  i. Phacomorphic glaucoma (swelling of the lens in intumescent stage of cataract).
  ii. Phacolytic glaucoma (leakage of lens protein in hypermature cortical cataract).
  iii. Associated simple glaucoma (primary angle closure or open angle glaucoma).

Treatment

  i. Raised tension is controlled medically before cataract surgery as it may result in expulsive haemorrhage during surgery due to increased pressure gradient. Trabeculectomy is performed prior to or along with cataract surgery. Iridectomy (peripheral buttonhole) alone may be done in case of narrow angle glaucoma. Following this cataract extraction is done in the routine manner.
  ii. Alternatively, trabeculectomy and cataract extraction can be combined.
  iii. Recent advanced procedures such as Argon laser trabeculoplasty (ALT) or iridotomy or laser filtration may be done.

Precaution

Following trabeculectomy, care is taken to make the corneo-scleral incision,
  i. In the upper part of the cornea, in front of the drainage area or filtering bleb.
  ii. Alternatively in the lower temporal part of the cornea, i.e. corneal section should be away from the bleb.

AFTER OR SECONDARY CATARACT

After or secondary cataract is an opacity which persists or follows after extracapsular lens extraction or discission (needling) of the lens. In both these operations, the posterior capsule and part of anterior capsule remains *in situ.*

Clinical Types

1. *Thin membrane*—It may remain following extracapsular lens extraction even with modern suction and infusion devices.

2. *Ring of Sommerring*—The new lens fibres are formed by the proliferation of anterior capsular cells. These are enclosed within the two capsule layers. It can get dislocated into the anterior chamber.

Fibrous membrane   Ring of Sommerring   Elschnig's pearls

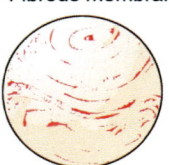 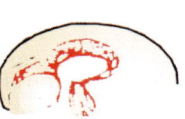 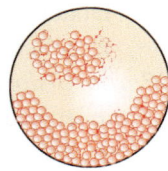

Clinical types of after cataracts

3. *Elschnig's pearl*—The subcapsular cells proliferate to form large balloon-like cells.
4. *Fibrous membrane*—It is usually formed when there is associated iritis.

Treatment

After cataract has to be removed if the vision is markedly impaired.
1. **Thin pupillary membrane** is removed by:
    i. Discission (needling), irrigation and aspiration.
    ii. Vitreous infusion suction cutter (VISC).
    iii. YAG laser capsulotomy or pupillary reconstruction.
2. **Thick pupillary membrane**
    i. It is cut into small pieces with Ziegler knife or vitreous scissors and is aspirated by VISC.
    ii. YAG laser capsulotomy or pupillary reconstruction.

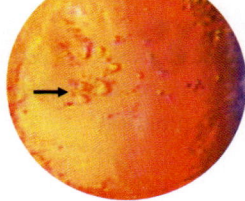

Elschnig's pearls

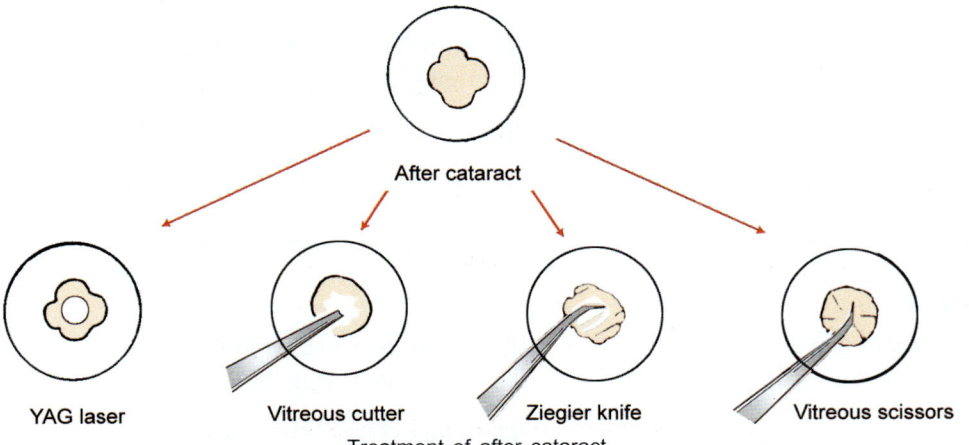

Treatment of after cataract

DISLOCATION OF LENS

The lens is displaced from its normal position due to complete rupture of the zonule.

Etiology

1. Congenital, e.g. Marfan's syndrome, homocystinuria, Marchesani's syndrome, Weill-Marchesani syndrome, hyperlysinemia, sulphite oxidase deficiency, etc.
2. Traumatic dislocation may occur following blunt or perforating injury.

Types

i. *Complete dislocation*—There is complete or total rupture of zonule hence the lens is dislocated,
   - In the vitreous or in the posterior chamber.
   - In the anterior chamber.
   - Under the conjunctiva.
   - Expelled out from the eye.
ii. *Partial dislocation (subluxation)*—Subluxation or tilting of the lens occurs due to partial rupture of zonule.

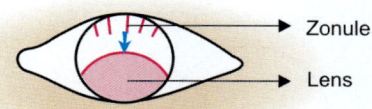

Subluxation of lens

Symptoms

1. There is blurred vision due to refractive error, i.e. aphakia or astigmatism.
2. Uniocular diplopia may be present in cases of partial dislocation (subluxated lens).

Signs

1. Iridodonesis—Tremulousness (tremors) of iris is present in both subluxated and dislocated lens.
2. The edge of lens and zonule are visible in subluxation of lens by the ophthalmoscope and slit-lamp examination.

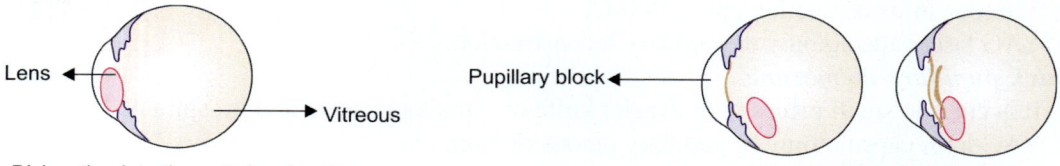

Dislocation into the anterior chamber

Dislocation into the vitreous

3. Dislocated lens is visible by naked eye or slit-lamp if it is in the anterior chamber.
4. The diagnosis can be confirmed by ultrasonography.

Complications

1. Secondary glaucoma may occur in cases of dislocation into the anterior chamber due to the angle closure.
2. Posterior chamber dislocations may result in pupillary block or phacolytic glaucoma.

Treatment

1. No treatment is required if the vision is good. It is similar to the old technique of 'couching'.
2. Remove the lens if it is opaque and if there is associated secondary glaucoma.

CONGENITAL ABNORMALITIES OF LENS

1. *Coloboma of lens*—A notch-shaped defect is seen in the inferior margin of lens.
2. *Ectopia lentis*—There is subluxation of lens usually 'upwards' or in the 'up and in' direction. It is bilateral usually. It is a hereditary condition. It may be associated with Marfan's syndrome and homocystinuria.
3. *Lenticonus*—The posterior surface of lens is conical, which results in myopia. It is typically seen in Alport's syndrome.

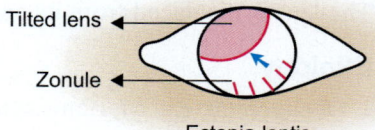

Ectopia lentis

MULTIPLE CHOICE QUESTIONS

1. Lens capsule is thinnest at the
   a. centre anteriorly
   b. laterally
   c. superior pole
   d. inferior pole
2. Congenital cataract is associated with all *EXCEPT*
   a. toxoplasmosis
   b. Lowe's syndrome
   c. galactosaemia
   d. glycogen storage disease
3. Diminished vision in daylight is seen in
   a. central cataract
   b. peripheral cataract
   c. zonular cataract
   d. none of the above
4. Cataracts are found in association with
   a. parathyroid deficiency
   b. myotonic dystrophy
   c. dinitrophenol toxicity
   d. all of the above
5. White pupillary reflex is seen in the all *EXCEPT*
   a. optic atrophy
   b. retinoblastoma
   c. total retinal detachment
   d. after cataract
6. Most common cause of blindness in India is
   a. trachoma
   b. vitamin deficiency
   c. glaucoma
   d. cataract
7. Postoperative flat anterior chamber may be due to
   a. pupillary block
   b. leaking wound
   c. choroidal detachment
   d. all of the above
8. Expulsive haemorrhage may occur following
   a. blunt injury with hyphaema
   b. perforating injury
   c. lens extraction
   d. panophthalmitis
9. The etiology of complicated cataract includes all *EXCEPT*
   a. disciform keratitis
   b. iridocyclitis
   c. retinitis pigmentosa
   d. retinal detachment
10. Displaced lens is seen in all, *EXCEPT*
    a. Marfan's syndrome
    b. Marchesani's syndrome
    c. Laurence-Moon-Biedl syndrome
    d. Homocystinuria
11. The most common complication in exfoliation of the lens capsule is
    a. iritis
    b. conjunctivitis
    c. glaucoma
    d. optic neuritis
12. Ideal site for intraocular lens implantation is
    a. in the anterior chamber
    b. transfix in the pupillary margin
    c. in the posterior chamber
    d. behind the posterior lens capsule
13. Polyopia is a symptom of
    a. cortical cataract
    b. cupuliform cataract
    c. radiation cataract
    d. electrical cataract

14. Ring of Sommerring is a type of
    a. congenital cataract
    b. complicated cataract
    c. after cataract
    d. traumatic cataract
15. Attack of acute congestive glaucoma can occur in
    a. incipient stage of cortical cataract
    b. intumescent stage
    c. immature stage
    d. mature stage
16. Burst Morgagnian cataract may cause
    a. secondary glaucoma
    b. iritis
    c. both
    d. none
17. Elschnig's pearls arise from
    a. anterior capsule of lens
    b. posterior capsule of lens
    c. cubical cells underneath lens capsule
    d. none of the above
18. Diagnostic criteria of immature cataract includes
    a. greyish lens
    b. presence of iris shadow
    c. black shadow visible against red fundal glow
    d. all of the above
19. Which of the following congenital or developmental cataract can also be acquired
    a. coronary
    b. polar
    c. suture
    d. coralliform
20. Lens derives its nourishment from
    a. air
    b. aqueous humour
    c. vitreous
    d. perilimbal capillaries
21. After cataract is seen after following operations
    a. lensectomy
    b. extracapsular lens extraction
    c. vitrectomy
    d. intracapsular lens extraction
22. Intraocular lenses are generally made of
    a. prolene
    b. PMMA
    c. HEMA
    d. silicone
23. Rosette-shaped cataract is a feature of
    a. traumatic cataract
    b. diabetic cataract
    c. coronary cataract
    d. complicated cataract
24. Polychromatic lustre is typically seen in the following cataract
    a. anterior polar cataract
    b. complicated cataract
    c. traumatic cataract
    d. diabetic cataract
25. Lensectomy is an operation whereby
    a. lens is removed
    b. nucleus and anterior capsule are removed
    c. lens and anterior vitreous phase is removed
    d. none of the above
26. YAG laser is used in the treatment of
    a. diabetic retinopathy
    b. open angle glaucoma
    c. after cataract
    d. retinal detachment

27. Following are associated with zonular cataract *EXCEPT*
    a. IUGR
    b. rickets
    c. dental anomalies
    d. diabetes
28. After cataract operation, lenses are prescribed after
    a. 2 weeks
    b. 4 weeks
    c. 6 weeks
    d. 12 weeks
29. Most common type of cataract following radiation is
    a. anterior subcapsular
    b. posterior subcapsular
    c. diffuse cataract
    d. tear drop cataract
30. Late complication of vitreous loss during cataract surgery.
    a. updrawn pupil
    b. retinal detachment
    c. corneal oedema
    d. any of the above

ANSWERS

1—a	2—d	3—a	4—d	5—a
6—d	7—d	8—c	9—a	10—c
11—c	12—c	13—a	14—c	15—b
16—c	17—c	18—c	19—b	20—b
21—b	22—b	23—a	24—b	25—c
26—c	27—d	28—c	29—b	30—d

CHAPTER 11
The Vitreous

APPLIED ANATOMY

The vitreous is an inert, avascular, transparent, jelly-like structure which serves only optical functions. It consists of a delicate framework of collagen and hyaluronic acid. It is a hydrophilic gel which becomes "fluid" when its protein basis is coagulated due to,
- *Advancing senile age.*
- *Degenerations, e.g. as in high myopia.*
- *Chemical and mechanical trauma.*

Attachments

1. It is attached anteriorly to the lens (Hyaloid capsular ligament of Wieger) and ciliary epithelium in front of the ora serrata. The part of the vitreous about 4 mm across the ora serrata is known as the "base of vitreous," where the attachment is strongest.
2. It is attached posteriorly to the edge of the optic disc and macula lutea (foveal region) forming ring-shaped structure around them.

Age Changes in the Vitreous

The vitreous undergoes significant physical and biochemical changes with aging.
1. *At birth*—The Cloquet's canal runs straight from lens to the optic disc. It contains the primary vitreous.

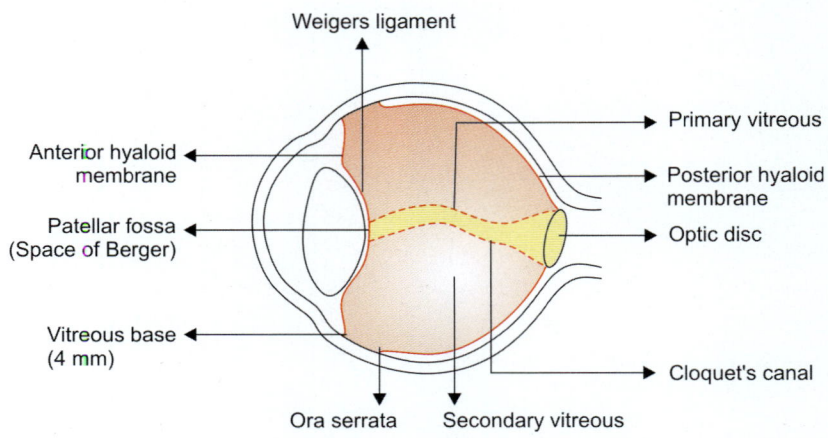

Structures of Vitreous

Diseases of the vitreous

  i. Opacities in the vitreous,
 ii. Vitreous bands and membranes,
iii. Persistent hyperplastic vitreous,
 iv. Vitreous haemorrhage,
  v. Vitreous loss,
 vi. Vitreous inflammation,
vii. Vitreous detachment

2. *In young persons*—The vitreous gel is homogeneous but its fibres become coarse with the process of advancing age.
3. *In old age and in high myopes*—The secondary vitreous liquefies (syneresis) and shrinks, producing a vitreous detachment, vitreous and retinal haemorrhage and retinal break.

Function

The vitreous forms one of the refractive media of the eye.

The vitreous does not have any blood vessels. It derives nutrition from the surrounding structures like choroid, ciliary body.

OPACITIES IN THE VITREOUS

Opacities in the vitreous may result in marked visual impairment due to 'floaters' or visual loss.

Etiology

1. **Developmental causes**—The opacities are usually located in the Cloquet's canal and are remnants of the hyaloid system.
2. **Degenerative causes**
    i. *Muscae volitantes*—These are black spots floating in front of the eye due to minute opacities in the vitreous. They look like small mosquitoes. They are seen in normal persons. They do not cause any disturbance of vision and are harmless.
   ii. *Asteroid hyalosis*—These are unilateral spherical minute, white bodies of calcium soaps resembling snowball. They are suspended in an essentially normal vitreous. It is seen in the elderly and affects both sexes. It is associated with diabetes mellitus and hypercholesterolaemia. It is asymptomatic therefore no treatment is required usually. A pars plana vitrectomy may be considered if vision is markedly reduced.
  iii. *Synchysis scintillans*—There is deposition of freely floating, highly refractive cholesterol crystals in the lower part of fluid vitreous. It affects damaged eyes which have suffered trauma or inflammation. Golden shower is seen during the movements of the eye. No treatment is indicated.
   iv. *Amyloid degeneration*—It is a rare bilateral systemic disease with deposition of amyloid in the vitreous and other parts of the body. Retinal detachment and secondary glaucoma may occur at a later stage. It can be treated by pars plana vitrectomy.

v. *Other causes*—These include the following common causes:
- Senile degeneration
- High myopia
- Retrolental fibroplasia
- Wagner's disease
- Ehlers-Danlos syndrome
- Marfan's syndrome
- Chronic cyclitis
- Diabetes and Eale's disease
- Neoplasm.

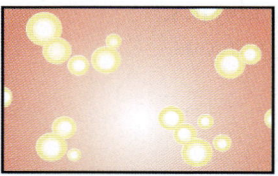

Asteroid bodies

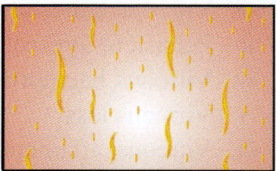

Synchysis scintillans

VITREOUS BANDS AND MEMBRANES

Vitreous bands and membranes are formed after posterior detachment of the vitreous. They consist of hyalocytes, fibrocytes and endothelial cells of the capillaries. They cause oedema, haemorrhage and hole formation in the retina. This is followed by tractional retinal detachment. The central vision is impaired. Metamorphopsia and flashes of light (photopsia) may be seen. Pars plana vitrectomy with epiretinal stripping is the treatment of choice.

PERSISTENT HYPERPLASTIC VITREOUS

Etiology
There is failure of primary vitreous structure to regress after birth.

Symptoms
- White reflex is seen in the pupillary area shortly after birth.
- There may be presence of associated cataract, glaucoma, microphthalmos, intraocular (vitreous) haemorrhage.

Diagnosis
It is diagnosed by computerized tomography scanning (CT scan).

Treatment
- Early removal of cataract and retrolental tissue must be done.
- *Lensectomy*—Lens is aspirated with excision of retrolental membrane along with anterior vitrectomy by VISC (vitreous infusion suction cutter) via pars plana approach. Visual prognosis is usually poor.

VITREOUS HAEMORRHAGE

Types
There are two types of vitreous haemorrhage :
1. *Preretinal or subhyaloid haemorrhage*—The haemorrhage occurs between the retina and the vitreous. The blood remains fluid, red in colour and moves with gravity forming boat-shaped figure in the macular area due to peculiar ring-shaped attachment of vitreous around the macula.

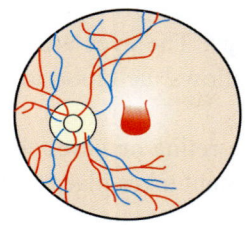 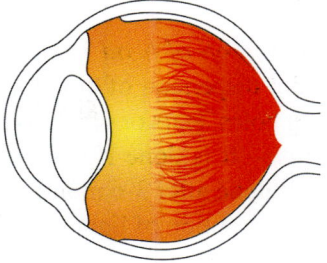

Subhyaloid haemorrhage   Large intravitreal haemorrhage

2. **Intravitreal haemorrhage**—The haemorrhage may get absorbed or degenerate to form a white fibrous tissue mass.

Etiology

The common causes of vitreous haemorrahage are as follows:
1. Trauma—By contusion or penetrating injury.
2. Vitreous retraction—Vitreous fibrous band or membrane retraction.
3. Central retinal vein thrombosis.
4. Eale's disease—It is due to retinal vasculitis and periphlebitis.
5. Malignant hypertension often results in large intravitreal haemorrhage.
6. Blood dyscrasias—Leukemia, sickle cell anaemia, purpura, etc.
7. Diabetes mellitus—It is common in diabetic proliferative retinopathy.

Symptoms

1. Black spots or cloud may be seen in front of the eye.
2. There is impaired vision. It may be reduced to perception of light.

Signs

1. *Fundus examination*
    i. A faint or no red reflex is seen.
    ii. Grey opacities may be present in the vitreous.
2. *Slit-lamp examination*—Fresh blood or clotted blood may be seen in the vitreous.

Complications

1. Complicated cataract may occur.
2. Retinal atrophy may be present due to haemosiderosis.
3. Retinal detachment may occur due to organised fibrous tissue bands.
4. Profound visual loss may be present leading to complete blindness.

Investigations

B scan ultrasonography is helpful in identifying fibrovascular proliferations on the retinal surface and associated tractional or rhegmatogenous retinal detachment.

Basic Ophthalmology

Treatment

1. *Bed-rest with elevation of head* is advised in the initial stage. The eyes are bandaged so that there is minimum dispersion of blood in the vitreous. This allows the blood to settle down and helps in locating holes, tears or phlebitis.
2. *Photocoagulation*—It is done if new vessels are seen in the retina or vitreous.
3. *Vitrectomy*—It is done after 3-6 months if no visual improvement takes place and when vision is reduced to only perception of light or hand movements.

Prognosis

- Small haemorrhages are usually absorbed.
- Large or recurrent haemorrhages may lead to retinitis proliferans.

VITREOUS LOSS

Etiology

Accidental vitreous loss may occur during surgery on the lens, cornea and iris. The vitreous may herniate only in the anterior chamber or may escape outside the eye.

Signs

1. Corneal oedema may be present due to endothelium damage.
2. Updrawn pupil is usually seen due to attachment of vitreous bands to the pupillary margin and corneoscleral section.
3. Macular oedema may be associated with massive vitreous loss.

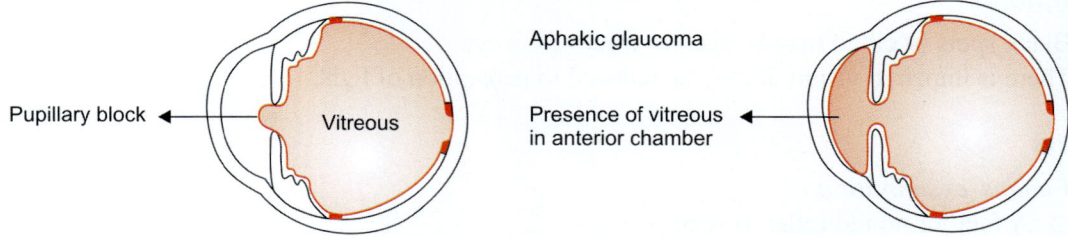

Pupillary block glaucoma

4. There may be presence of fibrous bands in the vitreous later on.
5. Aphakic glaucoma may occur at a later stage due to pupillary block or due to presence of vitreous in the anterior chamber causing angle closure.

Treatment

Anterior vitrectomy by vitreous infusion suction cutter (VISC) or vitreous scissors is performed through a large corneal section after removal of the lens. It is also useful for accidental vitreous loss which may occur during aphakic keratoplasty.

Prophylaxis

Intraocular pressure is kept low preoperatively by the administration of acetazolamide and application of digital pressure, Flieringa ring, pinky ball, etc.

VITREOUS INFLAMMATION

Vitreous is an excellent culture medium for the growth of bacteria and fungus leading to *endophthalmitis* and *vitreous abscess* formation.

In addition to bacteria and fungi, vitreous abscess with intense eosinophilia may be seen with parasitic infections such as *Taenia*, microfilaria, Toxocara canis, etc.

The response of the vitreous to infection is characterized by,

i. *Liquefaction of vitreous gel (synchysis)*
ii. *Opacification of vitreous*
iii. *Shrinkage of vitreous (syneresis)*

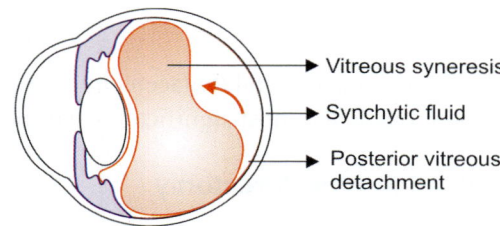

Shrinkage of vitreous and detachment

The presence of white blood cells results in the laying down of fibrous connective tissue and capillary proliferation. This leads to the formation of fibrous bands and cyclitic membrane. Cyclitic membrane often leads to total retinal detachment due to contraction.

VITREOUS DETACHMENT

1. Posterior Vitreous Detachment (PVD)

It refers to separation of cortical vitreous from the retina anywhere posterior to vitreous base (3-4 mm wide attachment to ora serrata)

Synchysis—There is associated vitreous liquefaction.

Syneresis—There is collapse of the vitreous due to collection of synchytic fluid between the posterior hyaloid membrane and the internal limiting membrane of the retina.

Incidence

- It is common above the age of 65 years.
- It may occur in eyes with senile liquefaction with development of a hole in the posterior hyaloid membrane, e.g. aphakia, high myopia.

Symptoms

Photopsia or flashes of light and floaters are seen.

Signs

- Biomicroscopic examination of vitreous shows collapsed vitreous behind the lens. There is an optically clear space between detached posterior hyaloid phase and the retina.
- An annular opacity (Weiss ring or Fuchs ring) representing the ring shaped attachment of vitreous to the optic disc is pathognomic of PVD.

Complications

These include retinal breaks, haemorrhage, vitreous haemorrhage, cystoid maculopathy, etc.

2. Detachment of Vitreous Base and Anterior Vitreous

This usually occurs after blunt trauma. There may be associated vitreous haemorrhage, anterior retinal dialysis and dislocation of lens.

VITRECTOMY

Removal (excision) and replacement of the vitreous is known as vitrectomy. Vitrectomy or excising the vitreous is the most significant advancement in the surgical management of vitreous diseases.

Indications for Vitrectomy

1. Persistent vitreous opacity
    i. Haemorrhage
    ii. Vitreous membrane and bands
    iii. Preretinal membranes
2. Complications of cataract extraction
    i. Loss of vitreous
    ii. Vitreous touch with bullous keratopathy
    iii. Incarceration of vitreous in wound with traction.
    iv. Malignant glaucoma
    v. Removal of intraocular lens or nucleus from the vitreous cavity.
3. Endophthalmitis with vitreous abscess.
4. Trauma
    i. Removal of non-magnetic intraocular foreign body.
    ii. Removal of subluxated or dislocated lens.
5. Complicated retinal detachment
    i. Massive vitreous traction by fibrovascular bands.
    ii. Giant retinal tear
    iii. Retinal dialysis.
6. Congenital cataract (lensectomy).
7. Persistent hyperplastic primary vitreous.

Preoperative Investigations

1. Vision—Perception to light and accurate projection of rays (PLPR) are important. A patient is submitted to vitrectomy when his visual acuity is at least hand movements.
2. Evaluation of retina
    i. Structural integrity is tested by ultrasonography (USG).
    ii. Functional integrity is tested by electroretinography (ERG). In cases with hazy media, bright flash ERG may be used.
3. Fluorescein angiography denotes the status of the vascular system.
4. Specific investigations, are done to confirm the diagnosis of the underlying disease, e.g. diabetes mellitus, Eale's disease, bleeding disorders, etc.

Techniques

The term "vitrectomy" implies the cutting of formed vitreous gel which is responsible for producing various complications. A variety of vitrectomy units are available. All instruments perform vitreous cutting and aspiration under microscopic control with the help of fiberoptic illumination, e.g. vitreous infusion suction cutter (VISC), vitreous cutter, vitreous stripper, etc.

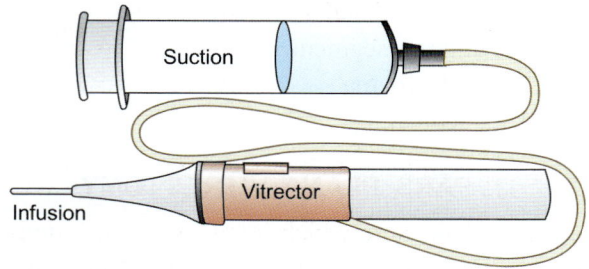

Vitreous infusion suction cutter (VISC)

There are two main types of vitrectomy techniques:
1. Anterior vitrectomy
2. Pars plana vitrectomy

1. ANTERIOR VITRECTOMY

It is also known as open sky vitrectomy. This is performed through the limbus or a large corneal section after removal of the lens. It is useful for vitreous loss during lens extraction and aphakic keratoplasty. The following are the two main methods:
  i. *Sponge vitrectomy*—Vitreous is cut off by using small triangular cellulose sponges (or cotton swabs) and de Wecker's scissors until adequate amount of vitreous is removed.
  ii. *Automated vitrectomy*—Vitreous is excised from the anterior chamber with the help of vitrector (VISC) or an equivalent instrument. The anterior chamber is reconstituted with an air bubble.

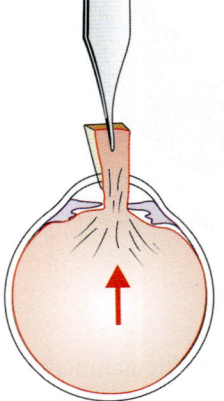
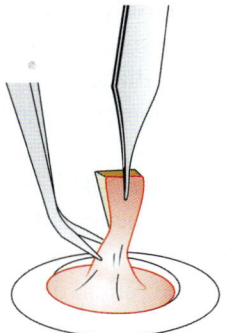

Anterior vitrectomy

Indications

1. Vitreous loss during lens extraction—Vitreous loss is managed by clearing the vitreous from the incision and the anterior chamber.
2. Vitreous loss occurring during aphakic keratoplasty.
3. Removal of a dislocated lens associated with vitreous loss.
4. Removal of a large foreign body associated with vitreous loss.
5. Vitreous complications in the anterior segment
    i. Vitreous "touch" with corneal oedema
    ii. Aphakic pupillary block glaucoma.

2. PARS PLANA VITRECTOMY

It is an intraocular microsurgical procedure which involves the insertion of instruments through a very small incision in the pars plana into the vitreous cavity. Vitrectomy through the pars plana approach is the best established procedure. It has many advantages namely,

i. It avoids both anterior segment and retinal complications as the approach is through the pars plana.
ii. There is no danger of scleral collapse as the system is a closed one.
iii. Lens removal is not necessary as is required in case of anterior vitrectomy.
iv. Operative trauma is minimal as smaller incisions are used.

The aim of pars plana vitrectomy are the following :
i. *Removal and replacement of vitreous gel*
ii. *Repair of retinal detachment along with photocoagulation.*

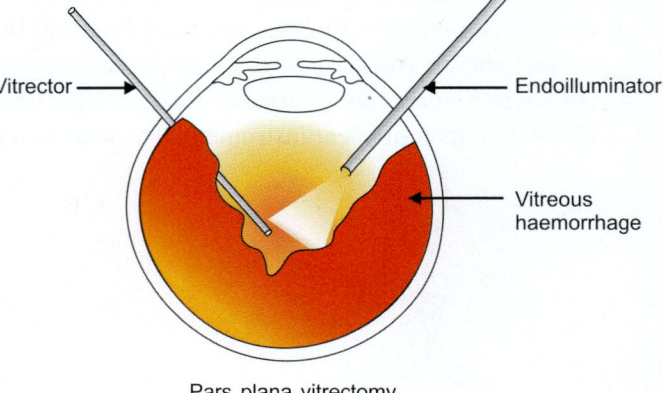

Pars plana vitrectomy

Indications

1. Persistent large vitreous opacities affecting useful vision.
2. Severe persistent vitreous haemorrhage, e.g. diabetes, hypertension.
3. Fibrous membranes in the vitreous cavity.
4. Massive preretinal proliferation of fibrous tissue, e.g. diabetic retinopathy.
5. Tractional retinal detachment involving the macula.
6. Combined tractional and rhegmatogenous (with retinal break) retinal detachment.
7. Any opacity in the anterior segment such as after cataract and pupillary membrane.
8. Large intraocular foreign body in the posterior segment.
9. Endophthalmitis and vitreous abscess.

Technique

It is performed through a surgical microscope allowing coaxial illumination and fine movements by X-Y coupling. Special planoconcave lenses are placed on the cornea to provide a clear image of the posterior third of the eye.

Microscope attachments allow re-inversion of the image seen.

Three sclerotomies of 20-gauge size are made at the pars plana, 3-3.5 mm away from the limbus and are use for
1. In one, an infusion line is inserted for balanced salt solution.
2. In the second, a fibreoptic light source provides endoillumination.
3. Through the third, a vitrectomy instrument for suction and cutting of the vitreous is inserted.

Any abnormalities in the vitreous can be cleared bimanually under direct vision using the vitrectomy instrument and the endoilluminator as support when needed. Once the visibility of the retinal is restored, the cause for the vitreous disturbance is treated.

VITREOUS SUBSTITUTES

The vitreous replacement is necessary for restoration of intraocular pressure, and repositioning of the retina in retinal detachment surgery.

An ideal vitreous substitutes should be:
- Optically clear
- Biologically inert
- Having a high surface tension.

Various substances have been tried to replace vitreous after vitrectomy such as;
  i. *Liquid*—Normal saline, BSS (balanced salt solution), silicone oil, hyaluronic acid, sodium hyaluronate (Healon), perfluorocarbon liquids (PFCL), etc. Silicon oil allows better controlled retinal manipulations during operation
  ii. *Gas*
   - Air is still the most commonly used intraocular gas. It causes internal tamponade, i.e. it replaces the retina firmly against the sclera.
   - Sulfur hexafluoride (SF_6)—It doubles its volume and lasts for approximately 10 days
   - Perfluoropropane (C_3F_8)—It quadruples its volume and last for about 28 days
   - Octafluorocyclobutane (C_4F_8).

They are used as 40% mixture with air for restoration of normal intraocular pressure.

Combining agents available for tamponade provide better support to superior and inferior retina simultaneously e.g. semifluorinated alkanes with silicone oil, fluorosilicone and silicone oil and 30% F_6H_8 with 70% polydimethyl siloxane 1000.

The purpose of using these vitreous substitutes is;
1. To expand or replace vitreous volume.
2. To replace opaque vitreous with optically clear material.
3. To provide internal tamponade, i.e. it pushes back the retina to its normal position in retinal detachment surgery.
4. To mechanically separate epiretinal tissue from the retina.

MULTIPLE CHOICE QUESTIONS

1. Vitreous is attached to the following structures *EXCEPT*
   a. retina
   b. lens
   c. ciliary epithelium near ora serrata
   d. optic disc
2. Which of the following is not a source of nutrient to cornea
   a. air
   b. aqueous humour
   c. perilimbal capillaries
   d. vitreous humour
3. Asteroid hyalitis is
   a. clinically symptomless
   b. bilateral usually
   c. crystalline spherical bodies
   d. all of the above
4. Synchysis scintillans is seen in eyes which have suffered
   a. trauma
   b. inflammatory disease
   c. both
   d. none
5. The causes of vitreous degeneration include
   a. myopia
   b. cyclitis
   c. amyloidosis
   d. all of the above
6. Subhyaloid haemorrhage occurs between
   a. retina and vitreous
   b. within vitreous
   c. behind retina
   d. none of the above
7. The treatment of vitreous haemorrhage includes all *EXCEPT*
   a. bed-rest with elevation of head
   b. photocoagulation
   c. lensectomy
   d. vitrectomy
8. The complications of vitreous bands and membranes are
   a. retinal oedema
   b. retinal hole formation
   c. retinal detachment
   d. all of the above
9. Clinical features of vitreous loss include
   a. aphakic glaucoma
   b. updrawn pupil
   c. macular oedema
   d. all of the above
10. Vitreous abscess is commonly due to all *EXCEPT*
    a. penetrating injuries
    b. postoperative infection
    c. hordeolum internum
    d. septicaemia
11. Common causes of vitreous haemorrhage include all *EXCEPT*
    a. trauma
    b. Eale's disease
    c. diabetic retinopathy
    d. choroiditis
12. Synchysis scintillans is due to
    a. asteroid bodies
    b. muscae volitantes
    c. cholesterol crystals
    d. amyloid degeneration
13. Vitrectomy is indicated in
    a. vitrious loss during cataract surgery
    b. retinal detachment associated with traction bands
    c. endophthalmitis
    d. all of the above

14. Features of asteroid bodies in vitreous include
    a. clinically innocuous
    b. calcium crystals
    c. usually bilateral
    d. all of the above
15. The vitreous contains
    a. hyaluxonic acid
    b. plasma protein and collagen
    c. a dilute solution of salts
    d. all of the above.

ANSWERS

1—d	2—d	3—d	4—c	5—d
6—a	7—c	8—d	9—d	10—c
11—d	12—c	13—d	14—d	15—d

CHAPTER 12

Glaucoma

Glaucoma is a chronic, progressive optic neuropathy caused by a group of ocular conditions which lead to damage of optic nerve with loss of visual function. The most common risk factor known is raised intraocular pressure.

Normal intraocular pressure	=	10–20 mm Hg (Schiotz)
Suspicious case	=	20–25 mm Hg (Schiotz)
Glaucoma	=	Above 25 mm Hg (Schiotz)
Hypotony	=	Below 10 mm Hg (Schiotz)

APPLIED ANATOMY

Pathophysiology of glaucoma revolves around the aqueous humor dynamics. The principal ocular structures concerned with it are the pars plicata part of the ciliary body, angle of anterior chamber and the aqueous outflow system.

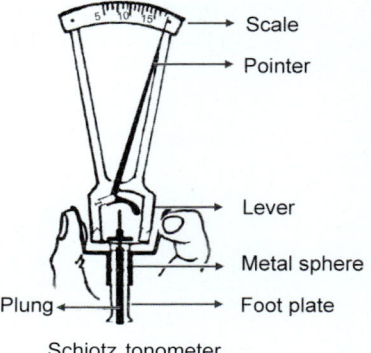

Schiotz tonometer

1. Ciliary Body

It is the main site of aqueous production. The shape of the ciliary body is like an isosceles triangle with its base forwards. Iris is attached to about the middle of the base of the ciliary body. The outer side of the triangle lies against the sclera with the suprachoroidal space in between.

Structure

The ciliary body consists of four layers namely,
1. *Ciliary muscles*—These are flat bundles of non-striated muscle fibres which are helpful in accommodation of the lens for seeing near objects.
2. *Stroma*—It consists of connective tissue of collagen and fibroblasts, nerves, pigments and blood vessels.
3. *Ciliary processes*—There are about 70 ciliary processes seen macroscopically. Suspensory ligament or zonule of Zinn is attached to them and the equator of the lens. Each finger-like process is lined by two layers of epithelial cells. The core of the ciliary process contains blood vessels and loose connective tissue. These processes are the main site of aqueous production.
4. *Epithelium*—There are two layers of pigmented and non-pigmented epithelial cells.

Parts

Ciliary body has two parts namely,
  i. *Pars plicata*—The anterior one-third of ciliary body (about 2 mm) is known as pars plicata. The ciliary processes are attached to this part. Pars plicata part of the ciliary body secretes aqueous humor

ii. *Pars plana*—The posterior two-third of ciliary body (about 4 mm) is known as pars plana. It is relatively avascular therefore posterior segment of the eye is entered through the pars plana incision 3-5 mm behind the limbus.

2. Angle of Anterior Chamber

It plays an important role in the process of aqueous drainage. It is formed by the root of iris, anterior most part of the ciliary body, scleral spur, trabecular meshwork and Schwalbe's line (prominent end of Descemet's membrane of cornea). The angle width varies in different
individuals and plays a vital role in the pathogenesis of different types of glaucoma. Clinically the various angle structures can be visualised by gonioscopic examination.

3. Aqueous Outflow System

It includes the trabecular meshwork, canal of Schlemm, aqueous veins and the episcleral veins.
1. *Trabecular meshwork*—It is a sieve-like structure through which aqueous humor gets filtered into the canal of Schlemm.
2. *Canal of Schlemm*—This is an endothelial lined oval channel present circumferentially in the scleral sulcus.
3. *Aqueous veins*—These are about 25-35 in number. They leave the canal of Schlemm at oblique angles to terminate into episcleral veins.
4. *Episcleral veins*—These are branches of anterior ciliary veins. There is pressure difference of about 5 mm Hg between the anterior chamber and the episcleral veins so that the aqueous drains continuously in them.

MAINTENANCE OF NORMAL INTRAOCULAR PRESSURE

The factors which maintain the normal intraocular pressures are:
1. The formation of the aqueous humor.
2. The outflow of the aqueous humor.
3. The pressure in the episcleral veins.

1. The Formation of the Aqueous Humour

The aqueous humor is a clear watery fluid filling the anterior chamber (0.25 ml) and posterior chamber (0.06 ml) of the eyeball. In addition to its role in maintaining normal intraocular pressure, it also plays an important role in providing nutrients and removing metabolites from the avascular cornea and lens.

For many years Leber's theory of simple filtration from the blood was generally accepted. However, the chemical analysis of the aqueous humor indicated that *ultrafiltration and secretion* are involved in the formation of the aqueous humor.

Aqueous humor is derived from the plasma within the capillary network of ciliary processes. The production of aqueous humor takes place by the ciliary epithelium by following mechanisms:
  i. *Secretion*—It is an active metabolic process
  ii. *Ultrafiltration*—Its rate is influenced by the level of blood pressure in the ciliary capillaries, plasma osmotic pressure and the level of intraocular pressure.

Blood-aqueous barrier—The system of semipermeable membranes separating the blood from the ocular cavity is known as the *Blood-aqueous barrier*.

2. The Outflow of the Aqueous Humor

The normal outflow takes place by two routes,
   i. *Angle of anterior chamber (conventional route)*
   ii. *Uveoscleral outflow (unconventional route)*

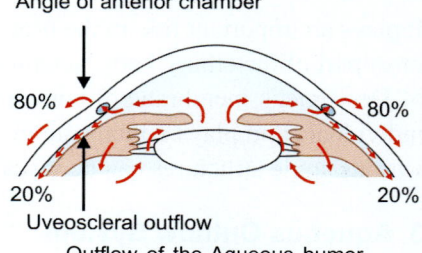
Outflow of the Aqueous humor

i. *Angle of anterior chamber (approximately 80%)*
   The aqueous is formed by the ciliary epithelium. It flows from the ciliary region to the posterior chamber. It then flows through the pupil into the anterior chamber and escapes through the drainage channels at the angle to the episcleral veins.

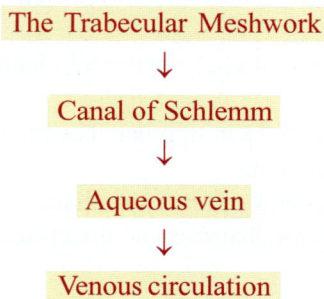

ii. *Uveoscleral outflow- (approximately 20%)* This is the second accessory exit through the ciliary body into the suprachoroidal space and choroid. It then passes into the episcleral tissue. This pathway is of importance particularly in buphthalmos.

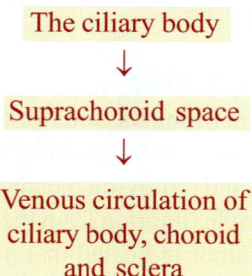

3. The Pressure in the Episcleral Veins

There is a pressure difference of approximately 5 mm Hg between the anterior chamber and the episcleral veins so that there is a continuous flow of aqueous into the venous system. In cases of orbital varicose veins or tumour, the venous pressure rises causing obstruction to the flow of aqueous.

GLAUCOMA

Etiology

The most important factor which causes rise of intraocular pressure is *obstruction to the drainage of the aqueous humor* through the:
  i. *Angle of the anterior chamber*
  ii. *At the pupil.*

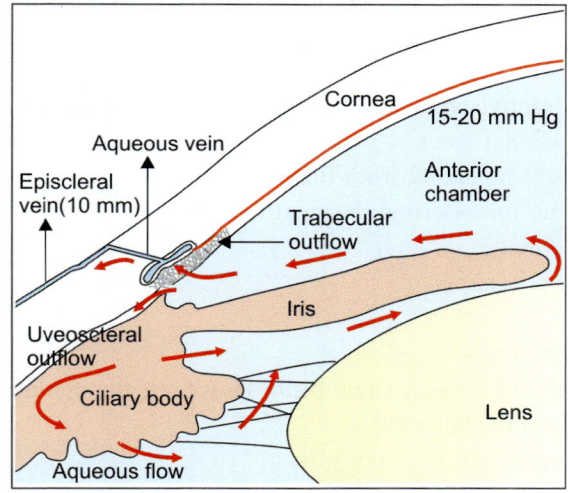

Mechanism of aqueous formation, flow and outflow pathways in the normal eye

Pathogenesis

The glaucomatous damage is attributed to a combination of factors which affect perfusion of optic nerve head.
1. *Mechanical changes*—The coats of the eye can withstand raised intraocular pressure except at the lamina cribrosa which is pushed backwards. This squeezes the nerve fibres within its meshes to disturb the axoplasmic flow.
2. *Vascular factors*—The perfusion of optic nerve head may be affected due to decreased blood flow in the capillaries and in annulus of Zinn which supply nutrition to the laminar and post-laminar optic nerve head.

Classification

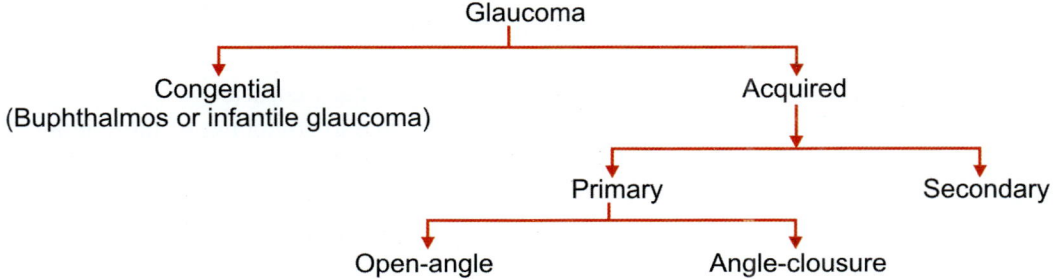

Absolute glaucoma—It is the end stage of all the above types of glaucoma where there is no perception of light and the person is blind. The intraocular tension is markedly raised.

CONGENITAL OR INFANTILE GLAUCOMA (BUPHTHALMOS, HYDROPHTHALMOS)

It is defined as glaucoma appearing between birth and the age of 3-4 years. There is raised intraocular tension present since birth. When the glaucoma presents at puberty, it is known as *Juvenile glaucoma*.

Etiology

It is usually of a simple obstructive type due to congenital abnormality at the angle of anterior chamber. It is transmitted as an autosomal recessive trait.
1. The iris is not completely separated from the cornea.
2. Persistence of embryonic mesodermal tissue at the angle.
3. Absence of canal of Schlemm.

Incidence

It occurs in about 1 in 10000 births
   i. *Age*—It is congenital and present since birth. However, the symptoms may manifest within 1-3 years of life (Infantile glaucoma)
   ii. *Sex*—Boys are affected more than the girls
   iii. It is usually bilateral.

Types

1. Congenital glaucoma—It manifests at birth.
2. Infantile glaucoma—It presents between 1-3 years.
3. Juvenile glaucoma—It presents around puberty.

Syndromes Associated with Infantile Glaucoma

1. *von Recklinghausen's disease*, i.e. generalised neurofibromatosis.
2. *Sturge-Weber syndrome*—The capillary naevus of face is associated with angiomatous conditions of the choroid and the brain.

Symptoms

1. Lacrimation is present due to corneal oedema and erosion.
2. Photophobia is associated with corneal involvement.
3. There is defective vision due to corneal oedema leading to hazy cornea.
4. There is enlargement of cornea and the eye as a whole, due to stretching of the sclera.

Signs

1. Enlargement of the eyeball as a whole is present with globular cornea.

2. There is corneal oedema and opacities due to endothelium damage and rupture of Descemet's membrane (Haabs' striae). These occur because Descemet's membrane is less elastic than the corneal stroma. Tears are situated in the periphery and are concentric with the limbus.
3. Deep anterior chamber with iridodonesis may be seen due to backward displacement of the lens. Iris may have atrophic patches in the late stages.
4. Lens is flattened and displaced backwards due to stretching of the zonule of Zinn.
5. Sclera becomes thin and bluish as the uveal tissue shines through it.

Diagnosis

1. *Raised intraocular pressure*—It is not raised markedly due to:
   i. Extensibility or stretching of the sclera
   ii. Uveoscleral outflow.
2. *Measurement of corneal diameter*—Corneal enlargement occurs along with the enlargement of the globe—buphthalmos (Bull-like eyes), specially when the onset is before the age of 3 years. A normal infant's cornea measures about 10.5 mm in diameter. A diameter of more than 13 mm confirms enlargement. The prognosis is usually poor when the diameter is more than 15 mm.
3. *Fundus examination*—The cupping of optic disc is seen due to stretching of the lamina cribrosa and raised tension. Optic atrophy usually sets in after the third year.
4. *Gonioscopy*—The angle of anterior chamber shows certain abnormalities.

Differential Diagnosis

i. Keratoglobus (megalocornea)—It is present since birth.
ii. Very high myopia—The eyeball is large as a whole.
iii. Raised intraocular pressure (IOP) in infants may be associated with:
- Retinoblastoma.
- Retinopathy of prematurity.
- Aniridia or absence of iris.
- Persistent primary hyperplastic vitreous.

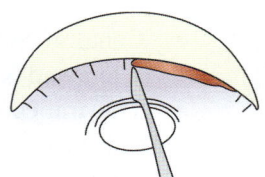

Goniotomy knife

DIFFERENCES BETWEEN CONGENITAL GLAUCOMA AND KERATOGLOBUS

CLINICAL FEATURES	INFANTILE GLAUCOMA	KERATOGLOBUS	HIGH MYOPIA
1. Intraocular pressure	Raised	Normal	Normal
2. Corneal opacity	Present	Absent	Absent
3. Optic disc cupping	Present	Absent	Absent
4. Angle of anterior chamber	Abnormal	Normal	Normal

Treatment

The treatment of congenital or infantile glaucoma is always *surgical*.

1. Medical Treatment

Systemic acetazolamide and mannitol IV along with local beta blockers, e.g. timolol maleate control the intraocular pressure preoperatively. Miotics are useless as they do not help in aqueous outflow.

2. Operative Treatment

i. Goniotomy
- A specially constructed knife is passed at the limbus.
- A Barkan goniotomy knife is swept across the angle of the anterior chamber in the opposite segment under direct gonioscopic observation.
- It opens up the blockage of the corneoiridic angle by the persistent embryonic tissue.

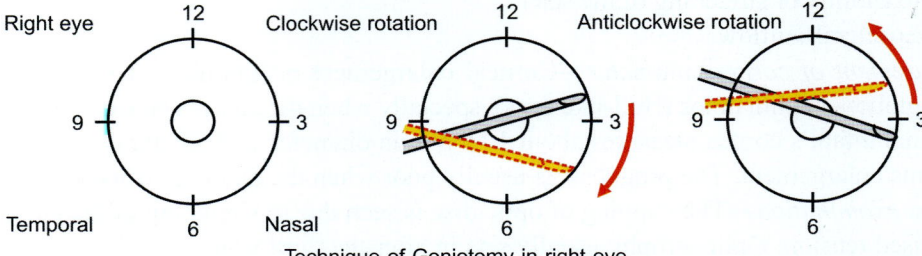

Technique of Goniotomy in right eye

ii. Trabeculotomy
- A small flap of conjunctiva and a partial thickness flap of sclera are made at the upper limbus
- Canal of Schlemm is exposed by making a vertical incision and dissection through the sclera and is identified.
- The trabecular meshwork is incised by passing a probe or lower prong of Harm's trabeculotome (the upper prong is used as a guide) into the canal and then rotating it into the anterior chamber to break the inner wall over one quarter of the canal.

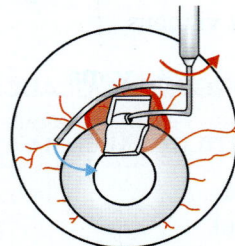

Harm's trabeculotome

- This is repeated on the other side also.
  It is often difficult to localise the Schlemm's canal. However it is useful in cases where goniotomy has failed or when the angle is not visible due to hazy cornea.

iii. Trabeculectomy
—If all forms of trabeculotomy fail then a trabeculectomy, a type of filtering operation may be considered.

PRIMARY OPEN ANGLE GLAUCOMA (POAG)

It is a chronic, slowly progressive condition with an insidious onset. This presents an entirely different clinical picture from the acute closed angle glaucoma.

Etiology

It has a genetic basis. There is sclerosis of the trabecular meshwork in any type of eye. The endothelial lining of the canal of Schlemm may also be sclerosed.

Incidence

i. *Age*—It affects 6-7th decade mainly.
ii. *Sex*—Both sexes are involved equally.
iii. It is a *bilateral* condition usually.
iv. *Rare*—It is more common and severe in black people than in white.

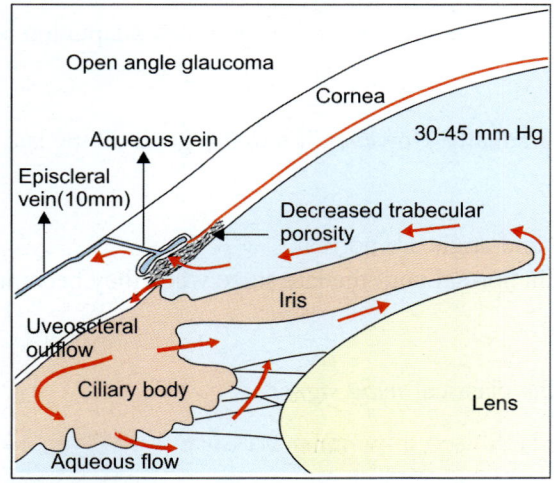

Mechanism of rise in intraocular pressure in open angle glaucoma

Mechanism of Primary Open Angle Glaucoma

There is increased resistance to the outflow of the aqueous humor offered by:
1. *The sclerosed trabecular meshwork*—Electron microscopic picture shows following changes in the trabecular meshwork. (i) Proliferation of endothelial lining with thickening of the basement membrane. (ii) Narrowing of intertrabecular spaces. (iii) Deposition of amorphous material in the juxtacanalicular tissue.
2. *The sclerosed endothelium lining of the canal of Schlemm*—This leads to narrowing or collapse of canal of Schlemm.

Associated Ocular Pathology

Following ocular diseases may be present in association with primary open angle glaucoma.

- High myopia
- Fuchs endothelial dystrophy
- Retinitis pigmentosa
- Retinal vessel occlusion
- Retinal detachment.

Symptoms

1. There is painless, progressive loss of vision. Due to its insidious onset, it is usually noticed when vision is completely lost in one eye and the other eye is seriously impaired.
2. Mild headache and eyeache may be present.
3. A defect in the visual field (noticed by an intelligent patient) is often present.
4. There is increasing difficulty in doing near work. Reading or close work is often difficult due to accommodative failure as a result of pressure upon the ciliary muscle and its nerve supply. There is frequent increase in the strength of presbyopic glasses.
5. Light sense is defective. Light minimum is raised and dark adaptation is slowed.

Signs

1. Visual acuity decreases gradually. However, it remains good till the late stage as the central field of vision persists.
2. Cornea is usually clear.
3. Anterior chamber depth and angle are normal.
4. Pupillary reactions remain normal until the late stage when they become sluggish.

Diagnosis

The diagnosis depends on the classical *triad signs:*

1. Raised intraocular pressure
↓
2. Cupping of the optic disc
↓
3. Visual field defects

Pathogenesis

1. **Raised tension**—In primary open angle glaucoma careful study and repeated observations of tension are required.
    i. Initially there is exaggeration of normal diurnal variation. A variation of intraocular pressure over 5 mm Hg (Schiotz) should always excite suspicion of glaucoma.
    ii. Later on there is permanent elevation of tension so that the normal basal level is not attained.
2. **Cupping of the optic disc**—*Pathogenesis of optic disc changes*—Both mechanical and vascular factors play a role in the cupping of the disc.

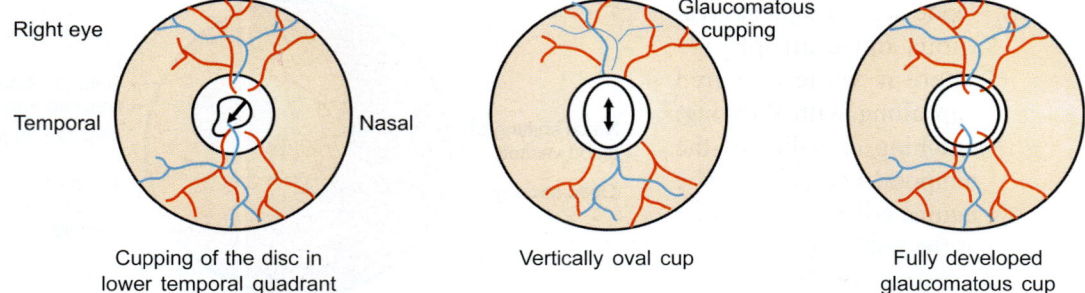

Cupping of the disc in lower temporal quadrant   Vertically oval cup   Fully developed glaucomatous cup

a. Mechanical effect of raised intraocular pressure forces the lamina cribrosa backwards and squeezes the nerve fibres within its meshes to disturb the axoplasmic flow.
b. Vascular factors—Ischaemic atrophy of the nerve fibres occur without corresponding increase of supporting glial tissue. As a result, large caverns or lacunae are formed (cavernous optic atrophy).
   i. The cupping of the optic disc usually starts as a focal enlargement in the lower temporal quadrant. However, it may enlarge in concentric circles
   ii. Vertically oval cup—It is due to the thinning of the lower margin of the optic cup at the 6 O'clock position.

Normal physiological cup   Glaucomatous cup

   iii. When fully developed it should be differentiated from the physiological cup.
   - Normal cup/disc ratio = 0.3.
   - Glaucomatous cup/disc ratio may vary from 0.6 to even 0.9, specially if in the vertical axis
   - An asymmetry between the two optic nerve heads of more than 0.2.

DIFFERENCES BETWEEN NORMAL PHYSIOLOGICAL CUP AND GLAUCOMATOUS CUP

CLINICAL FEATURES	NORMAL PHYSIOLOGICAL CUP	GLAUCOMATOUS CUP
1. Excavation	Nil	It reaches to the edge of the disc
2. Margins	Shelving	Steep
3. Lamina cribrosa	Normal position	Backward displacement
4. Retinal vessels	Continuity is intact.	Bayonetting sign—retinal vessels appear to be broken off at the margin of the cup.
5. Parallax	Nil	Marked in deep cup.
6. Pulsation of arteries	Nil	May be present when there is raised tension.

iv. Optic nerve atrophy (cavernous optic atrophy)—There is white coloured cup along with thinning, notching or pallor of the temporal neural rim. The lamina cribrosa is exposed at the bottom of the cup.
v. Laminar dot sign—Dot or slit-like openings of the lamina cribrosa are visible upto the margin of the cup. It is primarily due to vascular ischaemia leading to the degeneration of nerve fibres along with the direct mechanical pressure effect on the optic nerve head.

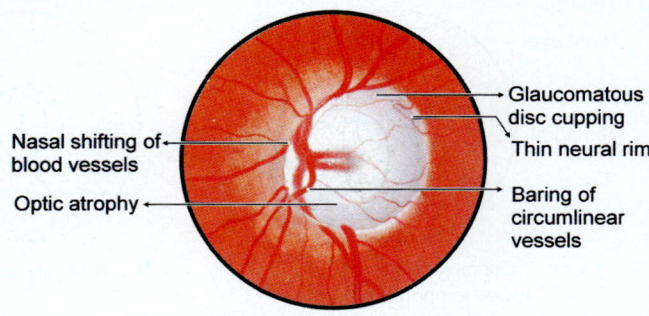

Glaucomatous optic atrophy

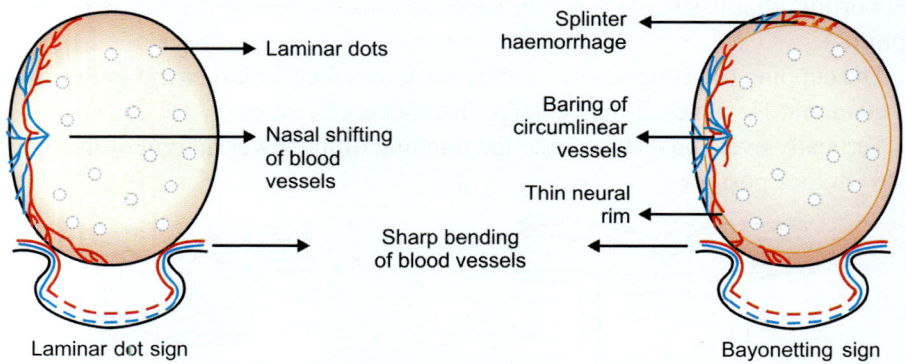

Laminar dot sign   Bayonetting sign

vi. Bayoneting sign—The retinal vessels appear to be broken off at the margin of the cup. There is double angulation of the blood vessels as they pass backwards and then turn along the steep wall of the excavation before angling again on to the floor of glaucomatous cup.
vii. There may be nasal shifting of retinal vessels along with baring of circumlinear vessels at the disc margin and 'overpass' of the central vessels.
viii. Splinter haemorrhages may be seen at the disc margin.
3. **Visual field defects** These run parallel to the changes in the optic disc.

Anatomy of the Retinal Nerve Fibres

The retinal nerve fibres are arranged in a precise pattern which forms the basis for the characteristic optic disc and visual field changes.
1. *Macular fibres*—These have straight course to the optic disc forming spindle-shaped papillomacular bundle. They get affected last with retention of central vision until the advanced stage of glaucoma.
2. *Nasal fibres*—These have relatively straight course to the optic disc.

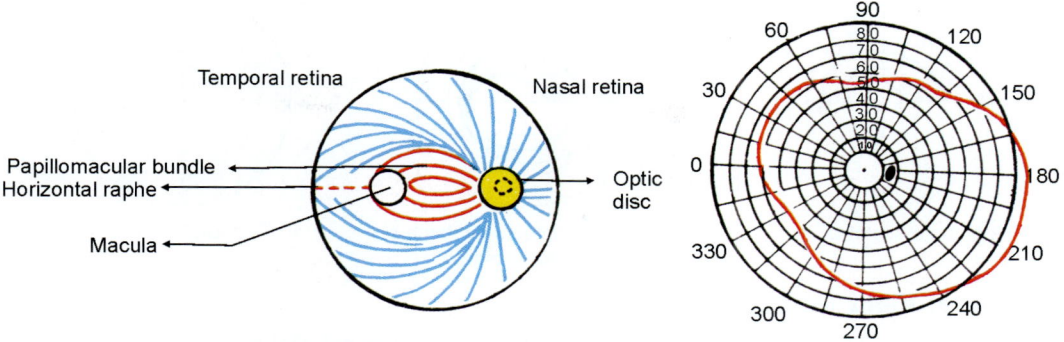

Arrangement of retinal nerve fibres   Extent of normal visual field-Right eye

3. *Temporal fibres*—They follow an arcuate path around the papillomacular bundle. There is an imaginary horizontal raphe dividing the superior and inferior part. These fibres are most sensitive to glaucomatous changes.

I. Central Field Defects (up to 30°)

It is preferably tested by automated instruments or Bjerrum's screen. Typical scotomas are seen in the central field which are as follows,

1. **Baring of the blind spot**—There is localised constriction of the central field to a very small test objects (1/2000). The central field curves inwards to exclude the blind spot. However, this sign is not pathognomonic of early glaucoma.

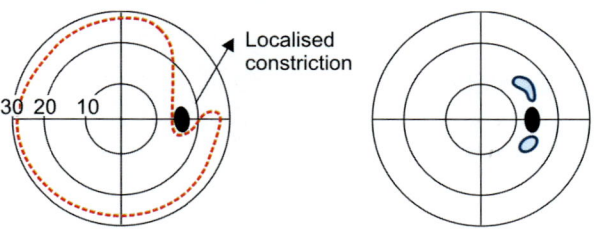 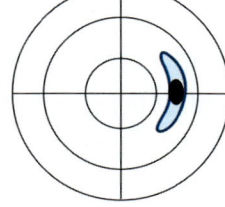

1. Baring of the blind spot   2. Small scotomatous areas   3. Seidel's sign

2. **Small scotomatous areas**—One or more scotomatous areas appear in the same isoptre. They are usually present above the blind spot.
3. **Seidel's sign**—There is a sickle-shaped extension of the blind spot above or below or both. The concavity of the sickle is directed towards the fixation point.
4. **Bjerrum's scotoma**
    i. Arcuate scotoma—An arc-shaped scotoma passes from the blind spot above the fixation point.
    ii. Annular or double arcuate scotoma—Two arc-shaped scotomas pass above and below the fixation point forming an annular or ring scotoma.
5. **Temporal-central islands**—Eventually temporal-central islands are present as the macular fibres get affected last.

270 Basic Ophthalmology

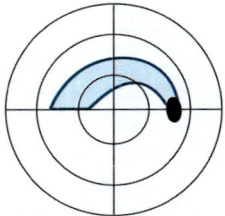 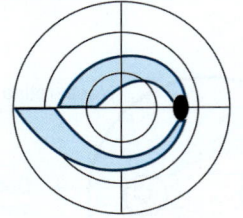 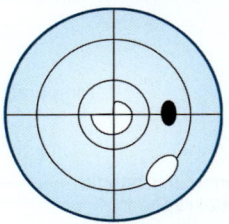

4. Bjerrum's arcuate scotoma
5. Double arcuate scotoma or annular scotoma
6. Temporal-central island

II. Peripheral Field Defects

1. *Roenne's step*—Usually the upper or sometimes lower nasal fields show sectorial defects. They have sharply defined horizontal edge which looks like a step.
2. *A paracentral area of temporal field persists eventually,* the central vision being abolished due to general contraction of the field of vision.

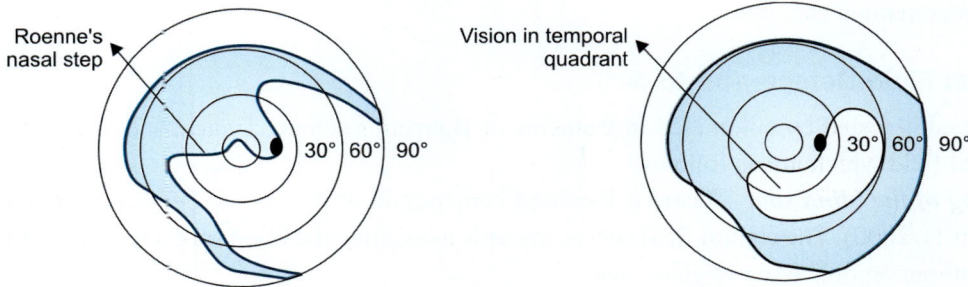

Peripheral visual field defects

Clinical Importance of Visual Field Defects

1. To establish the presence of disease.
2. To measure its progress.
3. To estimate its prognosis.
4. To assess the value and response to treatment.

Investigations

1. *Raised intraocular tension*—It can be measured by Schiotz tonometer or various types of applanation tonometers.
2. *Cupping of the optic disc*—It is seen by direct ophthalmoscopy or by slit-lamp biomicroscopy using a + 90 D or a + 78 D lens.
3. *Typical visual field defects*—Central field is tested by automated perimetry or Bjerrum's screen, whereas peripheral field is examined by Lister's or Goldmann's perimeter.
4. *Water drinking test*—The patient is asked to drink one litre of water before breakfast. This lowers the osmotic pressure of blood. If there is a rise of tension more than 6 mm Hg after 1/2 hour, it is suspicious of open angle glaucoma.

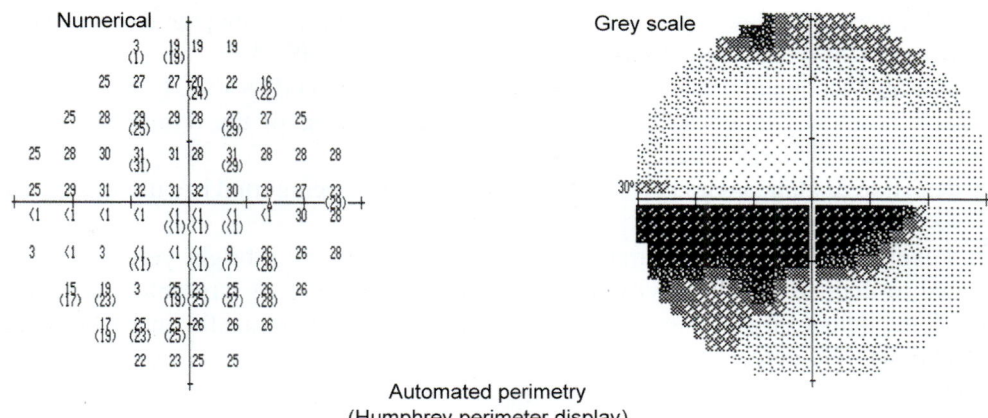

Automated perimetry
(Humphrey perimeter display)

5. *Tonography*—It is a graphic record of the intraocular pressure using electronic tonometer. However, it is of doubtful value in assessing the prognosis and the extent of blockage of drainage channels.

6. *Confocal scanning laser tomography (CSLT)*—The use of this exciting new technology allows the ophthalmologist to obtain a topographic image of optic nerve containing more than 2 million data points in less than 1 second. The image is generated through the transmission of laser beam and the computer synthesises data obtained from many different levels. The computer analyses the point data and produces three dimension images like a CAT scan of optic nerve head. CSLT is superior to stereo-photographs and are excellent tools to keep a record of topography.

   It is commercially available as *The Heidelberg retinal tomograph (HRT)*—It is a confocal laser scanning ophthalmoscope designed for three-dimensional imaging of the posterior segment of the eye. It provides highly accurate and reproducible images. It is useful in patients having or suscpected to have glaucoma.

7. *Optical coherence tomography (OCT)*—It provides high resolution cross-sectional images of the retina. It uses light from a superluminescent diode, analogues to B scan ultrasonography which uses sound waves. In glaucoma, it can be used to measure retinal nerve fibre layer thickness around optic nerve head and optic disc cupping.

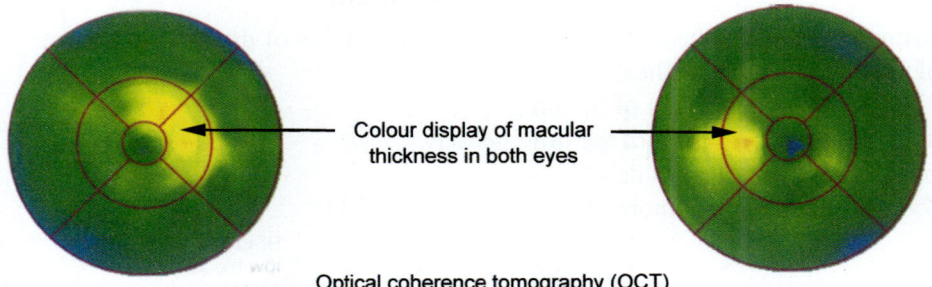

Optical coherence tomography (OCT)

8. *Nerve fibre layer analyser (NFLA) (Scanning laser polarimetry)*—A related new technology is also valuable to detect subtle changes before disc damage has actually occurred in glaucoma, NFLA determines the depth of nerve fibre layer by measuring retardation of light as it moves

through the nerve fibre layer. NFLA is a step forward in determining that optic nerve deterioration is occurring before it can be detected by visual field examination.

The current version of nerve fibre layer analyser is known as GD × VCC (Glaucoma Diagnosis × Variable Corneal Compensation). It estimates the thickness of the retinal nerve fibre layer (RNFL) in the peripapillay area.

9. Early detection of glaucomatous visual field changes is now being tried in a number of ways such as:
- Short wavelength (blue) light stimuli—In automated perimetry a bright yellow background is presented to depress the sensitivity of the green and red cones. A large blue target is used to measure the sensitivity of the short wave length system. It is useful in early detection of glaucomatous field defects.
- Frequency doubled stimuli
- Contrast detection techniques
- Motion detection and flicker frequency fields.

Treatment

Principle

The main aim of treatment is to prevent visual loss and visual field defect which result from high intraocular pressure. Regular supervision by tonometry and fundus photography if possible is advised to assess the progress of disease.

Methods

The treatment options available at present are medicines, laser or surgery to lower the intraocular pressure.
1. *Medical*—It is always the treatment of choice in the early stages.
2. *Surgical*—It is considered to be the last resort.
3. *Argon or diode laser trabeculoplasty (ALT or DLT)*—It is the most advanced technique.
4. *Recent advanced procedures*—These include laser filtration, seton valves, deep sclerotomy and viscocanalostomy.

I. Medical Treatment

Medical treatment is always the treatment of choice. Basic rules of drug treatment are:
i. Initial therapy is usually medical.
ii. Use the lowest concentration of the drug.
iii. Use the minimum frequency of the drug per day.
iv. Choose the drug with least side effects.
v. Combined drug therapy is more effective and convenient.

1. Local

1. *Pilocarpine* (0.5-4%) 2% eyedrops are applied four times a day. It is also available as 4% pilocarpine gel for night use soaked hydrophilic contact lens and ocuserts (pilo-20 and pilo-40) where it is slowly released.

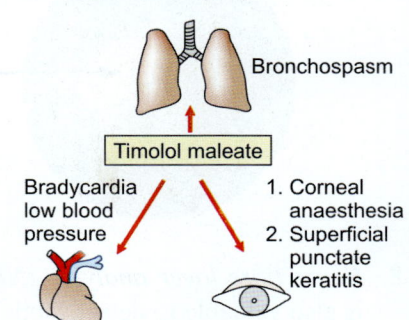

Side effects of timolol maleate

Mode of action—It increases aqueous outflow by miotic action. It is a cholinergic drug, supplementing the normal effect of acetylcholine. There is contraction of ciliary muscle which increases the facility of aqueous outflow through trabecular meshwork.

Side effects—There may be diminished night vision, iris cyst, miosis, myopic shift, brow ache, accomodative spasm etc. It is a safe drug.

2. *Beta-blockers*
   i. *Timolol maleate* (0.25-0.5%) eyedrops are applied twice daily. Timolol maleate gel is used once a day

Mode of action—It reduces aqueous secretion. It is a non-selective beta 1 and beta 2 adrenergic blocking agent. It does not alter the pupillary size.

Side effects—Bronchospasm, bradycardia, low blood pressure and corneal anaesthesia, depression and fatigue.

   ii. *Betaxalol* (0.5%) eyedrops are applied twice daily. It is a cardioselective beta-adrenergic blocking agent which has the advantage of having little effect on cardiopulmonary system. However, it is less effective than timolol and levobunolol.
   iii. The other non-selective beta adrenergic blockers are
   - *Levobunolol* (0.25-0.5%, 1-2 times a day)
     The action of levobunolol lasts the longest and therefore it is more reliable for once a day use than timolol.
   - *Carteolol* (1-2%, 1-2 times a day)
     It raises triglycerides and lowers high density lipoproteins the least. It is therefore best choice for patients with open angle glaucoma having associated hyperlipideamia or athero-sclerotic cardiovascular disease. It is similar to timolol in action.
   - *Metipranolol* (0.1-0.6%, 1-2 times a day)
     It is almost similar to timolol in all respects.

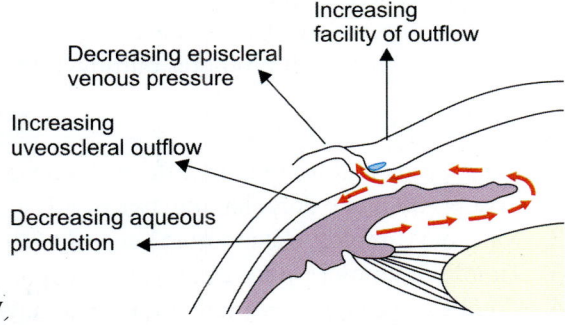

Measures to decrease intraocular pressure

3. *Adrenergic drugs*
   i. *Adrenaline (Epinephrine)* (1-2%) eyedrops are applied twice daily. It is an alpha and beta adrenergic agonist.
   Mode of action
   a. It reduces aqueous production due to vasoconstriction (α-adrenergic effect).
   b. It increases aqueous outflow by stimulation of β-receptors in the outflow system (β-adrenergic effect).
   Side effects
   Local—Conjunctival hyperaemia, allergic blepharoconjunctivitis, nasolacrimal obstruction, adrenochrome deposits in the conjunctiva, angle closure glaucoma and cystoid maculopathy.
   General—premature cardiac contractions and other arrhythmias.
   ii. *Brimonidine (Alphagan)* (0.2%, twice daily). It is an alpha-2 adrenergic agonist.
   Mode of action—It acts by reducing aqueous production and also by increasing uveoscleral outflow. It also has a neuroprotective effect.
   Side effects—Allergic conjunctivitis, xerostomia, drowsiness and fatigue may occur.

iii. *Apraclonidine* (0.5%, 1%)—It is also an alpha agonist. It is mainly used after laser surgery on the anterior segment to offset an acute rise in IOP. It is not suitable for long-term use because of tachyphylaxis and higher incidence of local side effects.
4. Topical carbonic anhydrase inhibitors
    i. *Dorzolamide* (2%, 2-3 times a day) It is a recently introduced topical carbonic anhydrase inhibitor. It is water soluble and has excellent corneal penetration
    Mode of action-It lowers intraocular pressure by decreasing aqueous secretion
    Side effect—It may cause allergic blepharo conjunctivitis.
    ii. *Brinzolamide* (1% three times a day)—It is similar to dorzolamide but there is lower incidence of ocular allergy.
5. *Prostaglandin and prostamide analogues* (prostaglandin F 2 alpha).
    Mode of action—They act by increasing uveoscleral outflow. They are additive with all other agents.
    i. *Latanoprost* (0.005% once a day)
    Side-effects—conjunctival hyperaemia, eyelash lengthening and hyperpigmentation of lashes, iris and periorbital skin. Anterior uveitis and cystoid macular oedema may occur in predisposed eyes, hence should be used with caution in uveitic glaucoma.
    ii. *Travoprost* (0.004% once a day)—It is similar to latanoprost but may have a superior ocular hypotensive effect.
    iii. *Bimatoprost* (0.03% once a day)—It is a synthetic prostamide analogue similar to prostaglandins. It promotes outflow through both uveoscleral and trabecular routes.

Combine Drugs Therapy

Combine preparations are more effective, convenient and improve patients' compliance.
1. Cosopt (timolol + dorzolamide) twice daily
2. Xalacom (timolol + latanoprost) once daily
3. TimoPilo (timolol + pilocarpine) twice daily
4. Combigan (timolol + brimonidine) twice daily
5. Duotrav (timolol + travoprost) once daily.

2. Systemic

Carbonic Anhydrase Inhibitors (CAI)

These drugs are not recommend for long-term use because of the side effects.

Dosage
  i. Tab acetazolamide 250 mg is given one to four times daily
  ii. Sustained action capsules of acetazolamide 250-500 mg (substitute) are given once or twice daily
  iii. Tab Methazolamide 50-100 mg is given twice daily.

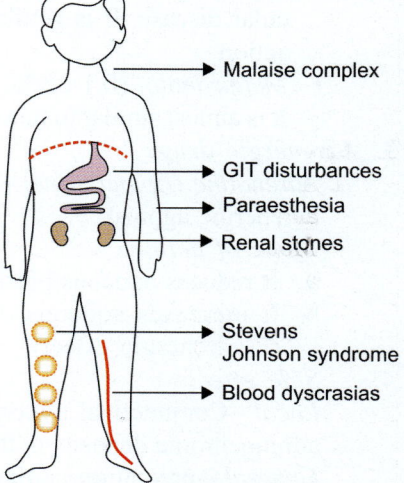

Side effects of acetazolamide

Mode of action—There is decreased formation of bicarbonates which causes less secretion of aqueous from the ciliary epithelium (diuretic effect is not a factor in the reduction of intraocular pressure).

COMMON TOPICAL ANTI-GLAUCOMA DRUGS

DRUGS	DAILY DOSE	MODE OF ACTION	SIDE EFFECTS
1. MIOTICS (PARASYMPATHOMIMETICS)			
i. Pilocarpine 1%, 2%, 4%	3-4 times daily	Ciliary muscle contraction, miosis, opens spaces in trabecular meshwork	Miosis and spasm, induced myopia, hyperaemia, risk of retinal detachment, cataract, iris cyst
2. SYMPATHOLYTIC DRUGS			
A. Nonselective beta blockers			
i. Timolol Maleate 0.25, 0.5%	Twice daily	Reduces aqueous secretion	Bronchospasm, bradycardia, arrhythmia, low blood pressure, corneal anesthesia
ii. Levobunolol 0.25%, 0.5%	Once daily	Reduces aqueous secretion	Same as timolol but with lesser ocular side effects
B. Selective beta blockers Betaxolol 0.5%	Twice daily	Reduces aqueous secretion	Same as timolol except no corneal anesthesia. Lesser pulmonary side effect.
3. SYMPATHOMIMETIC			
i. Epinephrine 1% Dipivefrine 0.1%	Twice daily	Increases aqueous outflow by their beta agonist action Reduce aqueous formation due to vasoconstriction	Irritation, conjunctival congestion, cystoid macular oedema
ii. Brimonidine 0.2%	Twice daily	Increases aqueous outflow and decreases aqueous secretion	Hyperaemia, foreign body sensation, allergy
iii. Apraclonidine 0.5%	2-3 times daily	Increases aqueous outflow and decreases aqueous secretion	Same as Brimonidine
4. PROSTAGLANDIN AND PROSTAMIDE ANALOGUES			
i. Latanoprost (Xalatan) 0.005%	Once daily	Enhances uveoscleral outflow	Hyperaemia, iris pigmentation, allergy, risk of cystoid macular oedema
ii. Travoprost (Travatan) 0.004%	Once daily	Enhances uveoscleral outflow	Conjunctival hyperaemia
iii. Bimatoprost (Lumigan) 0.03%	Once daily	Enhances both trabecular and uveoscleral outflow	More conjunctival hypercaemia but fewer headache and less iris hyperpigmentation
5. CARBONIC ANHYDRASE INHIBITOR			
i. Dorzolamide 2% (topical)	2-3 times daily	Decreases aqueous production	Allergy, superficial punctate keratitis, blurring dryness
ii. Brinzolamide 1%	2-3 times daily	Decreases aqueous production	Similar to dorzolamide but lower incidence of stinging and local allergy

Side effects—Paraesthesia, malaise complex, gastric irritation, renal stone formation, Stevens-Johnson syndrome and blood dyscrasias. It is supplemented by 1 g potassium daily as there is associate potassium loss.

3. Hyperosmotic Agents

Mode of action—These agents increased the plasma tonicity or osmolality to draw water out of the eyes. This results in lowering the intraocular pressure.

1. Oral
i. Glycerol (50% solution)—1.5 g/kg body weight. It is a sweet tasting sticky liquid. 30 ml of pure glycerol with equal amount of fruit juice is given stat and then 3 times daily.
ii. Isosorbide—1-2 g/kg body weight. It is metabolically inert so it can be safely given to diabetic patients. It does not cause nausea.

2. Intravenous
i. Mannitol (20%)—1-2 g/kg body weight. A 20% solution is given over 30-40 minutes
ii. Urea—1-2 g/kg body weight. A 30% solution in sugar used to be given. It is not used in recent times.

II. Surgical Treatment

Trabeculectomy, a filtering operation is done when the miotics and β-blockers fail to control the tension and the field defects progress.

III. Argon or Diode Laser Trabeculoplasty (ALT or DLT)

It is a safe, non-invasive and an out-patient department procedure. The average drop of intraocular tension is 8-10 mm Hg. It has dramatically changed the treatment of uncontrolled open angle glaucoma.

Mode of action—Discrete laser beam causes a shrinkage of the collagen on the inner surface of the trabecular ring, thereby, opening the intertrabecular spaces. This increases the aqueous outflow.

Argon Laser Trabeculoplasty (ALT)

Indications
1. Open angle glaucoma
   - Patients with insufficient response to topical treatment
   - Poor compliance to the medical treatment by patients
   - Elderly patients in whom laser therapy may postpone surgery to beyond life expectancy.
2. The intraocular pressures do not reach normal limits after filtration surgery.

Contraindication—Invisibility of the trabeculum (e.g. closed or narrow angle, blood obscuring the angle, hazy cornea), paediatric glaucoma, secondary glaucoma, previously failed ALT.

Extent—180°

Viewing power—The slit-lamp is utilised with a gonioscopic lens with 25-fold ocular viewing power.

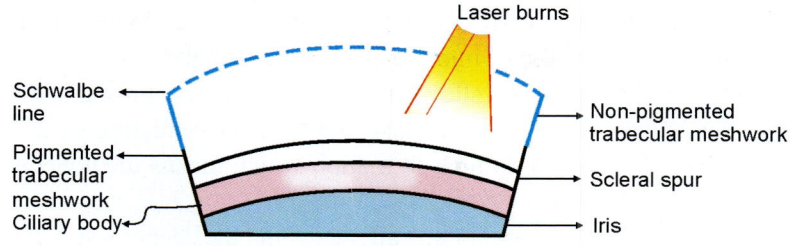

Placement of the argon-laser beam focus

Direction—The beam is to be focused at the junction between the pigmented and non-pigmented trabeculum.

Spot size—50 mm

Duration—0.1 sec

Energy—700-1500 mW (aim is to achieve transient blanching or bubble formation at the point of impact). Note that less pigmented angles require higher energy.

Number of burns—Approximately 100.

Diode Laser Trabeculoplasty (DLT)

This gives similar results to ALT but there is less disruption of blood-aqueous barrier.

IV. Recent Advanced Procedures

These are adviced when standard procedures fail.

1. *Laser filtration*—It is done with virtually any laser coupled to a fiberoptic delivery system. It produces a sclerostomy (opening in the sclera). The advantage over routine filtering operations are fewer complications by use of smaller or no incision.

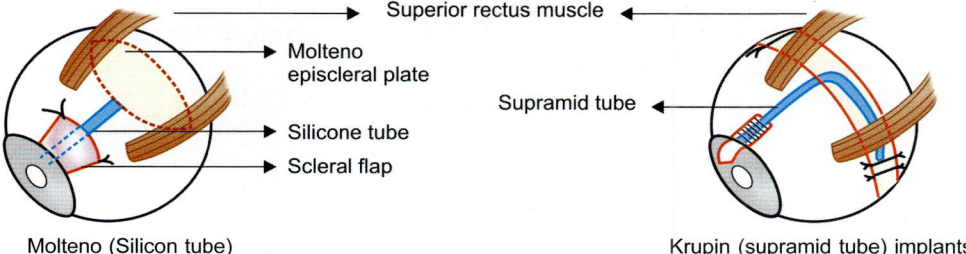

Molteno (Silicon tube)   Krupin (supramid tube) implants

2. *Seton valves*—These include filtration devices such as the Molteno (silicon tube) and Krupin (supramid tube) implants. It is a subconjunctival implant connected to a tube that enters the anterior chamber. Aqueous is shunted through the implant and diffuses away in the subconjunctival tissue. It is used in refractory glaucoma.
3. *Non-penetrating surgery*—The anterior chamber is not entered and the internal trabecular meshwork preserved. This reduces the incidence of postoperative overfiltration and hypotony. The two currently used procedures are:

a. *Deep sclerectomy*—A window is created in the Descemet's membrane which allows aqueous seepage from the anterior chamber into the collector channels.
b. *Viscocanalostomy*—This operation allows aqueous to percolate through an intact window in the Descemet's membrane into the scleral lake and then into Schlemm's canal and finally into the collector channels. There is no bleb formation which means the aqueous does not drain into the subconjunctival space.

It is similar to deep sclerectomy except that after excising the deeper sclera flap, high viscosity viscoelastic substance is injected into the Schlemm's canal.

NORMAL TENSION GLAUCOMA (NTG)

Definition

The term normal tension glaucoma, also referred to as low tension glaucoma is characterized by typical glaucomatous disc changes with visual field defects, with an intraocular pressure remaining constantly below 21 mm of Hg.

It is a variant of primary open angle glaucoma.

Incidence

1. The prevalence above the age of 40 years is approximately 0.2%
2. It is seen in about 16% of all cases of open angle glaucoma
3. Females are at a greater risk than males (2:1 ratio).

Etiology

The exact cause is not known.
It results due to vascular insufficiency of optic nerve head. This view is supported by presence of:
- Nocturnal systemic hypotension and overtreated systemic hypertension
- Migraine
- Reduced blood flow velocity in the ophthalmic artery and posterior ciliary arteries (as shown by transcranial Doppler imaging)
- Raynaud phenomenon—There is peripheral vascular spasm on cooling.

Diagnosis

1. Intraocular pressure IOP is constantly below 21 mm Hg
2. Open drainage angle on gonioscopic examination
3. Optic nerve head
   - It is usually larger than open angle glaucoma
   - Glaucomatous cupping and parapapillary changes are identical
   - Splinter haemorrhages and optic disc pits are more frequent than open angle glaucoma
4. Visual field defects—They are same as in primary open angle glaucoma. They tend to be closer to the fixation point, deeper, steeper and more localised.

Investigation

Perimetry should be done at 4-6 monthly interval to demonstrate progression before starting medical treatment. In some cases the visual field loss is stationary and treatment is not required.

Treatment

The risk factors necessary for treatment include:
- Progression of visual field loss
- Presence of disc haemorrhages
- Female patients
- Associated migraine.

The aim is to lower IOP by atleast 30%
1. *Medical*
   - Betaxolol—It is the drug of choice as it increases optic nerve blood flow along with lowering IOP.
   - Prostaglanding analogues, e.g. latanoplast tend to have a greater ocular hypotensive effect.
2. *Trabeculectomy*—It may be considered in atleast one eye if progressive visual field loss occurs inspite of low IOP.
3. Monitoring of systemic hypertension for 24 hours is done. If nocturnal drop of blood pressure is present, avoid high dose of antihypertensive medication.
4. Non selective topical beta blocker should not be used at bed time.

PRIMARY ANGLE-CLOSURE GLAUCOMA (PACG)

This is a condition in which the intraocular tension is raised due to the narrow or closed angle of the anterior chamber. There is obstruction to the outflow of the aqueous humor.

Etiology

It has a genetic basis. It is typically seen in eyes which are:
  i. *Small and hypermetropic eye*
 ii. *Anatomical narrow angle of the anterior chamber*
iii. *Shallow anterior chamber*
 iv. *Iris—lens diaphragm is pushed forwards.*

Small and hypermetropic eye

Incidence

  i. *Age*—It affects mainly in the 5th-6th decade
 ii. *Sex*—Women are usually affected (male: female ratio is 1:4)
iii. It is usually *bilateral* but one eye is involved first
 iv. *Personality*—Highly strung, anxious persons with unstable vasomotor system
  v. *Race*—It is common among Asians and Eskimos but rare in Africans and Caucasians.

Mechanism of Angle-closure Glaucoma

1. **Relative pupil block**—Normally pupillary margin just touches the anterior surface of the lens.

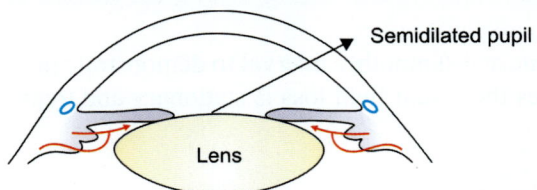

1. Pupillary block due to semidilated pupil

2. ***Physiological iris bombe***—On dilatation of the pupil there is crowding of the iris in the angle of anterior chamber causing obsruction to the flow of aqueous from the posterior to the anterior chamber at the level of the pupil. The iris bows forwards due to the increased pressure in the posterior chamber.

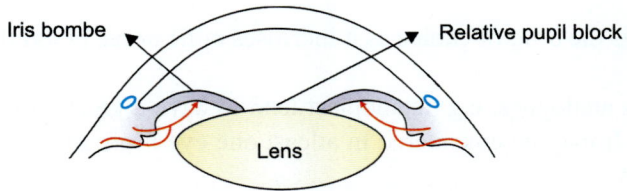

2. Physiological iris bombe

3. ***Irido-trabecular contact***—It totally cuts off the drainage channel by forming a false angle. It precipitates an attack of raised intraocular pressure (acute congestive attack).

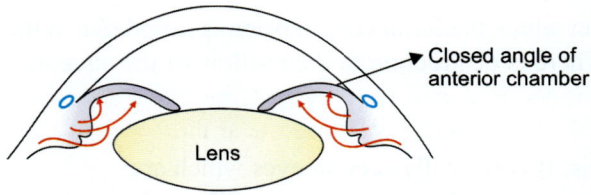

3. Irido-trabecular contact

Stages

The clinical course of the disease has been divided into five stages. The condition however does not necessarily progress from one stage to the other in an orderly sequence.

1. *Primary angle-closure glaucoma suspect (latent)*
2. *Subacute or intermittent primary angle-closure glaucoma*
3. *Acute primary angle-closure glaucoma*
4. *Chronic primary angle-closure glaucoma*
5. *Absolute primary angle-closure glaucoma*

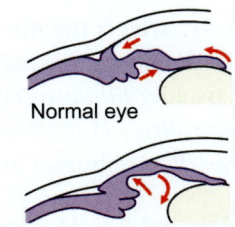

Mechanism of closed angle glaucoma

1. PRIMARY ANGLE-CLOSURE GLAUCOMA SUSPECT (LATENT)

The term essentially implies to an anatomically predisposed eye.

Clinical Features

1. Symptoms are absent.
2. Slit lamp examination.
   i. Axial anterior chamber depth is less than normal or decreased
   ii. Iris-lens diaphragm is convex in shape
   iii. Close proximity of the iris to cornea in the periphery.
3. Gonioscopy shows an 'occludable' angle (less than 20 degrees). The pigmented trabecular meshwork is not visible (Shaffer grade 1 or 0) without indentation or manipulation in at least three quadrants.

Diagnosis

1. *Dark room test*—It is a provocative test. The patient is asked to lie down in a dark room, in the prone (face downwards) position for 1 hour without sleeping. A rise in IOP of 8 mm Hg or more in the presence of closed angle is diagnostic.
2. *Mydriatic test* (0.5% tropicamide)—It is usually not preferred because this is not physiological.

Primary angle-closure glaucoma suspect is a retrospective diagnosis. It is confirmed in one eye during an attack of acute congestive angle closure in the other eye usually.

Investigations

1. van Herrick method—Slit-lamp grading of the angle can be used with fair accuracy when a gonioscope is not available. An optical section of the peripheral cornea and anterior chamber is made with the illumination and viewing arms at 60 degrees to each other. The viewing arm is perpendicular to the cornea using a magnification of × 15. The peripheral anterior chamber depth (PACD) is compared to the adjacent corneal thickness (CT) and the presumed angle width is graded as shown below:

   Grade 4 (Wide open angle)   : PACD = 3/4 to 1 CT
   Grade 3 (Mild narrow angle)   : PACD = 1/4 to 1/2 CT
   Grade 2 (Moderate narrow angle)   : PACD = 1/4 CT
   Grade 1 (Extremely narrow angle)   : PACD < 1/4 CT
   Grade 0 (closed angle)   : PACD = Nil.

   This is an approximate and subjective assessment.

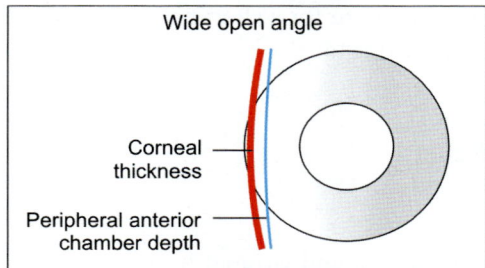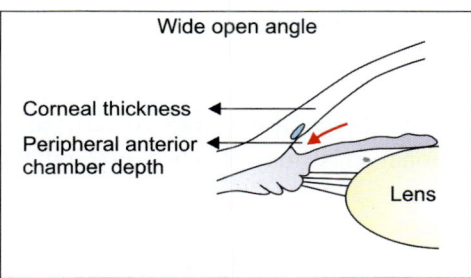

van Herrick method of slit-lamp grading of angle of anterior chamber

2. *Orbscan II ultrasonography*—Objectively the anterior chamber can be measured optically by the pachymetry attachment of a slit-lamp or by Orbscan II ultrasonography.

It is a corneal topography mapping system which combines scanning slit with placido disc technology.

Course

Clinical course without treatment may be as follows:
- Intraocular pressure (IOP) may remain normal
- Acute of subacute angle-closure may occur
- Chronic angle-closure glaucoma may develop without passing through acute or subacute stages.

Treatment

Prophylactic peripheral laser iridotomy in both eyes will prevent an acute attack. If untreated, the risk of acute pressure rise during the next 5 years is approximately 50%.

2. SUBACUTE (INTERMITTENT) PRIMARY ANGLE-CLOSURE GLAUCOMA

There are occasional attacks of raised intraocular pressure with unilateral blurring of vision, coloured halos, mild headache and browache. In between the recurrent attacks the eyes are free from symptoms.

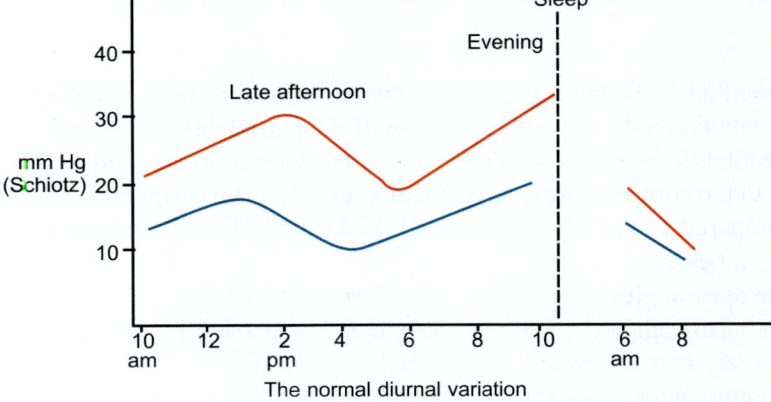

The normal diurnal variation

Intermittent angle closure occurs in an anatomically predisposed eye in which physiological factors such as reading in dim illumination or watching television in a dark room precipitates a pupillary block due to mydriasis. This causes a sharp rise in intraocular pressure for a short period of time followed by a spontaneous resolution of the pupillary block possibly due to:
  i. *Rest*
  ii. *Sleep* (As the pupil becomes constricted)
      Emotional stress may also be a precipitating factor.

Symptoms

  i. *Blurring of vision*—This occurs due to corneal oedema and stromal haze.

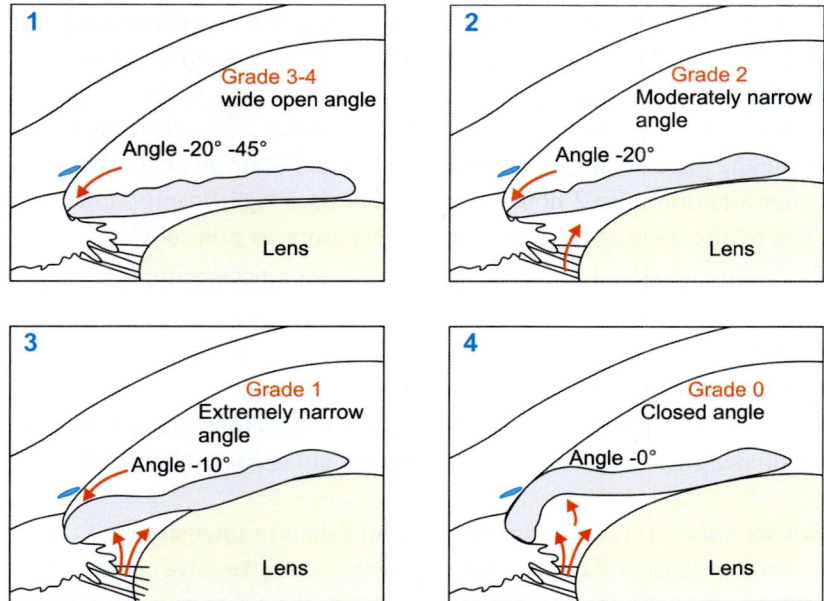

Becker and Shaffer classification of angle of anterior chamber

ii. *Coloured halos around lights*—There is accumulation of fluid in the corneal epithelium and corneal lamellae which alters the refractive conditions of the cornea. As halos are seen as coloured rings around lighted bulb, they are observed only after dark. The colours are distributed as in the spectrum of rainbow with red colour being outside and violet inner most.
iii. *Mild headache and browache*—This is mainly due to raised intraocular tension.
iv. *In between the recurrent attacks*—The eyes are free from symptoms.

Course
Some eyes may develop an acute attack or may progress into chronic primary angle-closure glaucoma.

Diagnosis
Diagnosis in the early stages (angle-closure suspect and intermittent or subacute angle-closure) is important since adequate treatment at this stage is easy and certain to prevent the loss of vision.
1. History of seeing coloured halos around light bulb with blurred vision. If the patient gives a vague history, the halo can be demonstrated by him on looking through a thin layer of lycopodiun powder enclosed between two glass plates made up as a trial lens.
2. Gonioscopy
   - Presence of narrow angle of the anterior chamber is seen
   - There is narrow angle recess with clumping of pigments in the angle
   - Occasional peripheral anterior synechiae may be present.
3. Provocative tests- Rise in tension can be tested by the provocative tests even if the tension is normal.

284 Basic Ophthalmology

   i. *Dark room test*—The patient lies awake in the prone (with face downward) position in a dark room for 1 hour. The pupil dilates and if the rise in tension is more than 8 mm Hg (Schiotz), it is pathological.
   ii. *Mydriatic test*—A weak mydriatic (0.5% tropicamide, 2.5% phenylephrine) is sometimes used to dilate the pupil with great care as it may precipitate an acute attack. A rise in tension is noted after a period upto 2 hours. The tension rises significantly. Full miosis is achieved after the test by the instillation of pilocarpine eyedrops as precaution.

   This test is strictly nonphysiologic and has significant false negatives.

Differential Diagnosis

1. *Iritis*—This has already been discussed on page no 173.
2. *Lenticular halos*—These are typically seen in early cataractous changes in the lens. The two may be differentiated by Fincham's test. A stenopaeic slit is passed before the eye across the line of vision.
   i. *Glaucomatous halo*—It remains intact but diminished in intensity.
   ii. *Lenticular halo*—It is broken up into segments which revolve as the slit is moved. It is typically seen in the case of incipient cataract due to the prismatic effect of the wedge-shaped peripheral cortical opacities where the halos "make and brake".
3. *Halo in conjunctivitis*—This is due to the sticking of conjunctival discharge on the cornea. It disappears on washing the discharge.

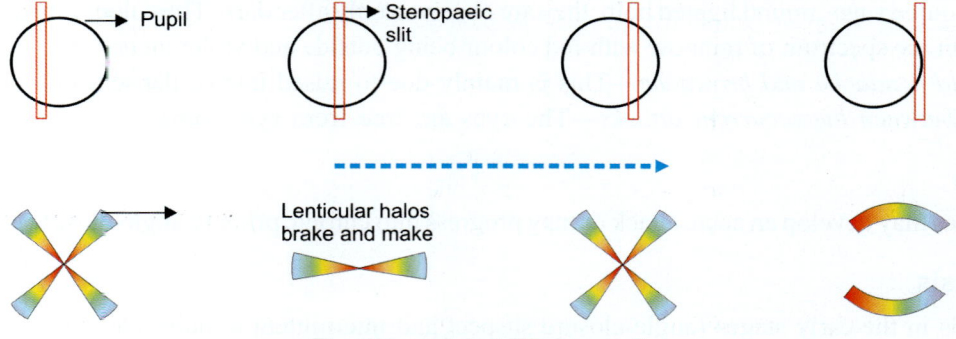

The stenopaeic test (Fincham test)

Treatment

Prophylactic peripheral laser iridotomy is performed in both eyes of all the patients because if untreated the risk of acute pressure rise during the next 5 years is very high (50% approximately).

3. ACUTE PRIMARY ANGLE-CLOSURE GLAUCOMA

Acute or congestive angle-closure glaucoma is *always* associated with the sudden closure of the angle of anterior chamber with marked elevation of intraocular pressure and congestion (red eye). It is a sight-threatening emergency.

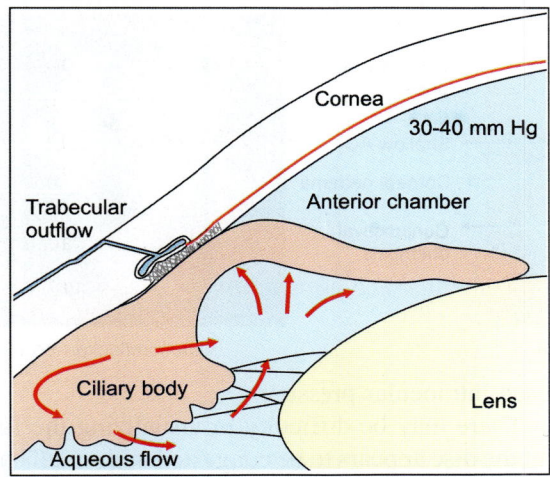

Mechanism of the rise in intraocular pressure in angle-closure glaucoma

Pathogenesis

The crisis is due to acute ischaemia associated with liberation of prostaglandin-like substances. If the attack lasts for several hours or days, irreversible damage may occur to the ocular tissues.

Symptoms

1. Severe unilateral headache, nausea, vomiting and prostration are often associated. It is often mistaken for an acute abdomen or appendicitis.
2. There is sudden onset of intense unbearable pain in the eye due to stretching of the sensory nerves. It radiates along the branches of the 5th nerve.
3. There is marked dimness of vision. It may be reduced to only hand movement or perception of light. It is mainly due to ischaemia due to optic neuropathy and partially due to corneal oedema stasis and increased permeability of the capillaries.
4. Redness, lacrimation and photophobia are present due to corneal oedema erosion and conjunctival and ciliary congestion.

Signs

1. There is oedema of the lids and conjunctiva (chemosis).
2. There is marked conjunctival and ciliary congestion (red eye).
3. Cornea is cloudy (oedematous) and insensitive. Accumulation of the fluid occurs in all the layers of the cornea. This is due to the imbibation of fluid in the cornea caused by the dysfunction of the 'endothelial pump' as a result of raised intraocular pressure.
4. Anterior chamber is very shallow as the iris gets pushed forwards.
5. Iris pattern is lost and may be discoloured. Atrophic patches (white or grey coloured) may be seen due to ischaemia.
6. Pupil is moderately dilated and vertically oval. Light and accommodation reflexes are absent.
7. Lens—Glaucoma fleckens are small greyish white anterior subcapsuler opacities seen in the lens in the pupillary area. They are due to atrophy of the newly formed lens fibres. They are diagnostic of previous attack of acute congestive glaucoma.

Vertically oval pupil

Vertically oval pupil

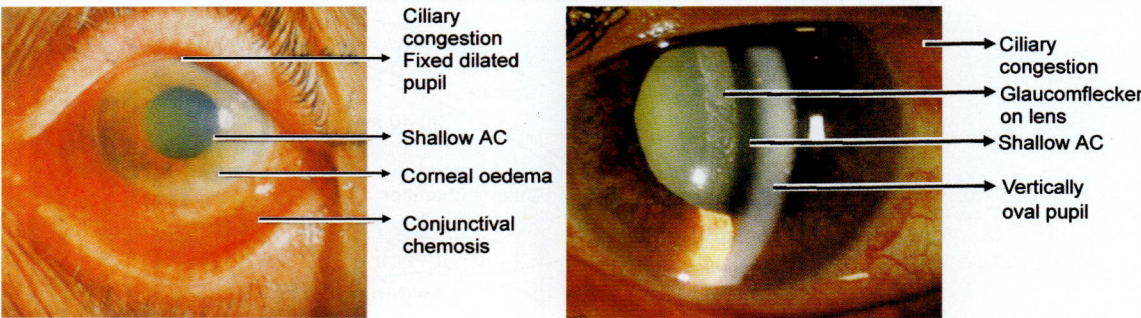

Acute congestive glaucoma   Glaucomflecken on lens

8. There is markedly raised intraocular pressure.
9. Fundus examination—There may be difficulty in visualizing the fundus due to hazy cornea. There is no cupping but the disc appears to be congested with small haemorrhages. Spontaneous pulsation of the central retinal artery may be seen.
10. Gonioscopy—It reveals abnormally narrow angle of the anterior chamber with or without anterior synechiae. Peripheral anterior synechiae (organized exudates) occur as a result of prolonged and repeated acute congestive attack. Initially there is iridocorneal contact but later on it becomes iridotrabecular.
11. The fellow eye usually has a shallow anterior chamber with a narrow angle.

Complications

Acute ischaemic neuropathy may occur leading to total visual loss. The perfusion of optic nerve head is affected due to decreased blood flow in the capillary and in annulus of Zinn which supplies nutrition to the laminar and post-laminar optic nerve head.

Course

1. There may be spontaneous improvement but after each attack,
    i. The visual acuity is lowered
    ii. The visual field contracts irregularly
    iii. False angle of anterior chamber is formed due to peripheral anterior synechiae.
2. It usually passes into the stage of chronic primary angle-closure glaucoma as the angle becomes slowly and progressively closed.

Treatment

Although the treatment of primary angle-closure glaucoma is essentially surgical, the initial treatment is medical in order to control the raised tension. After controlling the raised intraocular pressure, laser iridotomy or surgical peripheral iridectomy (PBI) should be performed when the eye is quiet.

I. Medical Treatment

It is useful in lowering the raised tension particularly in the acute congestive attack preoperatively. The patient should be positioned supine (lying straight) to allow the lens to shift posteriorly.

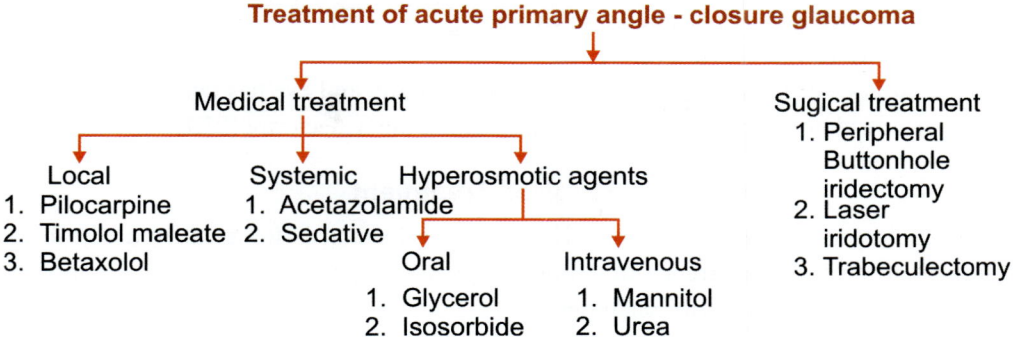

1. Systemic

1. *Full sedation* is attained. Strong analgesics (even injection pethidine) and antiemetics may be given.
2. *Carbonic anhydrase inhibitors*—It reduces the formation of aqueous by inhibiting the action of carbonic anhydrase enzyme. Thus, there is decreased formation of bicarbonates. Acetazolamide 500 mg intravenously and 500 mg orally and/or intravenous mannitol is given after making sure that the patient is not suffering from cardiovascular disease. Later acetazolamide 250 mg may be given orally four times a day.
   a. This reduces the raised intraocular pressure
   b. It relieves ischaemic changes in the iris
   c. It also decreases the corneal oedema.
3. *Pressure with moist cotton swab* can be applied on the central part of the cornea if the pupil remains blocked. This helps to mechanically push the iris away from the cornea.

2. Local

1. *Pilocarpine (2%)*—It should be started half to one hour after commencement of systemic treatment, i.e. after the IOP is lowered a bit. At higher pressure, iris sphincter is ischaemic and unresponsive to pilocarpine.
   Initially pilocarpine is instilled every 30 minute and later hourly till maximum miosis is achieved. Thereafter it is used four times daily. Ocuserts and gel are also available for prolonged action. This is effective in pulling the iris away from the angle and opening the drainage channels.
   Mode of action—It increases aqueous outflow by miotic action.
2. *Timolol maleate*—Initially 0.25-0.5% eyedrops are instilled frequently. Thereafter it is used twice daily.
   Mode of action—It reduces the aqueous secretion from the ciliary epithelium.
3. Betaxolol and other non-selective beta adrenergic blockers may also be used.

3. Hyperosmotic Agents

Initially 20% IV mannitol (1-2 g/kg) over 45 minutes or 50% oral glycerol (1 g/kg) or isosorbide may be given to lower the raised tension. They act by drawing water out of the eye and thus reducing the IOP.

i. The osmotic pressure of plasma is increased
ii. This draws water out of the eye.

When the intraocular pressure has been reduced medically and eye has become quiet, the further treatment is laser iridotomy or surgical peripheral buttonhole iridectomy (PBI).

II. Surgical Treatment

It is *always* indicated for permanent cure. However, the tension is lowered by medical treatment before surgery to prevent occurrence of expulsive haemorrhage. The choice of operation depends on the state of the angle of anterior chamber.

A careful gonioscopic examination is necessary in deciding the percentage of angle closure by peripheral anterior synechiae (PAS) before considering the type of surgery :

i. If the angle closure by PAS is less than 50%, then a laser iridotomy or surgical iridectomy should be sufficient.
ii. If the angle closure by PAS is more than 50%, a filtration operation, e.g. trabeculectomy is preferred.

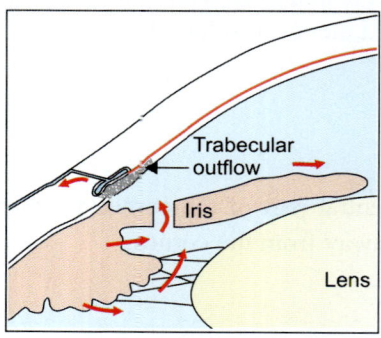

Laser iridotomy or peripheral iridectomy

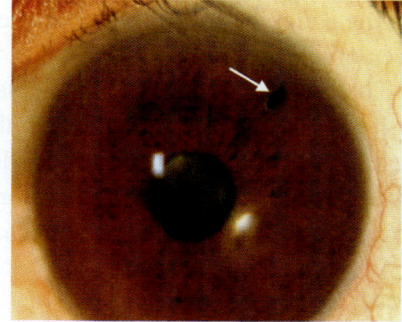

Nd: YAG Laser iridotomy

1. **Laser iridotomy** (Nd:YAG) or surgical peripheral buttonhole iridectomy (PBI)
   This is useful in cases where the peripheral anterior synechiae are present in less than 50% circumference of the angle of anterior chamber. In general, Nd: YAG (neodymium yttrium-aluminium-garnet) laser iridotomy is superior to surgical iridectomy in the treatment of most forms of pupil-block glaucoma. Nd: YAG is the best as it can be used in all types of irides.

   Technique
   A drop of topical pilocarpine is instilled frequently 30 minutes before laser therapy. This helps to keep the peripheral iris tight and straight relatively.

   A crypt in the iris is noted. The laser with an anterior offset is then used to make an opening measuring 150-200 microns in size is made in the periphery of iris. The power used varies from 3 to 6 mJ.

   By making a hole in the periphery of iris, pupillary block is relieved permanently. It re-establishes communication between posterior and anterior chambers so it bypasses the pupillary block and controls the raised IOP. Posterior chamber aqueous pressure is thus relieved by :

i. Aqueous flowing through this extraopening into the anterior chamber
ii. The peripheral iris falls away from the trabecular meshwork.

Laser iridotomy is effective in about 75% of eyes. Unresponsive cases may require trabeculectomy.

Postoperative management—Steroids and anti-glaucoma treatment is given for 5-7 days to control the inflammation and rise in IOP.

Advantages
- It is a non-invasive procedure and chances of infection are nil
- It is a relatively painless, out-patient department procedure
- It is cheap in cost to the patient.

Disadvantages
- Laser is not widely available as it is costly
- It is difficult to perform iridotomy in presence of corneal oedema and flat anterior chamber
- It may cause endothelial burns
- Iridotomy hole may be blocked by scar tissue later on.

2. **Trabeculectomy**—It is done when extensive peripheral synechiae are present (more than 50% angle closure). It is a type of filtering operation. A partial thickness of a part of limbus (trabecular meshwork and canal of Schlemm) is excised under a scleral flap.

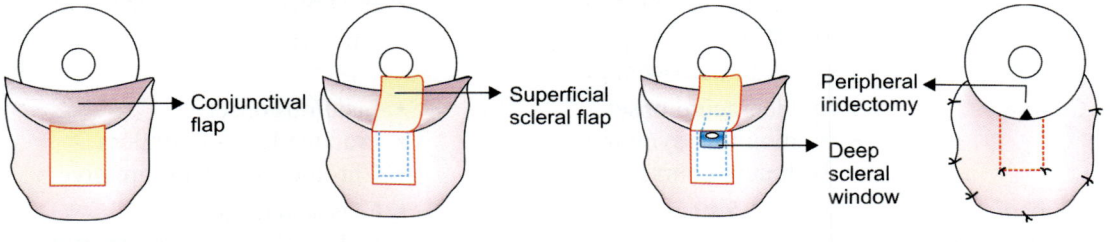

1. Conjunctival flap   2. Scleral flap   3. Trabeculectomy   4. Conjunctival suture

Technique
1. A conjunctival flap is dissected anteriorly 10 mm away from the limbus in the upper part of cornea (12 O'clock position).
2. A 5 × 5 mm area with base at the limbus is marked on the bare sclera.

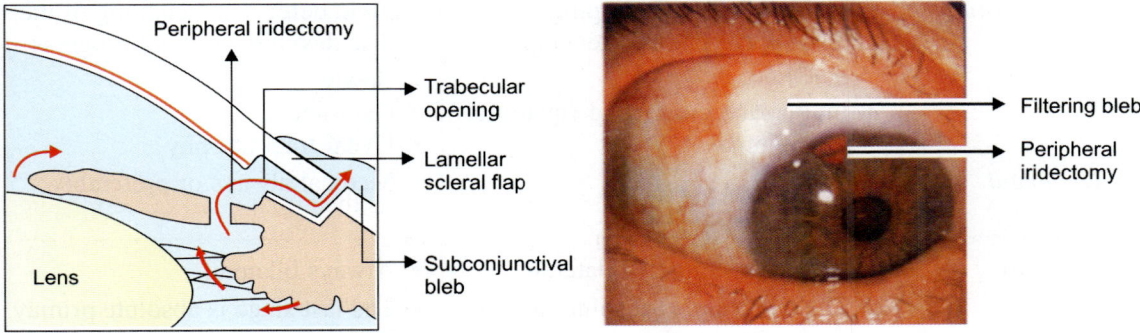

Conjunctival filtering bleb following trabeculectomy

3. The superficial flap of the sclera measuring 5 × 5 mm is dissected anteriorly upto the limbus.
4. A deeper scleral window 2 × 4 mm is cut and a peripheral iridectomy done.
5. The superficial scleral flap is repositioned and sutured. The conjunctival flap is also sutured.
6. The aqueous seeps out from the anterior chamber into the scleral window → It passes in between the two scleral flaps → It flows into the subconjunctival space. This forms a small 'bleb' or swelling under the conjunctiva.

Postoperative management Topical broad spectrum antibiotic drops and ointment, cycloplegic and corticosteroids are given for a period of 2-3 weeks.

Prophylaxis—The fellow or the second eye should be treated by laser iridotomy or surgical peripheral buttonhole iridectomy (PBI) as soon as possible as the condition is always eventually bilateral.

DIFFERENCES BETWEEN PRIMARY ANGLE-CLOSURE AND OPEN ANGLE GLAUCOMA

CLINICAL FEATURES	PRIMARY ANGLE-CLOSURE	PRIMARY OPEN ANGLE
1. *Type of patient*	• Women • 5-6th decade • Anxious, excitable habit • Unstable vasomotor system	• Either sex • A decade later in 6-7th decade • Nil • In subjects of sclerosis
2. *Type of eye*	• Small hypermetropic eye with narrow angle	• Any type of eye
3. *Course*	• Sudden acute onset • Premonitory symptoms • Turbulent course	• Insidious onset • Practically symptomless • Chronic, slowly progressive
4. *Clinical features*	Typical 5 stages: i. Primary angle-closure glaucoma suspect (latent) ii. Subacute or Intermittent iii. Acute primary angle-closure iv. Chronic primary angle-closure v. Absolute primary angle-closure	• Classical triad signs: i. Raised intraocular pressure ii. Cupping of the optic disc iii. Visual field defects
5. *Complications*	• Field defects and cupping of the disc appear late but develop rapidly • Intercalary, ciliary and equatorial staphyloma	• Field defects and cupping of the disc develop early but progress slowly • Cataract • Uveal tract atrophy
6. *Treatment*	• Surgical always Initially medical	Medical always or preferably
Similarity	1. Always eventually bilateral. 2. The end stage is absolute primary angle-closure glaucoma.	• Always bilateral • The last stage is absolute primay angle-closure glaucoma.

4. CHRONIC PRIMARY ANGLE-CLOSURE GLAUCOMA

In this stage the angle of the anterior chamber becomes slowly and progressively closed resulting in diminution of vision. It is associated with eyeache and headache.

Pathogenesis

Type 1(Creeping)—It is caused by gradual and progressive closure of the angle by synechiae over atleast 180 degrees. It always starts superiorly and progresses circumferentially.

Type 2 (Subacute)—It is caused by synechial angle closure as a result of subacute (intermittent) attacks secondary to the pupillary block.

Type 3 (Mixed)—It is caused by combination of primary open angle glaucoma (POAG) with narrow angles. It may be associated with long term use of miotics.

Clinical Features

1. There is diminution of vision associated with eyeache and headache.
2. The eye is irritable and the visual acuity is always impaired.
3. Circumcorneal ciliary congestion is present around the limbus as reddish blue zone.
4. Intraocular pressure is permanently raised when about two-third or more circumference of the angle is closed by peripheral anterior synechiae.
5. Typical scotomatous defects are seen in the visual field.
6. Cupping of the disc appears for the first-time. Thus, it simulates the clinical features of open angle glaucoma. Pallor and shallow temporal shelving may be also seen.

Diagnosis

1. *Gonioscopy*—It shows variable amount of angle closure.
2. *Fundus examination*—Cupping of the disc appears for the first-time. Thus, it simulates the clinical features of primary open angle glaucoma.

Treatment

As extensive peripheral anterior synechiae have been formed; miotics, surgical peripheral iridectomy (PBI) or laser iridotomy are of no use at this stage as they are unable to open drainage channels.

Therefore after lowering the raised intraocular pressure with β-blockers, acetazolamide and hyperosmotic agents ; a filtration surgery (trabeculectomy) should be done.

1. Laser iridotomy alone or along with medical therapy may be tried.
2. Trabeculectomy is necessary when the above treatment fails to control raised IOP.
3. Prophylactic laser iridotomy should be done in the fellow eye.

5. ABSOLUTE PRIMARY ANGLE-CLOSURE GLAUCOMA

The chronic phase if untreated, with or without the intermittent subacute attacks, gradually passes into the final stage of absolute glaucoma.

The eye is completely blind with markedly increased intraocular pressure.

Symptom

Painful blind eye with no perception of light (no PL) is the most prominent symptom.

Signs

1. Ciliary congestion is present around the limbus.
2. Cornea is clear and insensitive with
    i. Vesicles (bullous keratopathy) may be seen
    ii. Filaments (filamentary keratopathy) may be present.
3. Anterior chamber is very shallow.
4. The iris is atrophic (white patches) and may have a broad zone of pigment around the pupil (ectropion of the uveal pigment) due to fibrosis of the iris tissue.
5. The pupil is grey instead of jet black, dilated and vertically oval.
6. The tension is usually very high and the eyeball is as hard as stone.
7. There is deep cupping of the optic disc.

Complications

1. *Atrophic bulbi*—The eye is completely blind with no perception of light. The intraocular pressure is raised usually. Ocular structures like cornea, iris, anterior chamber can be easily identified unlike in phthisis bulbi. The eyeball is of normal size and shape.

    Essentially it is a histopathologial diagnosis, whereby the cytoarchitecture of the eye is maintained in the blind eye.
2. *Phthisis bulbi*—It is due to degeneration of the ciliary body whereby its secretory functions are decreased or abolished. This results in marked hypotony and drooping of the upper eyelid. The eyeball is shrunken and ocular structures cannot be identified clearly. Phthisis bulbi is essentially a clinical diagnosis.

    In phthisis bulbi, in addition to atrophy there is disorganisation of the ocular cytostructure in the blind eye.
3. *Staphyloma*—The intercalary, ciliary and equatorial staphyloma are formed as a result of raised tension and the degeneration and thinning of scleral tissue.
4. *Rupture of the eyeball* may occur even from slight injury.

DIFFERENCES BETWEEN ATROPHIC BULBI AND PHTHISIS BULBI

CLINICAL FEATURES	ATROPHIC BULBI	PHTHISIS BULBI
1. Size of eyeball	Normal	Sunken
2. Ocular structures—Cornea, iris, anterior chamber, etc.	They can be easily identified	They cannot be appreciated clearly
3. Drooping of upper eyelid	Nil	Present due to lack of support.
4. Visual acuity	Blind eye (no PL)	Blind eye but some vision may be present in the initial stages
5. Intraocular pressure	Normal or raised	Reduced (marked hypotony)
6. Common causes	Absolute glaucoma	• Perforated corneal ulcer • Perforating ocular injury • Endophthalmitis • Panophthalmitis

Treatment
Pain is relieved by the following procedures:
1. *Retrobulbar injection of 1.5 ml procaine 4% (local anaesthetic) is given.* Wait for 7 minutes and then inject 1-2 ml alcohol 80%. Firm pad and bandage are applied for 24 hours. This results in the paralysis of ciliary ganglion and relieves pain.
2. *Absolute thrombotic glaucoma*—Pain may be relieved by atropine 1% drops together with dexamethasone 0.1% drops applied twice daily.
3. *Filtering operations* done alone are rarely effective. Use of adjunctive mitomycin C or 5 fluorouracil (5-FU) both cidal to fibroblasts is more helpful in lowering the tension. It is comparable to full thickness procedures.
4. *Partial destruction of the ciliary body*—It may be done by :
    i. Cyclodiathermy using surface electrodes may result in necrosis of scleral tissue and staphyloma formation
    ii. Cyclocryopexy application through the conjunctiva over the ciliary body (90°-180°). It causes tissue necrosis and often results in patients discomfort and ocular inflammation. It can cause marked hypotony if applied over more than 180°
    iii. Application of intense ultrasound to produce focal lesions of the sclera (over the pars plana). It is a more desirable procedure as it is effective, more predictable and pain free
    iv. Nd: YAG laser cyclodestruction or diode laser cycloprotocoagulation may be done.
5. *Enucleation*—Excise the eye in cases of unbearable painful blind eye as a last resort.

SECONDARY GLAUCOMA
Secondary glaucoma occurs due to a specific anomaly or disease of the eye.

Etiology
1. *Inflammatory glaucoma*—Hypertensive uveitis is due to the dilation of uveal blood vessels and blockage of the angle by plasmoid aqueous and exudate.
2. *Postinflammatory*—It occurs due to the,
    i. Blockage at the pupil by the annular posterior synechiae or occlusiopupillae
    ii. Blockage at the angle of anterior chamber by the peripheral anterior synechiae and organised exudate.
3. *Perforation of cornea*—It can occur as a result of ulcer, trauma or operative wounds causing formation of the peripheral anterior synechiae.
4. *Massive intraocular haemorrhage*—It may occur,
    i. *In the anterior chamber (hyphaema)* following a blunt injury
    ii. *In the vitreous*—The iris-lens-diaphragm gets pushed forwards
    iii. *Neovascular glaucoma* results commonly due to thrombosis of the central retinal vein and rubeosis iridis in diabetes mellitus.
5. *Lens*—It occurs in the ,
    i. *Phacomorphic glaucoma—Intumescent stage* (swollen lens) of senile cortical cataract

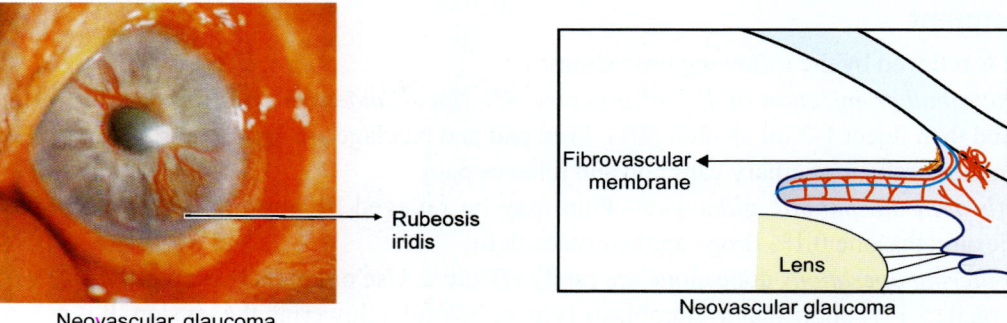

Neovascular glaucoma

ii. *Anterior dislocation of lens*—The lens may block the angle of anterior chamber
iii. *Phacoanaphylaxis*—There is hypersensitivity reaction to lens protein postoperatively
iv. *Phacolytic glaucoma*—It occurs in cases of hypermature cataract due to leakage of lens protein through the capsule
v. *Aphakia*—There may be pupillary block or vitreous may fill the anterior chamber.
6. **Intraocular tumour**—It usually results due to the infiltration of the angle or by direct pressure effect of the tumour mass on the angle of the anterior chamber.
7. **Venous obstruction**—This leads to raised venous pressure which decreases the drainage of aqueous in the episcleral veins as in,
   i. Orbital inflammation
   ii. Large orbital tumour
   iii. Arteriovenous communications
8. **Obstructive glaucoma**—There is organic blockage of the angle of anterior chamber due to
   i. *Inflammatory exudates* resulting in peripheral anterior synechiae formation
   ii. *Neoplasm* may infiltrate the angle or cause direct pressure
   iii. *Degeneration*
      a. In glaucoma capsulare there are degenerative changes and exfoliation of the anterior lens capsule and anterior uvea. The flakes block the trabecular meshwork
      b. In pigmentary glaucoma there is pigment dispersion which blocks the angle.
   iv. *Epithelialisation of the anterior chamber*—It occurs following perforating injury to the cornea or after cataract surgery. The conjunctival epithelium grows inside the anterior chamber and blocks the angle.

Treatment

Treat the basic underlying cause of raised tension.

APHAKIC GLAUCOMA

It is a type of secondary glaucoma which occurs following extraction of the lens.

Etiology

It occurs after cataract surgery due to:
  i. Delayed formation of anterior chamber—This results in the formation of peripheral anterior synechiae. It may occur due to choroidal detachment or leaking section
  ii. The vitreous protruding through the pupil in the anterior chamber may cause pupillary block
  iii. Presence of vitreous in the anterior chamber blocks the angle.

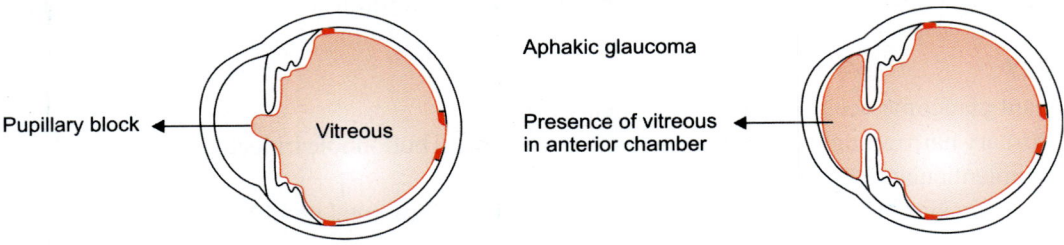

Aphakic glaucoma

Symptoms

1. There is severe pain in the eyes and headache due to raised intraocular tension.
2. There is gradual dimness of vision due to pressure atrophy of the optic disc.
3. Photophobia and lacrimation may occur due to corneal oedema and erosion.

Signs

1. There is raised intraocular tension.
2. Cornea may be hazy due to corneal oedema as a result of endothelial damage.
3. Cupping of the optic disc may be present.
4. Associated visual field defects may be present.

Treatment

1. *Trabeculectomy with vitrectomy* is a useful procedure. Trabeculectomy is preferably done in lower temporal quadrant to facilitate the drainage of aqueous by gravity.
2. *Cyclodialysis*—A cyclodialysis spatula is passed in the suprachoroidal space and rotated around 180°. This facilitates the uveoscleral outflow. It is not very useful.
3. *Cyclocryopexy*—A single row of cryoprobe application is done over 90°-180° of the circumference of the eyeball in the ciliary region (3-4 mm behind the limbus). It produces trans-scleral freezing and partial destruction of the ciliary body.

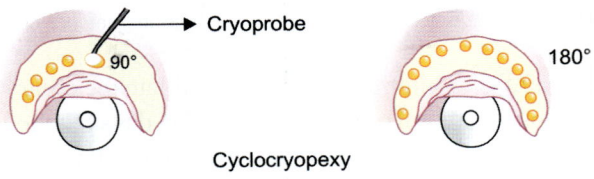

Cyclocryopexy

4. *Trans-scleral or transvitreal photocoagulation* of the ciliary processes under direct vision causes partial destruction of the ciliary body. This results in decreased formation of the aqueous.
5. *Therapeutic high intensity ultrasound* is a more desirable approach in many cases because it is an effective, more reliable and pain-free procedure.

MALIGNANT GLAUCOMA

Malignant glaucoma is a rare condition which may occur as a complication of any intraocular surgery.

Etiology

Malignant glaucoma occurs typically in patients with
  i. Primary narrow angle glaucoma operated for peripheral buttonhole iridectomy or trabeculectomy (ciliolenticular block)
  ii. Aphakic eyes following vitreous phase disturbance (ciliovitreal block).

Pathogenesis

1. It is believed that following intraocular operation, the tips of the ciliary processes rotate forward and press against the equator of the lens in phakic eyes (ciliolenticular block) or press against the anterior phase in aphakic eyes (ciliovitreal block)
2. This blocks the normal flow of aqueous which is diverted posteriorly and collects as aqueous pockets in the vitreous.
3. Thus the anterior chamber becomes flat and IOP is markedly raised.

Signs

1. There is persistent flat anterior chamber following any intraocular operation.
2. There is markedly raised IOP in early postoperative period.

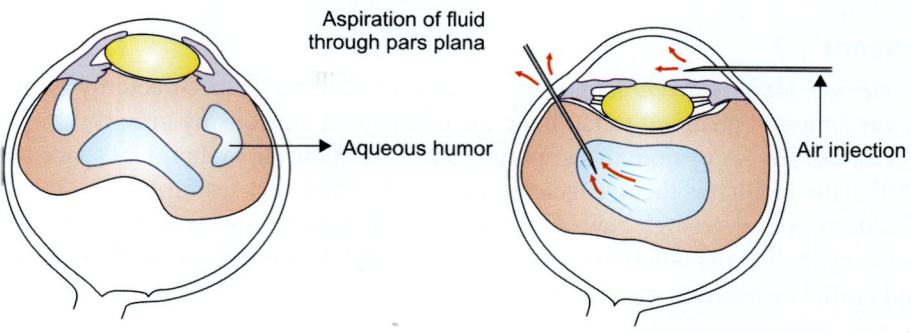

Pockets of aqueous in the vitreous

Aspiration of fluid and air injection in the anterior chamber

Treatment

1. *Medical therapy*—Atropine drops or ointment is applied to dilate the ciliary ring. Acetazolamide, timolol maleate and intravenous mannitol may be given for 5-6 days but they are seldom effective.
2. *Surgical therapy*—Aspiration of fluid from the vitreous cavity along with vitrectomy is done through a pars plana incision. This is followed by air injection in the anterior chamber.

MULTIPLE CHOICE QUESTIONS

1. Aqueous humor formation occurs by all means *EXCEPT*
   a. ultrafiltration
   b. active secretion
   c. passive diffusion
   d. de nove synthesis
2. Large haemangioma of lids and cheek along with glaucoma is seen in
   a. von Recklinghausen's disease
   b. Sturge-Weber syndrome
   c. von Hippel-Lindau disease
   d. none of the above
3. Glaucoma may be secondary to all the following *EXCEPT*
   a. iritis
   b. dislocation of lens
   c. hyphaema
   d. occlusion of short ciliary artery
4. Regarding buphthalmos, which is correct
   a. boys are affected more than girls
   b. bilateral
   c. trabeculotomy is the treatment of choice
   d. all of the above
5. Rainbow halo around light is seen in
   a. early stages of closed angle glaucoma
   b. early stages of cataract
   c. acute mucopurulent conjunctivitis
   d. all of the above
6. Primary acute congestive glaucoma manifests as
   a. cupping of disc
   b. pinpoint pupil
   c. hand movements vision
   d. all of the above
7. The drug which is *NOT* used in open angle glaucoma
   a. epinephrine
   b. corticosteroids
   c. beta adrenergic blocker
   d. pilocarpine
8. Shallow anterior chamber is seen in
   a. adherent leucoma
   b. after trabeculectomy
   c. closed angle glaucoma
   d. all of the above
9. Glaucoma after cataract extraction may result from
   a. pre-existing glaucoma
   b. development of peripheral anterior synechiae
   c. pooling of fluid behind the anterior hyaloid membrane
   d. all of the above
10. Rapid change in presbyopic correction is a classical feature of
    a. neovascular glaucoma
    b. open angle glaucoma
    c. closed angle glaucoma
    d. glaucoma capsulare
11. All of the following field defects are characteristic of glaucoma *EXCEPT*.
    a. arcuate scotoma
    b. ring scotoma
    c. baring of blind spot
    d. binasal quadrantinopia
12. Which of the following is contraindicated in primary glaucoma
    a. atropine
    b. pilocarpine
    c. adrenaline
    d. eserine
13. Coloured halos are not seen in
    a. accommodation
    b. narrow angle glaucoma
    c. steroid induced glaucoma
    d. phakogenic glaucoma

14. Stony hard eye is seen in
    a. infantile glaucoma
    b. chronic open angle glaucoma
    c. absolute glaucoma
    d. none of the above
15. Treatment of malignant glaucoma is
    a. timolol maleate
    b. pilocarpine
    c. corticosteroids
    d. vitreous aspiration
16. Laser is used in
    a. Angle-closure glaucoma
    b. open angle glaucoma
    c. retinal detachment
    d. all of the above
17. Cupping of the disc is not a feature of
    a. megalocornea
    b. chronic open angle glaucoma
    c. chronic angle-closure glaucoma
    d. buphthalmos
18. Intercalary staphyloma occurs at
    a. equator
    b. area extending upto 4 mm from limbus
    c. at the vortex vein perforation site
    d. limbus
19. Most common presenting feature of a patient with primary open angle glaucoma is
    a. eyeache
    b. headache
    c. coloured halos
    d. chronic deterioration of vision noticed suddenly
20. Drugs used in primary open angle glaucoma include
    a. timolol maleate
    b. atropine
    c. steroids
    d. none of the above
21. Clinical features of absolute glaucoma include all EXCEPT
    a. completely blind eye
    b. pain
    c. shallow anterior chamber
    d. constricted pupil
22. Peripheral anterior synechia occurs in
    a. open angle glaucoma
    b. closed angle glaucoma
    c. neovascular glaucoma
    d. none of the above
23. Provocative test for angle-closure glaucoma is
    a. dark room test
    b. water drinking test
    c. venous congestion test
    d. all of the above
24. Eyes prone to angle closure have all the following characteristics EXCEPT
    a. hypermetropic
    b. shallow anterior chamber
    c. large lens
    d. wide angle
25. Trabeculoplasty to reduce intraocular pressure in primary open angle glaucoma is done by
    a. YAG laser
    b. argon laser
    c. excimer laser
    d. CO_2 laser
26. 100 day glaucoma is seen in
    a. central retinal artery occlusion
    b. central retinal vein occlusion
    c. steroid induced
    d. primary open angle glaucoma

27. Visible retinal arterial pulsation is a feature of
    a. cenral retinal artery occlusion
    b. normal eye
    c. central retinal vein occlusion
    d. raised IOP pressure
28. Increased ocular pressure in Buphthalmos causes all the following EXCEPT
    a. streching of sclera
    b. corneal vascularisation
    c. corneal curvature promisence
    d. Rupture of Descemet's memebrane
29. Pain in absolute glacoma is best relieved by
    a. analgesics
    b. retrobulbar injection of alcohol
    c. Trabeculectomy
    d. Miotics
30. In acute angle-closure, prophylactric treatment of choice for the other eye is
    a. Nd:YAG laser, iridotomy,
    b. peripheral irodotomy
    c. pilocarpine instillation
    d. retrobulbar alcohol injection
31. Treatment of choice for congenital glaucoma is
    a. drugs
    b. goniotomy
    c. cyclodialysis
    d. trabeculectomy
32. Treatment of choice in primary open angle glaucoma is prime
    a. cyclodialysis
    b. iridectomy
    c. cyclodiathermy
    d. medical

ANSWERS

1—d	2—b	3—d	4—d	5—d
6—c	7—b	8—d	9—d	10—c
11—d	12—a	13—a	14—c	15—d
16—d	17—a	18—b	19—d	20—a
21—d	22—b	23—a	24—d	25—b
26—c	27—c	28—b	29—a	30—a
31—b	32—d			

CHAPTER 13

The Retina

APPLIED ANATOMY

Retina is the inner most layer of the eye and is derived from neuroectoderm. Retina is a thin membrane extending from the optic disc to the ora serrata in front. It varies in thickness from 0.4 mm near the optic nerve to 0.15 mm anteriorly at the ora serrata.

Ora Serrata

It is the anterior termination of the retina where it is continuous with the epithelium of the ciliary body.

Macula Lutea (Yellow Spot)

It is an area 1.5 mm in diameter situated at the posterior pole, about 3 mm to the temporal side of the optic disc.

Fovea Centralis

It is a small depression in the centre of the macula. The cones predominate in this area. The fovea is the most sensitive part of the retina.

Structure

It is composed of two main layers with a potential space in between the layers:
   i. The outer retinal pigment epithelium
   ii. The inner neural layer.

Retina consists of ten layers namely,
1. *Layer of pigment epithelium*—A single layer of hexagonal cells containing melanin pigment is situated on the outer aspect of retina.
2. *Layer of rods and cones*—These are the end organs for visual sensation.
3. *External limiting membrane*—It lies between rods and cones and outer nuclear layers.
4. *Outer nuclear layer*—It consists of nuclei of rods and cones.
5. *Outer plexiform layer*—It consists of arborizations of the axons of rods and cones nuclei with the dendrites of the bipolar cells.
6. *Inner nuclear layer*—It consists of nuclei of bipolar cells.
7. *Inner plexiform layer*—It consists of synapses of the axons of the bipolar cells with the dendrites of the ganglion cells.
8. *Layer of ganglion cells*—Large ganglion cells are present in this layer.
9. *Nerve fibre layer*—These are axons of the ganglion cells. These fibres are non-medullated and are continued as optic nerve fibres.
10. *Internal limiting membrane*—It separates the retina from vitreous.

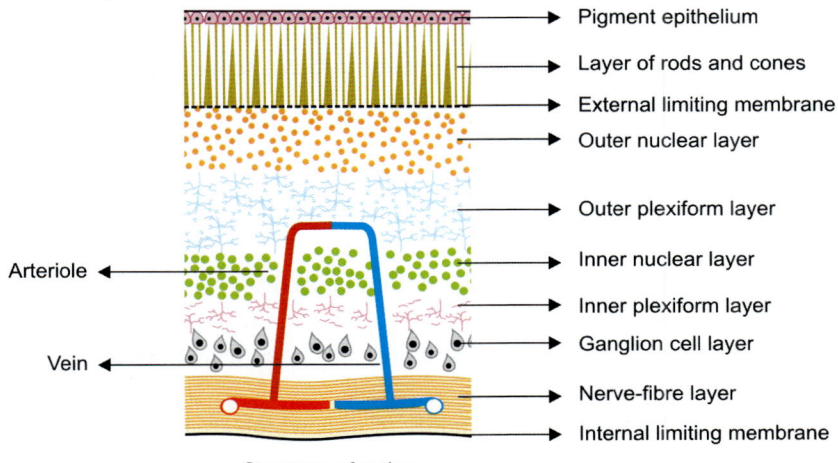
Structure of retina

Blood Supply

1. The choriocapillaris of the choroid supplies the pigment epithelium, the layers of rods and cones and the outer nuclear layers.
2. Central retinal artery supplies rest of the layers of the retina. It is a branch of the ophthalmic artery and is an end artery. It enters the optic nerve on its lower surface 15-20 mm behind the globe. The normal artery : vein ratio is 2 : 3

Nutritional support for the sensory retina comes largely from the Muller cell which spans almost the entire thickness of the retina.

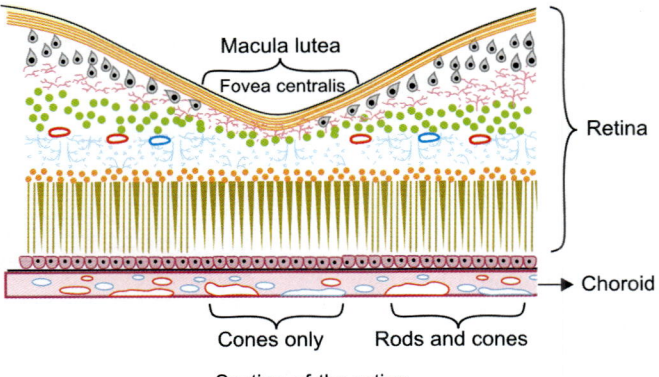
Section of the retina

Venous Drainage

1. The inner layers drain into the central vein of the retina.
2. The outer layers drain into the vortex veins through the choriocapillaris.

Functions

Visual functions are classified under the term light sense, form sense and colour vision.

Retinal functions are tested by the following tests :
  i. Visual acuity
  ii. Visual fields
  iii. Colour vision
  iv. Dark adaptation.
  v. Electroretinogram (ERG) and electro-oculogram (EOG).

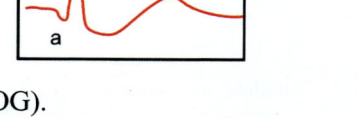

The visual impulses reach occipital cortex after 124 m sec following retinal stimulation.
  1. The central part (macula lutea) consists mainly of cones which are responsible for vision in the day light and for colour vision.
  2. The peripheral part of retina consists mainly of rods which are responsible for vision at night.

DISEASES OF THE RETINA

1. **Inflammations**
   i. Periphlebitis retinae (Eale's disease)
   ii. Central serous retinopathy
   iii. Exudative retinopathy of Coats' (Coats' disease)
   iv. Photoretinitis.

2. **Vascular Lesions**
   i. Haemorrhage
   ii. Central retinal artery occlusion
   iii. Central retinal vein occlusion.

3. **Retinopathies due to Systemic Diseases**
   i. Hypertensive retinopathy
   ii. Toxemia of pregnancy
   iii. Diabetic retinopathy.

4. **Degenerations**
   i. Senile macular degeneration
   ii. Retinitis pigmentosa.

5. **Tumour**
   Retinoblastoma.

6. **Retinal Detachment**

7. **Congenital Anomaly**
   Coloboma of retina and choroid.

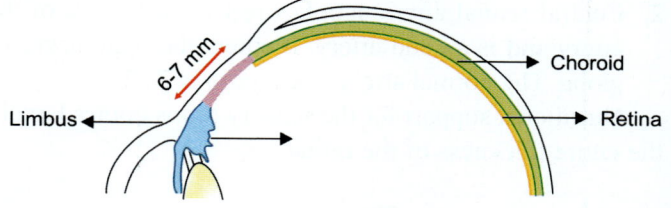

Applied anatomy of retina

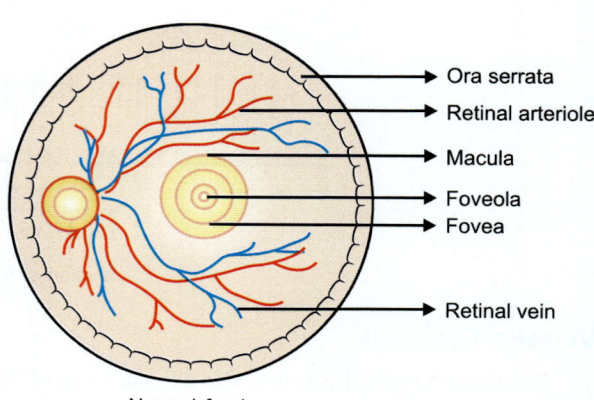

Normal fundus

INFLAMMATIONS OF THE RETINA
Periphlebitis Retinae [Eale's Disease]

Eales disease is an idiopathic, inflammatory peripheral retinal vasculopathy which presents with recurrent vitreous and retinal haemorrhages in young males.

Etiology

There is periphlebitis, i.e. inflammation of the wall of the retinal veins commonly associated with tuberculosis (tuberculoprotein hypersensitivity).

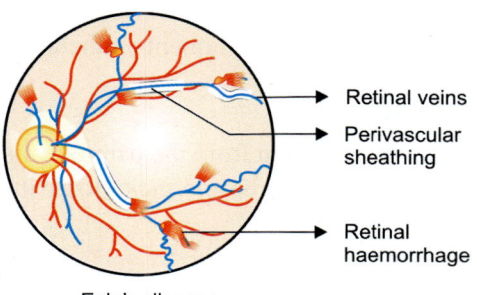

Eale's disease

Incidence

Age—Young adults (20-30 years) are affected commonly.
Sex—It occurs in males usually. It is a bilateral condition.

Symptom

Usually none but there may be sudden impairment of vision due to vitreous haemorrhage.

Signs

1. Peripheral retinal veins appear thickened, tortuous and congested.
2. Perivascular sheathing of veins is usually present.
3. Peripheral neovascularisation is seen at the juction of perfused and non perfused areas of the retina. Retinal haemorrhages may be seen near the veins.
4. A large vitreous haemorrhage may occur all of a sudden.

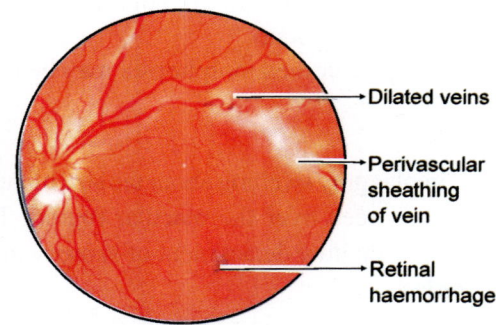

Fale's disease

Complications

1. Loss of vision may occur due to recurrent haemorrhages and vitreous opacities.
2. Retinitis proliferans—It follows large vitreous haemorrhage leading to fibrous tissue proliferation.
3. Tractional retinal detachment may occur eventually.
4. Rubeosis iridis, glaucoma and cataract may develop in late stages.

Treatment

1. Treat the underlying cause of inflammation, e.g. tuberculosis or septic foci.
2. Systemic corticosteroids are helpful in controlling the inflammation in early vasculitic stage.
3. Photocoagulation of leaking areas prevents retinal hypoxia.
4. Vitrectomy with division of fibrous bands is recommended in cases of retinitis proliferans.

Prognosis

It is bad if the condition is bilateral and in cases of recurrence.

CENTRAL SEROUS RETINOPATHY (CSR)

It is characterized by a localised detachment of the sensory retina at the macula secondary to local defect in the retinal pigment epithelium. It is a typical example of macular oedema.

Etiology

There is exudation from the parafoveal or choroidal capillaries due to angiospasm and hyperpermeability which may be allergic or toxic in nature. This results due to vasomotor instability.

Incidence

Healthy young male adults are usually affected.

Symptoms

1. There is transient and sudden impairment of central vision or visual acuity.
2. Black patch is seen in front of the patient's eyes (positive scotoma).
3. Micropsia or metamorphopsia may be present.

Signs

1. Circular grey swelling about the size of the optic disc is seen over the macular region. This is due to shallow detachment of sensory macular retina.
2. There may be ring-shaped reflex or "halo" around the swelling.

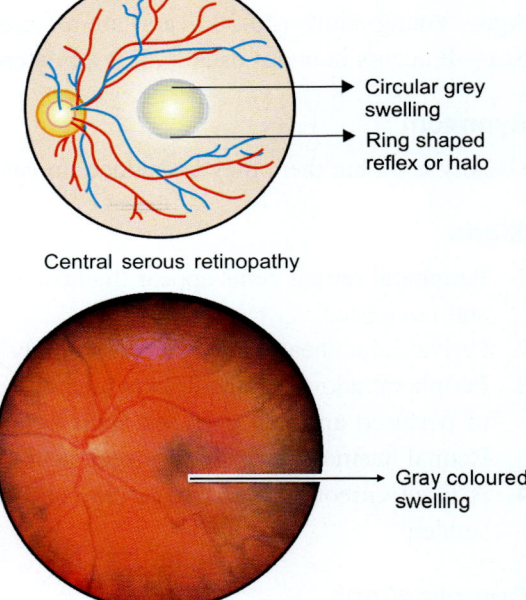

Central serous retinopathy

Central serous retinopathy

Complications

There may be geographic atrophy of pigment epithelium and choriocapillaries, fibrovascular scar formation and tears in the retinal pigment epithelium.

Diagnosis

Fluorescein angiography—It reveals leakage of dye through a defect in the Bruch's membrane into the subretinal space. Two patterns are commonly seen.
1. Ink-blot pattern—There are small hyperfluorescent spots which gradually increase in size.
2. Smoke-stack pattern—There is a small hyperfluorescent spot which spreads vertically like a smoke stack and then gradually spread laterally to look like mushroom or umbrella.

Treatment

1. Reassurance is the only treatment in majority of patients as 80-90 percent cases resolve spontaneously within 4-12 weeks.
2. Photocoagulation is effective in controlling the exudation process in long standing cases with marked loss of vision or recurrent cases.

Prognosis

It is usually good in majority of cases.

EXUDATIVE RETINOPATHY OF COATS (RETINAL TELANGIECTASIA)

It is a congenital anomaly of the vasculature of the retina.

Etiology

This is the most severe form of retinal telangiectasia with intraretinal and subretinal exudation.

Incidence

It is common in young boys who are otherwise apparently healthy.
It is often unilateral.

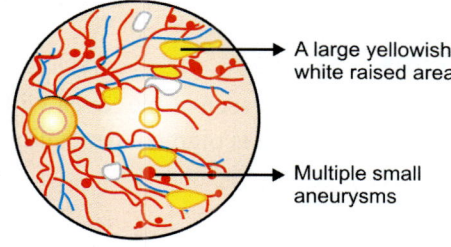

Exudative retinopathy of Coats

Symptoms

1. White reflex (leucocoria) is seen in the pupillary area.
2. There is associated impaired vision.

Signs

1. A large yellowish-white raised area or several smaller areas are seen posterior to the retinal vessels. At times cholesterol crystals are seen embedded in the exudates.
2. The retinal vessels are markedly dilated, tortuous and engorged.
3. Multiple small aneurysms are seen all over the fundus.
4. Fluorescein angiography—Retinal vessels show abnormal coarse, net of dilated capillaries, irregular aneurysmal dilatation and leakage of dye.

Complications

1. Retinal detachment may occur due to marked exudation.
2. Secondary or neovascular glaucoma results due to rubeosis iridis.
3. Complicated cataract occurs in posterior cortex due to disturbance to the nutrition of lens.

Differential Diagnosis

- A similar clinical picture may be seen in angiomatosis or von Hippel-Lindau disease.
- A similar disease may occur in older patients.
- Retinoblastoma—There is rapid progression and it usually occurs in children below 4 years.

Treatment

1. In the early stage, treatment with photocoagulation or cryotherapy may be successful in preventing progression of the disease process and improving symptoms.
2. No treatment is effective in later stages.

PHOTORETINITIS (Retinitis from Bright Light)

Retinitis from bright light occurs after exposure of the eyes to bright sunlight as in looking at the eclipse of the sun unguarded (eclipse blindness), exposure to the flash of the short circuiting of a strong current. Almost all the visible rays and many infrared rays (wavelength above 700 nm) are absorbed by the pigment epithelium causing severe retinal burn.

Symptoms

There is persistence of after-image which leads to positive scotoma.

Signs

1. A pale spot is seen at the fovea with a brown ring around it.
2. Later on there is pigment deposition and retinal hole formation at the foveal region.

Prophylaxis

- Glasses impervious to infrared and ultraviolet rays should be used while looking at solar eclipse.
- Light source must be seen by reflection from a mirror or not at all.

Treatment

No treatment is effective. Guarded prognosis is given although improvement often occurs with corticosteroids.

VASCULAR LESIONS OF THE RETINA
RETINAL HAEMORRHAGES

Etiology

i. *Trauma*—Blunt or penetrating injury of the eye is a common cause.
ii. *Venous obstruction*, e.g. as in central retinal vein occlusion.
iii. *Vascular retinopathies* due to diabetes, hypertension, toxemia of pregnancy, nephritis.
iv. *Blood dyscrasias* such as anaemia, purpura, leukemia, etc.

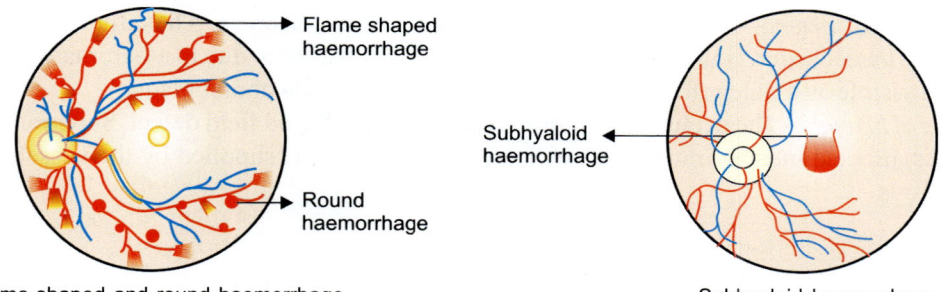

Flame-shaped and round haemorrhage   Subhyaloid haemorrhage

Types

1. *Intraretinal haemorrhage*—When the haemorrhage from the retinal vessels is small and situated within the retinal tissue, it is known as intraretinal haemorrhage.
    i. *Flame-shaped*—It occurs when the haemorrhage is in the nerve fibre layer.
    ii. *Round or irregular shape*—It occurs when the haemorrhage is in deeper layers, i.e. in the outer part of the inner nuclear layer (Duke-Elder).
2. *Preretinal or subhyaloid haemorrhage*—It occurs when a large vessel bleeds. The blood breaks the internal limiting membrane and the haemorrhage lies between the retina and vitreous. It commonly occurs in the macular area and is globular or boat-shaped. However, due to gravity the upper margin becomes horizontal after a few days as a result of sedimentation of red blood cells.
3. *Vitreous haemorrhage*—Large retinal haemorrhage breaks into the vitreous. It may lead to proliferation of fibrous tissue.

Course

The haemorrhages are usually absorbed in due course of time.

CENTRAL RETINAL ARTERY OCCLUSION

It is an ocular emergency. There is obstruction to the arterial circulation of the retina.

Etiology

It is usually due to an embolus or thrombosis along with spasm of the artery. It commonly occurs in cases of hypertension, arteriosclerosis, atherosclerosis, temporal arteritis or Buerger's disease.

Pathogenesis

Arterial ischaemia results in the:
   i. Infarction of the inner two-third of the retina.
  ii. Reflex constriction of the whole retinal arterial blood vessels.
 iii. Stasis in the retinal capillaries.

Site of Occlusion

The common site of origin of embolus is from common carotid artery in the neck, aorta or endocardium of the heart.

1. *Central retinal artery*—The occlusion occurs at the lamina cribrosa. Thus, the entire retina is affected. The occlusion is usually at the bifurcation. It is invariably due to atheromatous embolus which is visible as a pale refractile body within the artery (Hollenhorst plaque).
2. *Peripheral branch*—The occlusion results in typical sector-shaped field defect. Superior temporal branch is affected most commonly. The distal area of the retina supplied by the vessel becomes oedematous.

Symptoms

1. There is sudden, complete and permanent loss of vision.
2. At times some central vision may persist due to presence of cilioretinal artery which supplies the macular area.
3. Amaurosis fugax—In the early stage, there is sudden but transient loss of vision. The recovery of vision is due to the dislodgement of embolus into the peripheral arterioles.

Signs

1. Fundus Examination

i. *In complete block*
- The arteries are extremely thin and may not be visible.
- The veins are usually normal except at the disc where they are contracted.
- The retina becomes opaque and milky white specially near the disc and macula.
- Cherry red spot is seen at the fovea centralis. Choroid is seen through the thin fovea.
- Optic disc is pale due to ischaemia.

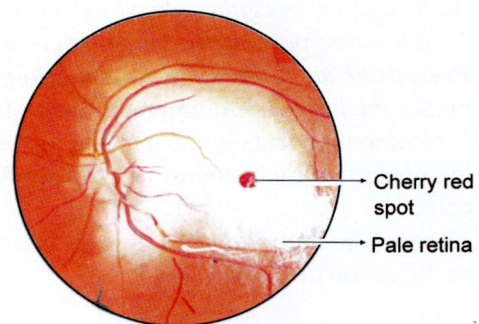

Central retinal artery occlusion

ii. *In partial or incomplete block*
The column of venous blood may break into red beads separated by clear interspaces which move to and fro (cattle truck appearance) by gentle pressure on the eyeball.
iii. *Obstruction of a branch*—Sector-shaped retinal pallor results with narrowing of one branch. Superior temporal branch is affected most commonly at the bifurcation.

2. Pupil

It is widely dilated and does not react to light.

Differential diagnosis of cherry red spot
i. *Tay-Sachs disease*
ii. *Niemann-Pick disease*
iii. *Myoclonus*
iv. *Berlin's oedema*
v. *Macular hole or haemorrhage.*

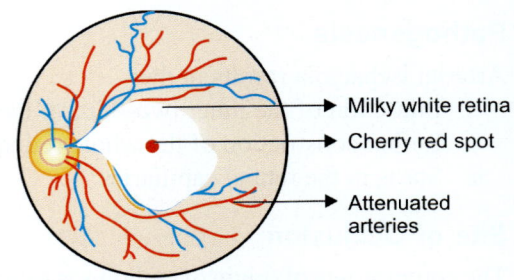

Central retinal artery occlusion

Complication
1. Complete blindness may occur due to cystic or disciform degeneration of the macula.
2. It may cause thrombotic or neovascular glaucoma due to retinal ischaemia.

Treatment
It is an ophthalmic emergency. Prompt treatment is essential as anoxic retina is irreversibly damaged in about 90 minutes.

It is usually ineffective. In early stages the aim of the treatment is to relieve spasm and to remove the embolus into a peripheral branch of central retinal artery.

1. *Vasodilators*, e.g. amyl nitrate inhalation, injection of acetylcholine into Tenon's capsule immediately has been advised but with little success.
2. *Massage the globe along with IV acetazolamide*—This helps in dislodging the embolus mechanically.
3. *Paracentesis*—It produces immediate hypotony causing vasodilatation.
4. *Inhalation of 95% oxygen and 5% carbon dioxide mixture.*
5. *Panretinal photocoagulation with argon, krypton, diode, etc. laser prevents neovascularisation.*

RETINAL VEIN OCCLUSION

There is obstruction to the venous circulation of the retina due to thrombosis or embolus.

Etiology
i. It commonly occurs in elderly persons with cardiovascular diseases such as hypertension, arteriosclerosis, atherosclerosis and diabetes.
ii. In young persons it is usually caused by infective periphlebitis (branch occlusion) and local causes such as orbital cellulitis or facial erysipelas.
iii. Chronic open angle glaucoma may be a contributing factor.

Pathogenesis

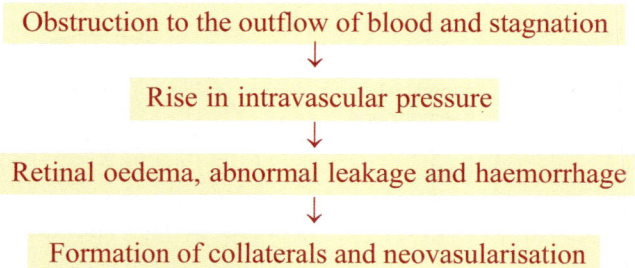

Site of Occlusion
It is just behind the lamina cribrosa where artery and vein share a common sheath. A peripheral branch alone may be involved.

Symptom

There is sudden onset of impaired vision. However, the loss of vision is not so sudden as in central retinal artery occlusion.

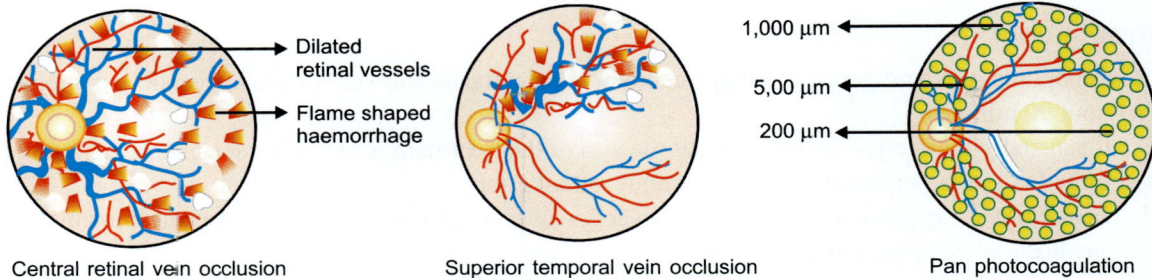

Central retinal vein occlusion   Superior temporal vein occlusion   Pan photocoagulation

Signs

i. *In complete block*
   - Retinal veins are markedly dilated, engorged and tortuous.
   - Retina is covered with multiple extensive haemorrhages (tomato splash appearance) along with cotton wool exudates.
   - Neovascularisation, i.e. tortuous new vessels are seen upon the disc and retina due to collateral circulation in the later stage.
   - The typical fundus picture is sometimes called "blood and thunder fundus".
   - Eventually retina becomes atrophic with fine pigmentary changes.

ii. *In branch vein occlusion*
   - Oedema and haemorrhages are limited to the area supplied by the vein. The superior temporal vein is most commonly affected.

Complications

1. Secondary neovascular glaucoma occurs at a later stage (usually within 3 months or 90 days) due to sclerosis and neovascularisation at the angle of anterior chamber (rubeosis iridis). It is rare in branch vein thrombosis.

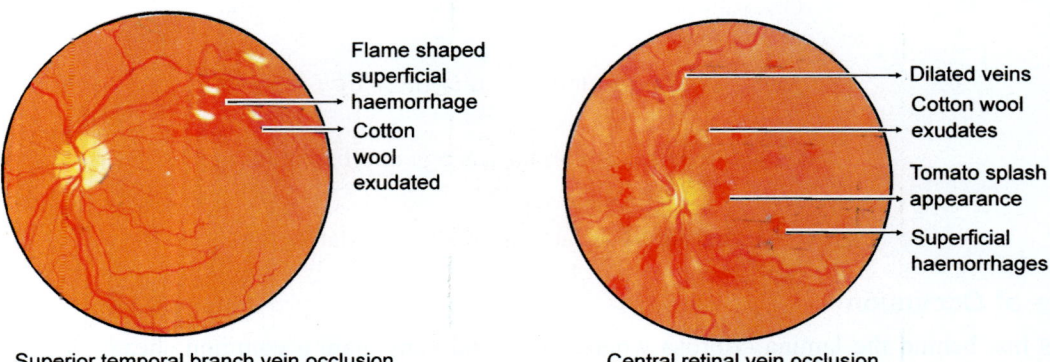

Superior temporal branch vein occlusion   Central retinal vein occlusion

2. Large vitreous haemorrhage and subhyaloid haemorrhage may occur.
3. Maculopathy leads to further diminution of vision at a later stage.
4. Complete blindness develops eventually.

Treatment

It should be started as early as possible.
1. No treatment is effective if the blockage has become complete. Anticoagulants and steroid can be tried under medical control.
2. Neovascular glaucoma can be prevented by panphotocoagulation of the retina or cryoapplication if the media is hazy. Panretinal photocoagulation should be given early when most of the intraretinal blood is absorbed.

HYPERTENSIVE RETINOPATHY

Hypertensive retinopathy refers to the fundus changes occurring in patients suffering from hypertension. Hypertension is the most common vascular disease but visual loss secondary to hypertensive retinopathy is rare unlike diabetes mellitus.

Predisposing Factors

The following factors influence the development of hypertensive retinopathy,
1. *Severity of hypertension*—It is reflected by the vascular changes and retinopathy.
2. *Duration of hypertension*—It is indicated by the degree of arteriosclerotic changes and retinopathy.
3. *Age of the patient*
   a. In young—The primary response to systemic hypertension is narrowing of the retinal arterioles due to 'spasm'.
   b. In aged—The response to systemic hypertension depends on the amount of pre-existing 'involutional sclerosis' or replacement fibrosis.

Pathogenesis

Essential hypertension with sustained elevation of blood pressure results in
   i. Thickening of the arteriolar wall.
  ii. Fibrinoid necrosis of smooth muscles and endothelium of the vessels.
 iii. Leakage of plasma and blood.

I. Hypertensive Retinopathy

The fundus picture is characterised by the following:
1. *Vasoconstriction*—Narrowing of the retinal arterioles is related to the severity of hypertension. It occurs in pure form in young persons but it is affected by the pre-existing involutional sclerosis in the older patients. It may be focal or generalized.
2. *Arteriolosclerosis changes*—These manifest as changes in arteriolar reflex and A-V crossing changes. These result from thickening of the vessel wall. They are reflection of the duration of hypertension. In aged patients, arteriolosclerotic changes are already present (involutional sclerosis).

3. *Increased vascular permeability*—This results from retinal ischaemia (hypoxia) and is responsible for haemorrhages, exudates (soft and hard) and retinal oedema.

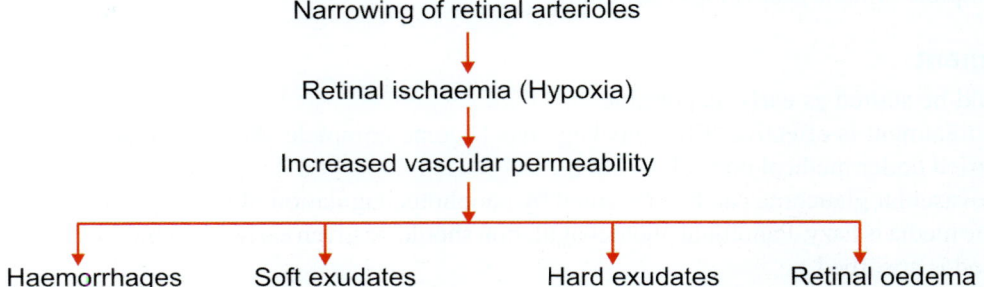

II. Hypertensive Choroidopathy

This typically occurs in young patient experiencing acute hypertension, such as patient with pre-eclampsia, eclampsia or accelerated hypertension.

The fundus examination may show the following features:
1. *Elschnig spots* are small, black spots surrounded by yellow halos which represent focal choroidal infarcts.
2. *Siegrist streaks* are flecks which are arranged lineraly along the choroidal vessels.
3. *Exudative retinal detachment* may occur specially in toxaemia of pregnancy.

Classification

I. Keith Wagner and Barker (1939)

Keith, Wagner and Barker (1939) have classified hypertensive retinopathy into four grades on the basis of ophthalmoscopic characteristics. It correlates directly with the degree of hypertension and inversely with the prognosis for survival of patients. It helps in assessing the hypertensive damage to the heart, brain and kidneys.

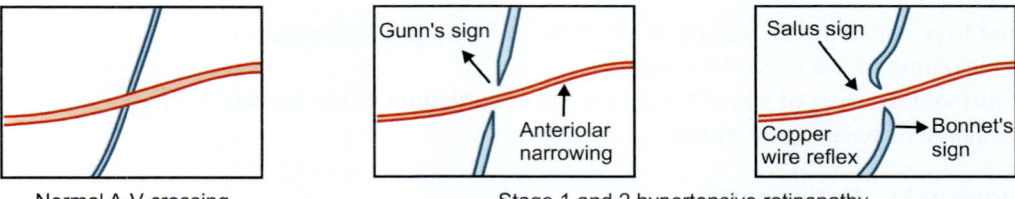

Grade 1

Mild to moderate narrowing or sclerosis of the retinal arterioles is present. These patients have benign essential hypertension with adequate cardiorenal function.

Grade 2

1. There is moderate to marked narrowing of retinal arterioles.
2. Copper wire reflex—When the transparent arterial wall becomes thick and reflects light, the reflex looks wider and burnish copper coloured.

3. Typical arteriovenous crossing changes are present.
   i. Marcus Gunn's sign—The apparent constriction or nipping of the vein where it is crossed over by the rigid artery is known as the Gunn's sign.
   ii. Bonnet's sign—Occasionally there is 'banking' in the vein distal to the A-V crossing.
   iii. Salus sign—A 'S' -shaped deviation of the vein occurs at the A-V crossing.

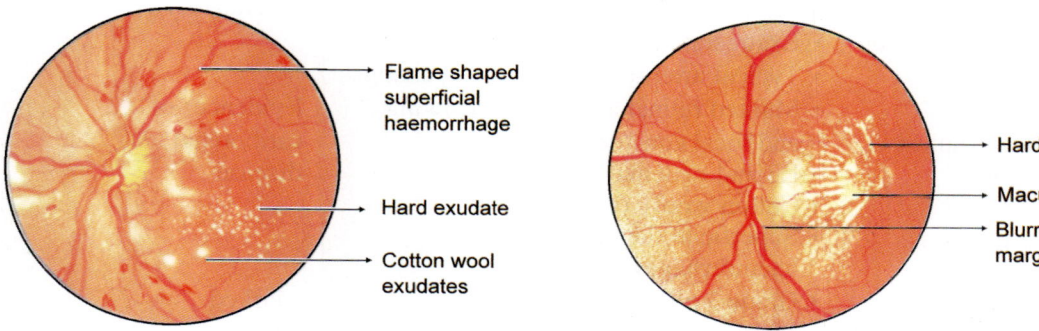

Hypertensive retinopathy grade 3

Hypertensive retinopathy grade 4

Grade 3
1. There is retinal arteriolar narrowing and focal constriction
2. Silver wire reflex—Marked thickening of the arterial walls causes all the light to reflect and the artery looks brilliant white.
3. Retinal oedema may be present due to extravasation of fluid.
4. Cotton wool or soft exudates consisting of fibrin and protein are scattered all over the fundus. They consist of grey-white patches measuring about 0.5 disc diameter.
5. Superficial flame-shaped haemorrhages are present in the nerve fibre layer.

Prognosis—The life expectency of these patients is about 2 years if untreated.

Grade 4 (Malignant hypertension)
1. All the changes seen in stage three are present.
2. Macular star is formed due to accumulation of hard exudates in the outer plexiform layer.
3. Papilloedema is pathognomonic of this stage.

Prognosis—These patients have grave prognosis and their life expectancy is one year if untreated.

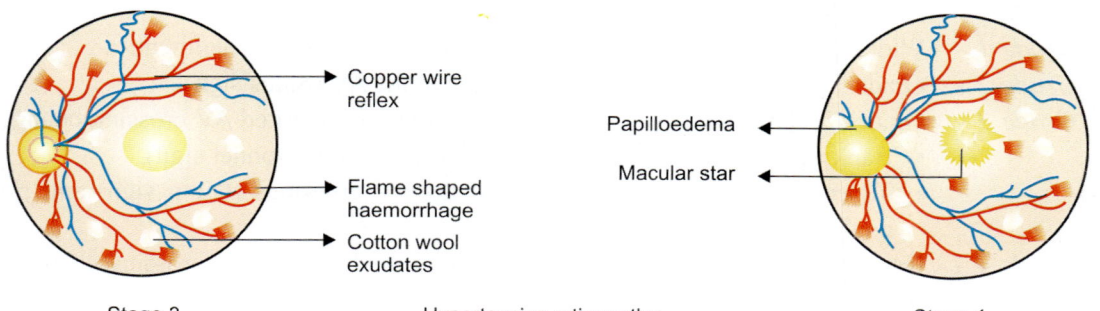

Stage 3

Hypertensive retinopathy

Stage 4

CLASSIFICATION OF HYPERTENSIVE RETINOPATHY
(KEITH, WAGENER AND BARKER-1939)

GRADES	FUNDUS EXAMINATION	CARDIORENAL FUNCTION
Grade 1 Mild hypertension	Mild to moderate narrowing or sclerosis of the arterioles	Normal
Grade 2 Moderate hypertension	• Moderate to marked arteriolar sclerosis • Exaggeration of light reflex • Typical arteriovenous crossing changes	Satisfactory
Grade 3 Hight and sustained hypertension	• Marked retinal arteriolar narrowing and focal constriction • Retinal oedema • Cotton wool / (soft) exudates • Superficial flame-shaped haemorrhages	Evidences of cardiorenal disease
Grade 4 Malignant hypertension	• Grade 3 plus • Macular star • Papilloedema	Marked Cardiorenal damage

This classification is still in use today and is widely accepted.

II. *Scheie's Classification*

The retinal changes of hypertension and arteriolar sclerosis are graded separately according to Scheie's classification.

A. *Hypertensive features*

Grade 0 - Normal fundus.
Grade 1 - Narrowing of smaller retinal arterioles. There is no focal constriction.
Grade 2 - Severe narrowing with localized irregular constriction of the arterioles.
Grade 3 - Narrowing and focal irregularities of arterioles, retinal haemorrhage and exudates.
Grade 4 - All changes in grade 3 along with neuroretinal oedema, and / or papilloedema.

B. *Arteriolo-sclerotic features*

These changes develop if the hypertension is present over a period of many years, and are mainly seen in aged individual.

Grade 0 - Normal fundus.
Grade 1 - Widening of arteriolar light - reflex with simple venous concealment.
Grade 2 - Grade 1 changes with deflection of veins at the AV (Salus sign).
Grade 3 - Grade 2 changes with 'copper wire' arterioles and marked AV crossing changes.
  • Banking of veins distal to arteriovenous crossings (Bonnet sign).
  • Tapering of veins on both sides of the AV crossings (Gunn sign) and right-angled deflection of veins.
Grade 4 - Grade 3 changes with 'silver wire' arterioles and marked AV crossing changes.

Clinical Types
Clinically, hypertensive retinopathy may occur in four forms as follows:
1. **Simple hypertension without sclerosis**
    - It is seen in young patients with elastic retinal arterioles
    - Generalized constriction of the arterioles which appear pale, straight with acute branching
    - Superficial flame-shaped haemorrhages and cotton wool exudates may be present.
2. **Hypertension with involutionary sclerosis**
    - It occurs in elderly patients above 50 years with typical features of arteriosclerotic retinopathy
    - There is localized constriction and dilatation of vessels with thickening of vessel wall
    - Changes at the arteriovenous crossings are diagnosis (Gunn's sign)
    - There is deposition of hard exudates
    - Retinal haemorrhages without any oedema may occur.
3. **Hypertension with arteriolar sclerosis (diffuse hyperplastic)**
    - It is seen in younger patients
    - There is chronic glomerulonephritis and the classical ophthalmic picture is known as 'albuminuric' or 'renal' retinopathy
    - The vessels are narrow and tortuous with nicking at arteriovenous crossing
    - Multiple retinal haemorrhages are seen with oedema, diffuse cotton wool exudates (early), and hard exudates (later) usually forming macular star
    - Vision is seriously impaired.
4. **Malignant hypertension**
    - There is rapid progression of hypertensive state in patients with relatively young arterioles i.e. without any sclerosis
    - There is associated renal insufficiency (Hypertensive nephroretinopathy)
    - There is marked arteriolar narrowing with generalized oedema with soft and hard exudates resulting in papilloedema, macular star along with superficial flame-shaped haemorrhages
    - The visual prognosis is grave unless controlled medically.

Treatment
It depends on the cause. Energetic treatment with antihypertensive drugs results in remarkable improvement of the fundus picture.

THE TOXEMIA OF PREGNANCY
This occurs late in pregnancy, i.e. in the 9th month usually. It has many characteristics of hypertensive retinopathy.

Classification
There are three stages :
1. *Stage of angiospasm*
    - This occurs as a result of liberation of toxins.
    - There is narrowing of the retinal arteries usually the nasal branch.
    - Spasmodic contractions of the arteries may be seen.

2. *Stage of sclerosis of vessels*—This is dependent on the severity of hypertension.
3. *Stage of retinopathy*
    - Multiple superficial and deep haemorrhages may be present.
    - Retinal oedema and profuse exudation is seen all over the fundus.
    - Retinal detachment occurs due to massive exudation and haemorrhage.

Complications
1. There may be complete loss of vision in the stage of retinopathy.
2. Loss of life of the mother and fetus is a very serious complication.

Treatment
1. Adequate general antenatal care should be given to the expecting mother.
2. Control of high blood pressure with rest, sedation, salt restriction, diuretics and antihypertensive drugs is a must.
3. Timely induction of labour is essential. Termination of pregnancy is advised in cases of severe retinopathy not responding to treatment.

DIABETIC RETINOPATHY

Diabetic retinopathy refers to the retinal changes that occur in patients with diabetes mellitus. With increase in life expectancy in diabetic patients, the incidence of diabetic retinopathy has increased.

It is the leading cause of blindness particularly in the affluent society. It is common after the disease has lasted approximately 10 years. It usually occurs in patients after the age of 20 years. It affects young or old alike, for it is the diabetic age and not the actual age that is important.

Presence of retinopathy is not related to the prognosis of diabetes and expectancy of life. It is often associated with arteriosclerotic and hypertensive retinopathy.

Predisposing Factors
The following factors influence the occurrence of diabetic retinopathy,
1. *Duration of diabetes*—It is the single most determining factor. Approximately 50% of diabetic patients develop retinopathy after 10 years and about 80% after 15 years. It is seen much more frequently in insulin dependent diabetes mellitus.
2. *Heredity*—Diabetes is transmitted as a recessive trait. The effect of heredity is more marked in the proliferative retinopathy.
3. *Severity of diabetic retinopathy* is usually related to the
    i. Duration of the diseases
    ii. Adequacy of blood sugar control.
4. *Hypertension/pregnancy*—When there is associated hypertension or pregnancy it may enhance the changes of diabetic retinopathy.

Pathogenesis

1. Essentially, it is a microangiopathy affecting retinal precapillary anterioles, capillaries and venules. Characteristic changes in capillaries include:
    i. There is damage to the endothelial cells.
    ii. There is loss of intramural pericytes which are normally persent in the basement layers.
    iii. Basement membrane is thickened and fragmented.

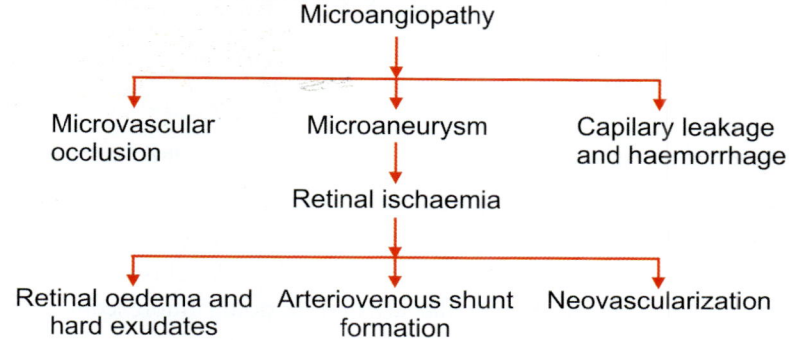

Pathogenesis of diabetic retinopathy

2. Microangiopathy results in microvascular occlusion, microaneurysm, capillary leakage and haemorrhages.
3. This leads to retinal ischaemia (retinal hypoxia) and retinal oedema.
4. Retinal hypoxia in turn causes formation of hard exudates, arteriovenous shunt formation and neovascularisation.

Classification

I. Eva Kohner's Classification

There are main three types of retinopathy according to Eva Kohner's classification :
1. Background retinopathy
2. Preproliferative retinopathy
3. Proliferative or neovascular retinopathy.

EVA KOHNER'S CLASSIFICATION OF DIABETIC RETINOPATHY

BACKGROUND RETINOPATHY	PREPROLIFERATIVE RETINOPATHY	PROLIFERATIVE RETINOPATHY
i. Capillary microaneurysm ii. Dot and blot haemorrhages iii. Hard exudates—Maculopathy iv. Venous changes—Dilatation, loop, coil and varicose formation v. Maculopathy—Focal, diffuse, ischaemic	Soft exudate	i. Neovascularisation ii. Vitreous haemorrhage iii. Retinal detachment

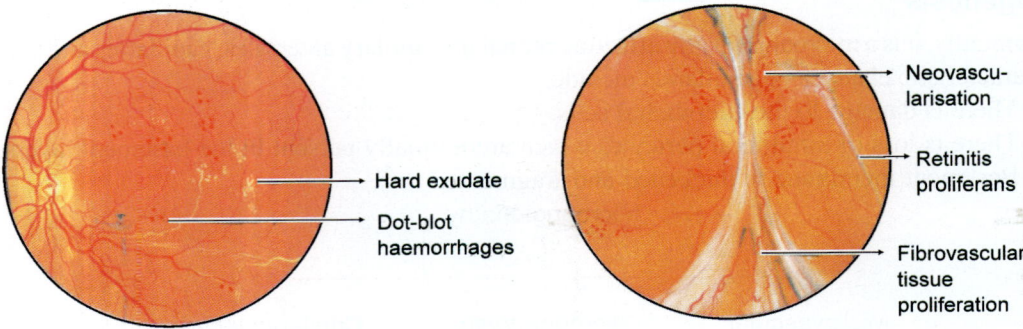

Advanced background diabetic retinopathy   Diabetic retinopathy - Proliferative

1. **Background retinopathy**—It usually affects the posterior pole.
    i. *Microaneurysms*—These are the most characteristic ocular lesions. It affects the smaller blood vessels by damaging the capillary wall. They look like cluster of grapes at the end of vascular twigs particularly in the macular area while doing fluorescein angiography. They consist of round or oval dilatation ranging from 20-200 nm in size. They are seen on the venous side of capillary net work at the inner nuclear layer.
    ii. *Haemorrhages*—Round-shaped 'dot and blot' deep haemorrhages occur due to rupture of microaneurysms in the inner nuclear layer.
    iii. *Hard exudates*—These are seen all over the posterior pole. They are white or yellow coloured, waxy looking patches of exudates containing hyaline and lipid with clear-cut and often serrated margins. They are situated between the inner plexiform and inner nuclear layers.
    iv. *Venous changes*—These include fusiform dilatation, loops, coiling and varicosity.
    v. *Diabetic maculopathy*—Involvement of the fovea by oedema and/or hard exudates is the most common cause of visual impairment in diabetic patients. It is of three types : focal, diffuse and ischaemic.
        a. Focal—There are well circumscribed leaking areas associated with complete or incomplete rings of hard exudates. Exudates have predilection for the perifoveal area.
        b. Diffuse maculopathy—There is generalised leakage from the dilated capillaries. Cystoid macular oedema is seen fequently.
        c. Ischaemic maculopathy—This is characterized by reduced visual acuity with relatively normal appearance of the macula. Fluorescein angiography confirms the diagnosis.

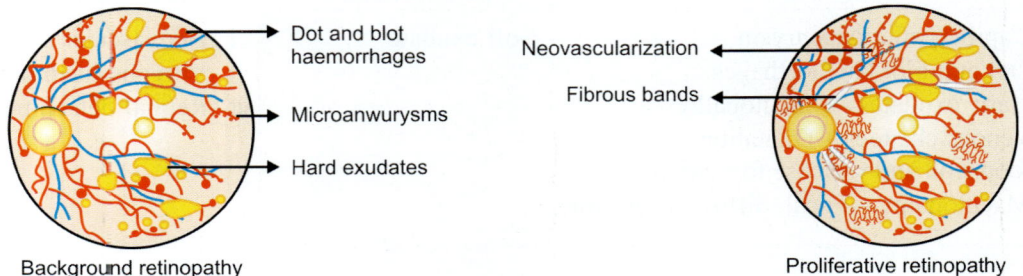

Background retinopathy   Proliferative retinopathy

2. **Preproliferative retinopathy**—Multiple cotton wool or soft exudates are present due to retinal ischaemia as a result of capillary occlusion in the nerve fibre layer. There is an interruption of the axoplasmatic transport.
3. **Proliferative retinopathy**—This is common in 'labile' diabetics between 3-4 decades. This is usually superimposed on simple background retinopathy.
    i. Neovascularisation arises from the optic nerve head and along the large vessels.
    ii. This is the most common cause of spontaneous *vitreous haemorrhage*.
    iii. Vitreous traction may cause retinal separation or tractional *retinal detachment*.

II. Early Treatment for Diabetic Retinopathy Study (ETDRS) Classification

1. Nonproliferetive retinopathy (NPDR)
    i. Mild
    ii. Moderate
    iii. Severe
    iv. Very severe
2. Proliferative retinopathy
    i. Early or without high-risk characteristics
    ii. With high-risk characteristics
3. Maculopathy
    i. Clinically significant macular edema (CSME)
    ii. Clinically nonsignificant macular edema (Non-CSME)
4. Advanced diabetic eye disease.

1. Nonproliferative Diabetic Retinopathy (NPDR)

   i. *Mild*—A few microaneurysms, retinal haemorrhages and hard exudates are seen in one or two quadrants.
   ii. *Moderate*—Above findings are seen in two or three quadrants.
   iii. *Severe*
      a. Above findings are present in all four quadrants.
      b. Atleast one of the following typical signs is also present:
         • Cotton wool spots
         • Irregular venous calibre
         • Intraretinal microvascular anomalies
   iv. *Very severe*
      a. Same as above
      b. Atleast two or three typical signs are present.

2. Proliferative Diabetic Retinopathy (PDR)

   i. *Early or without high-risk characteristics*
   Retinal neovascularisation—Not at disc but elsewhere (NVE) is seen.

ii. *With high-risk characteristics*
   a. Epi or peripapillary neovascularisation at disc (NVD) with or without epiretinal or vitreous haemorrhages is present.
   b. NVE with preretinal or vitreous haemorrhages is seen.

3. Maculopathy
   i. *Clinically significant macular oedema (CSME)*
      One of the following feature is seen on slit-lamp examination with +90, +78 or +60 D lens.
      a. There is thickening of the retina at or within 500 μm of the centre of the macula.
      b. Hard exudates are present at or within 500 μm of the centre of the macula
      c. • There are zones of retinal thickening of one disc area (1500 μm) or larger.
         • Any part of these zones is within one disc diameter of the centre of the macula.
   ii. *Fluorescein angiographically* diabetic maculopathy can be classified into four types:
      a. Focal exudative maculopathy
         • There are microaneurysms, haemorrhages, hard exudates arranged in a circinate pattern with macular oedema
         • Fluorescein angiography reveals focal leakage with adequate macular perfusion.
      b. Diffuse exudative maculopathy
         • There is diffuse retinal oedema, thickening at or around the macula with few hard exudates
         • Fluorescein angiography reveals diffuse leakage at the posterior pole.
      c. Ischaemic maculopathy
         • There are microvascular blocks resulting in marked visual loss
         • Microaneurysms, haemorrhages, mild or no macular oedema with few hard exudates may be seen. At times, macula may look relatively normal despite reduced visual acuity
         • Fluorescein angiography shows areas of non perfusion in the form of enlargement of foveal avascular zone (FAZ)
      d. Mixed maculopathy
         • There are combined features of ischaemic and exudative maculopathy.

4. Advanced Diabetic Eye Disease
It is the end result of uncontrolled proliferative diabetic retinopathy. There is marked visual loss due to neovascular glaucoma, vitreous haemorrhage and tractional retinal detachment.

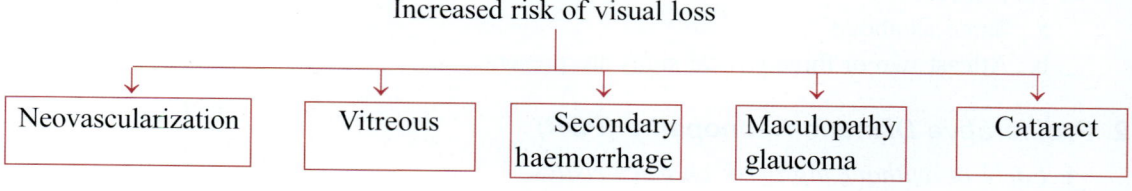

Prognosis

It is usually bad. The central vision is profoundly affected if the macular area is involved. There is increased risk of visual loss over 2 years period in cases of vitreous haemorrhage, neovascularisation, secondary glaucoma, cataract formation and maculopathy.

Investigations

1. Direct and indirect ophthalmoscopy—Whole circumference of the retina is examined carefully particularly the central part.
2. Fluorescein angiography and coloured fundus photographs should be taken as a record.

MANAGEMENT OF DIABETIC RETINOPATHY

TYPES OF RETINOPATHY	THERAPY	INDICATIONS
1. Background	Control of diabetes and regular review	All
2. Maculopathy—Clinically significant macular oedema (CSME)	Focal photocoagulation	Discrete areas of leakage seen on fluorescein angiography
3. Diffuse leak around macula (Circinate)	Grid laser Focal photocoagulation	
4. Preproliferative retinopathy	Frequent review	
5. Proliferative retinopathy	Panretinal photocoagulation	Neovascularisation elsewhere (NVE) / Neovascularisation of the disc (NVD)
6. Advanced diabetic eye disease	Vitreoretinal surgery with photocoagulation	• Persistent vitreous haemorrhage • Tractional retinal detachment

Treatment

1. Adequate medical control with low fat and antidiabetic drugs reduces the ocular and systemic complications.
2. Laser application—Photocoagulation by argon or diode lasers is used as follows:
    i. Panretinal photocoagulation (PRP) is indicated in severe cases of preproliferative and proliferative diabetic retinopathy. It reduces retinal ischaemia which in turn prevents further neovascularisation and vitreous haemorrhage.
    ii. Direct photocoagulation may be carried out to ablate the neovascularisation. It involves applying laser burns to microvascular lesions in the centre of rings of hard exudates located between 500 to 3000 μm from the centre of the fovea.
    iii. Focal argon laser burns are applied to individual microvascular formations in the centre of the hard exudate ring in focal exudative maculopathy.

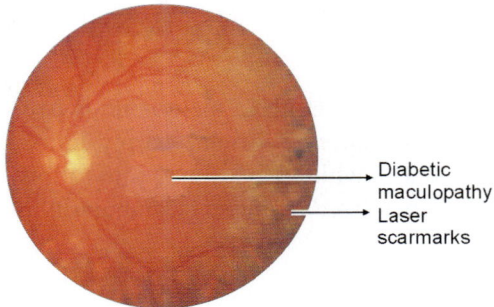

Laser scars following panretinal photocoagulation

iv. Grid pattern laser burns are applied in diffuse exudative maculopathy located more than 500 μm from the centre of the fovea and 500 μm from the temporal margin of the optic disc.
3. Vitrectomy with photocoagulation—It is useful in tractional retinal detachment, vitreous haemorrhage and proliferative vitreoretinopathy.
4. Surgical treatment—Associated retinal detachment also needs surgical repair.

AGE-RELATED MACULAR DEGENERATION (ARMD)

It is also called senile macular degeneration. It is an age-related, bilateral, non-hereditary degeneration. It involves the choriocapillaris, Bruch's membrane, retinal pigment epithelium and photoreceptors. It is the most common cause of permanent central visual loss in the elderly in developed countries.

Etiology

It is caused by sclerosis of the arteries which nourish the retina depriving it of oxygen and other nutrients. Predisposing factors include heredity, age, nutrition, smoking, hypertension and excessive exposure to sunlight.

Types

There are two types of senile macular degeneration:
 i. *Exudative (wet)*—There is presence of serous fluid (exudate) or haemorrhage.
 ii. *Non-exudative (dry)*—There is absence of fluid or exudate. It is atrophic degeneration.

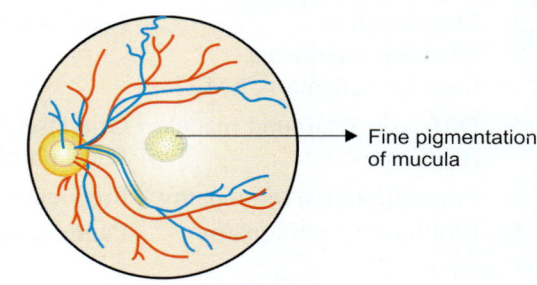

Senile macular degeneration

Symptoms

1. *Diminution of vision*—It can be gradual in atrophic (dry) type or a sudden painless loss of vision occurs in exudative type.
2. *Metamorphopsia*—Distorted vision may be seen, i.e. straight line appears wavy, bent or fuzzy.
3. There is difficulty in reading due to shadowed areas in the central visual field.

Signs

1. Drusen of Bruch's membrane is one of the early findings seen in the macular region. Drusen looks like small, bright, sharply defined circular points lying below the retinal vessels. These bright yellow-white masses may join to form larger round masses.
2. Generalized pigmentary granularity may be present all over the fundus.

Treatment

It is not effective usually.
 1. Wet senile macular degeneration
 • Photocoagulation of choroidal neovascular membrane may be helpful.
 • Photodynamic therapy (PDT), transpupillary thermal therapy (TTT) Argon green laser photocoagulation and anti-angiogenic therapy which include intravitreal steroids and anti-vascular endothelium growth factor (anti VEGF) are currently under trial.

- Surgery—Submacular surgery for removal of subfoveal CNV, macular translocation surgery are currently being evaluated.
2. Dry senile macular degeneration.
    - Antioxidants possibly prevent or delay the progression.
    - Strong near adds or low vision aids are useful.

PIGMENTARY RETINAL DYSTROPHY (RETINITIS PIGMENTOSA)

It is slow degenerative, hereditary disease of the retina involving the rods and cones. It appears as a recessive trait and usually occurs due to consanguinity of the parents.

Incidence
- It is a bilateral affection usually. The course is slow, chronic and progressive.
- It begins in childhood and causes blindness in middle and advanced age.

Symptoms
1. Defective vision in the dusk (night blindness) is an early complaint.
2. There is gradual constriction of the visual fields resulting in small central tubular vision.

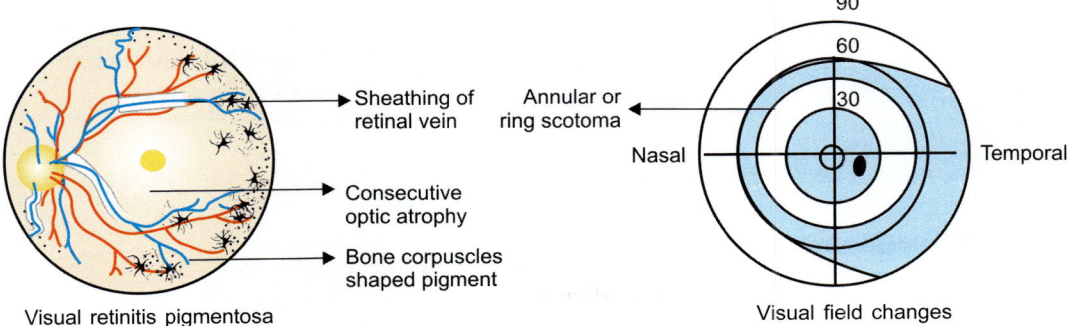

Visual retinitis pigmentosa

Visual field changes

Signs
1. *Fundus examination*
    - The retina is studded with jet black spots (pigments) which resemble bone corpuscles with a spidery outline. It affects the equatorial region first.
    - *The retinal blood vessels*—Both arteries and veins, become extremely attenuated and thread-like. The retinal veins, *never* the arteries, may have a sheath of pigment for part of their course.

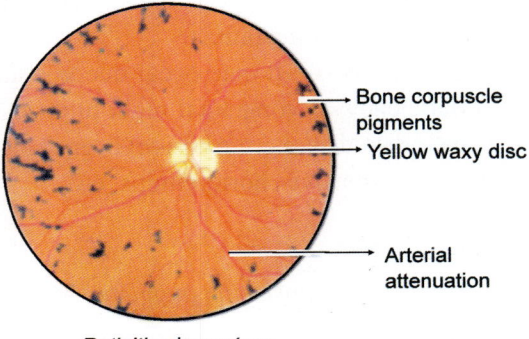

Retinitis pigmentosa

- *The optic disc*—It shows features of consecutive optic atrophy, i.e. pale, wax-like, yellowish appearance.
2. *Visual fields*
    - Annular or ring scotoma is present which leads to tubular vision.
    - There is complete blindness in the later stage.
3. *Dark adaptation* is increased due to rods dysfunction.
4. *The electroretinogram (ERG) and electro-oculogram (EOG)* are markedly subnormal or completely extinguished early in the disease.

Complications

1. Posterior cortical (complicated) cataract may be present.
2. Consecutive optic atrophy occurs eventually.

Associated dystrophies or degenerations
1. Systemic
    i. *Laurence-Moon-Biedl syndrome*
       Obesity, Hypogenitalism, Mental defect, Polydactyly.
    ii. *Usher's syndrome*
       Deafness
       Patients are both deaf and blind.
2. Ocular
    i. *Myopia*
    ii. *Conical cornea*
    iii. *Open angle glaucoma.*

Differential diagnosis of night blindness (nyctalopia)
1. Vitamin A deficiency
2. Liver diseases, e.g. cirrhosis
3. Retinitis pigmentosa
4. Congenital night blindness
5. Extensive chorioretinitis
6. Oguchi's disease

Differential Diagnosis

1. *Congenital syphilis*—It may produce a similar picture but there is typical 'pepper and salt' fundus with black and white spots seen in the periphery. Pepper and salt fundus may also be seen in rubella infection.
2. *Night blindness*—It may occur due to vitamin A deficiency, as congenital night blindness in hepatic disorders, e.g. cirrhosis of liver, Oguchi's disease, extensive chorioretinitis, etc.

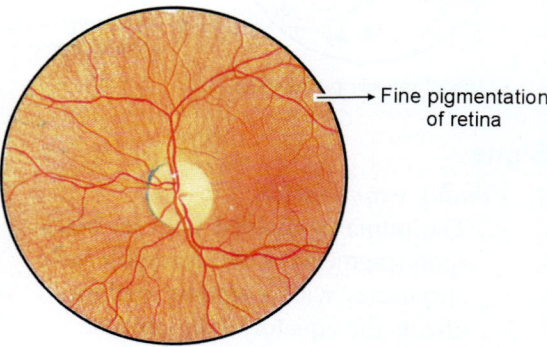

Pepper and salt fundus

Types

1. *Retinitis pigmentosa sine pigmento*—It has same symptoms but there is no visible pigmentation of retina.
2. *Retinitis punctata albescens*—There is same history and symptoms with the retina showing hundreds of small white pigments distributed uniformly. It may be stationary or progressive.

3. *Central or inverse pigmentary degeneration*—It involves the posterior pole predominantly.
4. *Uniocular and atypical form*—There is variation in amount and distribution of pigments.

Treatment

It is always unsatisfactory.
1. Low vision aids may be useful.
    i. Near vision—Hand and stand magnifier.
    ii. Telescopes—Monocular or binocular telescope of various magnification.
    iii. Electronic aids—Closed circuit television.
2. Genetic counselling is advised. There should be no consanguinous marriages.

Prognosis

The central vision steadily becomes very poor in advanced life.

5. TUMOURS OF THE RETINA RETINOBLASTOMA (GLIOMA RETINAE)

It is a common congenital malignant tumour of the retina occurring in early childhood. It is due to the proliferation of neural cells which have failed to evolve normally.

Incidence

1. It is common in infants and young children (2-4 years). Approximately, 1 in 20,000 live births.
2. Occasionally, it may remain quiescent and manifest in the 5th or 6th year or even later.
3. Heredity—It has autosomal dominant inheritance therefore children of the same family are usually affected (approximately 6%). However, sporadic cases occur by somatic mutation. Chromosomal abnormalities such as deletion of long arm of chromosome-13 and trisomy-21 may be present.
4. It is unilateral usually but about 25% cases, the second eye is affected.

Pathology

Retinoblastoma is a tumour derived from neurosensory retina. High power microscopic examination shows two different types of cellular characteristics.
1. Poorly differentiated, small to medium sized round cells with large hyperchromatic nuclei and scanty cytoplasm along with necrosis. It resembles the nuclear layer of the retina.
2. Well-differentiated tumour cells may be arranged in two special forms:
    a. Rosettes
    b. Fleurettes.

   a. Rosettes
    i. *Flexner-Wintersteiner rosettes*—These rosettes are specific for retinoblastoma. Single layer of columnar cells are arranged around a clear central lumen.
    ii. *Homer Wright rosettes*—These are not specific for retinoblastoma. The tumour cells are arranged radially around a central core of neural fibres. This type of cell arrangement can also be seen in neuroblastoma and medulloepithelioma.

iii. *Pseudorosettes*—Sometimes tumour cells are clustered around blood vessels in necrotic retinoblastoma. These are called 'pseudorosettes'.

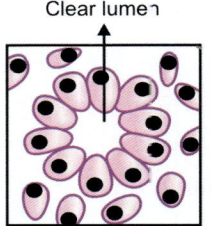
Flexner-Wintersteiner rosettes

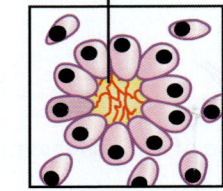
Homer Wright rosettes

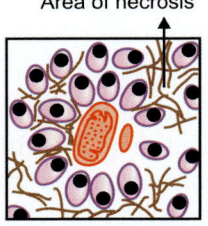
Pseudo–rosettes

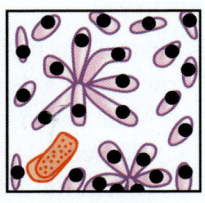
Fleurettes

b. Fleurettes

These are highly specific for retinoblastoma. There is flower bouquet type aggregation of tumour cells.
3. Other histological features include presence of necrosis and calcification.

Symptoms

1. Leucocoria—Peculiar yellow or white pupillary reflex called the "amaurotic cat's eye" is usually noticed by the parents. It is the most common presentation. It is due to reflection of light from the yellow-white mass in the retrolental area.
2. Squint usually convergent is the second most common presenting symptom.
3. Nystagmus is seen in bilateral cases.
4. Severe-pain may be present due to raised intraocular pressure.
5. Enlargement of the globe with protrusion of the eyeball is a common complaint.

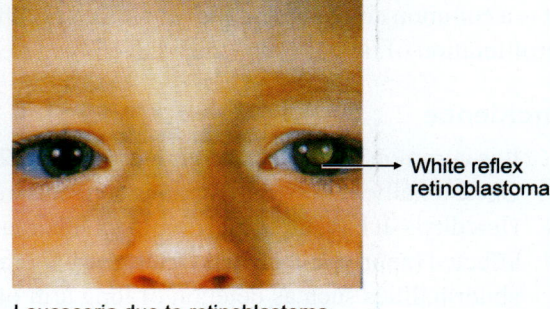
Leucocoria due to retinoblastoma

Signs

1. Multiple polypoid masses are seen in the fundus. There may be haemorrhages on the surface of the tumour at times.
2. The tumour mass may spread into the vitreous cavity.
3. Pseudohypopyon with esotropia (convergent squint) may be the presenting clinical feature.
4. The second eye may show a larger retinal tumour mass surrounded by numerous punctate satellites.

Types

There are two types of retinoblastomas:
1. *Glioma exophytum*—It grows outwards separating the retina from the choroid. It resembles detachment of retina.
2. *Glioma endophytum*—It grows inwards towards the vitreous.

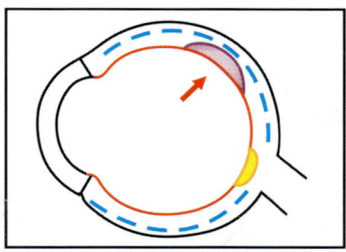
Exophytic retinoblastoma

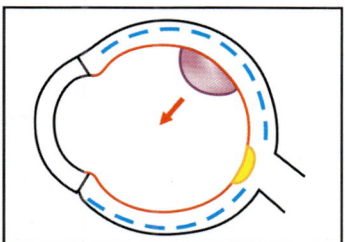
Endophytic retinoblastoma

Stages
There are four clinical stages:
Stage 1: *The quiescent stage*—It lasts from six months to one year.
Stage 2: *The glaucomatous stage*—There is enlargement of the globe, proptosis and severe pain associated with raised intraocular tension.
Stage 3: *The stage of extraocular extension*—The tumour bursts through the limbus followed by rapid growth.
Stage 4: *The stage of metastasis*—The tumour spreads by the:
   i. Lymphatics—Preauricular and cervical lymph nodes.
   ii. Direct extension—Cranial and other bones. Optic nerve and brain.
   iii. Bloodstream—It spreads by choroidal vessels. Most common sites are bone and liver.

Differential Diagnosis
In all cases atropine is instilled and thorough fundus examination of both eyes should be done under general anaesthesia to rule out bilateral involvement. The common causes of white pupillary reflex (leucocoria) in children include:
1. *Congenital cataract*—It is common in early childhood.
2. *Retinoblastoma*—It is the most common malignant tumour occurring in childhood.
3. *Pseudoglioma*—Several conditions in children give rise to similar signs and cause great difficulty in diagnosis.
   i. Inflammatory deposits in the vitreous following a plastic cyclitis or choroiditis.
   ii. Tuberculosis of the choroid specially the confluent type.
   iii. Toxocara infestation.
   iv. Congenital defects, due to persistent hyperplastic vitreous at the back of the lens.
   v. Retrolental fibroplasia.—It is common in premature babies due to hyperoxygenation.
4. *Other causes*
   i. Coats disease
   ii. Choroidal coloboma
   iii. Retinal dysplasia.

Diagnosis of Retinoblastoma
1. There is raised intraocular tension usually.
2. Lactic dehydrogenase and phosphoglucose isomerase enzyme levels are raised in the aqueous humor.

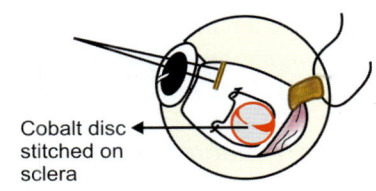
Cobalt disc stitched on sclera
Radiation by cobalt disc

3. *Plain X-ray orbit* —Calcification occurs in 75% cases of retinoblastomas.
4. *It is a progressive condition.*
5. *Ultrasonography, computerised tomography (CT scan) and MRI confirm the diagnosis.*

Treatment

1. *Enucleation*—Enucleation is the treatment of choice in clinical stage 1 and stage 2. Excision of the eye is done. The optic nerve should be cut as long as possible (atleast 10 mm) and cut end is examined microscopically for direct extension of tumour.
2. *Exenteration of the orbit*—It is done if there is conjunctival or orbital tissue extension, i.e. in clinical stage 3. It is a mutilating surgical procedure.
3. *Radiation and chemotherapy*—Retinoblastoma is a highly radiosensitive tumour. Radioactive cobalt disc is stitched to the sclera over the site of the nodule. A dose of 4000 rads is delivered to the summit of the tumour in one week in case of recurrence in the other eye. Brachytherapy with I^{125} may be used.
   It should be supplemented with Vincristine (50 mg/kg IV), Cyclophosphamide (20 mg/kg IV) and adriamycin (2 mg/kg IV) start and then at an interval of 3 weeks till 15 months. However, adriamycin should be discontinued after a total dose of 16 mg/kg has been given.
4. *Cryotherapy*—Cryotherapy by triple-freeze and thawing technique may be only useful for very small peripheral tumours situated anteriorly.
5. *Photocoagulation by argon laser or diode laser* can be considered in case of small tumour (less than 3 mm in diameter) which are situated behind the equator and recurrences.

Prognosis

1. It is always bad if untreated.
2. It is fair if the eye is removed before the onset of extraocular extension.
3. Prognosis is poor if the optic nerve is involved, tumour cells are undifferentiated and in 3rd and 4th clinical stages.
4. Spontaneous regression with massive necrosis and calcification may occur occasionally due to the immunological mechanisms.

RETINAL DETACHMENT
(SEPARATION OF THE RETINA)

Retinal detachment is a condition where there is separation of the two retinal layers, the retina proper and the pigmentary epithelium by the subretinal fluid.

Classification

It can be clinically divided into :
1. *Primary or simple (rhegmatogenous) detachment.*
2. *Secondary (non-rhegmatogenous) detachment.*

Simple (Rhegmatogenous) Detachment

It is always due to a break in the retina in the form of a hole or tear. This allows the fluid from the vitreous to seep through and raise the retina from its bed.

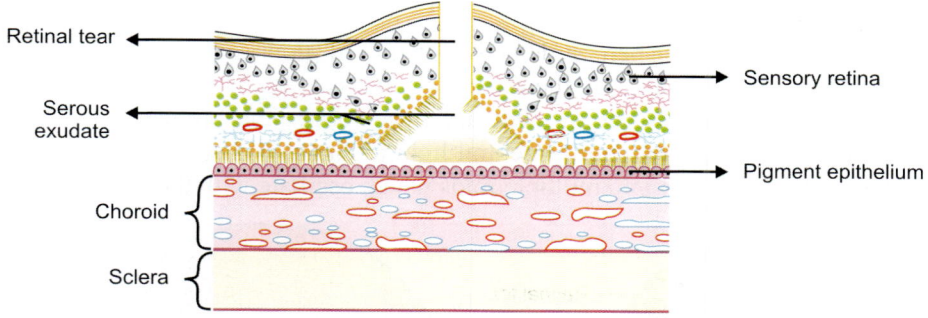
Primary retinal detachment

Mechanism of Detachment
i. Presence of retinal hole or tear due to retinal degeneration or trauma.
ii. Presence of degenerated fluid vitreous.
iii. A force sufficient to separate the retina and allow passage of fluid.

Secondary (Non-rhegmatogenous) Detachment
It is always secondary to the ocular diseases or pathology.

Mechanism of Detachment
1. *The retina being pushed away from its bed*
   i. Accumulation of fluid, e.g. blood (choroidal haemorrhage) or exudate (exudatives choroiditis or retinopathy).
   ii. Neoplasm, e.g. tumours of the choroid.
2. *The retina being pulled away from its bed*
   The contraction of fibrous tissue bands in the vitreous, e.g. as in plastic cyclitis, proliferative retinopathy or retrolental fibroplasia.

Symptoms
1. Premonitory symptoms like the transient flashes of light (photopsia), muscae volitantes and distortion of objects are common.
2. A shadow or cloud is seen in front of the eye.
3. There is profound dimness of vision.

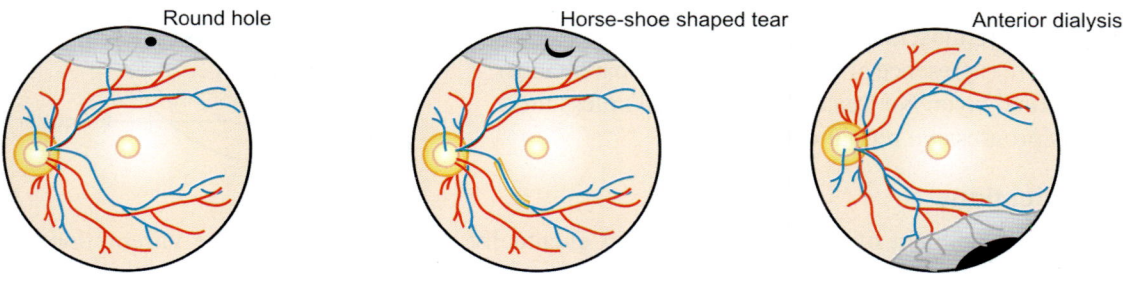
Retinal detachment

Signs

1. *Plane mirror examination*—There is defective or no red glow seen.
2. *Fundus examination*—It is done by the direct and indirect ophthalmoscope.
   - The detached retina looks greyish-white and raised above the surface.
   - The retinal vessels are dark with no central light reflex.
   - Detached retina is thrown into multiple folds which oscillate with the movement of the eye.

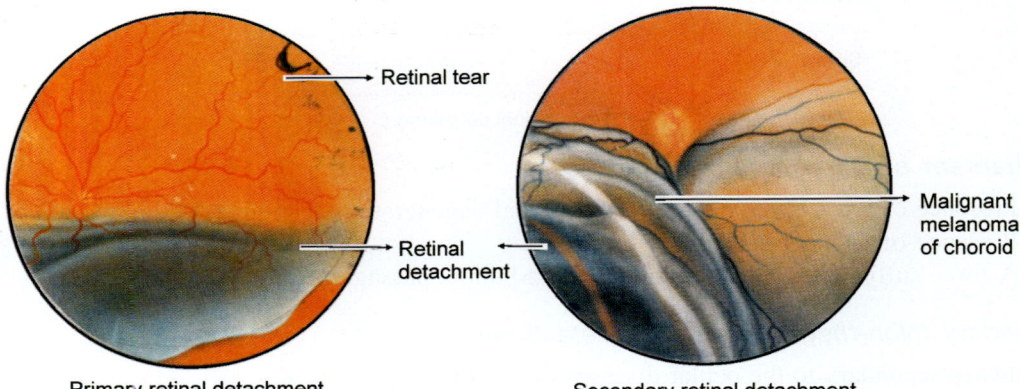

Primary retinal detachment
Secondary retinal detachment

- One or more holes or tear may be seen commonly in the upper temporal region.
- In total retinal detachment, the retina is funnel-shaped being attached to the disc and ora serrata. It is grey in colour.
- There may be associated degeneration, pigmentation and haemorrhage of the retina.

3. *Visual fields*—Scotomas are present corresponding to the area of the detached retina.
4. *Electroretinography (ERG)*—It is subnormal or absent.
5. *Ultrasonography* confirms the diagnosis of retinal detachment in cases when retina cannot be visualised, e.g. senile mature cataract, corneal opacity, vitreous opacities.

Differential Diagnosis

Senile Retinoschisis

There is splitting of the retina at the level of the inner nuclear and outer plexiform layers. It occurs in the lower temporal quadrant and progresses slowly.

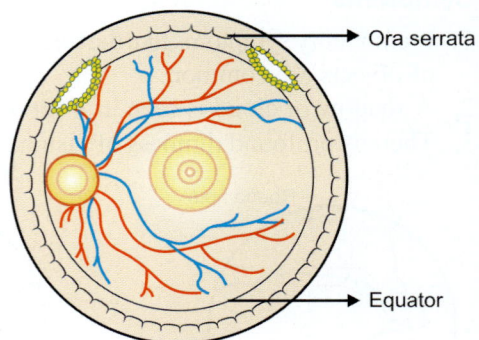

   i. There is presence of an absolute field defect in senile retinoschisis.
   ii. There is presence of immobile and transparent inner retinal layer. No treatment is required unless there is progressive retinal detachment.

Complications

1. Total detachment of the retina may occur eventually following proliferative vitreoretinopathy (PVR).

2. Complicated cataract is seen in the posterior cortex.
3. Chronic uveitis and phthisis bulbi may occur.

Treatment

Principle—The main principle of treatment is to approximate and adhere the torn part of the retina to an area of choroid by exciting aseptic inflammation.

1. **To seal retinal breaks**

   All the retinal breaks should be detected, accurately localised and sealed by producing aseptic chorioretinitis. This can be achieved by the following methods:

   i. *Photocoagulation*—Ideally a triple row of burns is placed around the break taking care to coagulate the area where sensory and pigment epithelial layers are still in opposition.

   ii. *Cryosurgery, i.e. cryopexy* is done to seal the retinal breaks by causing tissue necrosis.

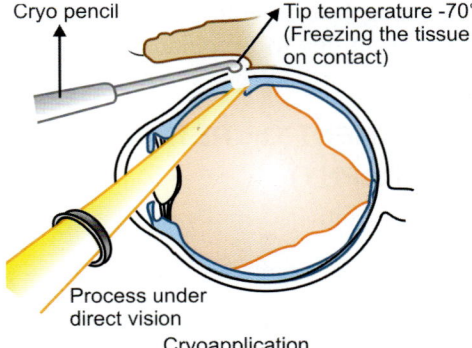
Cryoapplication

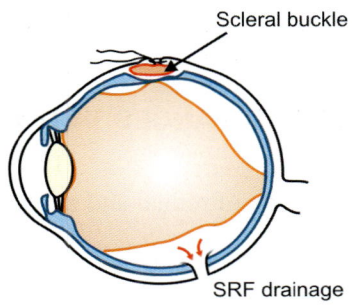
SRF drainage and scleral buckling

2. **To approximate the sclera, choroid and detached retina**

   i. *Scleral buckling*—Silicon band provides adequate mechanical support to overlying sclera.

   ii. *Drainage of subretinal fluid (SRF)* is required in long-standing cases.

   iii. *Pars plana vitrectomy*—It breaks the tractional band in the vitreous, thus, releasing the pull on the retina in cases of tractional retinal detachment.

   iv. *Pneumoretinopexy*—Air or other suitable gas such as SF6 or silicone oil is used as a vitreous substitute to produce internal temponade.

Prognosis

- The prognosis is bad if the simple detachment remains untreated due to the development of total detachment, complicated cataract and iridocyclitis.
- The prognosis is good if retina and vitreous are healthy and the patient is operated early.

COLOBOMA OF RETINA AND CHOROID

These are due to defective closure of the embryonic cleft. They are present in the lower part of the eye (typical) and may be associated with coloboma of the iris.

Symptoms

Central vision is bad and is associated with corresponding scotoma.

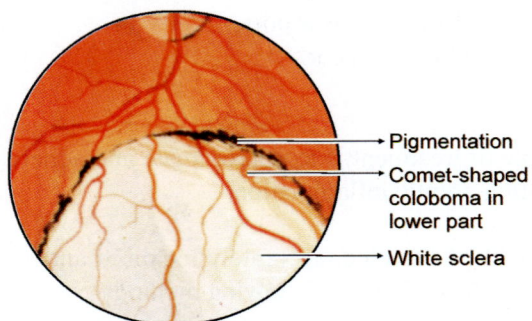
Retinal and choroidal coloboma

Fundus Examination

A typical coloboma is comet-shaped with rounded apex towards the disc. A few retinal and choroidal vessels are present on the surface. Ectatic coloboma may result due to irregular depression in the surface.

RECENT ADVANCES IN DIAGNOSIS AND MANAGEMENT OF RETINAL DISEASES (FLUORESCEIN ANGIOGRAPHY)

It is the study of retinal and choroidal vasculature using fluorescein.

Principle

It is based on the sensitivity of the recording film to the presence of fluorescent light from the dye. The fluorescein dye leaks freely from the normal choriocapillaris. However, it does not pass through healthy retinal pigment epithelium and retinal capillaries due to tight endothelial junction. Retinal capillaries (5-10 m) can be seen with this technique.

Method

The fluorescein is an alkali dye—sodium fluorescein. Its low molecular weight and high solubility in water allows rapid diffusion. About 5 cc of 10% solution of sodium fluorescein is injected intravenously in anticubital vein very fast through a wide bore needle.

The fluorescein can be observed directly by slit-lamp or ophthalmoscope and can also be photographed by a fundus camera. By sending light through an excitor filter (420-490 nm) for activation and by screening the emitted fluorescence through a barrier filter (510-530 nm), valuable informations of blood flow and perfusion are obtained.

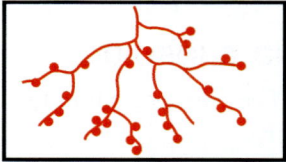
Out line of microaneurysms

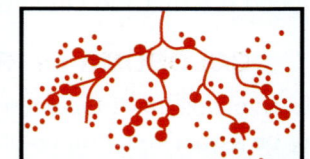
Leakage from microaneursms into retina

Fluorescein angiography

When the dye enters the eye within 8-11 seconds, there is at first a choroidal blush. It is followed by the passage through the retinal arterioles, the capillary bed and into the veins. The total retinal circulation time is 2-3 seconds.

It should be combined with fundus photography for permanent record and assessment.

Side Effects

1. Nausea and vomiting occur frequently.
2. Urticaria and allergy may occur occasionally.
3. Slight yellow skin discolouration for about 12-24 hours is usually seen.

Uses

It gives a clear idea of the integrity of the retinal vascular tree and choroidal circulation.

1. *Diabetic retinopathy*—It reveals neovascularisation, microaneurysms, rubeosis iridis and passage of dye into the vitreous (vitreous fluorophotometry).
2. *Neoplasms*—It outlines the abnormal dilated, engorged and tortuous vessels.
3. *Papilloedema*—It is useful in confirming the diagnosis by leakage and pooling of the fluorescein eye. Papillitis also shows many features of early papilloedema.
4. Retinitis pigmentosa and other retinal degenerations. It marks out the extent of retinal pigment epithelium atrophy.
5. *Choroidal disease*—It marks out area of choroidal neovascularisation.

INDOCYANINE GREEN ANGIOGRAPHY (ICG)

Indocyanine green stays within the choroidal circulation and is stimulated by a longer wavelength of light than fluorescein dye. This provides a better resolution of the choroidal vasculature, specially choroidal neovascular membranes (CNVM).

INVESTIGATIONS BY LASERS

There are more precise and objective ways of assessing the retina and optic nerve head morphology are available. They enable precise visualization of retina and optic nerve, layer by layer.
- Scanning laser ophthalmoscopy
- Scanning laser polarimetry
- Optical coherence tomography
- Scanning laser interferometry.

ULTRASONOGRAPHY

Principle

It is based upon pulse-echo technique. The ultrasonic frequencies in the range of 10 MHz are beamed into the ocular and orbital tissue. The reflected waves are converted into electrical potential and displayed on a oscilloscope (cathode ray tube).

A-Scan (Time Amplitude)

It traces a series of spikes on the oscilloscope. The height of each spike depends on the tissue's cellular composition. The distance between the spikes gives a measure of distance between intraocular structures.

This is useful in recording the axial length of the eye prior to doing intraocular lens implantation during cataract surgery.

B-Scan (Intensity Modulation)

The transducer is moved across the eye to obtain a two-dimensional picture of the ocular structures. B-scan is comparable to a histological section through the eye and orbit.

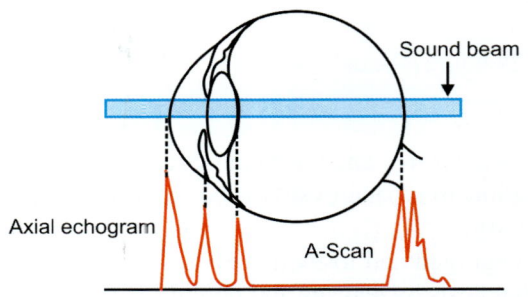
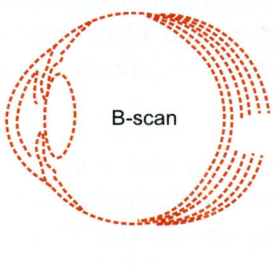

1. Detecting retinal detachment when there are vitreous or lenticular opacities.
2. To locate an intraocular foreign body which is radiotranslucent.
3. To locate intraocular tumours.

C-Scan

A strongly focused transducer scans a 4 cm square aperture in which eye is placed in the centre. It displays soft tissues in the coronal plane of the orbit.

CRYOSURGERY IN OPHTHALMOLOGY (CRYOPEXY)

Principle

The effect of freezing causes tissue necrosis, vascular occlusion and increased adhesion of the tissues.

Method

In cryopexy, a cold probe is applied to the tissue. The temperature of the cryoprobe has to be below the freezing point (–40°C) to have a desired effect. The temperature depends on the size of the tip, duration of the freezing process and the gas used.
1. The present cryosurgical units use freon, nitrous oxide or carbon dioxide gases as cooling agents.
2. The cryoprobes are available in different sizes, i.e. 1 mm for intravitreal use, 1.5 mm for cataract extraction, 2.5 mm for retina and 4 mm for cyclocryopexy.

Uses

1. *Lens*—The cryoextraction of the lens is the best technique for intracapsular lens extraction as it reduces the incidence of capsular rupture and vitreous loss.
2. *Retina*—The cryopexy seals retinal breaks in retinal detachment, flattens retinoschisis and destroys some small tumours such as angioma.
3. *Ciliary body*—The cyclocryopexy lowers the intraocular pressure by destroying some of the ciliary processes. It is useful in cases of absolute glaucoma and rubeosis iridis.

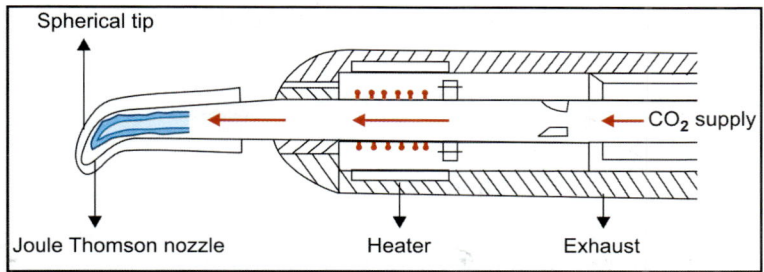
Cryoprobe-section through curved pencil

LASERS IN OPHTHALMOLOGY

Principle

The term "laser" means "light amplification by stimulated emission of radiation". The lasers produce highly coherent, monochromatic light. This light energy is converted into heat which is absorbed by the melanin pigment and haemoglobin in the eye.

Production of Laser Beam

In the laser system atomic environments of various types are stimulated to produce laser light which is the brightest existing light. A laser system consists of a transparent crystal rod or a gas or liquid-filled cavity constructed with a fully reflective mirror at one end and a partially reflective mirror at the other. Surrounding the rod or cavity is an optical or electrical source of energy that raises the energy level of the atoms within the cavity or rod to a very high and unstable level. This phenomenon is called 'population-inversion'. The atoms spontaneously decay back to a lower energy level, releasing the excess energy in the form of light which is amplified to an appropriate wavelength. Thus, laser is created mainly by two mechanisms:
  i. Population inversion in active medium
  ii. Amplification of appropriate wavelength of light.

COMMON TYPES OF LASERS	WAVELENGTH
1. Ruby laser (first laser)	550 nm
2. Argon laser	
• blue-green	488 nm
• pure green	518 nm
3. Krypton laser	647 nm
4. Nd-YAG laser (Neodymium: yttrium-aluminum-garnet)	
• single frequency	1064 nm
• double frequency (pulsed)	532 nm
5. Diode laser (Produced from semiconductor crystals. Lasing substance: Gallium-aluminum-arsanate)	810 nm
6. Excimer (Excited dimer) laser (Lasing substance: Argon fluoride)	193 nm

Types

Several types of lasers are available depending upon the type of atomic environment stimulated to produce the laser beam. Common types of lasers are as follows—Xenon arc laser, ruby laser, argon laser, krypton laser, YAG (yttrium-aluminum-garnet) laser, Neodymium ion laser, excimer laser, diode, tunable dye laser, erbium laser, etc.

TYPES OF LASER	ATOMIC ENVIRONMENT USED	LASER EFFECT
1. Argon	Argon gas	Photocoagulation
2. Krypton	Krypton gas	Photocoagulation
3. Diode	Diode crystal	Photocoagulation
4. Nd-YAG	A liquid dye or a solid compound of yttrium-aluminum-garnet and neodymium	Photodisruption
5. Excimer	Helium and fluorine gas	Photoablation

MECHANISM OF LASER EFFECTS AND THEIR THERAPEUTIC USES

1. Photocoagulation

The common lasers used in ophthalmic therapy are the thermal lasers. They depend upon absorption of the laser light by tissue pigments. The absorbed light is converted into heat, thus increasing the temperature of the target tissue high enough to coagulate and denature cellular elements.

Mode of Action

Argon, diode and krypton lasers, etc. are 'thermal lasers'.
Photocoagulation is effective in the treatment of ocular diseases by the following mechanisms,
1. *Production of scar tissue*, e.g. as in retinal detachment.
2. *Occlusion of the blood vessels*, e.g. as in diabetic retinopathy, haemangioma.
3. *Tissue atrophy*, e.g. in production of hole in iris as in closed angle glaucoma.
4. *Contraction of smooth muscles*, e.g. as in updrawn pupil.

Therapeutic Uses

1. *Eyelid lesions* such as haemangioma, small tumour, etc.
2. *Cornea*—It can be used for treating corneal vascularisation.
3. *Iris*—Laser coreoplasty or laser sphincterotomy can be done for updrawn pupil
   - Laser shrinkage of iris cyst.
4. *Glaucoma*
   - Laser iridotomy can be done for closed angle glaucoma (acute stage).
   - Argon laser trabeculoplasty (ALT) may be done for open angle glaucoma.
   - Laser goniopuncture is useful for congenital glaucoma.
   - Prophylactic pan-retinal photocoagulation is done to prevent neovascular glaucoma in patients with retinal hypoxia, e.g. central retinal vein occulsion.
   - Cyclophotocoagulation for absolute glaucoma by erbium laser.
5. *Retina and choroid*—They form the most important indications .
   i. *Diabetic retinopathy*—Panretinal photocoagulation (PRP) is done for proliferative retinopathy.
      - Focal or grid photocoagulation is done for exudative maculopathy.
   ii. *Retinal detachment*—Lasers are used for sealing retinal holes.
   iii. *Peripheral retinal vascular lesions*, e.g. Eale's disease, sickle cell disease, Coats diseases and retinopathy of prematurity can be treated.

iv. *Macula*—Central serous retinopathy, age-related macular degeneration.
v. *Intraocular tumours* can be successfully treated, e.g. small retinoblastoma, malignant melanoma, choroidal haemangiomas.

Complications
Complications of laser photocoagulation include:
1. *Macula*—Accidental foveal burns, cystoid macular oedema, macular pucker, etc.
2. *Retina*—Preretinal fibrosis, traction retinal detachment, haemorrhage from retina and choroid and retinal hole formation may occur.
3. *Optic nerve*—Ischaemic papillitis may occur rarely.
4. *Lens and cornea*—Localised opacification of lens and accidental corneal burns.

2. Photodisruption
Nd-YAG laser is based on this mechanism and it exerts a cutting or incising effect on the tissues. It ionizes the electrons of the target tissue producing a physical state called 'plasma'. This plasma expands with momentary pressures as high as 10 kilobars exerting a cutting effect.

Uses
1. It is used for capsulotomy of thickened posterior capsule.
2. It is also used for membranectomy of pupillary membrane (chronic iridocyclitis).
3. Peripheral buttonhole iridectomy.

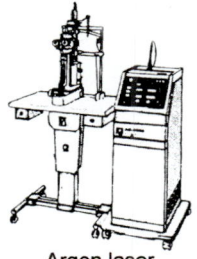
Argon laser

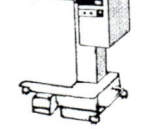
Nd-YAG laser

3. Photoablation
Laser based on this mechanism produce ultraviolet light of very short wavelength which breaks chemical bonds of biologic materials, converting them into small molecules which diffuse away. These lasers are collectively called excimer (excited dimer) lasers. These act by tissue modelling. Excimer, LASIK, pulsed holonium-YAG lasers, etc. act by tissue modelling.

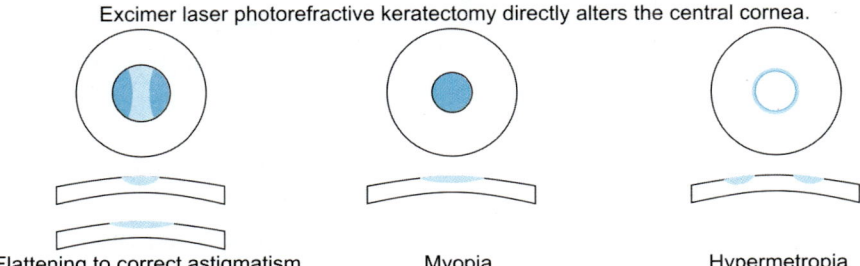
Excimer laser photorefractive keratectomy directly alters the central cornea.
Flattening to correct astigmatism   Myopia   Hypermetropia

Uses
1. It is used for photorefractive keratectomy (PRK) for correction of refractive errors.
2. It can be used for phototherapeutic keratectomy (PTK) for corneal pathology, e.g. band-shaped keratopathy.

MULTIPLE CHOICE QUESTIONS

1. After retinal stimulation the visual impulse reaches occipital cortex after
   a. 1 m sec
   b. 24 m sec
   c. 124 m sec
   d. 142 m sec
2. Retinal detachment is associated with
   a. malignant melanoma
   b. high myopia
   c. diabetic retinopathy
   d. all of the above
3. Retinoblastoma is
   a. most common in adults
   b. usually bilateral
   c. treated by evisceration
   d. all of the above
4. The late clinical features of retinitis pigmentosa include all *EXCEPT*
   a. normal vision
   b. waxy disc
   c. sheathing of disc vessels
   d. ring scotoma
5. Diabetic retinopathy is characterised by
   a. superficial haemorrhage
   b. perivasculitis
   c. microaneurysms
   d. A-V crossing changes
6. Toxoplasmosis usually affects
   a. iris
   b. ciliary body
   c. macula
   d. ora serrata
7. Salt and pepper appearance of fundus is seen in
   a. leprosy
   b. retinitis pigmentosa
   c. congenital syphilis
   d. toxoplasmosis
8. Cherry red spot is seen in
   a. chorioretinitis
   b. amaurotic familial idiocy
   c. central serous retinopathy
   d. all of the above
9. Flame-shaped haemorrhages are seen commonly in the retinopathy of
   a. diabetes
   b. hypertension
   c. retinitis pigmentosa
   d. all of the above
10. Rhegmatogenous retinal detachment is due to
    a. tumour
    b. retinal break
    c. vitreous traction
    d. proliferative retinopathy
11. The most common intraocular tumour in children is
    a. malignant melanoma
    b. retinoblastoma
    c. diktyoma
    d. medulloepithelioma
12. Roth's spots are seen in
    a. diabetes
    b. subacute bacterial endocarditis
    c. Eale's disease
    d. photoretinitis
13. Causes of secondary detachment are all *EXCEPT*
    a. intraocular tumour
    b. macular hole
    c. exudative choroiditis
    d. haemorrhage between retina and choroid

14. In Junius-Kuhnt's disease there is an early disciform degeneration of
    a. ciliary body
    b. pigment epithelium of macula
    c. suspensory ligament of lens
    d. none of the above
15. Retina after death becomes
    a. transparent
    b. white
    c. black
    d. red
16. Candle wax spots in the retina are seen in
    a. sarcoidosis
    b. toxocara
    c. syphilis
    d. cytomegalo inclusion virus
17. In retinitis pigmentosa pigmentation in retina starts at
    a. posterior pole
    b. anterior to equator
    c. equator
    d. the disc
18. The pathology of snow blindness involves the
    a. cornea
    b. iris
    c. retina
    d. optic disc
19. Nd:YAG laser wave is
    a. colourless
    b. red
    c. green
    d. blue
20. Ophthalmoscopically, the earliest sign of diabetic retinopathy is
    a. retinal haemorrhage
    b. microaneurysm
    c. soft exudate
    d. hard exudate
21. Pigmentary retinal dystrophy is associated with
    a. Laurence-Moon-Biedl syndrome
    b. Sturge-Weber syndrome
    c. Reiter's disease
    d. von Recklinghausen disease
22. The central retinal vein occlusion commonly occurs in persons with
    a. arteriosclerosis
    b. atherosclerosis
    c. orbital cellulitis
    d. all of the above
23. Neovascular glaucoma can be best treated by
    a. trabeculectomy
    b. pilocarpine
    c. panphotocoagulation of retina
    d. timolol maleate
24. The cardinal feature of stage 4 hypertensive retinopathy is
    a. arteriovenous crossing changes
    b. flame-shaped haemorrhage
    c. papilloedema
    d. soft exudate
25. The retinoblastoma can present itself as
    a. amaurotic cat's eye
    b. hypopyon with esotropia
    c. enlargement of the globe
    d. all of the above
26. Nyctalopia (night blindness) is seen in following except
    a. Oguchi's disease
    b. extensive chorioretinitis
    c. retinitis pegmentosa
    d. toxocariasis

27. Ring scotoma is seen in
    a. papilloedema
    b. macular oedema
    c. central retinal artery occlusion
    d. retinitis pigmentosa
28. Cattle truck appearance in fundoscopy is seen in
    a. central retinal artery occlusion
    b. central retinal vein occlusion
    c. hypertension
    d. diabetes
29. Photophthalmia is caused by :
    a. infrared rays
    b. ultraviolet rays
    c. slit-lamp examination
    d. trachoma
30. Which of the following is true of diabetic retinopathy
    a. always associated with hypertension
    b. seen only in uncontrolled diabetes
    c. incidence increases with duration of disease
    d. determines prognosis of disease.

ANSWERS

1—c	2—d	3—b	4—a	5—c
6—c	7—c	8—b	9—b	10—b
11—b	12—b	13—b	14—b	15—b
16—a	17—c	18—a	19—a	20—b
21—a	22—d	23—c	24—c	25—d
26—d	27—d	28—a	29—b	30—c

CHAPTER 14
The Optic Nerve

APPLIED ANATOMY

The Optic Nerve

It extends from the lamina cribrosa upto the optic chiasma.

The fibres of the optic nerve originate from the nerve fibre layer of the retina. All the retinal fibres converge to form the optic nerve about 5 mm to the nasal side of the macula lutea. The nerve pierces the lamina cribrosa to pass backwards and medially through the orbital cavity. It then passes through the optic foramen of the sphenoid bone, backwards and medially to meet the nerve from the other eye at the optic chiasma.

The optic nerve is covered with the meningeal sheaths, i.e. the pia mater, arachnoid mater and dura mater after it pierces the lamina cribrosa. These meningeal spaces are continuous with those in the brain.

The total length of the optic nerve is 5 cm. It can be divided into four parts :

Intraocular	—	1 mm
Intraorbital	—	25 mm
Intracanalicular	—	4-10 mm
Intracranial	—	10 mm (Duke-Elder)

Optic Disc

It represents the optic nerve head. It has only nerve fibre layer so it does not excite any visual response—"blind spot". It is a pink, oval or circular disc of 1.5 mm diameter. There is a depression in its central part which is known as the "physiological cup". It occupies the central one-third of the optic disc. Therefore, the normal cup: disc ratio is 1:3 or 0.3.

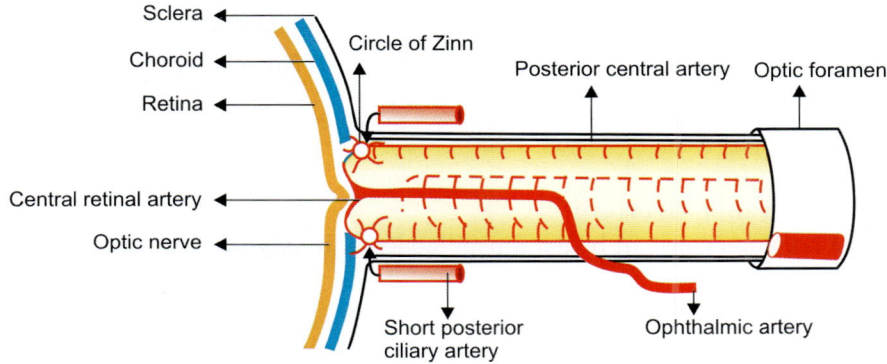

Blood supply of optic nerve

Blood Supply

The intraocular and intraorbital parts are supplied by the branches of the ophthalmic artery, short posterior ciliary arteries and central retinal artery forming circle of Zinn.

The *intracanalicular and intracranial parts* are supplied by the branches of the anterior cerebral artery and ophthalmic artery.

Venous Drainage

It is by the central retinal vein and superior and inferior ophthalmic veins.

Functions

1. Optic nerve is responsible for normal visual acuity and field of vision.
2. It also acts as a filter and functions as,
    i. Afferent pupillary pathway
    ii. Colour vision and light brightness appreciation.

DISEASES OF THE OPTIC NERVE

1. **Vascular disturbances**—Papilloedema.
2. **Inflammation**
    a. Acute
        i. Papillitis (optic neuritis)
        ii. Retrobulbar neuritis
        iii. Neuroretinitis
    b. Chronic—The toxic amblyopias.
3. **Degeneration**—Optic atrophy.
4. **Tumours**—Glioma, meningioma.
5. **Congenital anomalies**
    a. Coloboma
    b. Medullated nerve fibres.

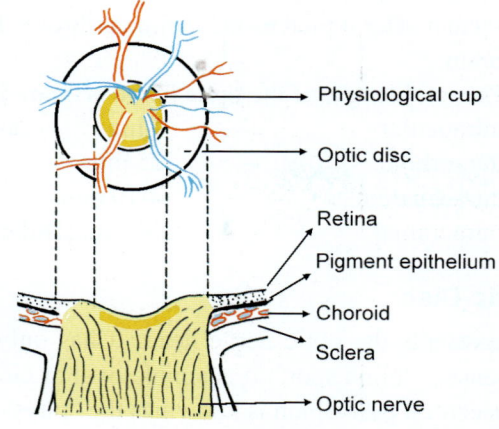

Fundus oculi examination

PAPILLOEDEMA (CHOCKED DISC)

It is a hydrostatic, non-inflammatory oedema of the optic disc. The optic disc swelling usually results from increased intracranial pressure and venous stasis.

Etiology

1. **Increased intracranial pressure**
   It is the most common cause of bilateral papilloedema. It may be associated with the following conditions:
   a. Intracranial space occupying lesions—These include space occupying lesions specially in the midbrain, parieto-occipital region and cerebellum. It may be a brain tumour, abscess, aneurysm,

subdural haematoma hydrocephalus, etc. The tumour of cerebellum, midbrain and parieto-occipital region produce papilloedema more repidly than the lesions involving other areas. The fast progressing lesions produce papilloedema more frequently and acutely than the slow growing lesions.

Foster-Kennedy syndrome—The frontal lobe, pituitary and middle-ear tumours such as meningiomata of the olfactory groove are sometimes associated with,
   i. Pressure atrophy of the optic nerve on the side of the lesion due to direct pressure.
   ii. Papilloedema on the other side due to the effect of generalized raised intracranial pressure.
   b. Systemic conditions include malignant hypertension, toxemia of pregnancy, cardiopulmonary insufficiency, blood dyscrasias and nephritis.
   c. Cerebral or subarachnoid haemorrhage can give rise to a papilloedema which is frequent and considerable in extent.
   d. Meningitis—It may be suppurative, syphilitic or tubercular.
   e. Encephalitis, cerebral oedema and encephalopathies.
   f. Pseudotumour cerebri—It is an important cause of raised intracranial pressure. It is a poorly understood condition, usually found in young obese women. It is characterised by chronic headache and bilateral papilloedema without any localising neurological signs.
2. **Orbit lesions**
The orbital space occupying lesions are frequently associated with papilloedema on the involved side such as tumours, orbital abscess and cellulitis, aneurysm of ophthalmic artery, pseudotumour and endocrinal exophthalmos.
3. **Ocular lesions**
These include marked ocular hypotony, acutely raised intraocular pressure, central retinal vein occlusion, anterior ischaemic optic neuropathy and uveitis.

Pathogenesis
1. It is due to venous stasis which results in the compression of the central retinal vein as it crosses the subdural and subarachnoid spaces.
2. There is vasodilatation at the disc due to hypoxia causing axoplasmic stasis.
3. The nerve fibres at the optic disc become swollen which degenerate later on.

Unilateral versus Bilateral Papilloedema
In majority of the cases with raised intracranial pressure, it is bilateral. Papilloedema due to ocular and orbital lesions is usually unilateral. However, unilateral cases as well as of unequal size do occur with raised intracranial pressure, e.g. Foster-Kennedy syndrome.

Symptoms
1. General symptoms include headache which is made worse by coughing, sneezing or straining.
2. Projectile vomiting (without nausea) is suggestive of raised intracranial pressure.
3. There are transient attacks of blurred vision (amaurosis fugax).
4. Central vision is affected only in late stages.

COMMON CAUSES OF BILATERAL AND UNILATERAL PAPILLOEDEMA

BILATERAL PAPILLOEDEMA	UNILATERAL PAPILLOEDEMA
1. Space occupying intracranial lesions.	1. Optic papillitis, neuroretinitis
2. Malignant hypertension, toxemia of pregnancy	2. Ocular hypotony
3. Head injury—cerebral oedema	3. Central retinal vein occlusion
4. Meningitis, encephalitis	4. Anterior ischaemic optic neuropathy
5. Intracranial vascular lesion—subarachnoid haemorrhage, cavernous sinus thrombosis, etc.	5. Leber's optic neuropathy
6. Blood dyscrasias—leukaemia, polycythemia, etc.	6. Optic nerve glioma or meningioma
7. Pseudotumour cerebri—with toxicity of drugs, like tetracycline, nalidixic acid, vitamin-A, oral contraceptives and corticosteroids	7. Orbital cellulitis
	8. Thyroid eye diseases
	9. Metastasis on the optic nerve head

Signs
1. **Fundus Examination**
   a. **Early changes**
      i. *Optic disc*—There is blurring of the disc margin.
         - Physiological cup gets filled up.
         - There is hyperemia of the disc with capillary dilatation.
         - The disc becomes gradually elevated (mushroom or dome-shaped) so that the vessels bend sharply over its margin. There is a difference of 2-6 D between the vessels at the top and those on the retina. By indirect ophthalmoscopy, a definite parallax can be elicited
         - Oedema gradually spreads to the surrounding retina.
      ii. *Vessels*—Veins are markedly congested, dilated and tortuous.
      iii. *Macula*—Macular star may be seen due to retinal oedema.
      iv. *General fundus*—Cotton wool soft exudates and both flame-shaped and punctate haemorrhages appear around the optic disc.
   b. **Late changes**
      i. *Postneuritic optic atrophy*—The disc becomes pale with blurred margin.
      ii. *Thickening of the perivascular sheaths lead to contraction of arteries.*
      iii. *Generalized retinal pigmentation may be present.*
2. **Visual Fields**
   - There is enlargement of the blind spot.
   - There is progressive contraction of the visual fields.
   - Complete blindness sets in eventually.
   - Associated neurological symptoms include headache, nausea and vomiting in cases of raised intracranial pressure.

Papilloedema
- Dome shaped disc
- Venous dilatation
- Blurred disc margins

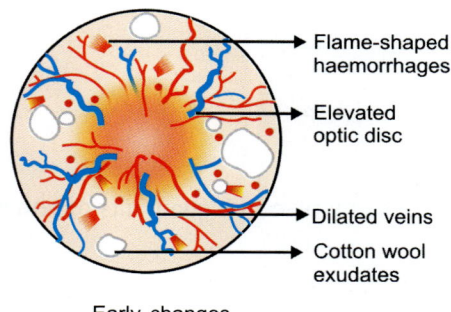

Early changes

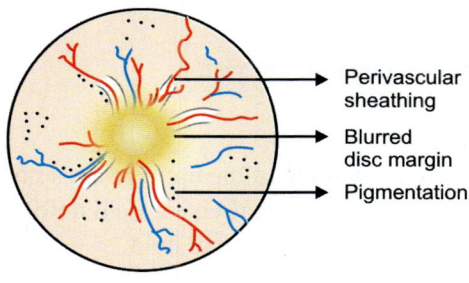

Late changes

Differential Diagnosis

Blurring of the optic disc margin is seen commonly in cases of:
1. Optic neuritis.
2. Pseudoneuritis—In hypermetropia the lamina cribrosa is small and the nerve fibres are heaped up.
3. Astigmatism.
4. Malignant hypertension.
5. Toxemia of pregnancy.
6. Central retinal vein occlusion.
7. Drusen of the nerve head—It is a typically bilateral and inherited condition.

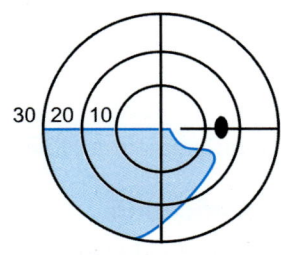

Papilloedema and oedematous retina

Treatment

It indicates raised intracranial pressure and a neurological emergency.
1. Treat the underlying cause of papilloedema.
2. Surgical decompression should be done early, i.e. before the visual field changes occur.
3. There is rapid recovery of vision after the decompression usually.

ANTERIOR ISCHAEMIC OPTIC NEUROPATHY (AION)

It is a condition of local anoxia of the anterior region of the optic nerve.

Etiology

It is due to the involvement of posterior ciliary artery and may be central retinal artery causing infarcts of the anterior part of the optic nerve and retina. It occurs commonly in,
   i. *Neglected acute attack of closed angle glaucoma*
  ii. *Severe anaemia*
 iii. *After a massive haemorrhage*
  iv. *Temporal arteritis.*

Altitudinal visual field defect in AION

Symptom
There is sudden loss of vision.

Signs
1. There is swelling of the optic disc resulting in optic atrophy.
2. Permanent altitudinal visual field defects are present. These involve two quadrants of either the superior or inferior visual field.

DIFFERENCES BETWEEN PAPILLOEDEMA AND PAPILLITIS

CLINICAL FEATURES	PAPILLOEDEMA	PAPILLITIS
1. *Incidence*	Bilateral	Unilateral
2. *Onset*	Gradual with slow progress	Sudden with rapid progress
3. *Visual acuity*		
Early	• Transient attacks of blurred vision	• Profound visual loss
Late	• Central vision is affected late	• Complete blindness
4. *Visual fields*	Enlargement of blind spot	Typically central scotoma
5. *Fundus examination*		
i. Optic disc	Difference of 2-6 D between the vessels on top of the disc and surrounding retina.	Difference is usually not more than 2-3D.
ii. Colour of disc	Reddish-grey	Marked hyperaemia
iii. Vessels	Marked venous dilatation, haemorrhages and exudates	Venous dilatation and exudates are less marked
iv. Macula	Macular star may be present	Macular fan may be present occasionally.
6. *Fluorescein angiography*	Vertical oval pool of dye due to leakage	Minimum leakage of dye
7. *Central nervous system involvement*	Presence of headache, projectile vomiting (raised intracranial pressure)	Presence of numbness, paresthesia, weakness and incoordination of limbs (demyelinating disease)
8. *CT scan and MRI*	Intracranial space occupying lesion can be detected	Demyelinating disorder can be seen

OPTIC NEURITIS

The inflammation of the optic nerve is known as optic neuritis.

Classification
It can be divided into two main types:
- Acute optic neuritis
- Chronic optic neuritis

The Optic Nerve

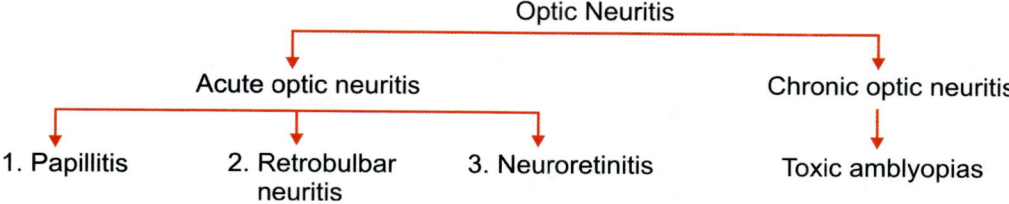

PAPILLITIS

Papillitis is an acute inflammation of the optic nerve head (papilla or optic disc) associated with rapid loss of vision. It is the ophthalmoscopically visible or anterior part of the optic nerve. It is often unilateral.

Etiology

1. *Multiple sclerosis is the most common cause.* It causes demyelination of the optic nerve.
2. *Other central nervous system diseases*
   - Neuromyelitis optica of Devic
   - Acute disseminated encephalomyelitis
   - Herpes zoster
   - Epidemic encephalitis
   - Poliomyelitis
   - Leber's disease
3. *Local causes*
   - Retinitis
   - Uveitis
   - Meningitis
4. *Endogenous causes*
   - Acute infections such as influenza, (measles, mumps, etc.)
   - Septic foci in teeth, tonsils, throat, etc.
   - Metabolic conditions, e.g. as in diabetes, anaemia, starvation.

> **Common causes of sudden loss of vision**
> 1. Optic neuritis—Papillitis, retrobulbar neuritis
> 2. Central retinal artery occlusion
> 3. Central retinal vein occlusion
> 4. Retinal detachment
> 5. Acute congestive glaucoma
> 6. Vitreous haemorrhage
> 7. Anterior ischaemic optic neuropathy (AION)
> 8. Cortical lesions—Trauma, vascular
> 9. Acute corneal hydrops as in keratoconus
> 10. Photo-ophthalmia—Eclipse and snow blindness, exposure to bright arc or flash light

Pathogenesis

There are inflammatory changes in the nerve (true optic neuritis) or in the sheath (perineuritis). There is infiltration and loss of myelin sheath. Finally, degenerative changes and reactionary gliosis occur.

Symptoms

1. Transient blurring of vision may be present initially.
2. Profound visual loss is the most important clinical feature.

3. There is usually unilateral involvement.
4. There is sudden onset and rapid progress of the disease process.
5. Complete blindness sets in rapidly in untreated cases.

Signs
1. *Pupil*—Direct light reflex is sluggish or absent as the afferent path is involved.
   - Indirect light reflex and near reflex are present.
2. *Fundus Examination*
   a. **Early changes**—These are similar to papilloedema. However, the disc swelling is usually upto 2-3D.
      i. Optic disc is hyperaemic with blurred margin.
      ii. The swelling spreads to the surrounding retina.
      iii. Retinal veins are tortuous and distorted.
      iv. Exudates are present at the disc and retina.
      v. Vitreous is cloudy with fine opacities.
      vi. Neuroretinitis—When the serious inflammation spreads from the disc towards the neighbouring retina, it is called neuroretinitis.

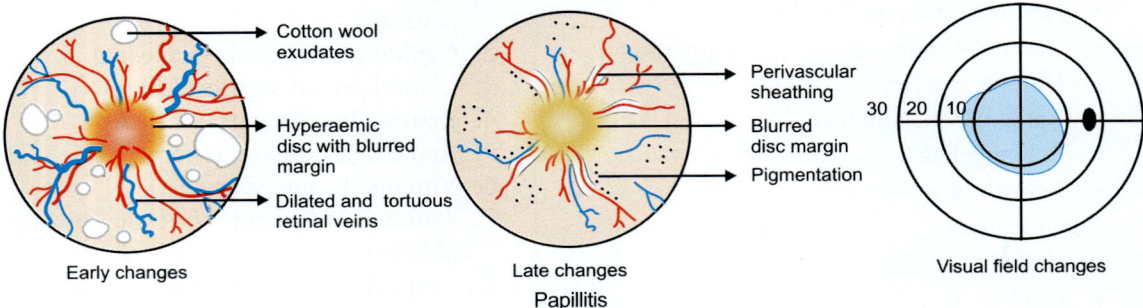

Papillitis

   b. **Late changes**
      i. Postneuritic atrophy sets in which is similar to papilloedema.
      ii. Disc margin is blurred.
      iii. Physiological cup gets filled up with organized fibrous tissue.
      iv. Perivascular sheathing is usually present.
3. *Visual Field Defects*—A generalized depression of the visual field is the most common of visual defect. Central, centrocaecal or paracentral scotoma may be present.

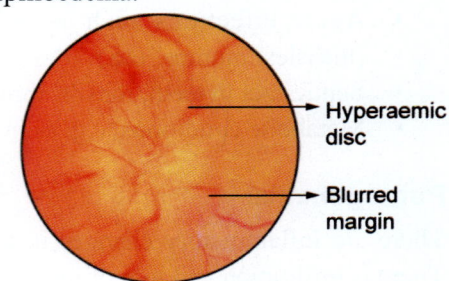

Papillitis

Treatment
1. Efforts should be made to find out and treat the underlying cause of papillitis.
2. There is no effective treatment for idiopathic and hereditary optic neuritis and that associated with demyelinating disorders.

3. Corticosteroids may help in early recovery.
   Optic neuritis treatment trial (ONTT) group has made the following recommendations for the use of corticosteroids.
   a. Oral prednisolone therapy alone is contraindicated in the treatment of acute optic neuritis, since it was not shown to improve visual outcome and recurrence rate is high with this regime.
   b. A patient presenting with acute optic neuritis should have MRI scan of the brain. If the brain shows lesions supportive of multiple sclerosis, the patient should receive immediate intravenous methylprednisolone (1 gm daily) for 3 days followed by oral prednisolone (1 mg/kg/day) for 11 days.
   c. Indications for intravenous methylprednisolone in acute optic neuritis patients with a normal brain MRI scan are:
      i. Bilateral simultaneous optic neuritis
      ii. Involvement of only good eye.
4. Vitamin B_1, B_6 and B_{12} injections are given in full doses. Hydroxycobalamine (B_{12}) acts as a detoxicating agent.

RETROBULBAR NEURITIS

It is an acute inflammation of the optic nerve situated behind the eyeball.

Symptoms
These are same as for papillitis.
Sudden, profound loss of vision is the most common presenting complaint.

Common causes of sudden painful loss of vision
1. Acute congestive glaucoma
2. Retrobulbar neuritis
3. Temporal arteritis

Signs
1. *Fundus examination*
   - "Neither the ophthalmologist nor the patient sees anything".
   - No ophthalmoscopically visible changes are seen.
   - If the lesion is situated near the lamina cribrosa, there is slight distension of the veins and attenuation of the arteries.
   - Temporal pallor of disc (due to involvement of papillomacular bundle) may be present occasionally.
2. *Local pain* on moving the eye is often present. There is tenderness over the attachment of the superior rectus muscle tendon.
3. *Marcus Gunn pupil*—There is lack of sustained constriction of the pupil to light in swinging flashlight test. It indicates an afferent pupillary defect. It is a diagnostic sign. Swinging flashlight test—A bright light is thrown on to one pupil and its constriction is noted. The light is rapidly transferred to the other pupil after 2-3 seconds. This process of swinging of light to and fro across the pupils is repeated several times so that there are equal impulses sent to the midbrain via the optic nerves.
4. *Field of vision*—Central, paracentral, sectorial scotomas or ring-shaped scotoma around fixation point may be present
5. *Early loss of colour vision and contrast sensitivity may be present* due to involvement of optic nerve.

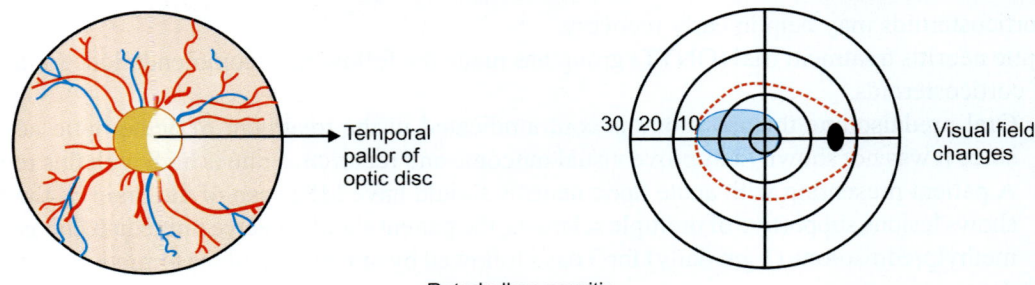

Retrobulbar neuritis

Complications
1. Recurrences are common specially in demyelinating diseases.
2. Complete blindness may occur eventually.

Differential Diagnosis
1. *Malingering*—It is seen in persons who hope to gain some advantage by pretending to be visually defective or handicapped. When one eye is said to be blind and there is absence of objective signs, following tests can be done.
    i. *A low convex or concave lens* (0.25 D) is placed before the 'blind eye' and a high convex lens (+ 10 D) is kept before the good eye. If the person can read distant types he is malingering.
    ii. *A prism* is placed base downwards before the 'good eye' and the patient is asked to look at a light source. If he sees two lights, he is malingering.
    iii. *Snellen's coloured types or FRIEND test*—The letters are printed in green and red. A red glass is placed before the 'good eye'. If the patient reads all the letters, he is malingering.
2. *Hysteria*—History of psychiatric illness is very important.
3. *Anterior ischaemic optic neuropathy (AION)*—There is sudden loss of vision due to ischaemia of anterior part of optic nerve.

Treatment
It is same as for papillitis.
1. Retrobulbar injection of dexamethasone is very effective.
2. Systemic corticosteroids are given in full doses.
3. Vasodilators (systemic or local) may be effective.
4. Vitamin B_1, B_6 and B_{12} administered in high doses are useful adjunct.

TOXIC AMBLYOPIAS
(CHRONIC RETROBULBAR NEURITIS)

These include a number of conditions in which optic nerve fibres are damaged by the exogenous poisons such as:
1. *Mild toxic agents*—Tobacco, ethyl alcohol, carbon disulphide, iodoform, etc. They produce central scotoma due to initial effect on papillomacular bundle.
2. *Severe amblyopia*—It is produced by quinine organic arsenic, etc. They produce marked peripheral contraction of the visual field or even blindness.

It is frequently bilateral and has a chronic course with permanent visual deterioration. These can be divided broadly into two groups mild and severe. The following toxic agents can be involved:
1. Tobacco
2. Ethyl alcohol
3. Methyl alcohol
4. Lead
5. Quinine
6. Chloroquine
7. Ethambutol
8. Oral contraceptives.

1. TOBACCO AMBLYOPIA

Etiology
It is caused by excessive use of tobacco by smoking and chewing. The toxic agent is the 'cyanide' found in tobacco leaves.

Incidence
1. Age—35-50 years age group is prone to get this disease.
2. It is a bilateral condition usually.

Predisposing Factors
1. General debility and malnutrition.
2. Digestive disturbances lead to malabsorption of vitamins.
3. Deficiency of vitamin B_{12} in dietary sources.
4. Associated alcoholism leads to deficient intake of vitamins and liver disorders.

Pathogenesis
There is degeneration of the ganglion cells of the retina specially in the macular region.

Symptoms
1. There is increasing fogginess of the vision.
2. Central vision is impaired so that there is difficulty in reading and doing near work.

Signs
1. *Fundus examination*—It is normal or it may show slight temporal pallor of the disc.
2. *Field of vision*—There are characteristic field defects in the central field.
    i. Central-caecal scotoma is present between the fixation point and the blind spot.
    ii. It gradually extends to the fixation point and the central vision is lost.

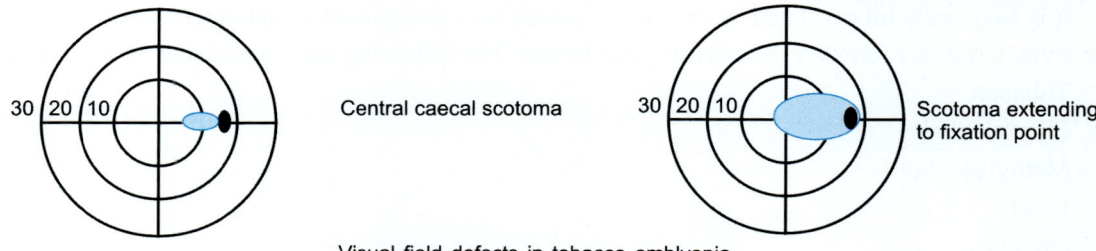

Visual field defects in tobacco amblyopia

Treatment
1. Complete withdrawal from tobacco and alcohol is a must.
2. General nutrition is improved.
3. Injections of vitamin B_1, B_6 and B_{12} are given in high doses. B_{12} injection 1000 mg are given intramuscularly biweekly × 3 weeks.

Prognosis
It is good if it is treated early and adequately.

2. ETHYL ALCOHOL

It usually occurs along with the tobacco amblyopia. However, it may occur alone.
    There is avitaminosis due to malnourishment and hepatic disorders.
    Alcoholic peripheral neuritis is often associated with ocular lesion.
    Symptoms, signs and treatment are same as for tobacco amblyopia.

3. METHYL ALCOHOL

Etiology
- It is caused by the intake of wood alcohol or methylated spirit.
- The toxic agent is the *formaldehyde* found in methyl alcohol.

Incidence
1. It usually occurs during prohibition.
2. It involves several persons at a time consuming the wood alcohol from the same source.

Pathology
There is degeneration of the ganglion cells of the retina.

Symptoms
1. *Acute form*—It causes nausea, headache, giddiness, coma and blindness.
2. *Chronic form*—The symptoms of acute form relapse with progressive loss of vision.

Signs
Fundus examination
1. The disc margin is blurred.

2. The blood vessels are markedly reduced in size.
3. Primary optic atrophy sets in the final stage.

Complications
Blindness and death occur due to acidosis occur eventually.

Treatment
1. *Immediate gastric lavage* is given to wash away the methy alcohol.
2. *Administration of alkali*—Soda bicarbonate is given by 5% intravenous drip or orally as there is acidosis.
3. *Ethyl alcohol* is given in small frequent doses, i.e. 90 cc every 3 hours × 3 days. It prevents acidosis and ocular symptoms.

Mode of action
1. Ethyl alcohol prevents oxidation of methanol to formaldehyde.
2. It competes with methanol for the same enzyme, i.e. alcohol dehydrogenase.

4. LEAD

It is rare nowadays as it is not being used in the pottery industry. The clinical features include those of optic neuritis, optic atrophy and retinopathy.

5. QUININE

It differs from tobacco amblyopia as it may cause total blindness with small dose of even 60 mg of quinine in susceptible cases.

Signs
1. The pupils are dilated and fixed.
2. Deafness and tinnitus may be associated.
3. Fundus examination shows pale and atrophic disc with contracted retinal vessels and oedema.
4. Visual fields are contracted causing tubular vision.

6. CHLOROQUINE

This is an antimalarial drug used in the treatment of lupus erythematosus and arthritis. The prolonged use of chloroquine may cause keratopathy, myopathy and retinopathy.

Fundus examination
1. A mild pigmentary disturbance leads to the characteristic "bullseye" lesion in the macular area.
2. There is widespread retinal atrophy with clumps of pigment and attenuated retinal vessels seen in the later stage.

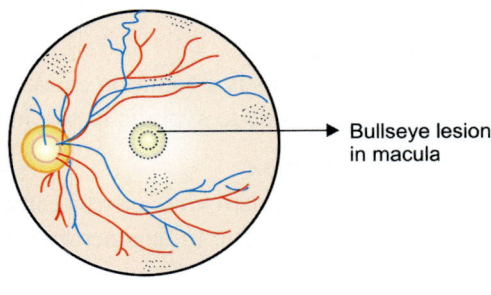

Chloroquine amblyopia

7. ETHAMBUTOL

Ethambutol is used in the treatment of tuberculosis. It may produce optic neuritis. The neuritis is reversible when the drug is stopped. The upper limit of safety dose is 15 mg/kg.

8. ORAL CONTRACEPTIVES

These are combination of progesterone and oestrogen. There is increased risk of vascular occlusion particularly in women who are suffering from hypertension, migraine or other vascular diseases. There may be infraction of optic nerve head.

OPTIC ATROPHY

It is an atrophic condition of the optic disc whereby the optic nerve is degenerated. A diagnosis of optic atrophy depends on:
  i. Pallor of the optic disc
  ii. Loss of visual acuity
  iii. Defect in visual field

Types
1. *Primary optic atrophy*
2. *Secondary optic atrophy*
3. *Consecutive optic atrophy*
4. *Postneuritic optic atrophy*
5. *Ischaemic optic atrophy*
6. *Toxic optic atrophy*
7. *Glaucomatous optic atrophy.*

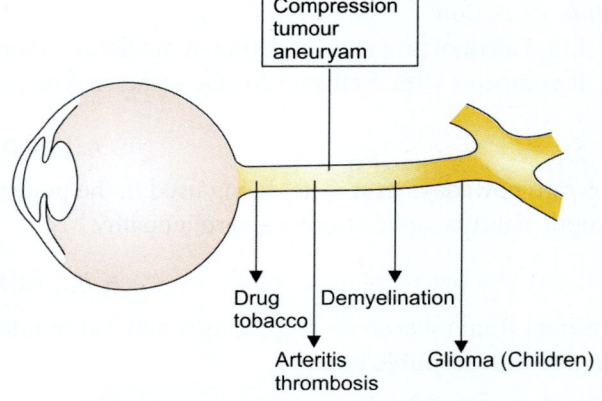

Common causes of optic atrophy

Pathogenesis
There is destruction of nerve fibres along with overgrowth of glial connective tissue.

1. Primary (Simple) Optic Atrophy
The lesion is proximal to the disc so there are no signs of local inflammation. It is associated with general disease usually of central nervous system.

Etiology
1. Multiple sclerosis is a common cause.
2. Tabes dorsalis due to syphilis is rare in recent times.

Fundus examination
1. Optic disc is greyish-white or white in colour with clear margin. There is shallow, saucer-shaped atrophic cupping due to degeneration of nerve fibres. The stippling of lamina cribrosa may be seen.
2. Retinal vessels and retina are normal.

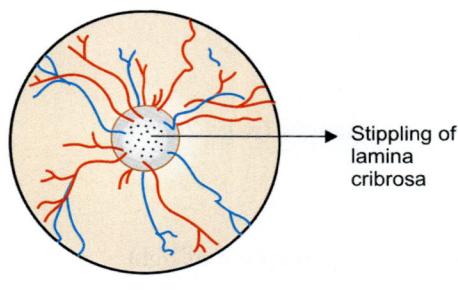
Primary optic atrophy

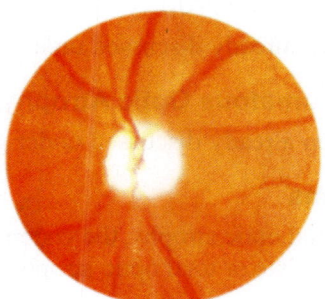
Primary optic atrophy

2. Secondary Optic Atrophy
Etiology
It follows any injury or direct pressure to the optic nerve from lamina cribrosa to the lateral geniculate body.

Fundus examination—It is same as for primary optic atrophy.

3. Consecutive Optic Atrophy
Etiology
Extensive retinal diseases cause ganglion cell destruction as occurs in retinitis pigmentosa and occlusion of central retinal artery.

Fundus examination
1. Disc is yellowish waxy in colour with less sharply defined margin.
2. Vessels are very much attenuated.

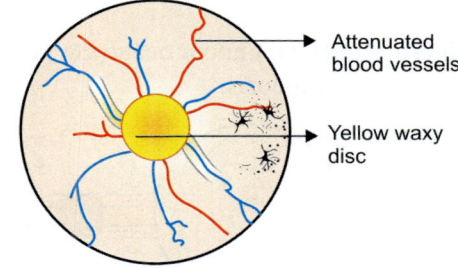
Consecutive optic atrophy

4. Postneuritic Optic Atrophy
Etiology
It follows after papilloedema and papillitis.

Fundus examination
1. Disc is pale along with blurred margin. The physiological cup is full.
2. Vascular sheathing is usually present.
3. Macular stippling may be seen.

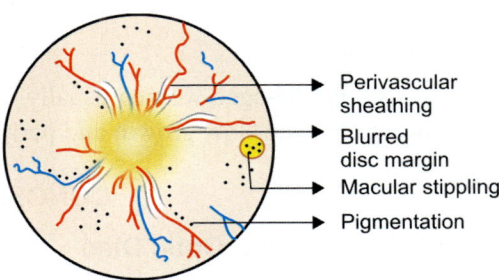
Postneuritic optic atrophy

5. Ischaemic Optic Atrophy
Etiology
It is due to the central retinal artery occlusion.

Fundus examination—Disc and macular area are pale. Retinal vessels are obliterated.

6. Toxic Optic Atrophy
It has been already discussed under toxic amblyopias (page 350).

7. Glaucomatous Optic Atrophy
It has been already discussed under glaucomatous optic disc changes (page 267).

Symptoms
1. In partial optic atrophy, the vision is markedly impaired.
2. In complete or total optic atrophy, the person is blind with no perception of light.

Signs
Pupil is dilated and fixed, i.e. not reacting to light.
Visual field shows concentric contraction with depression of central vision in initial stages with or without scotomata.

Treatment
- Treat the underlying cause in cases of partial optic atrophy.
- No treatment is effective once complete optic atrophy has set in.

TUMOURS

Glioma
It is a congenital tumour occurring in the age group of 2-5 years. It is slow growing and self-limiting with good prognosis.

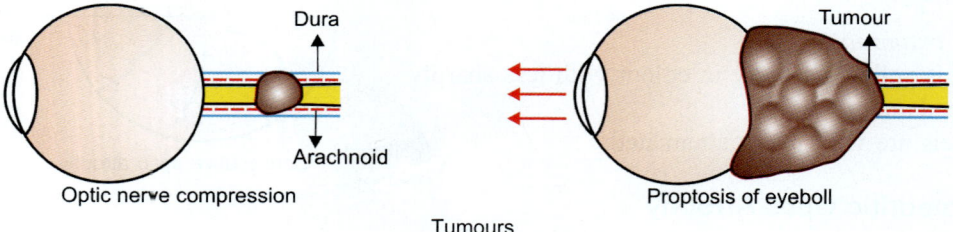

Tumours

Meningioma
It occurs in middle-aged women usually. There is early visual loss and proptosis. The prognosis is good because of the slow growth and peripheral situation of the tumour.

CONGENITAL ANOMALIES

1. Coloboma of the Optic Disc
Colobomas are bilateral in more than half the cases. It occurs in two forms:
i. *Inferior crescent*
   - This is a common form occurring due to incomplete closure of the embryonic fissure.
   - It occurs in hypermetropic and astigmatic eyes.
   - It may be ectatic.

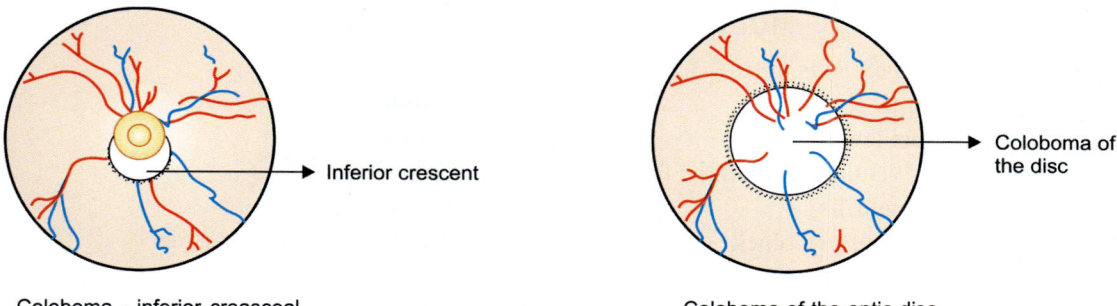

Coloboma - inferior creasceal   Coloboma of the optic disc

ii. *Coloboma of the disc*—There is a greater failure of the embryonic fissure to close. The apparent large disc is really the sclera. The vision is defective usually.

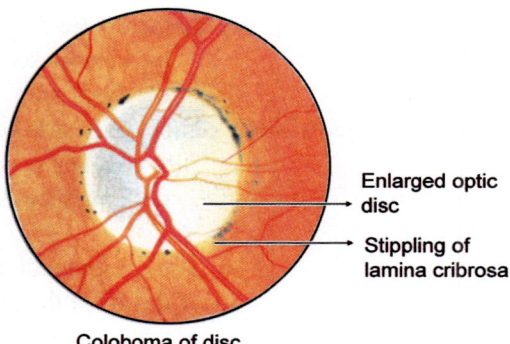

Coloboma of disc

2. Medullated (Opaque) Nerve Fibres

Normally the myelin sheaths of optic nerve stop at the lamina cribrosa. Occasionally patches of nerve fibres regain these sheaths after they have passed through the lamina cribrosa.

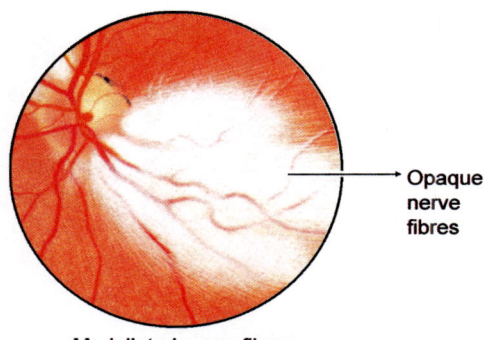

Medullated nerve fibres

They appear as white glistening patches with radially striated edges. They are continuous with the optic disc.

MULTIPLE CHOICE QUESTIONS

1. The optic nerve extends upto
   a. optic chiasma
   b. optic tract
   c. lateral geniculate body
   d. optic radiation
2. Sudden loss of vision occurs in the following *EXCEPT*
   a. retrobulbar neuritis
   b. papilloedema
   c. central retinal artery block
   d. central retinal vein occlusion
3. The characteristic sign of retrobulbar neuritis is
   a. hyperaemia of the optic disc
   b. ill-sustained pupillary reaction
   c. ciliary congestion
   d. optic atrophy
4. Consecutive optic atrophy is secondary to
   a. papilloedema
   b. papillitis
   c. diseases of retina and choroid
   d. glaucoma
5. In anterior ischaemic optic neuropathy, the characteristic defect is
   a. altitudinal field defect
   b. central scotoma
   c. centrocaecal scotoma
   d. nasal step
6. Unilateral papilloedema with optic atrophy on the other side comprises
   a. Devic's syndrome
   b. Weber's syndrome
   c. Foster-Kennedy syndrome
   d. Laurence-Moon-Biedl syndrome
7. Vision is grossly reduced in
   a. papillitis
   b. papilloedema
   c. pseudopapillitis
   d. all of the above
8. Characteristic "bullseye" occur due to
   a. ethambutol
   b. oral contraceptive
   c. lead poisoning
   d. chloroquine
9. Toxic amblyopia is most commonly produced by
   a. INH
   b. rifampicin
   c. ethambutol
   d. pyrazinamide
10. Enlargement of the blind spot occurs in
    a. papilloedema
    b. papillitis
    c. retrobulbar neuritis
    d. glaucoma
11. Blurring of the disc margin is seen typically in
    a. pseudoneuritis
    b. papillitis
    c. malignant hypertension
    d. all of the above
12. The normal cup: disc ratio is
    a. 1:2
    b. 1:3
    c. 1:4
    d. 2:4
13. Anterior ischaemic optic atrophy occurs due to
    a. neglected closed angle glaucoma
    b. severe anaemia
    c. temporal arteritis
    d. all of the above

14. The most common cause of papillitis is
    a. herpes zoster
    b. multiple sclerosis
    c. uveitis
    d. diabetes mellitus
15. The treatment of retrobulbar neuritis includes all *EXCEPT*
    a. retrobulbar injection of dexamethasone
    b. antibiotics
    c. vitamin B_1, B_6 and B_{12}
    d. vasodilators
16. The toxic agent in methyl alcohol poisoning is
    a. formaldehyde
    b. cyanide
    c. ethanol
    d. none of the above
17. The immediate treatment of methyl alcohol poisoning includes
    a. ethyl alcohol
    b. vitamin B_1, B_6, B_{12}
    c. antibiotics
    d. vasodilators
18. Yellowish waxy disc is seen typically in
    a. retinal detachment
    b. retinitis pigmentosa
    c. primary optic atrophy
    d. postneuritic optic atrophy
19. Marcus Gunn pupil is diagnostic of
    a. retrobulbar neuritis
    b. papillitis
    c. toxic amblyopias
    d. papilloedema
20. Postneuritic optic atrophy usually follows
    a. papilloedema
    b. papillitis
    c. both
    d. none
21. Gliomas of the optic nerve
    a. occurs in 2-5 years age group
    b. congenital
    c. self-limiting with good prognosis
    d. all of the above
22. Secondary optic atrophy occurs
    a. following injury or direct pressure to the optic nerve
    b. following extensive retinal disease
    c. following papilloedema and papillitis
    d. following central retinal artery occlusion
23. Differential diagnosis of retrobulbar neuritis includes
    a. hysteria
    b. malingering
    c. both
    d. none
24. Papilloedema can be differentiated from papillitis by the following features
    a. gradual onset with slow progress
    b. bilateral
    c. other signs of central nervous system involvement
    d. all of the above
25. The common causes of papilloedema include
    a. intracranial tumour
    b. grade 4 hypertensive retinopathy
    c. subdural haematoma
    d. all of the above

26. All are true of papilloedema EXCEPT
    a. vascular engorgement
    b. disc oedema
    c. Transient blurring of vision
    d. sudden painless loss of vision
27. Enlargement of blind spot is a sign of
    a. avulsion of optic nerve
    b. papillitis
    c. papilloedema
    d. retinal detachment
28. Treatment of methyl alcohol poisoing includes
    a. ethyl alcohol
    b. gastric lavage
    c. alkali administration
    d. all of the above
29. Consecutive optic atrophy occurs following
    a. retinitis pigmentosa
    b. central retinal artery occlusion
    c. both
    d. none
30. Anterior ischaemic optic neuropathy (AION) results due to
    a. severe anaemia
    b. temporal arteritis
    c. acute congestive glaucoma
    d. all of the above

ANSWERS

1—a	2—b	3—b	4—c	5—a
6—c	7—a	8—d	9—c	10—a
11—d	12—b	13—d	14—b	15—b
16—a	17—a	18—b	19—a	20—c
21—d	22—a	23—c	24—d	25—d
26—d	27—c	28—d	29—c	30—d

CHAPTER 15
Injuries to the Eye

The eyeball is well-protected by the bony orbit, the nose, the lids, eyebrows, eyelashes and a good cushion of fat behind the eyeball. The incidence of injury to the eye is high specially in the industrial towns. The common causes of injury in the children include playing with bow and arrow, throwing stones, ball, sharp pointed objects like pen, pencil, stick, etc. Chemical injuries are common in the laboratory and industry. Protective goggles are available for industrial workers.

An eye injury is an emergency and requires immediate medical or surgical treatment.

TYPES OF INJURY
1. *Extraocular foreign body*
2. *Chemical injuries and burns*
3. *Blunt injury (contusions)*
4. *Penetrating and perforating injury*
5. *Perforating injury with retained foreign body.*

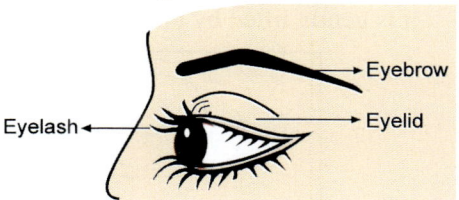

Side view of structures which protect the eye

EXTRAOCULAR FOREIGN BODY

Etiology
It is usually a small particle of coal, dust, emery (hard stone), steel and glass. At times wings of insect and husk of seeds may also involve the limbus.

Symptoms
1. There is sudden discomfort in the eye.
2. Reflex blinking due to foreign body sensation is very troublesome.
3. There is great irritation and gritty feeling if the foreign body is embedded in the cornea.
4. Lacrimation and photophobia are present in cases of corneal involvement.

Signs
1. There is marked reflex blepharospasm.
2. Foreign body is visible on the bulbar conjunctiva, limbus, cornea, sulcus subtarsalis and fornix by the naked eye, oblique illumination with a loupe or slit-lamp examination.
3. It may be single or multiple, superficial or deep.

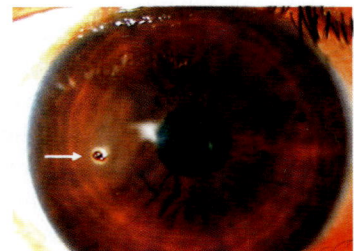

Superficial foreign body

Complications
1. Conjunctivitis may occur due to secondary bacterial infection.
2. Corneal ulcer may be present as a result of corneal erosion due to foreign body.

3. Brown ring or stain is left on the cornea by an embedded steel particle or emery.
4. Foreign body like sharp steel may penetrate into the anterior chamber.

Treatment

1. Do not rub the eyes—It is very important as the foreign body may penetrate in the deeper tissues.
2. Wash the eye with plenty of clean water.
3. If in the conjunctiva, it is picked up by a needle after application of local anaesthetic.

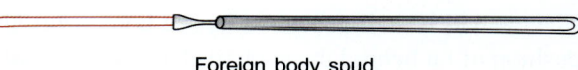

Foreign body spud

4. Foreign body spud—If in the cornea, it is gently scraped off with the foreign body spud with its blunt end.
5. Sharp needle (sterilized)—If the foreign body has penetrated in the superficial layers of cornea, it is gently lifted by the sideways motion or by liver action of a sharp needle.

Removal of superficial foreign body with needle

Prophylaxis

1. The tools with overhanging edges are banned.
2. Guards are put on machines used for grinding.
3. Protective goggles is a must for industrial workers.
4. Educative means are used such as "safety first" notices and lectures by the welfare officials in the factories.

CHEMICAL INJURIES AND BURNS

Etiology

1. The burn injury can be caused by hot water, steam, hot ashes, explosive powder, molten metals, etc. The chemical injury may be due to lime, acid, and alkali.
   - Alkali burns—The common alkalies responsible for causing injury are lime, caustic potash or caustic soda and liquid ammonia. These can cause considerable damage to the eye because they tend to penetrate deeper. They cause necrosis of the surface epithelium in a few seconds with occlusion of the limbal vasculature. This leads to a diminished vascularity of the anterior segment, corneal opacification and melting, cataract and symblepharon.
   - Acid burns—The common acids responsible are sulphuric acid, hydrochloric acid and nitric acid. These are less serious than alkalis burns because they coagulate the surface proteins and do not penetrate the eye.
2. Poison gases—Lacrimatory gases, phosgene, mustard, gas, arsenicals and other agents are used in war.

3. In *holi* festival (festival of colours), there is great danger of chemical injury to the eyes due to the presence of 'mica' in various coloured powders.

Symptoms
1. There is red eye with marked swelling of lids and conjunctiva.
2. Marked reflex blepharospasm is present usually.
3. Photophobia and lacrimation are present when there is corneal involvement.

Chemical burn – acid

Signs
1. There is severe congestion and chemosis of conjunctiva.
2. Marks of burn over surrounding skin are noticed.
3. Cornea is dull and opaque or may get sloughed off.
4. Fluorescein staining—It is positive and it demarcates the denuded epithelium.

Grading of Chemical Injuries
Grade I—Clear cornea and no limbal ischaemia.
Grade II—Hazy cornea but with visible iris details and less than one-third (120°) of limbal ischaemia.
Grade III—Total loss of corneal epithelium, stromal haze obscuring iris details and between one-third and half (120° to 180°) of limbal ischaemia.
Grade IV—Opaque cornea and more than half (> 180°) of limbal ischaemia

Complication
1. *Symblepharon*, i.e. adhesion of the lid to the globe due to conjunctival ulceration is a common complication. A glass rod well-coated with a lubricant or ointment is swept around the upper and lower fornix several times a day to break and prevent the formation of adhesions.
2. *Corneal ulcer* is usually present which may easily perforate.

Treatment
1. Immediately wash the eye thoroughly with plenty of clean water. Acid should be neutralized with dilute alkalies, e.g. soda bicarbonate solution. Alkalies can be neutralized with weak acids, e.g. boric acid or milk. Lime particles are picked up with a forceps and 1% EDTA (ethylene-diamine-tetra-acetic acid) is applied as a neutralizing agent.
2. If there is corneal erosion, treat it like a corneal ulcer.
3. If cornea is not involved, steroid drops and ointments should be used to prevent symblepharon formation and to reduce congestion and chemosis of the conjunctiva.
4. Conjunctivitis caused by lacrimatory gases is treated by irrigation with bland lotion, normal saline, 3% soda bicarbonate or clean water. Dark glasses are comforting.

BLUNT INJURY [CONTUSIONS]
Trauma by a blunt object like fist, ball, etc. can cause an injury from simple abrasion to the rupture of the globe.

MECHANICAL INJURY OF THE EYE

Closed globe injury	Open globe injury
Injury without full-thickness defect of the coats	Injury with full-thickness defects in the corneoscleral coat

1. Contusion—There is injury due to blunt trauma
2. Lamellar laceration—There is partial thickness wound of the coats due to a sharp object or blunt trauma
	1. Rupture—There is full-thickness wound of the eyeball due to blunt trauma
	2. Laceration—There is full-thickness outside to inside break in the ocular coats. It includes:
	  a. Penetrating injury—The object traverses the coats only once
	  b. Perforating injury—Both an entry and exit wound are present (earlier known as double perforation)

The ocular trauma classification group has proposed a new classification system for mechanical injuries to the eye.

1. Cornea
  i. *Simple or recurrent abrasions* of the cornea.
  ii. *Deep corneal opacity* is due to the oedema of corneal stroma and folds in the Descemet's membrane.
  iii. *Blood staining* of the cornea is due to associated haemorrhage into the anterior chamber with raised tension.
  iv. Partial or complete tear of the cornea.

2. Sclera
  i. *Rupture of the globe* may occur with prolapse of uveal tissue.
  ii. *This may lead to subconjunctival dislocation, expulsion or dislocation of lens in vitreous cavity.*
  iii. *Intraocular haemorrhage.*

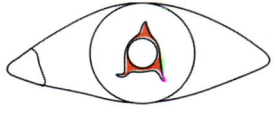
Radial laceration
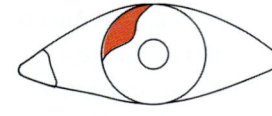
Anterior dialysis
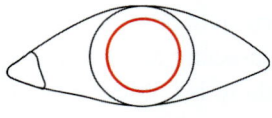
Aniridia

3. Iris and Ciliary Body
  i. *Traumatic miosis*—There is constriction of the pupil following trauma.
  ii. *Traumatic mydriasis*—There may be dilatation of pupil after trauma.
  iii. *Radiating lacerations* of iris may occur occasionally.
  iv. *Iridodialysis*—Iris is torn away from its ciliary attachment.
  v. *Antiflexion of iris*—In extensive iridodialysis, the pigmented portion of iris faces forwards.

vi. *Retroflexion of iris*—The whole iris is doubled back into the ciliary region (total inversion). Iris is invisible in this condition.
vii. *Aniridia or irideremia*—The iris is completely torn away from the ciliary attachment. It contracts and forms a minute ball which sinks to the bottom of the anterior chamber.
viii. *Cyclodialysis*—Ciliary body is ruptured near its anterior attachment and it may retract.
ix. *Hyphaema*, i.e. blood in the anterior chamber may be present.

4. Lens

i. *Vossius's ring*—Circular ring of stippled brown amorphous granules is seen on the anterior surface of the lens.
ii. *Traumatic cataract or concussion cataract*—Typical rosette-shaped cataract may form early or late, i.e. after 1-2 years in the posterior cortex usually. An accumulation of fluid marks out the star-shaped cortical sutures and lens fibres.

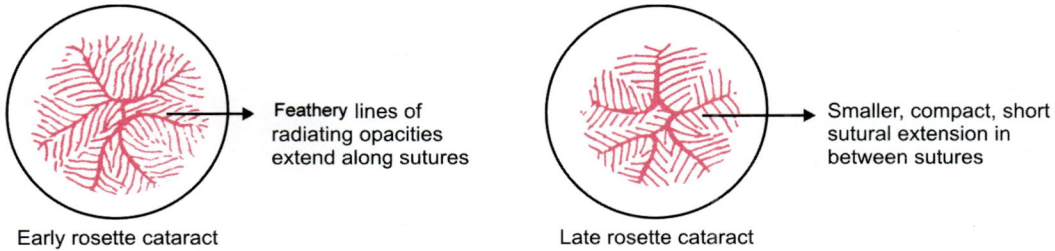

iii. *There may be dislocation* of the lens in the vitreous or anterior chamber.
iv. *Subluxation* of the lens may occur due to the partial rupture of zonule.

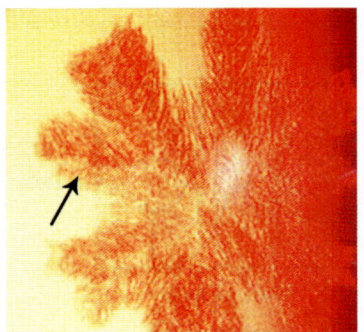

Traumatic Rosette cataract

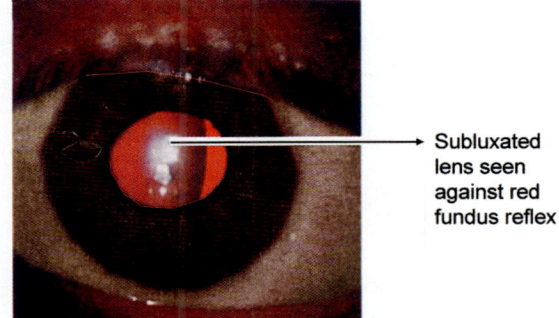

Subluxated lens following blunt injury

v. *There may be tear of the lens capsule* with absorption of the lens matter.
vi. Total lens opacification may occur.

5. Vitreous

i. *Clouds of fine pigmentary opacities* may be present in fluid vitreous.
ii. *Intravitreal haemorrhage* may occur occasionally.

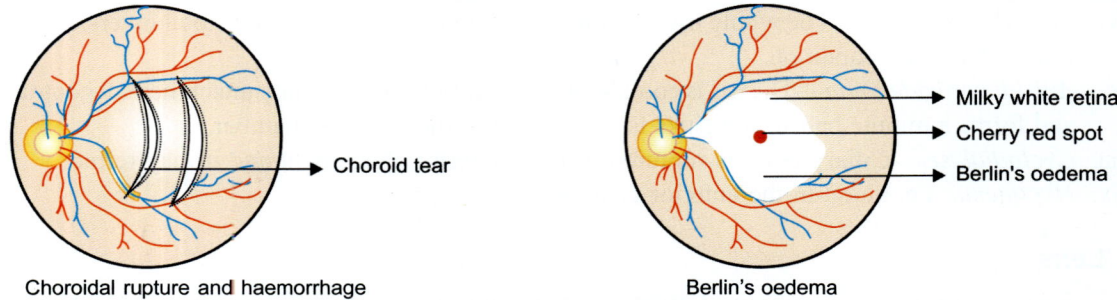

Choroidal rupture and haemorrhage   Berlin's oedema

   iii. *Vitreous herniation* in the anterior chamber causes secondary glaucoma.
   iv. *Vitreous loss* may occur in cases of globe rupture.

6. Choroid

   i. *Choroid rupture* may be single or multiple. It is situated on the temporal side usually. It is crescent-shaped and is concentric with the optic disc margin. The white coloured sclera shines through along with pigmentation at the edges.
   ii. *Choroidal haemorrhage* may be small or large.
   iii. *Choroidal detachment* may be present.

7. Retina

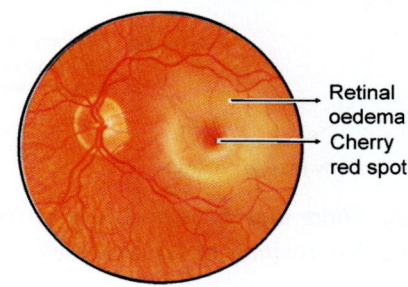

Commotio retinae (Berlin's oedema)

   i. *Macular oedema (Berlin's oedema or commotio-retinae)*—There is milky white cloudiness at the posterior pole with cherry red spot in the centre. It disappears after few days or may be followed by pigmentary deposits.

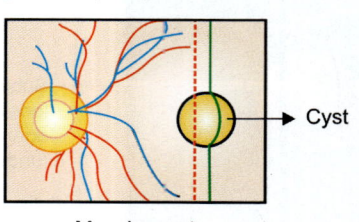

Macular cyst

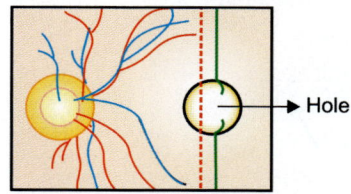

Macular hole

   ii. *Macular degeneration*—It may lead to macular cyst and hole formation.
   iii. *Retinal tear* may occur resulting in retinal detachment.
   iv. *Proliferative retinopathy* usually occurs following large haemorrhage in the vitreous. There is dense proliferation of fibrovascular tissue forming traction bands.

8. Optic Nerve

   i. *Optic atrophy* may occur due to injury to the optic nerve.
   ii. *Avulsion of optic nerve* can occur due to complete section of the nerve.

EFFECTS OF BLUNT INJURY ON LENS, IRIS, CILIARY BODY, CHOROID AND RETINA

LENS	IRIS	CILIARY BODY	CHOROID	RETINA
• Vossius ring • Traumatic cataract • Subluxation • Dislocation	• Miosis • Mydriasis • Hyphaema • Tear • Iridodialysis • Antiflexion • Retroflexion • Aniridia	• Spasm of accommodation • Cyclodialysis	• Rupture • Haemorrhage • Detachment	• Macular oedema • Macular degeneration • Tear • Detachment • Proliferative retinopathy (vitreous haemorrhage)

PENETRATING AND PERFORATING INJURY

Penetrating injury—There is single full-thickness break or wound of the eyeball caused by a sharp object such as knife, needle, iron particle, small stone, glass, etc.

Perforating injury—There is dual or double full-thickness break or wound (entrance and exit wounds) in the eyeball caused by sharp objects.

A perforating injury is likely to cause severe and serious damage to the eye due to the immediate trauma and the infection. It is an ocular emergency.

Laceration—There is outside - in injury of eyeball.

Rupture—There is inside - out injury of eyeball.

Signs of Perforation of the Eyeball

Any one or combination of the following suggest global perforation:
1. Decreased visual acuity
2. Marked hypotony or low IOP
3. Shallow anterior chamber or hyphaema
4. Alteration in pupil size, shape and location
5. Marked conjunctival oedema (chemosis)
6. Subconjunctival haemorrhage
7. Hole in the iris as confirmed by transillumination
8. Wound track in the corneal, lens or vitreous

Common sites for retention of an intraocular foreign body

Aim of Treatment

The main aim of the treatment is:
  i. To save the vision
  ii. To prevent the occurrence of the sympathetic ophthalmitis.

Principles of Treatment

It should be treated immediately by:
1. Proper suturing and apposition of the ocular tissues is done promptly. It is very important to free the uveal tissue from the corneal or corneoscleral wound.
2. Control and prevention of infection by suitable broad-spectrum antibiotics.
3. Close follow-up with topical antibiotics, atropine and corticosteroids is essential.

PERFORATING INJURY WITH RETAINED FOREIGN BODY

The foreign bodies which are likely to penetrate the eye and are retained include minute chips of iron and steel (90%), stone, glass, lead pellet, wood spicules, etc.

The retained foreign body causes damage to the eye depending on its size and velocity. The particles greater than 2 mm in size usually destroy eye and sight.

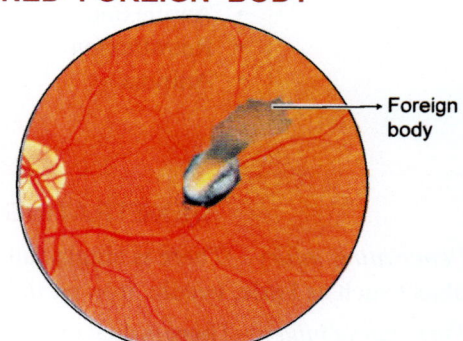

Intraocular metalic foreign body

Effects of Retained Foreign Body

1. *Mechanical effect*—The foreign body pierces cornea or sclera and falls to the bottom of the anterior chamber or is situated in the angle of anterior chamber.
   It may get lodged on the iris or pass into or through the lens into the vitreous. It may finally settle down in the retina. Occasionally, it may pierce the coats of the eye and stay in the orbital tissue which is known as the "double perforation". This results in hypotony.
2. *Infection*—It is introduced along with the foreign body. The small flying metallic particles are usually sterile due to the heat generated partly on their emission.
3. *Specific chemical action of the metals*—It varies with the chemical nature of the metal.
    i. *Inert metals*—Glass, plastic, porcelain, gold, silver, platinum, tantalum, etc.
    ii. *Little reaction with encapsulation*—Lead present in shot gun pellets becomes coated with carbonate.
    iii. *Local suppuration*—Aluminium, nickel, mercury, zinc, etc.
4. *Degenerative changes*—Iron and copper undergo electrolytic dissociation and get deposited throughout the eye. They cause degenerative changes known as siderosis bulbi and chalcosis respectively.

1. Siderosis Bulbi

It is due to the electrolytic dissociation of the iron metal by the 'current of rest' in the eye. Ferrous ion combines with cellular protein causing atrophy of the cells.

$$\text{Ferrous ion + cellular protein} \rightarrow \text{atrophy of the cells.}$$

Iron gets deposited in
   i. *Lens*—The anterior lens capsule wherein oval patches of rusty deposits are arranged radially in a ring. It corresponds with the edge of the dilated pupil. The lens becomes opaque eventually.

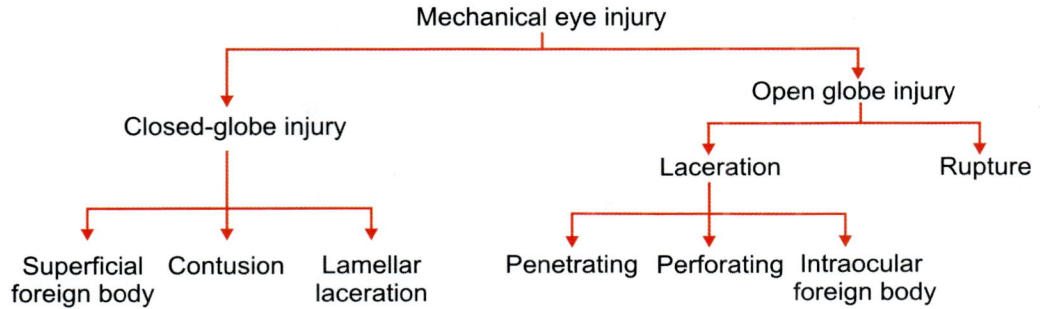

ii. *Iris*—It is stained greenish and later reddish-brown.
iii. *Retina*—Retinal degeneration occurs with the generalised deposition of pigment.
iv. *Secondary glaucoma* of chronic type occurs in late stage.
v. *Blindness* occurs unless the foreign body is removed early.

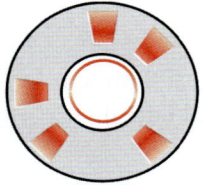

Siderosis bulbi

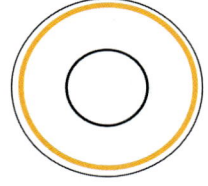

Kayser-Fleischer ring

Sunflower cataract

2. Chalicosis

A foreign body with pure copper content gives rise to a violent suppurative reaction with shrinkage of globe.

The heavily alloyed copper or brass foreign body (as from percussion caps) causes milder reaction called "chalicosis." Copper gets deposited in the cornea, lens and retina.

i. *Kayser-Fleischer ring*—There is deposition of copper in the deeper parts of periphery of cornea in the Descemet's membrane forming a golden brown ring.
ii. *Sunflower cataract*—The deposition of copper is in the form of petals of a flower and is brilliant golden green in colour.
iii. *Retina*—There are golden plaques deposited at the posterior pole which reflect the light with a metallic sheen.

Organic Materials

Wood splinter, other vegetable matter, eyelash or caterpillar hair produce proliferative reaction with formation of gaint cells.

Diagnosis and Localization of Intraocular Foreign Body

It is of extreme importance as the patient is often unaware that a particle has entered the eye. It should be localized upto the accuracy of 1 mm to avoid damage to intraocular structures. The various methods used for localization of an intraocular foreign body are:

1. *Slit-lamp examination and gonioscopy*—Search the wound of entry by loupe and slit-lamp. Gonioscopy is valuable in detecting minute foreign body in the angle. Localize the wound by the track and position of wound of entrance.

2. *Ophthalmoscopic examination*—Fundus examination under complete mydriasis.
3. *Radiographic examination*—The radiopaque foreign bodies are demonstrated by X-ray. Accuracy of localization of the order of 1 mm is essential.
    i. *Mackenzie-Davidson and Bromley method*—Two stereoscopic pictures at two fixed angle are taken with reference to a known opaque marker.
    ii. *Comberg method*—It relates the position of the foreign body to the leaded markings on a contact lens.

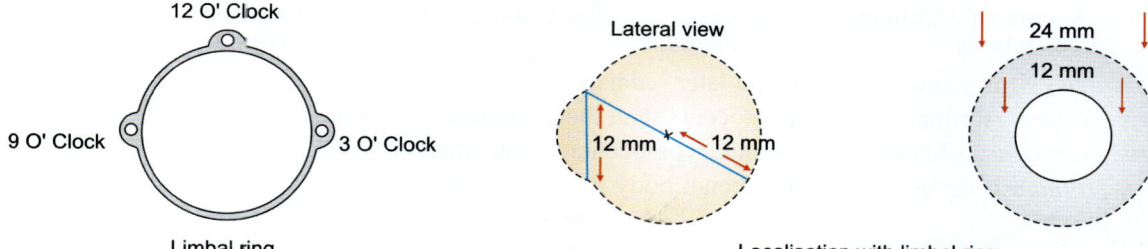

    iii. *Limbal ring method*—A thin metal ring (silver) is stitched to the conjunctiva at limbus at 3, 9 and 12 O'clock positions. Two exposures are essential—posteroanterior and lateral.
    iv. *Bone-free method*—Care is taken to avoid bone shadows.
4. **Electroacoustic location**—Any alteration in the secondary current produced by a metallic particle is noted by electroacoustic locators.
5. **Ultrasonography**—A scan localizes the foreign body in line with a probe. It is capable of localizing the foreign body with great accuracy.

Treatment

The composition of foreign body and its magnetic strength determine the type of treatment. Foreign body should be removed unless,
   i. It is inert and sterile.
   ii. Little damage has been done to vision.
   iii. The process of removal will invariably destroy sight.

Siderosis bulbi - rusty deposit on iris and lens

Methods of Removal

1. **Magnetic foreign body**—The magnetizable intraocular foreign body are more easily removed. Magnetic removal is recommended as early as possible by:
    a. **Hand magnet**—It is used when the distance from the particle is less than 2 mm.
    b. **Electromagnet**—It is used when the distance from the particle is more than 2 mm.
        i. *In the anterior chamber*—A small incision is given just inside the limbus. The positive pole of the hand magnet is placed over the foreign body (on outer surface of the cornea). It is moved towards the incision till the foreign body is drawn across the anterior chamber and removed.
        ii. *On the iris*—The part of the iris containing the foreign body must be abscissed with De Wecker's scissors.
        iii. *In the lens*—In case of cataract formation, discission and irrigation is done.

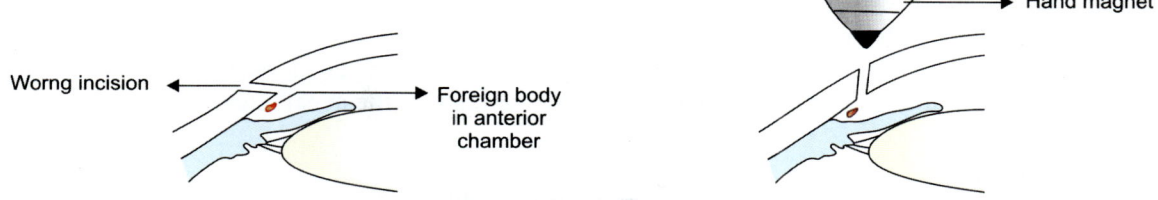

Removal of magnetic foreign body in the anterior chamber

   iv. *In the vitreous or retina*—A large or giant electromagnet is required for its removal. There are two routes of removal—anterior and posterior. Posterior route is preferred if the foreign body is large with irregular sharp edges as it causes less ocular damage.
      a. *Anterior route removal*—At first, the giant magnet drags the particle from the vitreous or retina into the posterior chamber. Then it passes through the pupil into the anterior chamber from where it is removed by hand magnet.

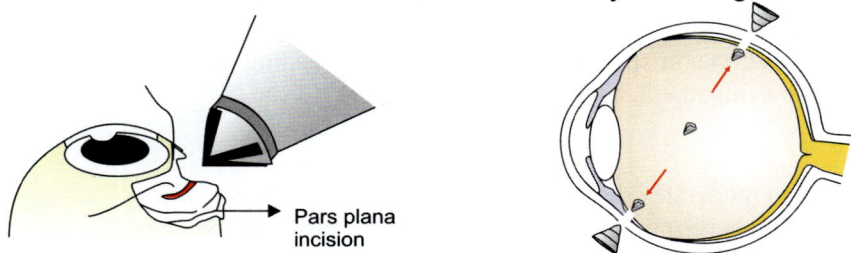

Removal of magnetic foreign body in the posterior chamber

      b. *Posterior route removal*—The ocular tension is lowered by IV mannitol or acetazolamide. The sclera is incised (concentric with limbus) as close to the foreign body as possible. After removing the particle cryoprobe is applied to the edges of wound to prevent retinal detachment.
2. **Non-magnetic foreign body**—The extraction of non-magnetic foreign body from the anterior segment of eye is easy in comparison to the posterior segment. If it is in the retina or vitreous it can be removed by special forceps through the pars plana incision under microscopic control.

SYMPATHETIC OPHTHALMITIS

It is a condition in which the normal eye gets seriously inflamed after injury to the other eye. It is rare in recent years due to better and early care of the injured eye and the use of corticosteroids and modern broad-spectrum antibiotics.

Etiology

- It always occurs after perforating wound specially when the ciliary body is involved and there is retention of the foreign body. Children are more susceptible.
- Wounds with incarceration of iris, ciliary body or lens capsule are dangerous.

Removal of non-magnetic foreign body in the posterior chamber

- It usually starts 4-8 weeks after injury to the first eye. The earliest reported case is after 9 days. It may be delayed for many months or years.
- It does not occur if the wound is sterile or actual suppuration has taken place.
- It is most probably due to allergic hypersensitivity reaction of the uveal tract.

Pathology

In the injured (exciting) eye—It is always plastic iridocyclitis.
In the normal (sympathizing) eye—It is also plastic iridocyclitis.

There is nodular aggregation of lymphocytes and plasma cells scattered throughout the uveal tract.

Dalen-Fuchs nodules are formed due to proliferation of pigment epithelium of iris and ciliary body with tissue invasion by lymphocytes and epithelioid cells.

Symptoms

1. Photophobia and lacrimation are the early presenting complaints.
2. There is impaired vision specially for near work or reading due to the involvement of ciliary muscles due to sympathetic irritation.

Signs

1. There is mild to moderate ciliary congestion and the eyeball is tender.
2. Keratic precipitates (kp) are present on the back of cornea (First sign).
3. Vitreous opacities are present usually.
4. Optic disc oedema may be seen occasionally.

Treatment

1. *Prophylactic*
    i. Early use of corticosteroids and modern antibiotics is of utmost importance.
    ii. Repair of the wound is done so as to free any incarcerations of uveal tissue or lens capsule.
    iii. Evisceration or Frill excision—Excision of the injured eye is done if there is no chance of saving useful vision.
2. *Curative*
    Treat it like a case of iridocyclitis with generous use of corticosteroids by all routes.
3. *Operative*
    In cases which have run their course and suffered severe organic damage and the eye has been quiet for many months.
    i. In milder case, optical iridectomy may be done.
    ii. In worst cases with perception of light and good projection of rays, lens may be extracted when the other eye is blind or has been removed.

Prognosis

- It is good if steroid therapy is commenced early.
- It is usually bad if the uvea is heavily infiltrated and inflammation has taken firm hold.

MULTIPLE CHOICE QUESTIONS

1. The most serious danger to vision is
   a. a blow to the eyeball
   b. fracture through optic foramen
   c. monocular proptosis
   d. Horner's syndrome
2. Most important complication of traumatic hyphaema is
   a. iridocyclitis
   b. iridodialysis
   c. blood staining of cornea
   d. siderosis bulbi
3. Enucleation is indicated in all *EXCEPT*
   a. retinoblastoma
   b. panophthalmitis
   c. ciliary staphyloma
   d. perforating injury of eye with no PL
4. Multitudes of brown amorphous granules of pigment lying on the anterior capsule of lens (Vossius's ring) is seen in
   a. iridocyclitis
   b. hyphaema
   c. closed angle glaucoma
   d. blunt trauma to the eye
5. The dreaded complication of penetrating eye injury is
   a. subluxation of lens
   b. ocular haemorrhage
   c. sympathetic ophthalmitis
   d. iridocyclitis
6. Lenticular rosette cataract formation is usually associated with
   a. concussion cataract
   b. complicated cataract
   c. diabetic cataract
   d. congenital cataract
7. 'Sunflower' cataract is characteristic of
   a. argyrosis
   b. siderosis
   c. chalcosis
   d. none of the above
8. Ophthalmia nodosa is seen in
   a. leprosy
   b. syphilis
   c. caterpillar hair in the eye
   d. granulomatous uveitis
9. A 16-year-old male comes with injury to the eye by a tennis ball, the following can be seen *EXCEPT*
   a. hypopyon
   b. hyphaema
   c. subluxation of lens
   d. subconjunctival haemorrhage
10. Intraocular foreign body with the most fulminant inflammation would be of
    a. copper
    b. iron
    c. lead
    d. aluminium
11. 'D'-shaped pupil is seen in
    a. iridocyclitis
    b. iridodialysis
    c. glaucoma
    d. dislocation of lens
12. Dalen-Fuch's nodules are seen in:
    a. sympathetic ophthalmitis
    b. phthisis bulbi
    c. absolute glaucoma
    d. pseudoxanthoma elasticum

13. Kayser-Fleischer ring is found in which layer of cornea.
    a. Bowman's membrane
    b. Descemet's membrane
    c. stroma
    d. endothelium
14. Following are inert foreign bodies in eye *EXCEPT*
    a. gold
    b. silver
    c. copper
    d. platinum
15. Berlin's oedema results due to
    a. syphilis
    b. toxocara
    c. cavernous sinus thrombosis
    d. trauma to eye

ANSWERS

1—b	2—c	3—a	4—d	5—c
6—a	7—c	8—c	9—a	10—d
11—b	12—a	13—b	14—c	15—d

CHAPTER 16
The Ocular Motility and Squint (Strabismus)

THE OCULAR MOTILITY

EXTRAOCULAR MUSCLES

There are six extraocular muscles in each eye which control their movements.

I. The Recti Muscles

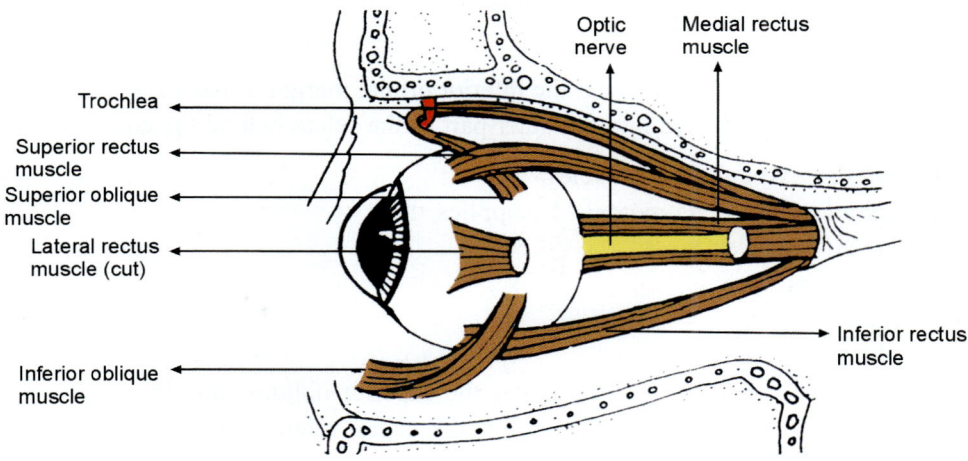

The extrinsic muscles of the eye

The *four recti muscles* originate from the common annular tendon of Zinn situated around the optic foramen at the apex of the orbit.

The recti muscles are inserted into the sclera by flat tendons at various distances from the limbus

1. Superior rectus—7.7 mm
2. Lateral rectus—7 mm
3. Inferior rectus—6.6 mm
4. Medial rectus—5.5 mm.

II. The Oblique Muscles

1. Superior oblique
2. Inferior oblique.

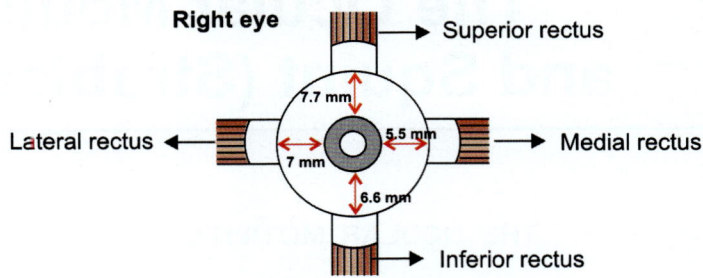

Insertion of recti muscle tendons in sclera

Superior oblique
It arises from the upper and inner margin of the optic foramen. It runs forwards to the upper and inner angle of the orbit. It passes through the trochlea (a fibrous pulley). It gets inserted into the upper and outer part of the sclera behind the equator.

Inferior oblique
It originates from the floor of the orbit near the inferior orbital margin. It passes outwards below the inferior rectus muscle. It is inserted into the outer part of the sclera behind the equator.

Nerve supply of the extraocular muscles
1. *The third cranial nerve (oculomotor)*—It supplies the:
    i. Superior rectus muscle
    ii. Inferior rectus muscle
    iii. Medial rectus muscle
    iv. Inferior oblique muscle.
2. *The 4th cranial nerve (trochlear)*—It supplies the superior oblique muscle.
3. *The 6th cranial nerve (abducens)*—It supplies the lateral rectus muscle.

Blood Supply

The blood supply is by the muscular branches of the ophthalmic artery.

Action of the Extraocular Muscles

These muscles rotate the eye around a 'centre of rotation'. This centre is situated 12-13 mm behind the cornea in a horizontal plane.
   Three types of movements are possible around the centre of rotation.
1. Movements around the vertical axis whereby eye is turned from side to side.
2. Movements around the horizontal axis whereby eye is turned upwards or downwards.
3. Movements around the anteroposterior axis whereby an involuntary movement of 'torsion' occurs.
    a. *Intorsion*—When the upper pole of the cornea rotates nasally.
    b. *Extorsion*—When the upper pole of the cornea rotates temporally.

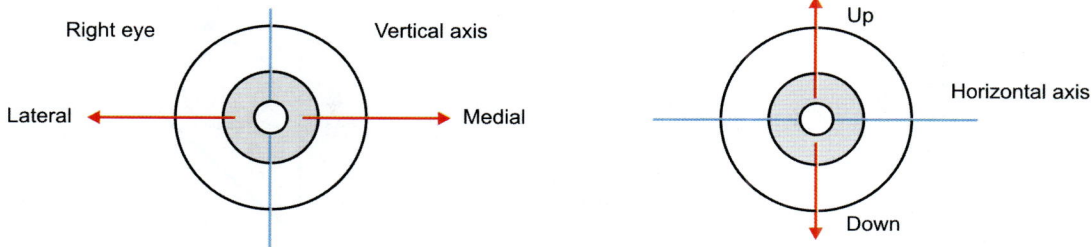

Action of the extraocular muscles

The lateral and medial walls of the orbit make an angle of 45° with each other. The orbital axis therefore forms an angle of 22.5° with both the lateral and medial walls. For the sake of simplicity this angle is usually regarded as being 23°. When the eye is looking straight ahead at a fixed point on the horizon with the head erect (primary position of gaze), its optical axis forms an angle of 23° with the orbital axis. The actions of the extraocular muscles depend on the position of the globe at the time of muscle contraction. The primary action of a muscle is its major effect when the eye is in the primary position and its subsidiary actions are the additional effects on the position of the eye.

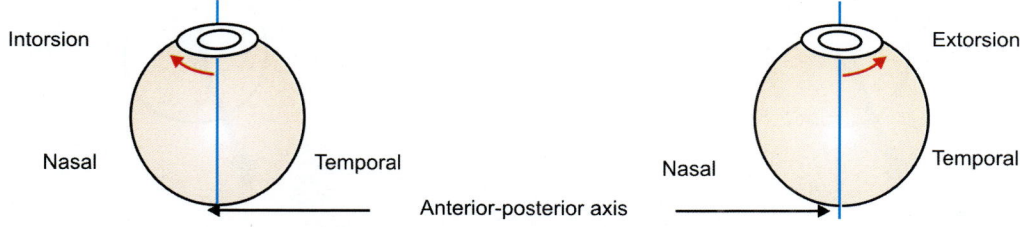

Right eyes viewed from above

Horizontal Recti (Medial and Lateral Rectus)

When the eye is in the primary position, the horizontal recti are purely horizontal movers around the vertical axis and have only a primary action.

Vertical Recti (Superior and Inferior Rectus)

The vertical recti run in the same line as the orbital axis and are inserted in front of the equator. For this reason they form an angle of 23° with the optical axis.

Superior Rectus

In the primary position, the primary action of the superior rectus is elevation. This movement occurs about the horizontal axis. The subsidiary actions of the superior rectus are adduction and intorsion.

When the globe is in a position of 23° of abduction, the optical and orbital axis coincide. In this position it has no subsidiary actions and can only act as an elevator. This is therefore the best position of the globe for testing the function of the superior rectus muscle.

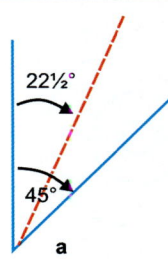 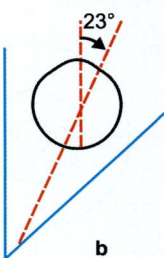

Applied anatomy of extraocular muscles

Superior oblique
The superior oblique is inserted behind the equator and it forms an angle of 51° with the optical axis. In the primary position, the primary action of the superior oblique is intorsion. This movement occurs about the vertical axis passing through the centre of pupil. In this position, subsidiary actions are depression and abduction.

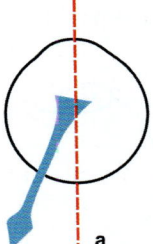 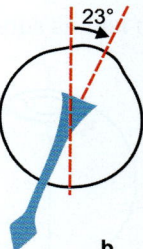

Actions of the superior rectus muscle

When the globe is in a position of 51° of adduction, the optical axis of the globe coincides with the line of pull of the muscle. In this position it can only act as a depressor. This is therefore, the best position of globe for clinically testing the action of the superior oblique muscle.

The action of the extraocular muscles can be thus summarized as follows:
1. All the recti muscles are *Adductors* except lateral rectus.
2. Both the oblique muscle are *Abductors*.
3. Both the superior muscles are *intortors*.
4. Both the inferior muscles are *extortors*.

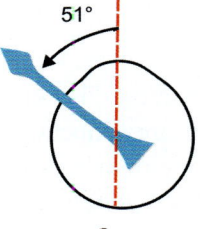 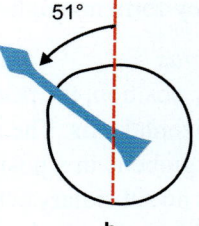

Actions of the superior oblique muscle

With this basic knowledge it is easy to work out the respective actions of the inferior rectus and inferior oblique muscles.

CONJUGATE MOVEMENTS OF THE EYEBALL

When both the eyes move together keeping their visual axis parallel, the movements are known as conjugate movements.

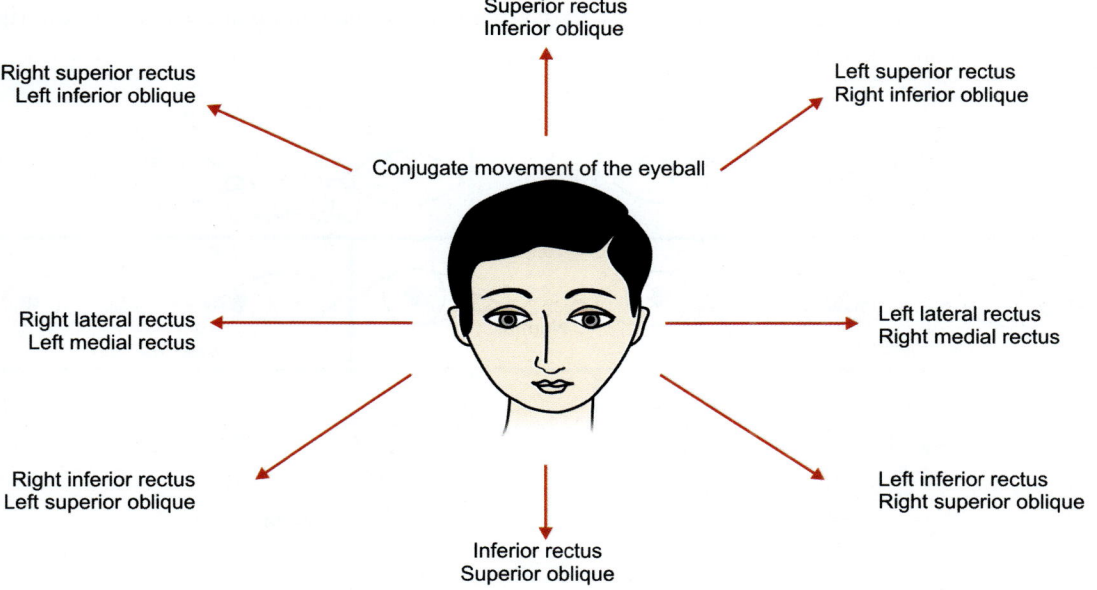

Conjugate movements of the eyeball

The Action of Extraocular Muscles in Binocular Movements

Every movement of the eyeball is a 'synkinesis' therefore:
- Abduction of one eye is always accompanied by adduction of the other.
- Elevation or depression of one eye is always accompanied by elevation or depression of the other.
- The only exception to this rule is bilateral abduction of the eye in convergence where both medial rectus contract together.

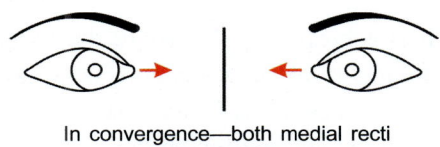

In convergence—both medial recti contract together

Synergist Muscles

The muscles which contract together or 'in pair' are called synergist muscles or 'yoke' muscles.

Antagonist Muscles

The muscles which suffer inhibition are called antagonist muscles.

CARDINAL POSITIONS OF GAZE

The six cardinal positions of gaze are dextroversion and laevoversion, dextroelevation and laevoelevation, dextrodepression and laevodepression. Although there are nine positions of gaze only six of these are cardinal.

When the eyes are moving into each of the six cardinal positions of gaze, a muscle of one eye is paired with a muscle of the opposite eye. For example, in dextroversion the synergist muscles are the right lateral rectus and the left medial rectus. In dextroelevation the synergist muscles are the right superior rectus and the left inferior oblique.

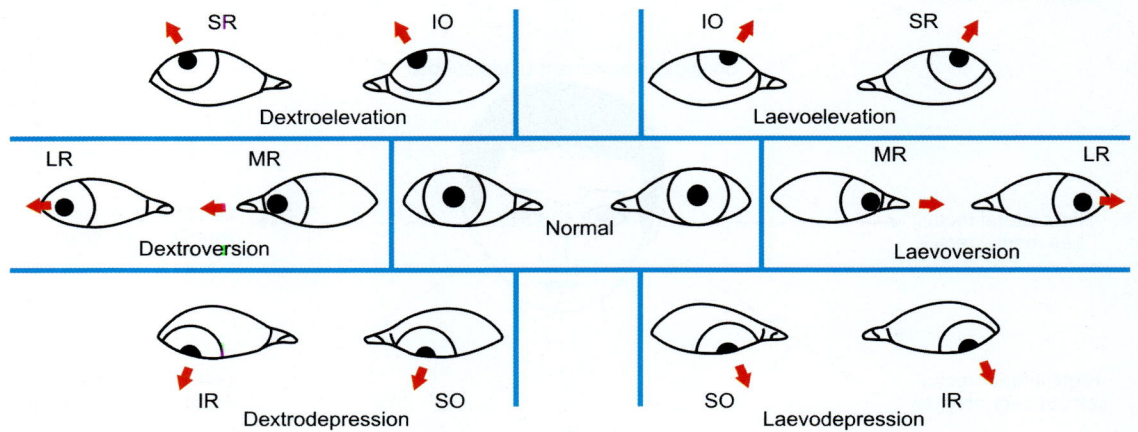

Six cardinal positions of gaze

THE NERVOUS CONTROL OF OCULAR MOVEMENTS

It is very complex being controlled by the nuclei of the 3rd, 4th and 6th cranial nerves situated in the midbrain, the intermediate centres and cerebral cortex.

BINOCULAR SINGLE VISION

It is achieved by the use of the two eyes together, so that separate and slightly dissimilar images arising in each eye are appreciated as a single image by the process of fusion. In addition to achieving single vision, this fusion results in stereopsis or three-dimensional vision. Binocular single vision is acquired and reinforced during the first few years of life.

It requires three factors for its development:
1. Reasonably clear vision in both eyes.
2. The ability of the visual areas in the brain to cause fusion of two slightly dissimilar images.
3. The accurate coordination of the two eyes for all directions of gaze. There must exist a precise physiological relationship between the two retinae (retinal correspondence) for achieving fusion.

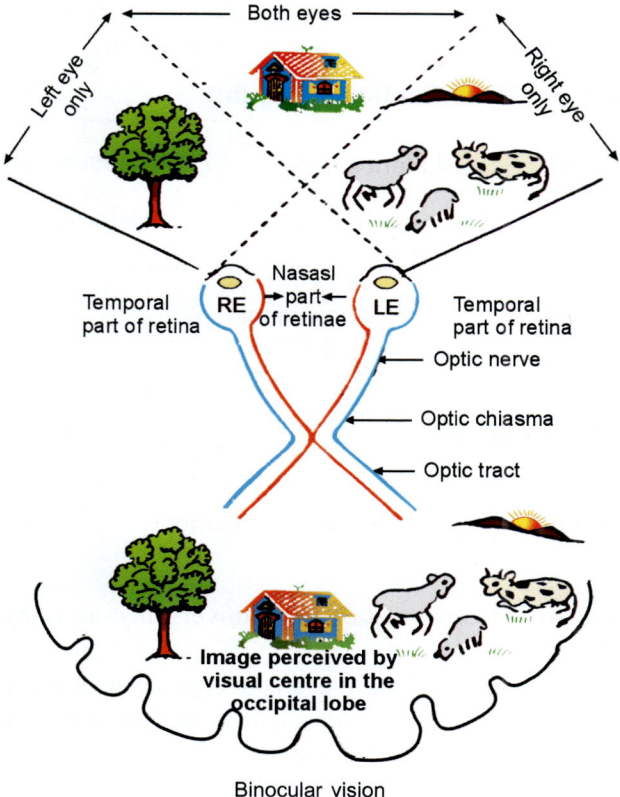

Binocular vision

SQUINT (STRABISMUS)

It is a condition when one eye deviates away from the fixation point (Duke-Elder). Under normal conditions both the eyes are in proper alignment.

I. APPARENT SQUINT

The presence of epicanthus and high errors of refraction simulate squint but in fact there is no squint.

II. LATENT SQUINT (HETEROPHORIA)

In latent squint, a tendency for deviation of the eyes is present when the fusion is broken. However, the eyes regain their normal alignment or position with fusion.

Types

Esophoria—There is a tendency for deviation of the eyeball inwards.
Exophoria—There is a tendency for deviation of the eyeball outwards.
Hyperphoria—There is a tendency for deviation of the eyeball upwards.
Cyclophoria—There is a torsional deviation of the eye.

Anisophoria—The deviation of the eyeball varies with the direction of gaze.
Orthophoria—There is no deviation of the eyes even when the fusion is broken.

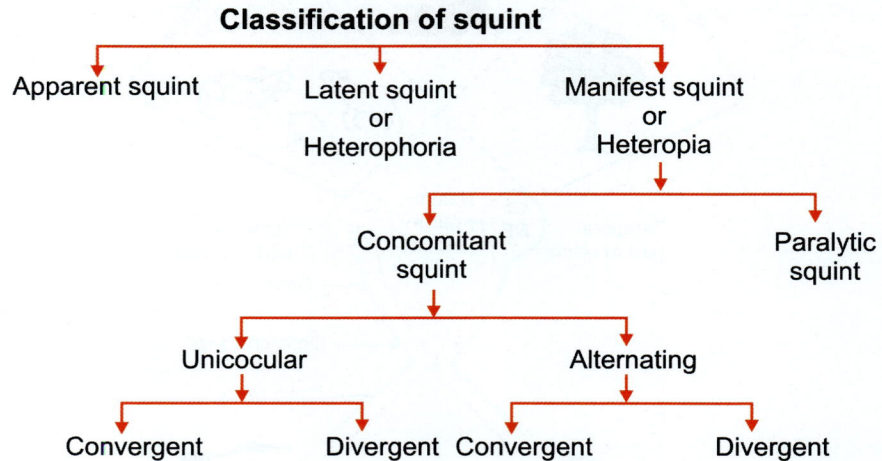

Etiology
1. Increased requirement for accommodation and convergence as in hypermetropia results in esophoria.
2. Decreased requirement for accommodation and convergence as in myopia results in exophoria.
3. Occupations requiring too much close work such as goldsmith, watchmakers.
4. General poor health, fatigue and advancing age.

Symptoms
1. There is eye strain and headache after prolonged near work.
2. There is blurring of prints and overlapping of words or lines while reading.
3. The patient complains of seeing double objects after close work for prolonged period (intermittent squint).

Diagnosis
It depends on abolishing fusion so that the eyes assume their position of rest by:
1. *Cover test*
2. *Maddox rod test*
3. *Maddox wing test*
4. *Prism vergence test.*

1. Cover Test

Principle
Fusion of the two eyes is abolished by covering one eye.

Method

The patient looks at a distant object.
- While observing one eye, cover and uncover the other eye. The movements of the observed eye and the eye under cover are noted.
- Repeat this process with the other eye and then alternately.

Interpretation

1. If there is no movement, patient has orthophoria.
2. If there is inwards movement on removing the cover the patient has exophoria.
3. If there is outwards movement on removing the cover the patient has esophoria.

2. Maddox Rod Test

Principle

This test is done to find out heterophoria for distance. It alters the appearance of the retinal image in one eye. There is no stimulation given to fusion.

Method

- The patient is seated 6 m from a spot of bright light in a dark room.
- A Maddox rod consisting of 4-5 cylinders of red glass fused side by side in a supporting disc is placed in front of one eye. The same effect is given by a disc of deeply grooved red glass (Maddox groove).
- The spot of light appears as a red line. If the cylinders are placed with their axis horizontal, the red line will appear vertical and *vice versa*.

Interpretation

If there is orthophoria, the bright spot will appear in the centre of the vertical red line.
1. *Type of heterophoria*: By the position of the vertical or horizontal line in relation to the spot of light, exact type of heterophoria is detected.
2. *Angle of deviation*: The strength of prism which is necessary to be placed in front of the Maddox rod or the other eye so that the red line and spot appear together; indicates the angle of deviation.
3. *Nature of deviation*: It is indicated by the position of the prism whether base in or base out.
4. *Amount of deviation* can be measured on a graduated tangent scale set on a wall.

3. Maddox Wing Test

Principle

The Maddox wing is an instrument that dissociates the two eyes for near fixation (one-third of a meter) and measures the amount of heterophoria.

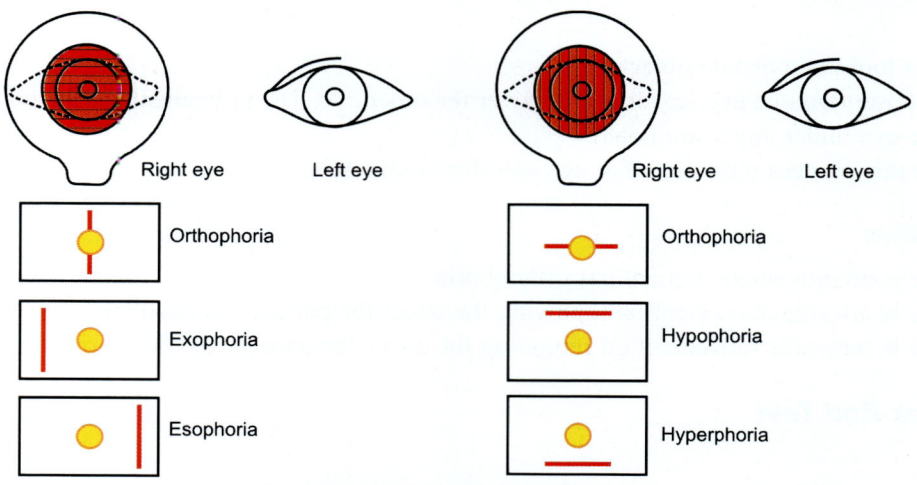

Maddox rod test for horizontal and vertical heterophorias

Maddox rod test

Method

The patient is asked to hold the Maddox wing and look through the two observation slits with both eyes open.
- The right eye sees a white arrow pointing vertically and a red arrow pointing horizontally to the left.
- The left eye sees the white figures in the horizontal lines and red figures in the vertical line. The figures are calibrated in degrees to read deviation.
- Ask the patient to read the figures corresponding to red and white arrows.

Interpretation

Any deviation indicates an esophoria, exophoria or hyperphoria which can be read on the scale.

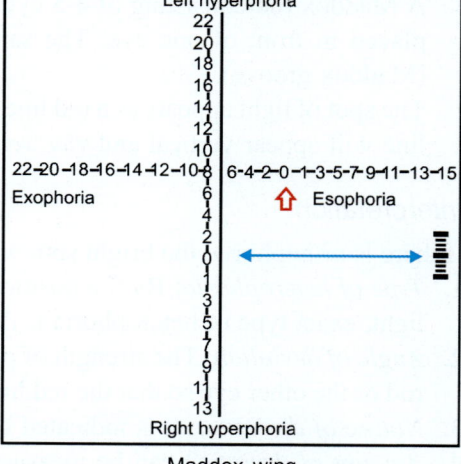

Maddox wing

4. Prism Vergence Test

Principle

The actual measurement of the deviation and strength of the muscles involved are tested. The muscles are forced to act with maximum effort against prisms.

Method

The patient is seated 6 m from a light source and looks at the Maddox tangent scale.
- The highest prism which can permit single vision gives the verging power.
- It is tested in different directions.

Interpretation

1. The normal converging power varies a great deal. It can be raised to 50 degrees (50°) or more. If it falls below 20 degrees, it is definitely insufficient.
2. The normal diverging power should be 4-5 degrees.

Treatment

1. The lower degrees of esophoria and exophoria cause no symptoms and need no special treatment.
2. Error of refraction is determined and corrected.
3. Exercises to increase the fusional reserve and convergence are advised.
    i. *Pencil exercise*: A pencil is held in the hand and brought slowly towards the nose until the tip appears double. The two images are then fused into a single image by an effort 8-10 times. This is repeated 3-4 times a day for several weeks.
    ii. *Exercise the weak muscles against prisms.*
    iii. *Exercise the weak muscle by the use of the synoptophore.*
4. Prisms can be prescribed in the spectacles. The base of the prism is kept towards the muscle to be helped.
5. Surgery of the affected muscle is done when deviation is large and is unaffected by the above treatment. Resection or recession of the muscle is done as the case may be.
6. General improvement of health and nutrition is necessary. Proper position, distance and illumination while doing near work is maintained with suitable breaks in between.

III MANIFEST SQUINT (HETEROTROPIA)

In manifest squint the deviation of eye is present as such. It is of two main types namely concomitant squint and paralytic squint.

1. CONCOMITANT SQUINT

It is a dissociation of the eyes wherein the deviation remains the same in all the directions of gaze (Duke-Elder).

Etiology

In concomitant squint the eyes are not in alignment but they retain their abnormal relation to each other in all the movements of the eye. The efferent pathway, i.e. nerve and muscle are normal. However, the afferent pathway is defective due to poor visual acuity as a result of:
    i. Defect in the eyes.
    ii. Breaking down of fixation and fusional reflex.

Types

1. *Uniocular concomitant squint:*
    i. Convergent concomitant squint
    ii. Divergent concomitant squint

2. *Alternating concomitant squint:*
   i. Convergent
   ii. Divergent.

1. Uniocular Concomitant Squint

When one eye deviates always and the normal eye takes up and maintains fixation, it is known as uniocular concomitant squint.

Concomitant convergent squint: In this condition one eye always deviates inwards while the other eye fixes an object. This develops typically in the early life before the binocular reflexes are firmly established, i.e. before the age of 6-8 years. It usually follows an attack of acute illness like measles or other debilitating disease.

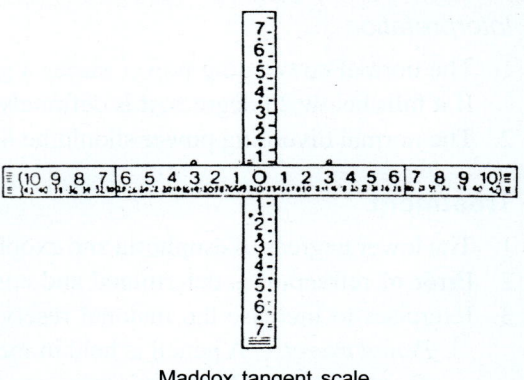

Maddox tangent scale

Etiology
1. *Defective vision:* It is usually seen in hypermetropia wherein excessive convergence and accommodation is needed.
2. *Congenital myopia:* Due to congenital myopia the child can only see objects close to the eyes. Thus he is used to excessive convergence causing convergent squint.
3. *Opacities in the media* such as cornea, lens, vitreous or ocular diseases result in the loss of fixation.
4. *Decompensation of esophoria.*

Concomitant divergent squint: In this condition one eye deviates outwards while the other eye fixes an object.

Etiology
1. *In myopia commencing at a later age:* When the vision in one eye is greatly reduced, it takes up the position of rest which is divergence. The better eye takes up the fixation.
2. *Complete loss of vision:* A blind eye diverges particularly in adults.
3. *Inherent neuromuscular coordination:* It usually starts at the age of 2-5 years.

2. Alternating Concomitant Squint

When one eye fixes, the other eye deviates either inwards or outwards and either of the eyes can take up fixation alternately, it is known as alternating concomitant squint.

The most important feature of alternating deviating eye is that of completely suppressed image in the brain so there is no diplopia.

Symptoms

- Usually there are no symptoms except cosmetic embarrassment to the patient.
- There is no diplopia as the image in the squinting eye is automatically suppressed. This suppression develops easily as concomitant squint usually occurs in young age group.
- The main feature of the concomitant squint is the failure of binocular vision.
- In uniocular concomitant squint, the vision in the squinting eye is usually defective.

Signs

There are two important signs:
1. The primary deviation is equal to the secondary deviation.
   Primary deviation: It is the angle of deviation of the squinting eye when the normal eye fixes an object.
   Secondary deviation: It is the angle of deviation of the normal eye under cover when the squinting eye fixes an object.
2. There is no limitation of movements of the eyeball in any direction usually. However, in cases of congenital weakness or paresis of the muscle, movements may be restricted.

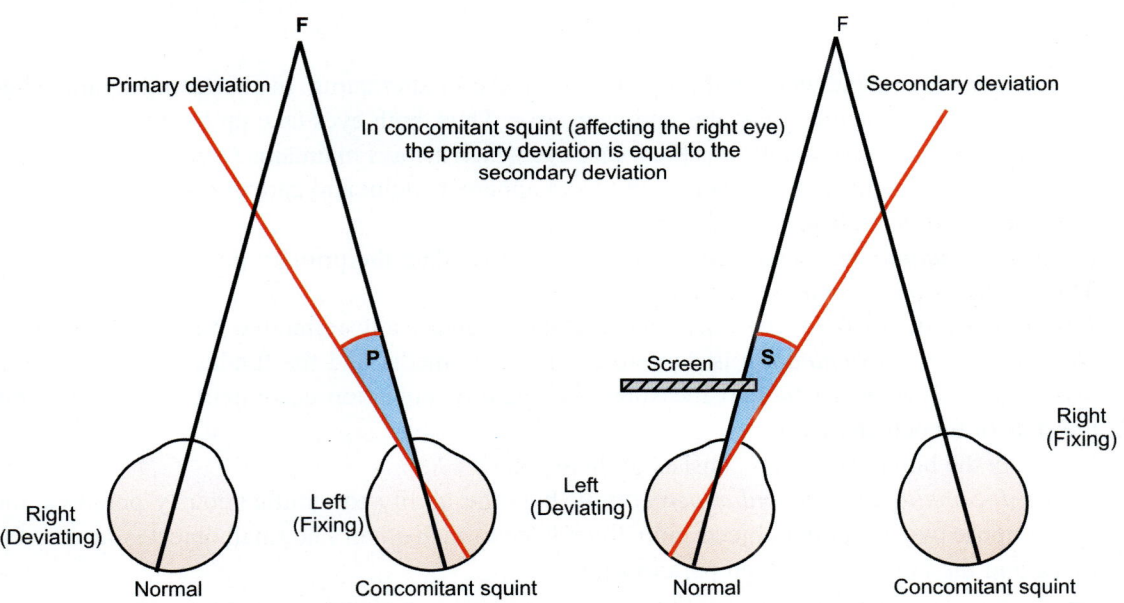

Primary and secondary deviation

INVESTIGATIONS

I. History

1. Age of onset
   - Accommodative squint usually become manifest at the age of 3-6 years.
   - The squint due to congenital paresis of muscles appear at a very early age.
   - The prognosis is better if the age of onset is late.
2. Any history of acute illness, head injury or mental shock?
3. Is the squint intermittent or constant?
4. Is there deviation of only one eye or alternate eye?
5. Family history of squint or refractive error is useful.

II. Examination

1. *Inspection*
   - Any deviation of left or right eye is noted.
   - The direction of the deviation whether inwards, outwards or vertical is noted.
   - Any opacity in the cornea or lens is noted.
   - Pupillary reactions are tested.
   - Hirschberg test—It is a quick and useful method to find out the angle of squint by the position of the corneal reflex when the light is thrown into the eye from a distance of about 50 cm.

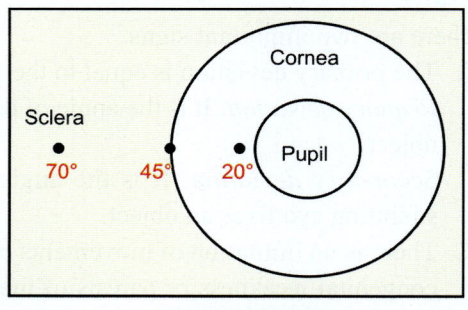

Hirschberg's test

2. *Cover test*
   i. It is done to find out whether the squint is uniocular or alternating. In alternating squint, when one eye fixes, the other deviates and *vice versa*. Thus, both eyes take up fixation alternately. In case of uniocular squint, it is the fixing eye which always maintains fixation.
   ii. It differentiates the concomitant squint from apparent squint and paralytic squint.

   In apparent squint: There is no deviation at all.

   In paralytic squint: The secondary deviation is greater than the primary deviation.

3. *Movements of the eyeball* are tested in all direction.
4. *Visual acuity is recorded and refraction* is done to detect any refractive error.
5. *Ophthalmoscopic examination* is done to examine the media and the fundus.
6. *Synoptophore (amblyoscope)*: It measures the angle of deviation accurately. It also finds out the state of binocular vision.

   Normally the binocular vision consists of three grades

   Grade 1–Simultaneous macular perception: It is the ability to simultaneously perceive and superimpose two dissimilar objects mutually related to each other. The small object is seen by the fovea and the larger one is seen parafoveally.

   Grade 2–Fusion: It is the ability of the two eyes to produce a composite picture from two similar objects each of which is incomplete in one small detail. The range of fusion is tested by moving the arms of the synoptophore so that both eye have to converge and diverge in order to maintain fusion.

   Grade 3–Stereopsis: It is the ability to obtain an impression of depth by the superimposition of the two pictures of the same objects taken from slightly different angles. It gives a three-dimensional view of the object.
   - Usually the accommodative squints have grade 1 binocular vision
   - The alternating squints do not possess any grade of binocular vision.

TREATMENT OF CONCOMITANT SQUINT

1. UNIOCULAR CONCOMITANT SQUINT

There are four main principles of treatment:
   i. Optical correction

ii. Occlusion
   iii. Orthoptic training
   iv. Operative methods

1. Optical

Error of refraction is corrected by prescribing suitable glasses. The squint of minor degree may be corrected by this treatment.

2. Occlusion

If there is not much improvement with corrected glasses, the normal eye must be kept constantly occluded by a suitable occluder for minimum of 3 months. This absolute occlusion helps the squinting eye to see with corrected glasses and the vision rapidly improves in that eye. The occlusion is most effective upto the age of 8 years.

3. Orthoptic Training

It is given to achieve binocular vision and to increase the range of stereoscopic fusion preoperatively and postoperatively.

4. Operative Methods

Principle of Surgery

The aim of surgery is to correct the misalignment of the eye and if possible, also to restore binocular single vision.

Indications

The surgical treatment is indicated when the squint is more than 10° even after wearing suitable glasses and orthoptic training for a reasonable time. It should be undertaken early, i.e. as soon as the child is able to do postoperative orthoptic exercises.

Technique

The three main types of operation are:
1. Weakening procedures that decrease the pull of a muscle.
2. Strengthening procedures that enhance the pull of a muscle.
3. The procedures that change the direction of the action of a muscle.

Methods

   I. *In convergent squint:*
      i. *If the deviation is 10° or less*: The medial rectus muscle is recessed or made weak by shifting its insertion backwards towards it origin. Usually 1 mm recession corrects about 2.5° of the angle of squint. The recession must not be more than 5 mm as convergence insufficiency may develop.

ii. *If the deviation is more than 10°*: The lateral rectus muscle is resected or made shorter by removing a portion of the muscle
      Usually 1 mm resection corrects about 2° of the angle of squint. The medial rectus muscle may also be recessed.
   iii. *If the deviation is very large*: Similar procedures should be carried out in the other eye.
II. In divergent squint
   The medial rectus muscle is resected or made strong. The lateral rectus muscle is recessed or made loose. In large deviations, a recession of the opposite lateral rectus may be necessary.

Medial rectus muscle recession
This surgical procedure involves weakening of the muscle by the following steps :
1. The muscle is exposed and two absorbable sutures are passed through the outer quarters of the tendon.
2. The tendon is disinserted from the sclera.
3. The amount of recession is measured and it is marked on the sclera with the calipers.
4. The stump is resutured to the sclera posterior to its original insertion.

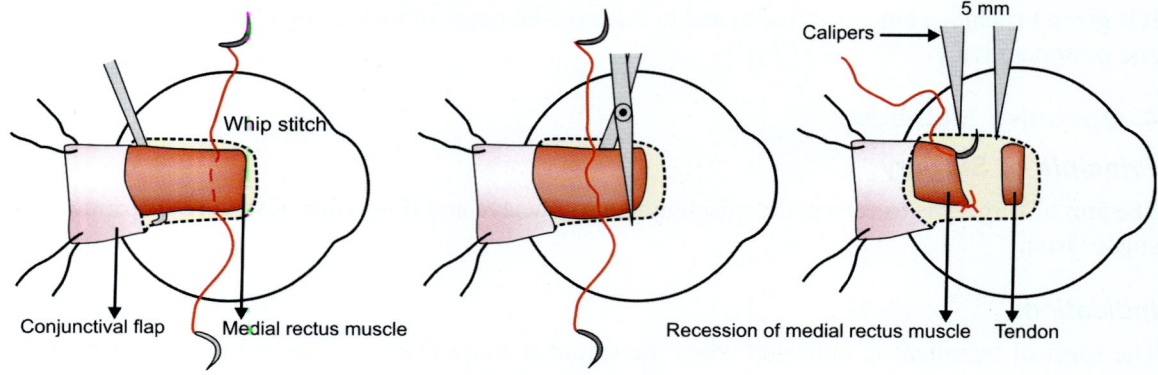

Recession of medial rectus muscle

Lateral rectus muscle resection
In this technique, the effective pull of the muscle is increased by making it shorter. The operation involves the following steps.
1. The muscle is exposed and two absorbable sutures are inserted into the muscle at a predetermined point posterior to its insertion.
2. The tendon is disinserted from the sclera.
3. The muscle anterior to the sutures is excised.
4. The stump is reattached to the original insertion.

Alternating Squint

1. The surgical correction is only for cosmetic purpose as the fusion does not develop.
2. The recession or resection of recti muscles is done depending on the type of squint.

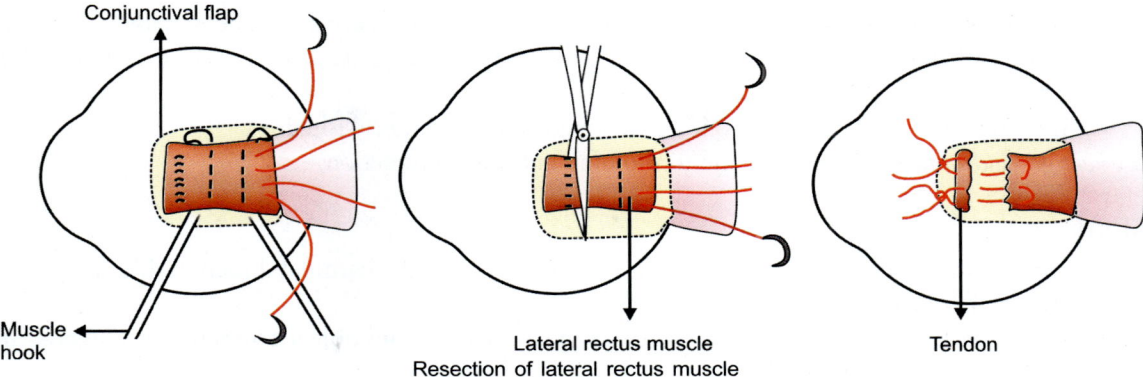

2. PARALYTIC SQUINT

In paralytic squint there is a deviation of the eye caused by the paralysis of extraocular muscles. The deviation of the eye varies in different directions of gaze.

Etiology

The afferent pathway is intact but the efferent pathway is defective. The lesion is situated at the level of lower neuron affecting the nuclei, the nerves or the muscles.
  i. *Lesions of the motor nerve nucleus:*
     - Congenital absence of the nucleus.
     - Inflammations such as encephalitis, disseminated sclerosis.
     - Degenerative and vascular lesions.
  ii. *Lesions of nerve trunk:*
     - Trauma by direct injury or by pressure.
     - Inflammations such as diabetes mellitus neuropathy
  iii. *Lesions of the muscle:*
     - Congenital absence or maldevelopment of the muscle.
     - Direct injury.
     - Myopathy.

Symptoms

1. *Diplopia or seeing double objects*: It is most marked in the direction of action of the paralysed muscle.
   - It may be crossed or uncrossed.

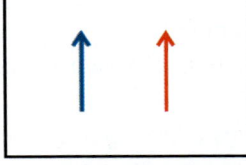

Paralysis of horizontally acting muscle

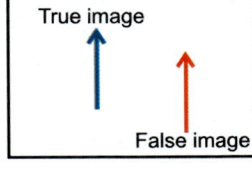

Paralysis of vertically acting muscle

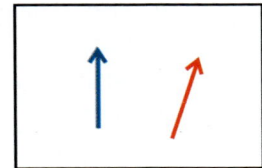

Paralysis of oblique acting muscle

Diplopia

- If the horizontally acting muscle is affected, the two images are seen side by side.
- If the vertically acting muscle is involved, one image appears at a slightly lower level than the other.
- If oblique muscle is involved one of the image appears slightly tilted.
2. *Vertigo and nausea*: These are due to diplopia and false projection.

Signs

1. *Limitations of movements*: Test the ocular movements in all the cardinal direction. If a muscle is paralysed, there will be limitation of movement.
2. *False orientation*: The patient is not able to grasp or point the object correctly on the side of action of paralysed muscle.
3. *Position of the head*: The patient's head and face is turned towards the direction of the action of the paralysed muscle.

Compensatory Mechanisms for Diplopia

There are three mechanisms by which a patient can compensate for double vision

1. *Suppression*: It is an adaptation which occurs mainly in children. It is produced subconsciously by an active neglect of the vision in the squinting eye by the visual cortex. When the fixing eye is covered, the squinting eye takes up fixation immediately.
2. *Strabismic amblyopia*: It occurs as a result of continuous monocular suppression of the deviated eye. There is unilateral impairment of vision even when the eye is forced to take up fixation. Eccentric fixation is a uniocular condition in which some part of the retina other than the fovea is used for fixation, and in which reorientation of sensory and motor functions may eventually occur so that the new area assumes a foveal type of visual fixation.
3. *Abnormal retinal correspondence (ARC)*: The retinal elements of the deviating eye assume an abnormal relationship with the fovea or other areas of the non-squinting eye. This occurs in young children with long-standing squint.

Investigations

History

Ask the patient about the onset and associated illness which may be the precipitating factor.

Examination

1. *Position of the eyes*: The deviation of the eyeball is noted.
2. *Position of the head*: Any tilting or abnormal position of the head is noted.
3. *Cover test*: The secondary deviation is more than the primary deviation. Each eye is covered and uncovered alternatively.
4. *Ocular movements*: The movements of the extraocular muscles are tested for each eye and both eyes together.
5. *Diplopia charting*: A spectacles containing a red lens for the right eye and a green lens for the left eye is worn by the patient. This dissociates the retinal images perceived by both the eyes.

Method: In a dark room a streak of light from a specially devised torch or a lighted candle is shown in the nine positions of gaze.
- The positions of the images seen by the patient are recorded upon a chart with nine squares—the red image with red pencil and green image with green pencil.
    i. The area of single vision and diplopia.
    ii. The distance between the two images.
    iii. The level of the two images.
    iv. The positions of the images, whether erect or tilted.
    v. The diplopia is crossed or uncrossed.

This test is purely subjective and patients are usually uncooperative. Therefore other investigations should be done.

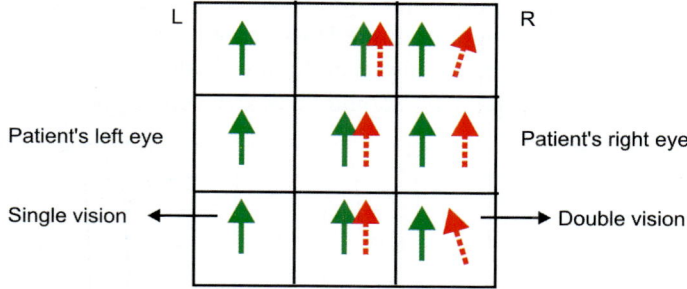

Diplopia chart for right lateral rectus palsy

6. *Worth's four dot test:*
   - The patient wears a red lens in front of his right eye which filters all colours except red. A green lens is placed in front of his left eye which filters all colours except green. Thus, he sees red and green colours with right and left eyes respectively.
   - He views a box with four lights—one red, two green and one white.

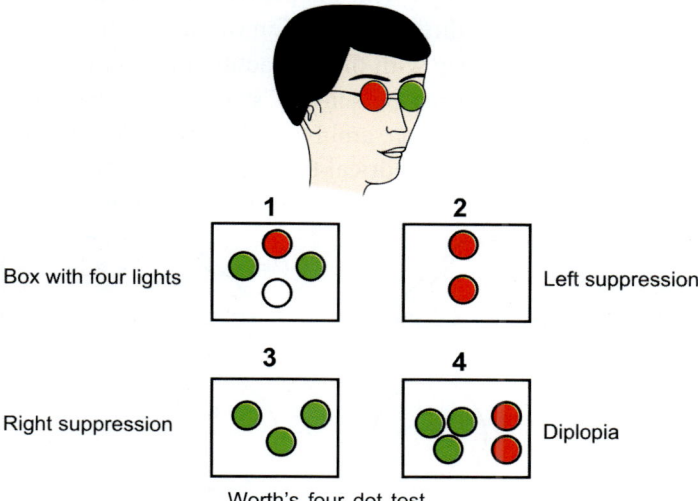

Worth's four dot test

- If the patient sees all four lights, he has normal fusion.
- If he sees two red lights, he has left suppression.
- If he sees three green lights, he has right suppression.
- If he sees that the green and red lights alternate, he has alternating suppression.
- If he sees two red and three green lights, he has diplopia.

7. *Hess screen:*
   Principle: Dissociation of retinal images of two eye is carried out by red-green goggles. The Hess screen test provides following informations:
   - A record of primary and secondary deviation.
   - In paralytic squint, it provides information about the progress of the case if taken at suitable intervals.

   Method: The patient wears red-green filter goggles and holds a green light projection pointer.
   - The surgeon holds a red light projection pointer which is used as a point of fixation.
   - The surgeon projects the red light onto the Hess screen.
   - The patient is asked to superimpose his green light onto the red light.
   - In normal condition, the two pointers should be nearly superimposed in all nine positions of gaze.

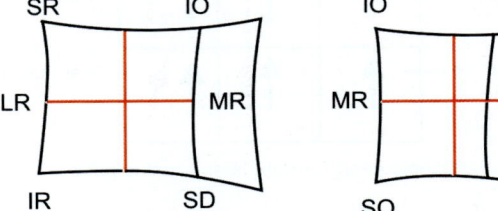

Hess chart in right lateral rectus palsy

Interpretation:
- The two charts are compared.
- The smaller chart indicates the eye with the paralysed right lateral rectus muscle. It shows greatest restriction in the main direction of action of the muscle.
- The larger chart indicates the eye with the overacting muscle, i.e. medial rectus muscle.

8. *Synoptophore (Amblyoscope):* It tests the sensory status of the eyes which includes grade of binocular vision, presence of suppression, amblyopia and retinal correspondence.
   The instrument consists of two cylindrical tubes with a mirrored right-angled bend. A +6.5 D lens is fixed in each eyepiece. The adjustments of the tubes are indicated on a scale.

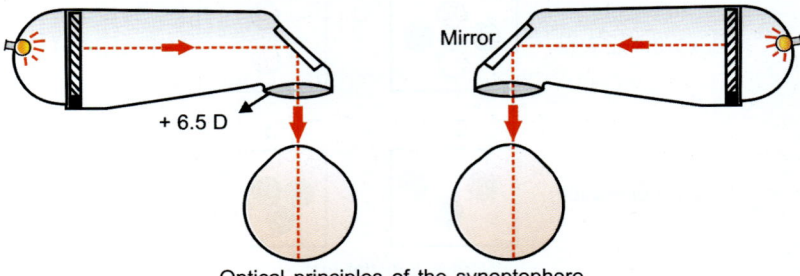

Optical principles of the synoptophore

1. Grades of Binocular Vision

Grade I: Simultaneous macular perception:
- Two dissimilar slides having pictures of a bird and a cage are introduced.
- If the patient can bring the bird in the cage and see both the objects, he has fusion of Grade I.

Grade II: Fusion: It is the ability to produce a complete picture from two similar but incomplete pictures. The classic example is two rabbits each lacking either a tail or a bunch of flowers. The range of fusion is tested by moving the arms of the amblyoscope so that the eyes have to converge or diverge in order to maintain fusion.

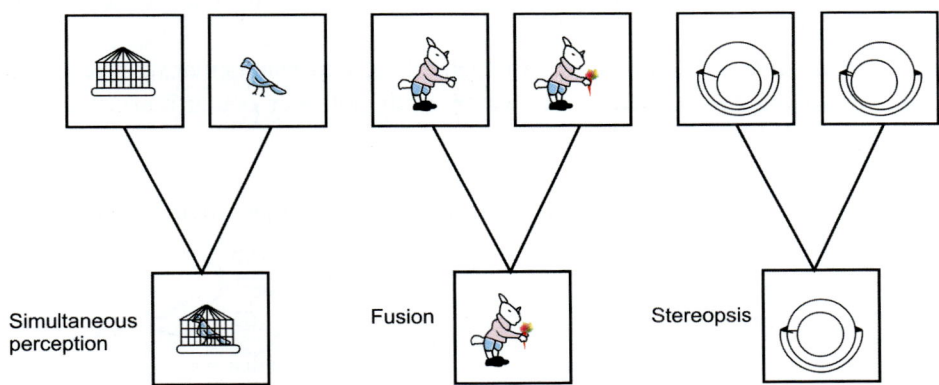

Three grades of binocular vision

Grade III: Stereopsis: The two test slides are devised to give an impression of depth. The classic example is the bucket which is appreciated in three-dimensions.

2. Suppression

The patient having suppression will see only one slide or alternate slide of Grade I binocular vision.

3. Retinal Correspondence

If the patient is able to superimpose the slides of Grade II binocular vision, he has a normal retinal correspondence. There is another test for testing the retinal correspondence—the after image test. This test domonstrates the visual direction of the two foveae.

After image test:
- The right fovea is stimulated by a vertical bright flash of light and the left fovea by a horizontal flash.
- The patient then draws the relative positions of the after images.
- If the two after images are seen as a cross, he has normal retinal correspondence.
- If he has abnormal retinal correspondence (ARC) or eccentric fixation, the two images will not cross.

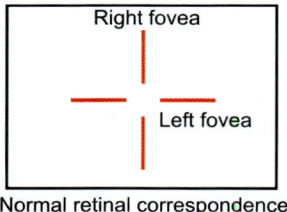
Normal retinal correspondence

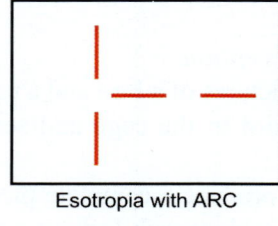
Esotropia with ARC

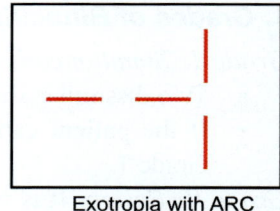
Exotropia with ARC

After image test

Types of Ocular Paralysis

1. *Total ophthalmoplegia*: A condition wherein all the extrinsic and intrinsic muscles of one or both the eyes are paralysed.
2. *External ophthalmoplegia*: A condition in which all the extrinsic ocular muscles are paralysed.
3. *Internal ophthalmoplegia*: A condition in which all the intrinsic ocular muscles are paralysed.

3rd Nerve Palsy

It supplies superior rectus, inferior rectus, medial rectus, inferior oblique, sphincter pupillae and ciliary muscles.

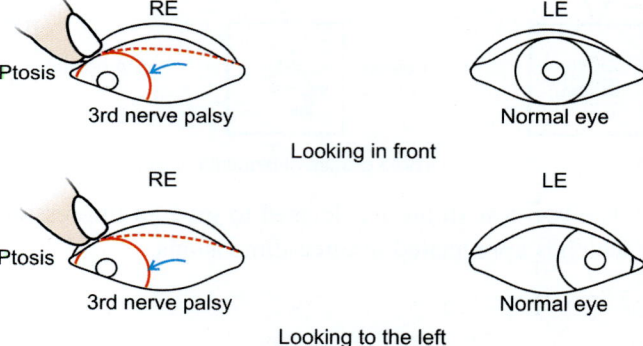

3rd nerve palsy – Right eye

- In complete paralysis, there is ptosis which prevents diplopia.
- There is limitation of upwards, downwards and inwards movements.
- Pupil is dilated and fixed and accommodation is completely lost.
- In incomplete paralysis, an individual muscle may be involved.

4th Nerve Palsy

The superior oblique muscle is paralysed causing restriction of downwards and inwards movement.

Unable to look downwards and towards normal side

4th nerve palsy – Right eye

6th Nerve Palsy

This is the most common type of ocular paralysis. Paralysis of the lateral rectus muscle causes limitation of outwards or lateral movement.

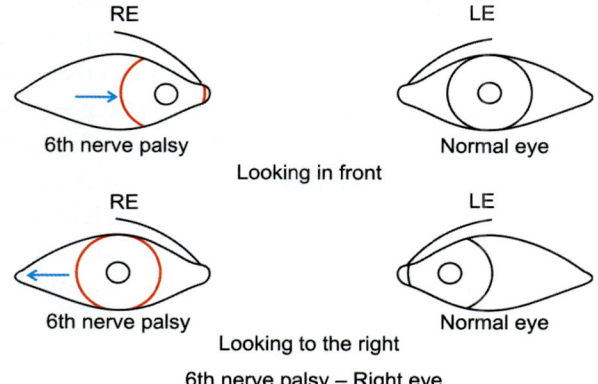

6th nerve palsy – Right eye

Treatment

There are three main principles of treatment:
1. *Treat the basic underlying cause.*
2. *Occlusion*: If the diplopia is troublesome, occlusion of the affected eye is done with an opaque disc or ground glass.
3. *Operative methods*: This should be undertaken after six months from the onset of paralysis as sufficient time must be given for recovery.
    i. The operative measure consists of recession or weakening of the antagonist muscle in the same eye with resection or strengthening of the paralysed muscle.
    ii. The recession of the opposite synergist muscle may be done.

NYSTAGMUS

It is the involuntary, symmetrical, synchronous, rapid oscillatory movements of the eyes. It is independent of the normal movements of the eyes which are not affected.

Etiology

It is a disturbance of ocular posture. The factors responsible for maintenance of ocular posture are the visual sensory pathway, the vestibular apparatus and the motor mechanisms which coordinate the sensory and motor functions.

1. *Ocular Nystagmus*

It is due to defect in maintaining fixation.
a. *Physiological:*
    i. *Optokinetic nystagmus*: It is seen when a person travels in a train and keeps on looking outside.

DIFFERENCES BETWEEN PARALYTIC AND CONCOMITANT SQUINT

	PARALYTIC SQUINT	CONCOMITANT SQUINT
1. Etiology	The afferent pathway and centres are intact but the efferent pathway breaks down • Traumatic or inflammatory lesion at the level of nuclei, nerve or muscle causes paralysis	The efferent pathway is intact but the afferent pathway and centres are defective • Due to poor visual acuity as a result of refractive error • The fixation and fusional reflexes are underdeveloped or broken down
2. Incidence	Adults usually	• Common in children and young adults
3. Signs and symptoms	1. Limitation of movement 2. Diplopia 3. False orientation 4. Abnormal position of head 5. Vertigo 6. Secondary deviation is more than primary deviation	Usually symptomless except cosmetic defect Primary and secondary deviations are equal on both sides
4. Investigations	1. Limitation of ocular movements 2. Cover test 3. Diplopia chart 4. Worth's four dot test 5. Hess screen 6. Synoptophore	1. Hirschberg's test 2. Cover test 3. Synoptophore
5. Treatment	1. Treat the basic cause 2. Optical-ground glass or occluder is used in cases of severe diplopia 3. Operative measures consist of resection of paralysed muscle with recession of the antagonist muscle of the same eye	1. Optical correction of refractive error 2. Occlusion of the good eye 3. Orthoptic exercises 4. Operative measures—It consists of recession or resection of appropriate muscles

    ii. *Latent nystagmus*: Nystagmus is not present when both the eyes are open. It becomes manifest on closing either eye.
- b. *Spontaneous:*
    - i. *Amaurotic nystagmus*: It is jerky or pendular type occurring in infants who are born blind and in whom macular fixation has not developed.
    - ii. *Amblyopic nystagmus*: It is due to interference with the development of macular fixation within the first 4 to 6 months of life, e.g. as in albinism, congenital total colour blindness or any opacity in the media.

iii. *Spasmus nutans*: Head nodding movement may occurs in children brought up in a very dim illumination.
iv. *Miner's nystagmus*: It is an occupational disease occurring in coal mine workers due to dim illumination. It is of rapid rotatory type.

2. Vestibular Nystagmus

i. It occurs in diseases of the internal ear, i.e. semicircular canals are involved.
ii. It can be produced in normal persons by rotatory movement, syringing the ear with cold water, etc.
iii. The nystagmus is jerky, fine, rapid and horizontal-rotatory.

3. Central Nystagmus

It is caused by lesions of the:
i. *Midbrain*: Disseminated sclerosis, encephalitis, vascular lesions.
ii. *Cerebellum*: Tumour, abscess. The nystagmus is jerky and is most commonly elicited on the lateral deviation of the eye.

4. Congenital Hereditary

It is hereditary and the cause is unknown.

Treatment

It is palliative like correction of refraction, use of smoked or tinted glass or contact lens in albinism and the treatment of any underlying disease.

Prognosis

Nystagmus tends to diminish with advancing age.

MULTIPLE CHOICE QUESTIONS

1. All the four recti originate from
   a. common annular tendon around optic foramen
   b. floor of orbit
   c. roof of orbit
   d. equator of eyeball
2. The 3rd cranial nerve supplies all muscles EXCEPT
   a. inferior oblique
   b. inferior rectus
   c. superior oblique
   d. superior rectus
3. Concomitant squint is distinguished from paralytic squint by all of the following EXCEPT
   a. there is no limitations of ocular movement
   b. head tilting is rare
   c. diplopia is rare
   d. the angle of deviation depends upon which eye is fixing
4. In paralytic squint deviation of the eye is present
   a. upwards
   b. inwards
   c. outwards
   d. in different directions of gaze
5. In Weber's syndrome there is a
   a. 3rd cranial nerve palsy
   b. 4th cranial nerve palsy
   c. 5th cranial nerve palsy
   d. 7th cranial nerve palsy
6. Alternating divergent squint is a form of
   a. concomitant squint
   b. paralytic squint
   c. apparent squint
   d. latent squint
7. Concomitant squint has a better prognosis if the onset is
   a. very early in life
   b. childhood
   c. at birth
   d. late in life
8. Anisophoria is the condition in which the deviation of the eyeball is
   a. upwards
   b. outwards
   c. downwards
   d. variable according to direction of gaze
9. The type of miner's nystagmus is
   a. rotatory
   b. lateral
   c. vertical
   d. none of the above
10. The vertical recti form an angle with the optical axis
    a. 45°
    b. 23°
    c. 51°
    d. 67°
11. The term 'intorsion' implies
    a. upper pole of cornea moves temporally
    b. upper pole of cornea moves nasally
    c. lower pole of cornea moves temporally
    d. lower pole of cornea moves nasally
12. In the primary position, the primary action of the superior rectus muscle is
    a. depression
    b. adduction
    c. elevation
    d. intorsion

13. 'Synergist muscles' are the extraocular muscles which act
    a. 'in pair'
    b. suffer inhibition
    c. both
    d. none
14. There are following cardinal positions of gaze
    a. 9
    b. 6
    c. 7
    d. 8
15. Binocular single vision requires all factors for its development EXCEPT
    a. clear vision in both eyes
    b. ability of the brain to cause fusion of two images
    c. accurate conjugate movements of the eyeball
    d. defective efferent pathway
16. Diplopia is a characteristic feature of
    a. uniocular concomitant squint
    b. alternating concomitant squint
    c. paralytic squint
    d. apparent squint
17. In Worth's four dot test the patient has diplopia if he sees
    a. only two red lights
    b. only two green lights
    c. green and red lights alternately
    d. two red and three green lights
18. Hess screen is a record of
    a. primary and secondary deviation
    b. heterophoria
    c. fusion
    d. retinal correspondence
19. Total ophthalmoplegia is a condition in which there is paralysis of
    a. all the extrinsic muscle of eyeball
    b. all the extrinsic and intrinsic muscles of the eyeball
    c. the optic nerve and extrinsic muscles of the eyeball
    d. none of the above
20. In concomitant squint
    a. the centre and afferent pathways are intact
    b. the efferent pathway is intact
    c. the efferent pathway is defective
    d. none of the above
21. Ptosis is typically caused in the paralysis of
    a. 3rd nerve
    b. 4th nerve
    c. 6th nerve
    d. 7th nerve
22. Concomitant convergent squint is seen in all EXCEPT
    a. hypermetropia
    b. opacities in the media
    c. congenital myopia
    d. paralysis of lateral rectus muscle
23. Different grades of binocular vision include all EXCEPT
    a. stereopsis
    b. simultaneous macular perception
    c. divergence
    d. fusion
24. Treatment of esophoria includes
    a. correction of error of refraction
    b. convergence exercises
    c. general improvement of health and nutrition
    d. all of the above

25. Concomitant divergent squint is seen in all EXCEPT
    a. myopia starting at a later age
    b. complete loss of vision
    c. paralysis of medial rectus muscle.
    d. inherent neuromuscular coordination
26. All are features of paralytic squint EXCEPT
    a. amblyopia
    b. abnormal head position
    c. unequal fixation
    d. vertigo
27. Action of right superior oblique is
    a. laevodepression
    b. laevoelevation
    c. dextrodepression
    d. dextroelevation
28. Exophoria is common in
    a. myopia
    b. hypermetropia
    c. aphakia
    d. presbyopia
29. In paralytic squint
    a. primary deviation > secondary deviation
    b. primary deviation < secondary deviation
    c. primary deviation = secondary deviation
    d. none of the above
30. Hirschberg test is used to detect
    a. squint
    b. field defect
    c. glaucoma
    d. optic atrophy

ANSWERS

1—a	2—c	3—d	4—d	5—a
6—a	7—d	8—d	9—a	10—b
11—b	12—c	13—a	14—b	15—d
16—c	17—d	18—a	19—b	20—b
21—a	22—d	23—c	24—d	25—c
26—a	27—a	28—a	29—b	30—a

CHAPTER 17
The Lids

APPLIED ANATOMY

The Eyelids

These are two movable folds of tissue situated above and below the front of each eye. There are short curved hair, the eyelashes situated on their free edges. The layers of tissue which form the eyelids are:
- A thin covering of skin.
- A thin sheet of areolar tissue.
- Three muscles—the orbicularis oculi, levator palpebrae superioris and Muller's muscle.
- A thin sheet of dense connective tissue, the tarsal plate, larger in the upper than in the lower eyelid. It supports the other structures.
- A lining of palpebral conjunctiva.

The Lid Margin

It is divided into rounded anterior and sharp posterior borders by the grey line. The eyelashes originate anterior to the grey line and ducts of the meibomian glands are located posterior to the grey line. Grey line is important in operations where the lid is split as it indicates the position of loose fibrous tissue between the orbicularis muscle and the tarsus.

Meibomian Glands (Tarsal Glands)

These are modified sebaceous glands about 20-30 in number embedded in the tarsal plate. They are directed vertically and open on the lid margin. Therefore vertical incision is given while incising the chalazion.

Zeis's Glands

These are also modified sebaceous glands attached to the hair follicles.

Moll's Glands

These are modified sweat glands which open in the hair follicles or directly in the lid margin.

Palpebral Fissure

The space between the two lids when the eye is open is known as the palpebral fissure or palpebral aperture.

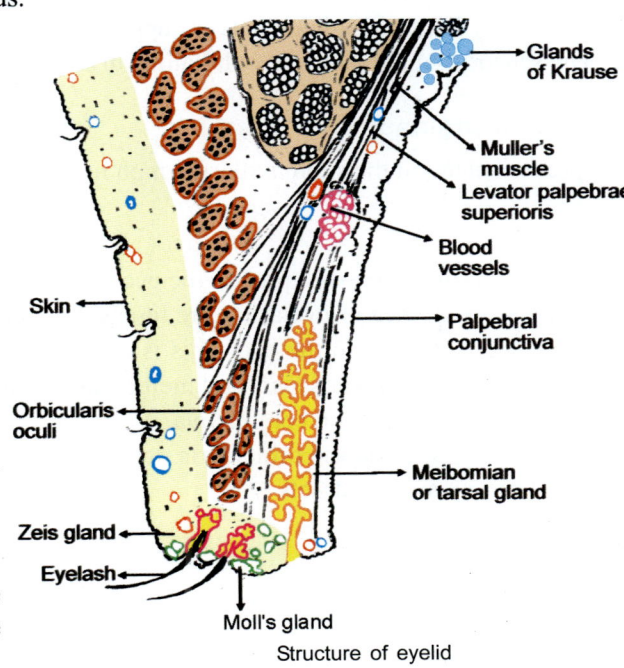

Structure of eyelid

The Outer Canthus
The outer or lateral angle of the palpebral fissure is called the outer canthus.

The Inner Canthus
The inner or medial angle of the palpebral fissure is called the inner canthus. A semilunar fold, the plica semilunaris with an elevation called the caruncle is situated in the inner canthus.

Blood Supply
It is supplied by the ophthalmic and lacrimal arteries by their medial and lateral branches. The venous drainage is through the ophthalmic vein.

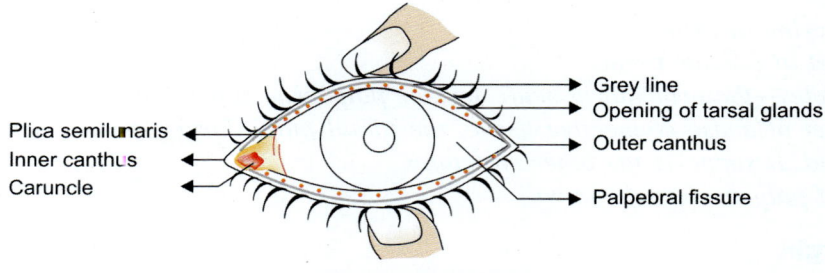

Structure of lid margin

Nerve Supply
1. The 7th nerve supplies the orbicularis oculi muscle. The 3rd nerve supplies the levator palpebrae superioris. The sympathetic nerves supply the Muller's muscle.
2. The sensory supply is by the ophthalmic division of the 5th cranial nerve.

Lymphatic Drainage
The preauricular and the submaxillary lymph nodes.

Functions
1. The eyelids and eyelashes protect the eye from injury. Reflex closure of the lids occurs when the conjunctiva, cornea or eyelashes are touched, when an object comes close to the eye or when a bright light shines into the eye. This is called the *conjunctival* or *corneal reflex*.
2. Regular blinking spreads tears and meibomian gland's secretions over the cornea which prevents drying of the cornea and conjunctiva.
3. The eyes close when the orbicularis oculi muscle contracts. The eyelids open when the levator palpebrae muscle contracts.

DISEASES OF THE LIDS
1. **Inflammation**
   - Blepharitis

- Hordeolum (stye)
- Chalazion (tarsal or meibomian cyst)
- Hordeolum internum

2. **Anomalies in the position of lids**
   - Trichiasis
   - Entropion
   - Ectropion
   - Symblepharon
   - Ankyloblepharon
   - Blepharophimosis
   - Lagophthalmos
   - Ptosis

3. **Tumours**
   - Xanthoma
   - Naevus or mole
   - Haemangioma
   - Neurofibromatosis
   - Squamous cell carcinoma
   - Basal cell carcinoma

4. **Congenital abnormalities**
   - Distichiasis
   - Coloboma
   - Epicanthus

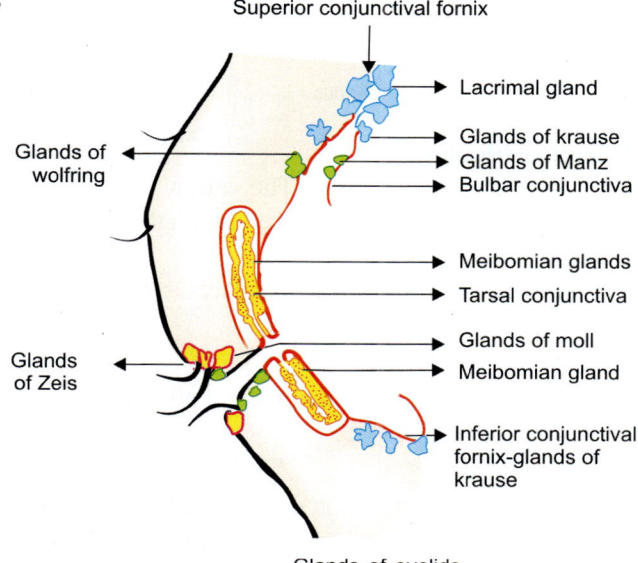

Glands of eyelids

INFLAMMATIONS

BLEPHARITIS

Blepharitis is a chronic inflammation of the lid margins.

Etiology

1. It follows chronic conjunctivitis due to *Staphyloccocus* in debilitated children usually who are living in poor hygienic conditions.
2. Parasites such as *Demodex folliculorum, Phthiriasis palpebrarum,* crab louse, head louse also cause blepharitis.

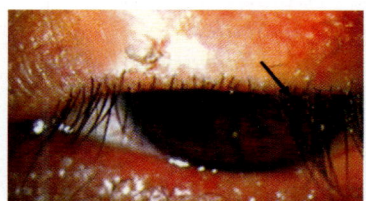

Squamous blepharitis

Types

1. **Squamous blepharitis**
   - It is due to abnormal metabolism and seborrhoea. It is usually associated with the dandruff of the scalp.
   - Numerous white coloured small scales accumulate among the eyelashes.
   - The eyelashes fall out readily but are replaced without distortion.
   - On removal of the scales, the underlying surface is hyperaemic.

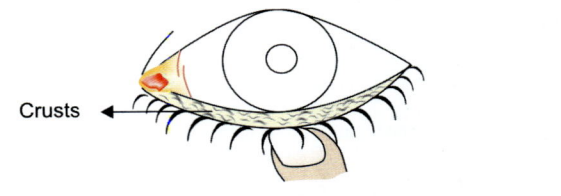
Squamous blepharitis

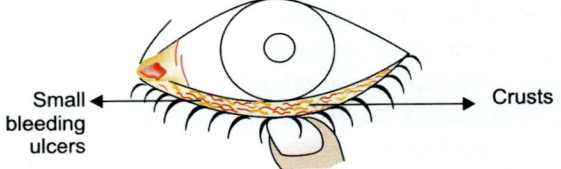
Ulcerative blepharitis

2. Ulcerative blepharitis
- It is an infective condition. The yellow crusts glue the lashes together.
- On removing the crusts, there are small ulcers seen around the bases of the lashes. These ulcers bleed easily.
- The eyelashes fall out being replaced by misdirected lashes.

Symptoms
Itching, redness, soreness, lacrimation and photophobia.

Sequelae
1. *Trichiasis*—This condition is due to misdirected eyelashes.
2. *Tylosis*—There is thickening or hypertrophy of the lid margin.
3. *Madarosis*—Absence of or scanty eyelashes as a result of destruction of the hair roots.
4. *Ectropion*—There is eversion of the lid margin due to the contraction of the scar tissue.
5. *Epiphora*—Constant watering of the eyes occurs as a result of ectropion which may lead to eczema of the skin.

Ulcerative blepharitis

DIFFERENCES BETWEEN SQUAMOUS AND ULCERATIVE BLEPHARITIS

	SQUAMOUS BLEPHARITIS	ULCERATIVE BLEPHARITIS
1. Clinical features		
i. Scales	White, fine and dry	Yellowing, coarse, and sticky
ii. Ulceration	Absent	Present
iii. Bleeding	Absent	Present
iv. Loss of eyelashes	Few and temporary	Permanent and almost all lashes are involved
2. Course	Mild	Progressive
3. Complications	Occasional	Usual and serious

Treatment
Local—The local treatment should be energetic in the ulcerative form.
  i. Removal of scales, crusts and diseased lashes is done by bathing the lid margin with 3% sodium bicarbonate lotion.
  ii. Epilation of loose and diseased eyelashes is advised.
  iii. Antibiotic drops and ointment are applied after culture and sensitivity.

General
  i. Improvement of general health and personal hygiene should be done.
  ii. Dandruff of the scalp is adequately treated.

STYE (HORDEOLUM)

Stye is an acute suppurative inflammation of one of the Zeis's glands.

Etiology

1. It is usually due to presence of staphylococci infection occurring in crops. It is often associated with boils, carbuncles and acne over face.
2. It is most common in young adults and debilitated persons.

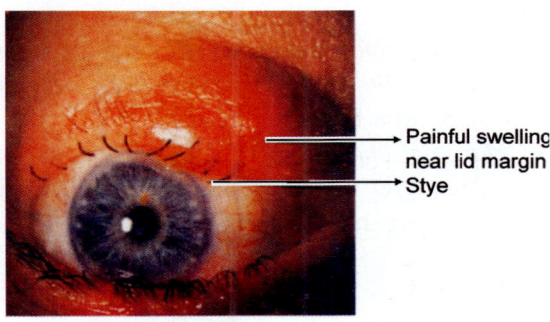

Symptoms

There is acute pain and tenderness over the inflamed Zeis's gland.

Signs

1. A localised painful and hard swelling is seen near the lid margin.
2. The lid margin is red and oedematous.
3. An abscess (yellow discolouration) may form which points near the base of the lash.
4. The pain subsides after evacuation of the pus.

Stye with lid swelling

Treatment

1. Hot fomentation applied frequently in the early stage is useful.
2. Evacuation of the pus by pulling the involved lash or incising the abscess is advised.
3. Antibiotic eyedrops and ointment are applied to control and prevent infection.
4. Systemic broad-spectrum antibiotics may be useful.
5. Analgesics and anti-inflammatory drugs control pain and inflammation.

CHALAZION (TARSAL OR MEIBOMIAN CYST)

Chalazion is a chronic granulomatous inflammation of the meibomian gland.

Etiology

1. It is probably due to chronic irritation caused by an organism of low virulence. The glandular tissue is replaced by granulation tissue containing giant cells predominantly.
2. It is often multiple in number occurring in crops.
3. It is more common in adults than in children.

Symptoms

1. There is no pain unless chalazion is secondarily infected.
2. There is disfigurement due to the presence of swelling in the lid.
3. It may be single or multiple in number.

Signs

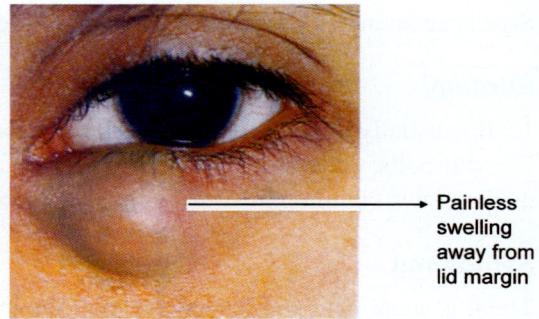

Painless swelling away from lid margin

1. A small non-tender hard swelling in the lid, slightly away from the lid margin is seen.
2. There are no signs of acute inflammation.
3. On everting the lid, the conjunctiva over the swelling is red or purple. It is grey in colour in later stages. It may be yellow when secondarily infected by pyogenic organisms.

Chalazion

Course

1. Complete spontaneous resolution may occur rarely.
2. The contents of the chalazion may be extruded through the conjunctiva occasionally which resembles a fungating mass.
3. *Marginal chalazion*—The granuloma is formed in the duct of the gland which projects as a reddish-grey nodule on the intermarginal strip.
4. *Recurrence* may occur in seborrhoeic dermatitis, acne rosacea and malignant change.

Treatment

1. It is incised and thoroughly scraped.
    - The conjunctiva and lid are anaesthetised with procaine.
    - The lid is everted and chalazion clamp is fixed at the site of maximum discolouration with the hollow side facing the conjunctiva.
    - A small vertical incision is given with a sharp blade over the conjunctival side.
    - The semifluid contents escape and walls of the cavity are thoroughly scraped with the chalazion scoop. The cavity is cauterized with carbolic acid to avoid recurrence.
    - Bleeding stops and usually no dressing is necessary.
2. Injection of triamcinolone directly into the chalazion may cause complete resolution.

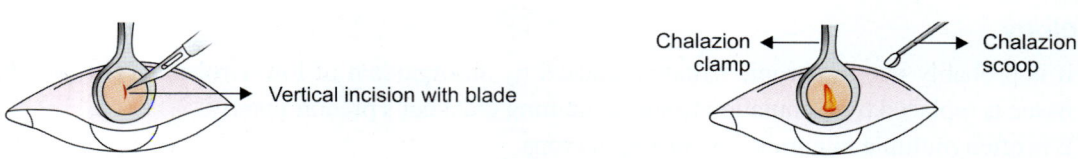

Incision and curettage of chalazion

DIFFERENCES BETWEEN STYE (HORDEOLUM), CHALAZION AND INTERNAL HORDEOLUM

	STYE (HORDEOLUM)	CHALAZION	INTERNAL HORDEOLUM
1. Onset	Acute	Chronic	Acute meibomian gland
2. Gland	Zeis's gland	Meibomian gland	Suppurative
3. Type of inflammation	Suppurative	Granulomatous	Severe pain
4. Symptoms	Acute pain and swelling	Painless Disfigurement	Yellow point seen on everting the lid
5. Signs	Localised, hard (pus) and tender swelling near the lid margin	Hard swelling away from lid margin	Vertical incision and drainage
6. Treatment	Hot fomentation Antibiotic and Removal of eyelash	Vertical incision and drainage	Antibiotic and analgesic

INTERNAL HORDEOLUM

It is an acute suppurative inflammation of the meibomian gland. It is uncommon.

Etiology

It occurs due to the secondary infection of the chalazion.

Symptoms

These are more violent than the stye because the gland is larger and it is embedded deeply in the dense fibrous tissue.

Signs

1. A yellow spot (pus) is seen shining through the conjunctiva on everting the lid.
2. It may burst through the duct, conjunctiva or the skin rarely.

Treatment

It is same as for the stye but the infected chalazion is incised vertically from the conjunctival side.

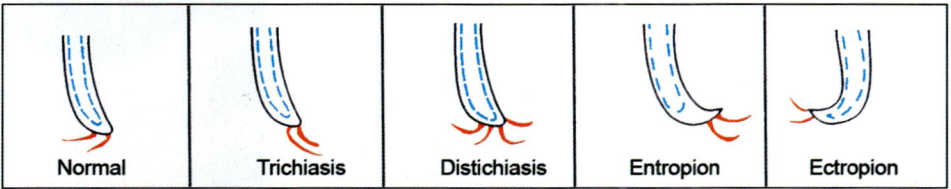

Section of the upper eyelid showing normal and abnormal position of tarsus and eyelashes

ANOMALIES IN THE POSITION OF LIDS

TRICHIASIS

Trichiasis is a condition where the eyelashes are misdirected backwards rubbing against the cornea. A few eyelashes or whole lid margin may be involved.

Etiology

1. Entropion due to cicatrization in stage IV of trachoma is a common cause.
2. Spastic entropion in old persons or due to tight bandaging may cause trichiasis.
3. Blepharitis specially the ulcerative form may result in trichiasis.
4. It may occur after recurrent stye.
5. Scars of the lid following burn, injury or operation may cause trichiasis.

Symptoms

1. There is foreign body sensation and photophobia due to corneal involvement.
2. Irritation, pain and lacrimation are very troublesome.
3. Conjunctival congestion is present usually.

Signs

1. Reflex blepharospasm and photophobia are seen in cases of corneal involvement.
2. Superficial corneal opacities are often present.
3. Ciliary congestion is often associated.

Complications

Recurrent erosion and corneal ulcer are common complications.

Treatment

1. *Isolated cilia*
    i. *Epilation* or removal of misdirected eyelash is repeated every few weeks.
    ii. *Electrolysis*—It is preferable as it causes destruction of hair follicle by a current of 3-5 mA for 10 seconds. It may be repeated every few months.
2. *Whole lid margin involvement*—Operative procedures as for entropion are employed.

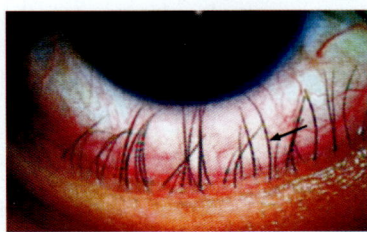
Trichiasis and corneal ulcer

ENTROPION

It is a condition in which the lid margin rolls inwards.

Types

There are two main types of entropion—spastic and cicatricial.

Spastic entropion

Etiology

1. *Spastic entropion*
    i. It is due to the spasm of the orbicularis oculi muscle as may occur after tight bandaging after operation or following chronic irritative corneal condition.
    ii. It commonly occurs in old people involving the lower lid.

2. *Cicatricial entropion*—It results due to contraction of the palpebral conjunctiva in:
    i. *Trachoma stage IV*
    ii. *Ulcerative blepharitis*
    iii. *Burns*
    iv. *Operations*
    v. *Diphtheritic membranous conjunctivitis.*

Symptoms and Signs

They are same as for trichiasis.

Entropion of lower lid with corneal scarring

Treatment

1. *Spastic entropion*—The basic cause of blepharospasm is treated:
    i. If it is due to prolonged and tight bonding, discontinue the application of bandage.
    ii. In senile patients the lower lid is pulled downwards by a strip of adhesive plaster.
2. *Cicatricial entropion*—It is treated by operative procedures.
    i. Resection of skin and muscle—Removal of an elliptical or spindle-shaped strip of skin and muscle 3 mm away from the lid margin corrects mild degree of entropion. It is the simplest procedure.

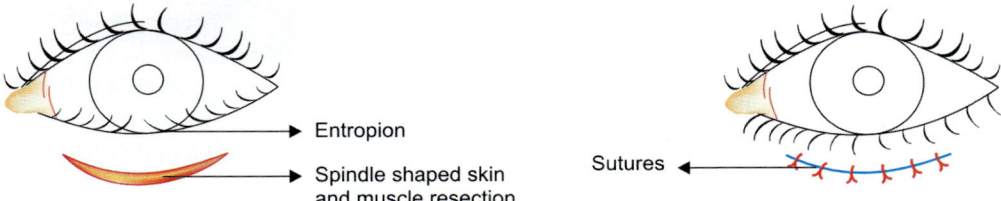

Skin and muscle resection

  ii. Resection of tarsus, skin and muscle—It gives support to the atrophic tarsus and atonic muscles as paring of the tarsal plate is done along with skin and muscle resection in this procedure.
  iii. Burow's operations—This procedure is done from the conjunctival side by everting the lid over a spatula. A horizontal incision is made through the conjunctiva, tarsal plate but not the skin along the whole lid margin 2-3 mm away from the posterior border of the lid.

   The temporal end of the strip may then be divided by a small vertical incision. The edge of the lid is kept everted during healing by a spindle-shaped pad of oiled skin, kept in position by sutures suitably applied.

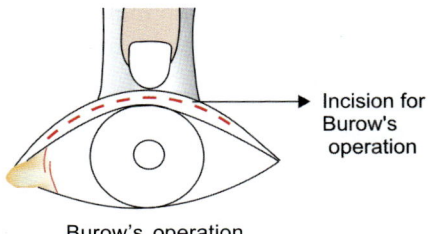

Burow's operation

ECTROPION

It is a condition in which the lid margin rolls outwards.

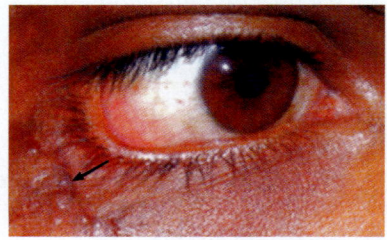
Cicatricial ectropion

Types
1. *Spastic ectropion*
   It occurs due to blepharospasm when lids are well-supported by the globe. It usually occurs in children and young persons.
2. *Mechanical ectropion*
   It occurs as a result of thickening of the conjunctiva, e.g. as in trachoma stage IV.
3. *Cicatricial ectropion*
   It may be due to several conditions such as chronic conjunctivitis, blepharitis, injury, burns, ulcers, etc.
4. *Senile ectropion*
   It is present in the lower lid due to the laxity of orbicularis oculi muscle and other tissues of lid.
5. *Paralytic ectropion*
   It occurs due to the paralysis of orbicularis oculi muscle.

Symptom

The most common symptom is epiphora, i.e. constant watering of the eyes.

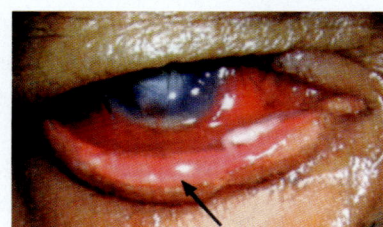
Senile ectropion

Signs
1. Conjunctiva becomes dry in appearance and thickened in texture.
2. Chronic conjunctivitis may be present due to exposure of the conjunctiva and cornea.
3. Corneal ulcer may develop (exposure keratitis).

Treatment
1. *Spastic ectropion*—The underlying cause of blepharospasm is treated.
2. *Cicatricial ectropion*—The aim of surgery is to free the lid margin from scar tissue and restore the lid to its normal position and function.
   i. *V-Y operation is done in mild cases.* A 'V'-shaped incision is made in the skin of the lower lid which includes the scar. The skin is excised and the wound is sutured in Y-shaped pattern thus correcting the ectropion.

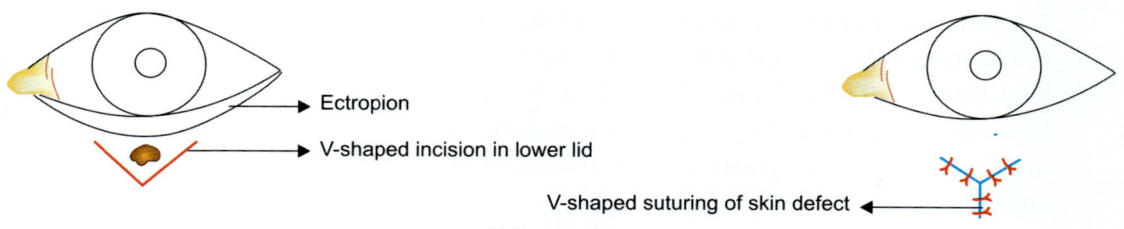
V-Y operation

ii. *Excision of scar tissue and application of skin graft* is useful in cases of extensive scarring. Split skin graft or full-thickness skin grafts are taken from the upper lid, behind the ear, inner side of upper arm or thigh.
3. *Senile ectropion*
   a. *Full-thickness shortening of the lid* is done by making an inverted house-shaped incision at least 5 mm away from the punctum and repairing it. This is useful if the ectropion is most marked in the middle portion of the lower lid.

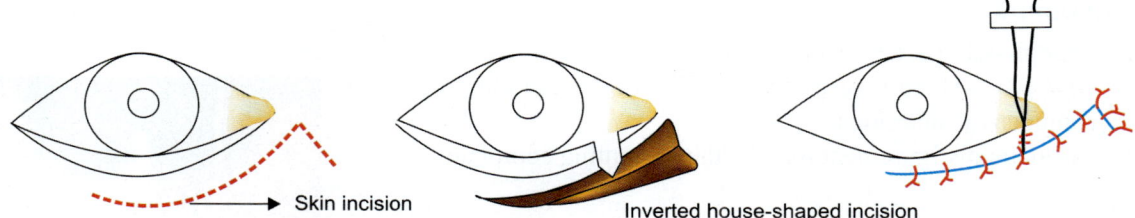

Full-thickness shortening of the lid

   b. *Kuhnt-Szymanowski procedure*—It is useful if the ectropion is severe and marked over the lateral half of the lower lid. It is modified by Byron Smith. A skin flap is prepared and a full-thickness shorting is done at the lateral canthus. The excess skin is removed and traction sutures applied.
4. *Paralytic ectropion*—Lateral tarsorrhaphy may be indicated. The palpebral aperture is shortened by uniting the lid margins at the junction of middle and outer one-third.

SYMBLEPHARON

It is a condition of adhesion of the lids to the globe.

Etiology

It is due to the formation of raw surfaces upon two opposite spots of the palpebral and bulbar conjunctiva, causing adhesion during the healing process. It is often due to :
   i. Burns due to heat or caustics
   ii. Ulcers
   iii. Diphtheria
   iv. Operations.

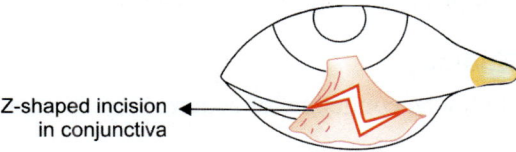

Z-plasty operation for symblepharon

Types
1. *Anterior symblepharon*—The lid margin is usually implicated.
2. *Posterior symblepharon*—The fornix is implicated so that the conjunctival surfaces are adhered to each other.
3. *Total symblepharon*—The fornix and lid margins are involved together. The lids are completely adherent to the eyeball. It is a rare condition.

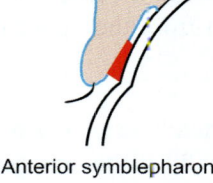 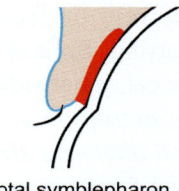

Anterior symblepharon   Posterior symblepharon   Total symblepharon

Types of symblepharon

Symptoms

1. Lagophthalmos, i.e. inability to close the lids properly is often present.
2. *Diplopia*—There is restricted mobility of the eye due to marked conjunctival adhesions.
3. Cosmetic disfigurement may be the presenting complaint.

Signs

Broad or narrow bands of fibrous tissue are seen stretching between lid and globe.

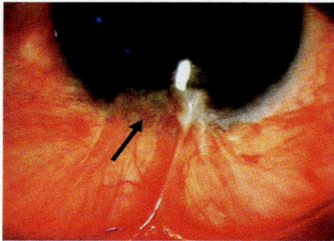

Symblepharon–traumatic

Treatment

1. *Prophylaxis*—Prevention is most important. It is achieved by applying eye ointment and moving a glass rod in the fornices several times a day. A therapeutic contact lens may be helpful.
2. *Mucous membrane graft*—The raw surfaces are covered by buccal mucous membrane graft or conjunctiva from the upper temporal quadrant of the same or opposite eye. It is difficult in cases of posterior symblepharon and broad bands. Therefore, great care is taken to prevent perforation of the globe.
3. *Z-plasty* operation can also be done.

ANKYLOBLEPHARON

It is a condition of the adhesion of the margins of the two eyelids. The adhesion may be partial or complete. It is usually associated with symblepharon.

Etiology

It may be congenital or acquired due to chemical burn, e.g. acid, alkali.

Treatment

Separation of the lid margins along with mucous membrane or conjunctival grafting is recommended.

BLEPHAROPHIMOSIS

It is a condition where the palpebral fissure appears to be contracted at the outer canthus.

Etiology

It may be congenital or acquired due to prolonged blepharospasm or epiphora.

Treatment

Canthoplasty, i.e. incision of the outer canthus is the treatment of choice. Apply a small artery forceps to the outer canthus. Wait for 2-3 minutes in order to achieve haemostasis. Then cut the outer canthus with a fine scissors or blade.

LAGOPHTHALMOS

It is a condition of incomplete closure of the palpebral aperture when eyes are shut.

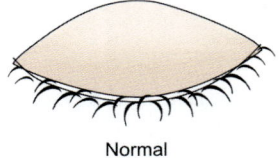
Normal

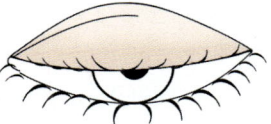
Incomplete closure of palpebral fissure on closing the eyes

Etiology
1. Congenital deformity of the lids.
2. Ectropion.
3. Proptosis.
4. Paralysis of orbicularis oculi muscle.
5. Absence of reflex blinking in extremely ill patients.

Complication
Exposure keratitis develops usually in the lower part of the cornea due to incomplete closure of lids.

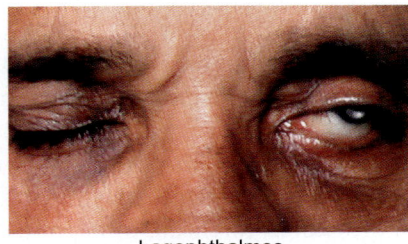
Lagophthalmos

Treatment
1. Application of antibiotic eye ointment and bandage during sleep is recommended.
2. Lateral tarsorrhaphy or paramedian tarsorrhaphy is done in neuroparalytic cases.

PTOSIS

It is a condition in which there is drooping of the upper lid below its normal position.

Etiology
1. *Congenital ptosis*—It occurs in about 80% of all cases. It is often bilateral. Heredity is an important factor. It is often due to:
    i. *Maldevelopment of the levator muscle.*
    ii. *Congenital weakness of the superior rectus muscle.*
    iii. *It may be associated with lid deformity like epicanthus.*
    iv. *Synkinetic ptosis* is seen in Marcus Gunn jaw winking phenomenon due to misdirected 3rd nerve or abnormal nervous communication between 3 and 5 cranial nerves. There is unilateral ptosis (winking) on movement of the jaw, i.e. on moving the pterygoid muscle.
2. *Acquired ptosis*
    i. *Neurogenic ptosis*—There is partial or complete paralysis of 3rd nerve.

ii. *Mechanical ptosis*—It is due to increased weight of the upper lid as a result of oedema, hypertrophy (trachoma) or tumour formation.
iii. *Myogenic ptosis*—It may be due to trauma to the levator muscle, muscular dystrophy and myasthenia gravis.
3. ***Pseudoptosis***—The appearance of ptosis is simulated due to lack of support of the upper lid in cases of microphthalmos, shrunken eyeball (phthisi bulbi) enophthalmos and empty socket.

Types

Classification of ptosis

1. Unilateral ptosis — Partial / Complete
2. Bilateral ptosis — Partial / Complete

Symptoms

1. There is no symptom if the pupil is not covered by the lid.
2. There is visual disturbance when the pupil is covered by the lid.
3. Cosmetic disfigurement is the most common complaint.
4. Compensatory changes may be present such as wrinkling of the skin of forehead, tilting of the head backwards and elevation of the eyebrow.

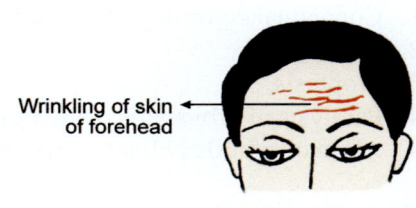

Wrinkling of skin of forehead

Ptosis

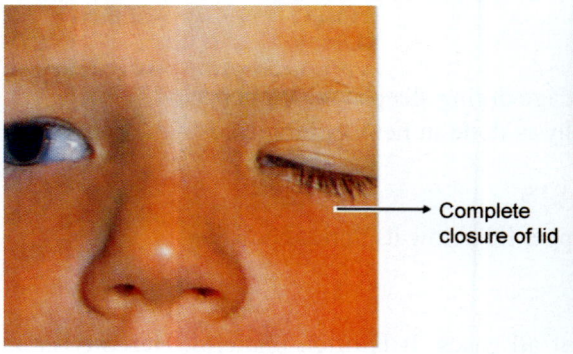

Complete closure of lid

Congenital ptosis

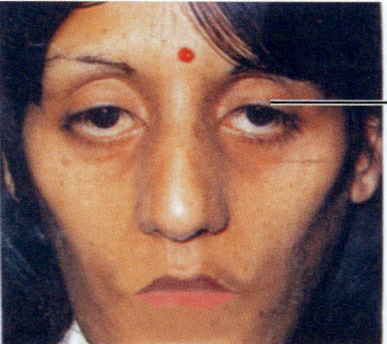

Partial drooping of lids
Bilateral ptosis

Bilateral ptosis - myasthenia gravis

Signs

1. The margin of the upper lid covers more of the cornea.
2. The palpebral fissure is narrower than normal.
3. There are no skin folds seen in the skin of the upper lid.
4. On an attempt to elevate the upper lid, there is elevation of the eyebrow and wrinkling of the skin of the forehead due to hyperaction of the frontalis muscle.
5. The head is lifted backwards so as to draw the lid upwards beyond the pupillary area.

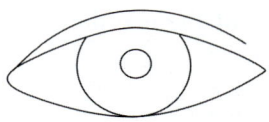
Normal eye

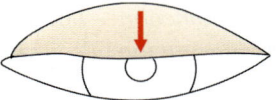
Narrow palpebral aperture
Ptosis

6. *Levator muscle function*
    i. This is tested by placing a thumb firmly against the patient's eyebrow to block the action of the frontalis muscle.
    ii. The patient is asked to look down as far as possible and then to look up.
    iii. The amount of excursion is measured by a scale and levator muscle function is graded as follows:

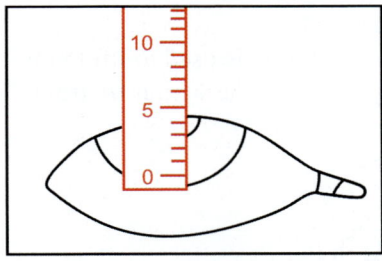 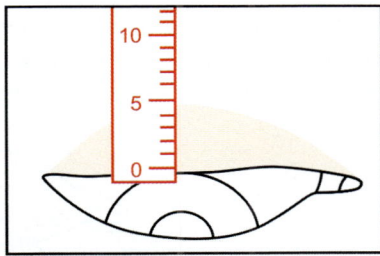

Measurement of levator muscle function

Normal—15 mm
Good—8 mm or more
Fair—5-7 mm
Poor—4 mm or less.

7. *Amount of ptosis*—In unilateral cases, vertical fissure on both sides is measured. The difference in measurement of both the eyes indicates the degree of ptosis.
    i. Mild ptosis—The difference in measurement is 2 mm.
    ii. Moderate ptosis—The difference in measurement is 3 mm.
    iii. Severe ptosis—The difference in measurement is 4 mm or more.
    A drawing should be made or ideally a photograph should be taken in
      a. Primary position
      b. Up—gaze
      c. Down—gaze.

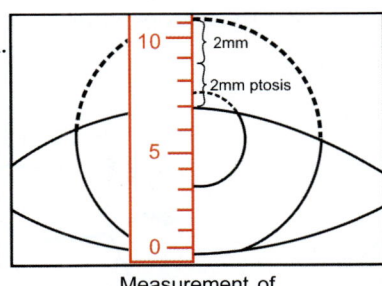
Measurement of vertical palpebral fissure

8. The other investigations include
    i. *Ocular mobility*—It is done to test the action of extraocular muscles.
    ii. *Corneal sensitivity*—If the cornea is insensitive, ptosis correction will result in corneal ulceration.
    iii. *Marcus Gunn jaw winking phenomenon*—There is unilateral ptosis on movements of the jaw as a result of misdirected 3rd nerve.

iv. *Bell's phenomenon*—The upwards and outwards rolling up of the eye during sleep or on forcibly closing the lids is known as the Bell's phenomenon.

Treatment
1. In case of paralysis of the 3rd nerve, the underlying cause is treated. In complete paralysis of 3rd nerve operation is usually contraindicated due to intolerable postoperative diplopia.
2. In cases of incurable paralysis, congenital and mechanical ptosis, the deformity can be relieved by suitable operation. The ideal age for surgery is 4-5 years but it can be done early in cases of complete bilateral ptosis.

Principle
There are three main techniques available for the correction of ptosis:
  i. If the levator muscle action is good, it may be shortened.
  ii. If the levator muscle is paralysed, the superior rectus muscle is used to lift the lid.
  iii. If both levator and superior rectus muscles are paralysed, the action of frontalis muscle is utilized.

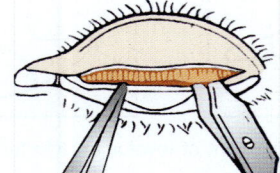

Blaskovics operation (conjunctival side)

Technique
1. *Resection of levator muscle*—If the levator muscle is not completely paralysed, the levator muscle may be shortened by the resection of the muscle.
    i. Blaskovics operation is done from the conjunctival side.
    ii. Everbusch operation is done from the skin surface.

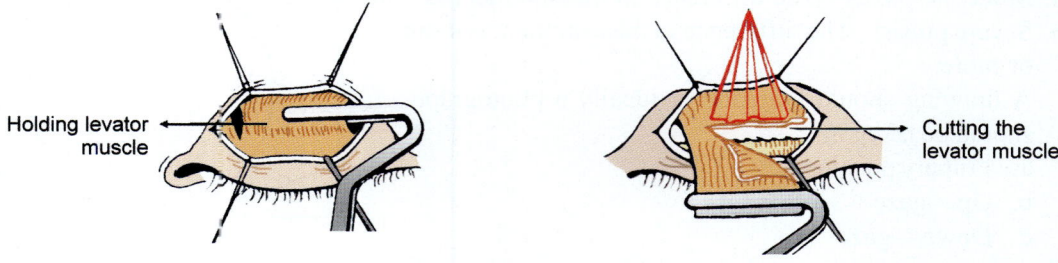

Everbusch operation (skin side)

   iii. Fasanella-Servat operation—The levator muscle is shortened along with excision of 4-5 mm of the tarsal plate. Muller's muscle and palpebral conjunctiva.
2. *Motais operation*—If the levator muscle is paralysed, the superior rectus is pressed into service to elevate the lid.

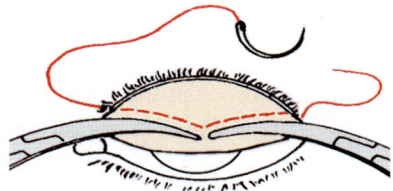

Fasanella-Servat operation

3. *Hess's operation*—If both levator palpebrae superioris and superior rectus muscles are paralysed, action of frontalis muscle is used in raising the lid by passing silk mattress sutures in tarsal plate.

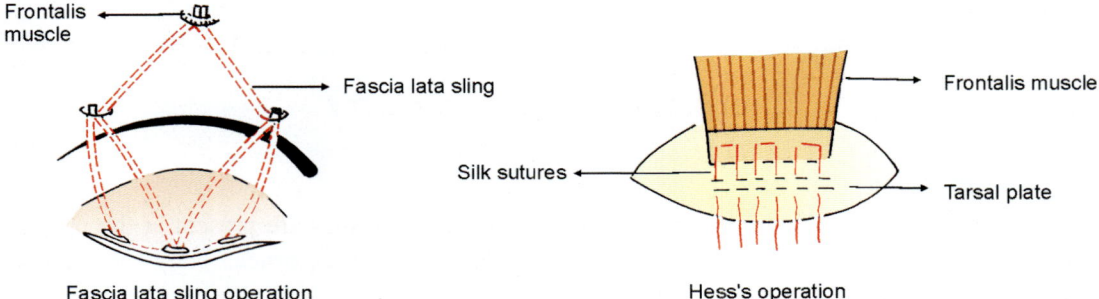

Fascia lata sling operation　　　　　　　Hess's operation

4. *Fascia lata sling operation*—Three incisions are made in the upper lid about 4 mm from the lid margin. Three more deep incisions are made above the eyebrow as shown in the diagram. The fascial strips are drawn through the lid openings and secured tightly by 5.0 chromic catgut at each eyebrow incision.

TUMOURS OF THE LIDS

The xanthoma, naevus, haemangioma and neurofibroma are benign tumours of the lids.

1. Benign Tumour

  i. **Xanthoma**
     These are often bilateral, symmetrical, slightly raised yellow plaques situated near the inner canthus. They are common in elderly women and diabetics with excess cholesterol formation.
 ii. **Haemangioma**
     It occurs as a localized capillary angioma or cavernous angioma. The lid may be affected along with the facial angioma as in Sturge-Weber syndrome.
iii. **Mole (naevus)**
     It occurs at the lid margin, involving both skin and conjuncitva. It is removed by excision as it may turn malignant.
 iv. **Neurofibroma**
     It is usually of plexiform type affecting the upper lid as in von Recklinghausen's disease or generalized neurofibromatosis. The thickened nerves can be felt through the skin as hard cords.

2. Malignant Tumour

i. Squamous cell carcinoma
It affects the elderly persons usually. It is seen at the edge of the lid (transition zone) where the characteristic of epithelium changes. It starts as a nodule which ulcerates. The preauricular lymph nodes are often enlarged.

Treatment—It is excised completely.

ii. Basal cell carcinoma (Rodent ulcer)
It is the most common malignant tumour of the lid. It is seen in the lower lid near the inner canthus usually. It is locally malignant. The epithelial growth spreads under the skin in all directions. It invades and destroys the lids, orbit and bone.

Treatment—If small, it is excised completely. If large, it can be treated with radiation therapy.

CONGENITAL ABNORMALITY

1. Distichiasis
It is a rare condition where one or more extra rows of eyelashes are present at the opening of meibomian glands. These are directed backwards towards the cornea. They rub against the cornea causing corneal erosion.

2. Coloboma
There is a triangular notch in the upper lid margin near the nasal side usually. Coloboma of the iris or accessory auricle may be associated.

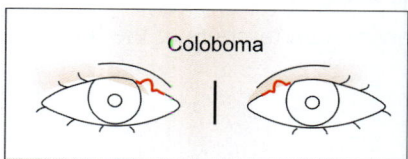

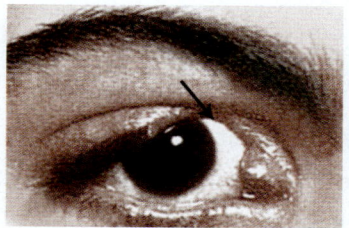

Coloboma

3. Epicanthus
It is a bilateral condition which may be associated with ptosis. A triangular fold of skin covers the medial canthus. The eyes appear to be far apart. It can be corrected by plastic surgery.

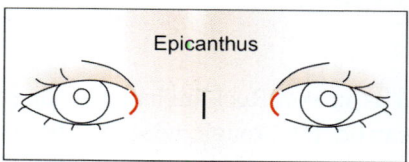

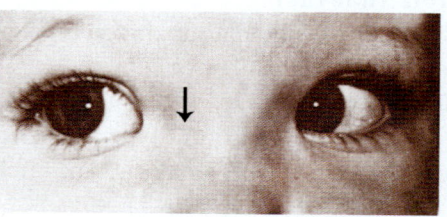

Epicanthus

MULTIPLE CHOICE QUESTIONS

1. Outrolling of the conjunctiva of the eyelid is called
   a. coloboma
   b. pterygium
   c. ectropion
   d. none of the above
2. Distichiasis is
   a. an extra row of eyelashes
   b. central fusion of eyelid
   c. white coloured lashes
   d. absence of lashes
3. Chalazion is a chronic inflammatory granuloma of
   a. meibomian gland
   b. Zeis gland
   c. Moll's sweat gland
   d. Wolfring gland
4. A semilunar fold of skin, situated above and sometimes covering the inner canthus is known as
   a. coloboma of lid
   b. epicanthus
   c. cryptophthalmos
   d. microblepharon
5. Hordeolum externum is an inflammation of
   a. lid margin
   b. tarsal plate
   c. meibomian gland
   d. Zeis gland
6. Lagophthalmos is the condition of
   a. incomplete closure of the palpebral aperture
   b. drooping of the upper eyelid below its normal position
   c. lid margin rolls outwards
   d. none of the above
7. Tylosis is
   a. hypertrophy and thickening of eyelid margin
   b. inversion of eyelid
   c. senile eversion of eyelid
   d. distortion of cilia
8. Skin grafting of upper lid should be done ideally from
   a. a split skin graft
   b. a full-thickness graft from behind the ear
   c. a full-thickness graft from forehand
   d. forehead rotation flap
9. Regarding lagophthalmos which is correct
   a. incomplete closure of palpebral aperture
   b. seen in extensively ill or morbid patients
   c. cornea is exposed and keratitis sets in
   d. all of the above
10. Paralytic ptosis is due to
    a. complete or partial 3rd nerve palsy
    b. 4th nerve palsy
    c. 6th nerve palsy
    d. 7th nerve palsy
11. Blepharitis is an inflammation of
    a. lid
    b. eyelashes
    c. lid margin
    d. Moll's gland
12. The most common complication of lagophthalmos is
    a. suppurative conjunctivitis
    b. exposure keratitis
    c. entropion
    d. trichiasis

Nerve Supply
1. *Sensory nerve*—The lacrimal branch of the ophthalmic division of the 5th nerve.
2. *Sympathetic supply*—The carotid plexus of the cervical sympathetic.
3. *Secretomotor fibres*—These are derived from the facial nerve via the sphenopalatine ganglion.

TEARS

Tear is a secretion from the lacrimal gland. It is slightly alkaline and consists mainly of water, small quantities of salts, such as sodium chloride, sugar, urea, protein and lysozyme, a bactericidal enzyme. The secretion of tear does not begin before 3-4 weeks after birth. The average normal secretion of tears is 0.5-2.2 ml. The normal pH of tear is 7.5.

The Tear Film
The fluid which fills the conjunctival sac consists of 3 layers namely:
1. *Mucous layer*—A hydrated layer of mucoproteins secreted by the goblet cells, crypts of Henle and glands of Manz.
2. *Aqueous layer*—It consists of tears secreted by the lacrimal gland and accessory lacrimal glands, e.g. glands of Krause and Wolfring.
3. *Lipid layer*—It consists mainly of cholesterol, esters and lipid being secreted by the meibomian glands and Zeis glands.

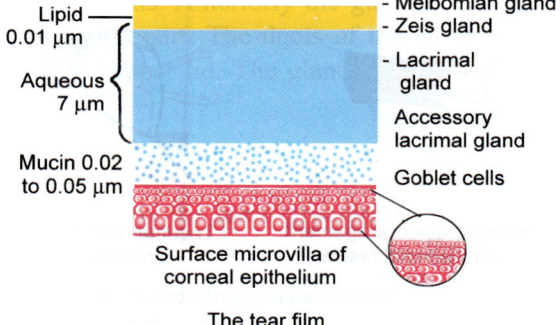

The tear film

Functions
The surface of the eyeball must remain wet for comfort and normal functioning. The tear film spreads over the surface of corneal epithelium by gravity, capillary action and blinking of the eyelids.
1. It washes away irritating material, e.g. dust and grit. It contains protective substances such as lysozyme, immunoglobulin, lactoferrin, compliments.
2. The bactericidal lysozyme (muramidase) prevents microbial infection.
3. The oiliness of this mixed fluid delays evaporation and prevents drying of the conjunctiva and cornea.

Normally, the rate of secretion of tears keeps pace with the rate of drainage. When a foreign body or other irritant enters the eye, the secretion of tears is greatly increased and the conjunctival vessels dilate. Secretion of tears is also increased in emotional stress states.

I. Diseases of the lacrimal gland
1. Acute dacryoadenitis
2. Dacryops
3. Mikulicz's syndrome
4. Tumours.

II. Diseases of the lacrimal passages
1. Congenital anomalies of the puncta and canaliculi
2. Dacryocystitis—acute and chronic.

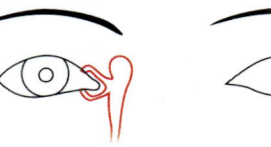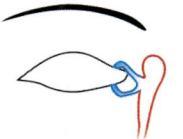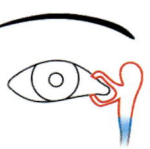

Elimination of tears by lacrimal pump mechanism

ACUTE DACRYO-ADENITIS

It is an acute inflammation of the lacrimal gland.

Etiology

It is a rare condition occurring in association with mumps, influenza, infectious mononucleosis, etc. sometimes leading to suppuration and fistula formation.

Symptom

There is marked pain, redness and swelling in the upper and outer angle of the orbit along with excessive watering of the eye.

Signs

1. A tender swelling is present at the outer part of the upper lid spreading towards the temple and cheeks.
2. There is congestion and chemosis of the conjunctiva in upper part.
3. Preauricular glands may be enlarged and tender.

Complications

1. Suppuration leads to abscess and fistula formation.
2. There may be cystic degeneration and atrophy of the gland resulting in dry eye.

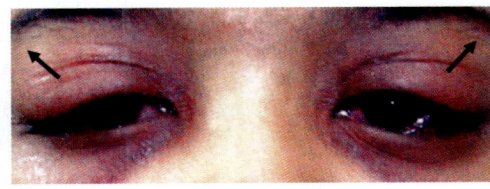

Acute dacryo-adenitis – Both eyes

Differential Diagnosis

It should be differentiated from lid abscess, stye, suppurative chalazion, acute purulent conjunctivitis, orbital cellulitis and osteomyeliltis of frontal bone.

Treatment

1. Hot compresses are applied several times a day.
2. Systemic broad-spectrum antibiotics are given in full doses.
3. Incision and drainage is done in cases of abscess formation.

DACRYOPS

It is a cystic swelling of the lacrimal gland due to retention of lacrimal secretion as a result of blockage of one of the lacrimal ducts.

MIKULICZ'S SYNDROME

There is symmetrical enlargement of the lacrimal and salivary glands (parotid glands) usually with lymphoid tissue hyperplasia. The etiology is unknown but it is seen in uveoparotid inflammations.

TUMOURS

Benign Tumour

The most common tumour is pleomorphic adenocarcinoma (mixed tumour). The benign mixed tumour usually occurs in middle life. It presents as a slowly progressive painless swelling in the upper lid. It may result in mechanical ptosis. It should be excised.

Malignant Tumour

The malignant tumour presents with a short history and pain. If malignant, radical surgical removal is necessary.

CONGENITAL ANOMALIES OF THE PUNCTA AND CANALICULI

Occasionally the puncta may be absent or constricted. There may be two puncta in a lid, both opening into the same canaliculus. Sometimes a groove is found instead of a canaliculus. The canaliculus may be occluded by other causes such as scar, foreign body (eyelash) or after prolonged use of IDU (iododeoxyuridine) eyedrops for viral affections.

Treatment

1. Punctum dilator is inserted in the punctum.
2. An opening is made and canaliculus knife is introduced in the punctum.

DACRYOCYSTITIS

Dacryocystitis is the inflammation of the lacrimal sac.

Classification

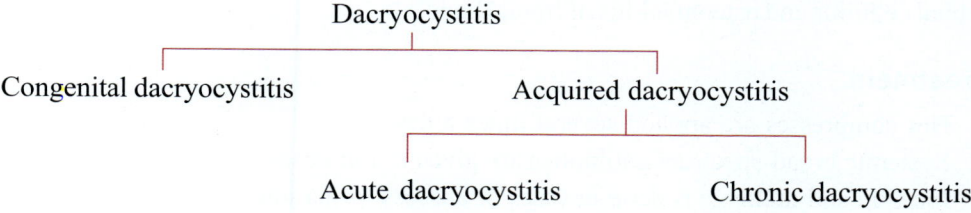

CONGENITAL DACRYOCYSTITIS
(DACRYOCYSTITIS IN THE NEWBORN)

Inflammation of the lacrimal sac in the newborn may present as an acute or chronic process.

Etiology

There is failure in canalization of the nasolacrimal duct, the lumen being blocked by epithelial debris. It may be a bilateral condition.

Symptom

1. There is epiphora or continuous watering of the eyes usually evident in 2nd week of life. Normally, the tears are secreted after 3-4 weeks after birth.
2. There may be purulent discharge or conjunctivitis in infected cases.

Signs

1. Stricky mucopurulent discharge and persistent epiphora are two important signs.
2. There is regurgitation of mucopurulent discharge on pressure over the sac area.

Treatment

1. Conservative treatment is indicated in early cases.
   i. *Massage over the lacrimal sac area* and clean the discharge several times a day. This constitutes the treatment of congenital nasolacrimal duct block up to 6-8 weeks of age. Method—Teach the mother to apply pressure over the sac area by the thumb. Then bring the thumb downward pressing towards the ala of the nose. This is repeated 3-4 times thrice daily. Massage increases the hydrostatic pressure in the sac and helps to open up the membranous occlusions. It should be carried out at least 3 times a day to be followed by instillation of antibiotic drops.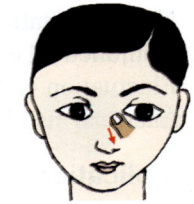

      Massage with thumb
   ii. *Broad-spectrum antibiotic* eyedrops are instilled frequently after expressing the contents of the sac by pressure over the sac area. Most cases (90%) are cured by this treatment.
2. Surgical treatment—*Aim*—To recanalise the nasolacrimal duct.
   i. Probing of the nasolacrimal duct.
   ii. Intubation with silicone tube—This may be performed if repeated probing is a failure. The silicone tube should be kept in the nasolacrimal duct for about six months.
   iii. Balloon dilatation of the duct may be tried.
   iv. Dacryocystorhinostomy (DCR) operation. When the condition fails to respond up to 4 years of age, DCR operation should be performed.

Probing of Nasolacrimal Duct

If there is no improvement after three months, probing of the nasolacrimal duct is performed through the upper punctum under general anesthesia. Great care is taken to avoid injury to the walls of the duct as it may cause fibrosis or infection.

3. *Atonic sac*—The contents of the atonic sac can be evacuated by external pressure only.
4. Lacrimal abscess may occur following probing or spontaneously due to pyogenic infection.
5. Lacrimal fistula may occur if the abscess bursts open repeatedly. The fistulous track is lined by the epithelium which prevent healing.

Investigations

1. Nasal examination is important to exclude deviation of septum, growth and atrophic rhinitis to judge the success of DCR operation.
2. Radiological examination—The lacrimal passage is visualized radiographically by :
    i. Dacryocystography (DCG) is done using lipiodol, urografin, conray, iodized oil, etc. It outlines the lacrimal excretory passage. X-ray is taken immediately and after 10-15 minutes to find out the size of the sac and site of obstruction.
    ii. Subtraction macrodacryocystography with canalicular catheterization is a more accurate diagnostic technique.
    iii. Radioactive tracer containing sulphur is instilled into the conjunctival sac and its excretion is visualized by gamma camera.

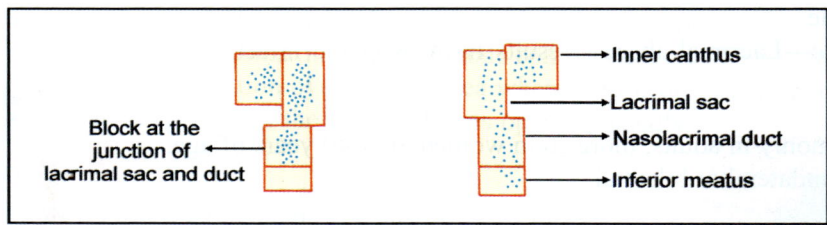

Gamma camera images

Treatment

1. **In recent cases**
   Repeating syringing of the nasolacrimal duct and frequent instillation of antibiotic drops is indicated in recent cases. It is indicated for two purposes:
      i. *Diagnostic*—It confirms the block in the lacrimal passage.
      ii. *Therapeutic*—Syringing is curative in early cases by separating the oedematous mucosal walls sticking together and by clearing the mucosal debris.
   Principle—It reduces the swelling of the inflamed mucosa and restores the patency of lacrimal excretory passage by clearing the epithelial debris.
   Method
      i. Conjunctival sac is anaesthetized by frequent instillation of topical xylocaine or other suitable local anaesthetic.
      ii. Punctum is dilated with the Nettleship's punctum dilator.
      iii. Lacrimal sac is syringed out 2-3 times using 24-26 gauge cannula attached to 5 cc syringe filled with normal saline and antibiotic drops are instilled.

Syringing through lower punctum

- Syringing is repeated daily initially and later twice weekly.
- After a few days the fluid may pass freely into the nasal duct.

2. **In recalcitrant cases**—The following surgical procedures are advised:
   i. *Dacryocystectomy*—The lacrimal sac is excised completely in elderly persons specially if the lacrimal sac is fibrosed.
   ii. *Dacryocystorhinostomy*—It is a nasal drainage operation performed in young and adult patients. It is the treatment of choice in most cases as it cures the persistent epiphora. The sac must be of normal size in order to anastomose it with the healthy nasal mucosa.
   iii. *Insertion of special tubes*, e.g. Lester-Jones tube, Pawar's cannula in the lacrimal sac facilitates the drainage of tears into the nasal cavity.

Dacryocystectomy (DC)

A complete excision of the lacrimal sac is done in this procedure. Thus, the lacrimal sac is removed as a whole.

Method

1. The lacrimal sac and the area surrounding it is anaesthetized by an injection of local anaesthetic.
2. A curved incision 2 mm above the medial palpebral ligament, 3 mm to the nasal side of inner canthus and 4 mm downwards and outwards is given. It coincides with the surface marking of the anterior lacrimal crest.
3. Orbicularis muscle is split along the incision line.
4. Lacrimal fascia is exposed and incised.
5. Lacrimal sac is freed by blunt dissector and drawn forwards. It is twisted 2-3 times and torn away from the nasal duct.
6. The upper end of the nasal duct is curetted and cauterized with carbolic acid.
7. Orbicularis muscle is sutured with catgut and the skin is sutured with continuous subcuticular sutures preferably for cosmetic purpose.

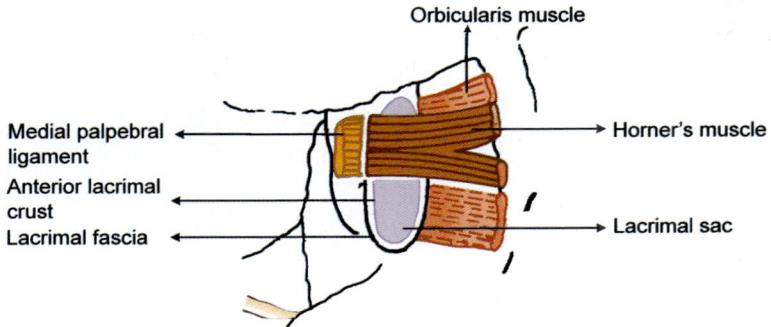

Normal position of lacrimal sac in lacrimal fossa

Complication
Epiphora may persist for sometime and then it gradually wears off.

Dacryocystorhinostomy (DCR)
It is a nasal drainage operation. It has the advantage over dacryocystectomy as there is no epiphora or watering of eyes postoperatively.

Method
- The nasal fossa of the same side is packed with cocaine or xylocaine and adrenaline.
- The canaliculi are dilated and lacrimal sac is irrigated with warm saline.
- The early steps are same as for excision of the sac.

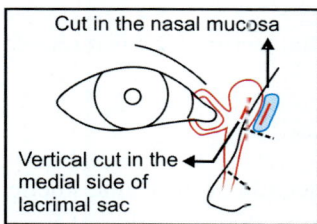
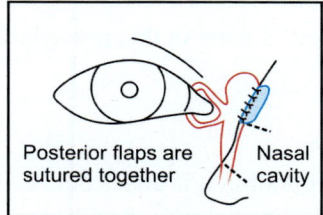
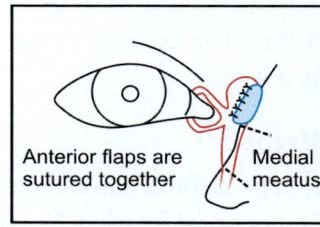

Dacryocystorhinostomy

- The periosteum over the lacrimal crest is incised and lacrimal bone is exposed.
- The bony crest is removed with a gouge and hammer and nasal mucosa is exposed.
- The nasal mucosa of the middle meatus is anastomosed with the medial wall of the sac by making vertical incisions in them.
- Syringing is done to test the patency of the passage after 1-2 days postoperatively.

Complications
i. *Haemorrhage*—Intranasal bleeding may occur from the nasal mucosa which requires nasal packing for 24 hours.
ii. *Failed DCR*—Small bony opening is the most important cause. Other causes include, improper suturing, postoperative infection, nasal pathology such as polyp, etc.

MULTIPLE CHOICE QUESTIONS

1. Epiphora occurs in
   a. iritis
   b. trachoma
   c. chronic dacryocystitis
   d. acute congestive glaucoma
2. The syndrome consisting of symmetrical enlargement of lacrimal and salivary gland is
   a. Sjögren's syndrome
   b. Mikulicz's syndrome
   c. Sturge-Weber syndrome
   d. Vogt-Koyanagi syndrome
3. All the following are serous acinous glands EXCEPT
   a. lacrimal gland
   b. glands of Krause
   c. meibomian gland
   d. salivary gland
4. Occlusion of canaliculus commonly occurs due to
   a. IDU eyedrops
   b. eyelash
   c. scarring
   d. all of the above
5. Solids in tear include
   a. soduim chloride
   b. protein
   c. sugars
   d. all of the above
6. The most common tumour of the lacrimal gland is
   a. basal cell carcinoma
   b. squamous cell carcinoma
   c. mixed tumour
   d. malignant melanoma
7. The accessory lacrimal glands are
   a. glands of Krause
   b. glands of Wolfring
   c. both
   d. none
8. The tear film has
   a. mucous layer
   b. aqueous layer
   c. lipid layer
   d. all of the above
9. The nasolacrimal duct opens in the nose at
   a. superior meatus
   b. middle meatus
   c. inferior meatus
   d. nasal septum
10. The sequela of chronic dacryocystitis includes
    a. lacrimal abscess
    b. atonic sac
    c. panophthalmitis
    d. all of the above
11. All are mucin-deficiency diseases EXCEPT
    a. vitamin A deficiency
    b. Stevens-Johnson syndrome
    c. trachoma
    d. exposure keratitis
12. Pleomorphic adenoma of the lacrimal gland
    a. may undergo squamous metaplasia
    b. biopsy is taken before deciding treatment
    c. may require exenteration
    d. all of the above

13. The choice of treatment of congenital dacryocystitis is
    a. syringing and probing
    b. dacryocystectomy
    c. DCR
    d. none of the above
14. Tears are produced in the newborn after
    a. 1 week
    b. 2 weeks
    c. 3 weeks
    d. 4 weeks
15. The treatment of dry eye is
    a. artificial tears
    b. vitamin A
    c. gelatin plugs
    d. all of the above

ANSWERS

1—c	2—b	3—c	4—d	5—d
6—c	7—c	8—d	9—c	10—d
11—d	12—d	13—a	14—d	15—d

CHAPTER 19

The Orbit

APPLIED ANATOMY

The two orbits are two pyramidal-shaped bony cavities situated on either side of the nose or midline of face. The apex is represented by the optic foramen and the base by the orbital margins of the frontal and maxillary bones. The average volume of orbit is approximately 30 cc.

1. Orbital Walls

The surfaces of each orbit (roof, floor, medial and lateral wall) are composed of seven bones: ethmoid, frontal, lacrimal, maxillary, palatine, sphenoid and zygomatic bones. The thinnest of these bones is the lamina papyracea over the ethmoid sinuses along the medial wall.

2. Orbital Apertures

I. *Superior orbital fissure*: It is located between the greater and lesser wings of the sphenoid. Structures passing through the fissure include:
   i. 3rd, 4th, and 6th cranial nerves
   ii. 5th cranial nerve—ophthalmic division.
   iii. Sympathetic nerve fibres
   iv. Orbital veins
   v. Recurrent branch of ophthalmic artery.

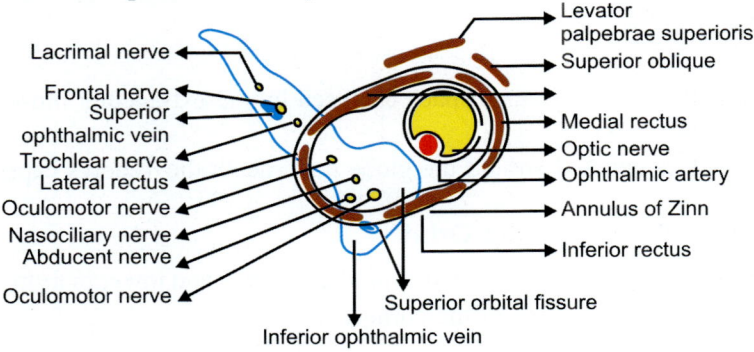

Superior orbital fissure and optic foramen

II. *Optic foramen and canal:*
   a. Optic canal (5-10 mm long): It is located in the lesser wing of sphenoid. It transmits following structures:
      i. Optic nerve
      ii. Ophthalmic artery
      iii. Sympathetic nerves.
   b. Optic foramen: It is the orbital end of optic canal. It measures 6 mm in diameter.

III. *Inferior orbital fissure*: It is situated in the lower part of the orbital apex. It transmits following structures:
  i. Fifth cranical nerve—maxillary division
  ii. Zygomatic nerve
  iii. Inferior ophthalmic vein.

3. Surgical Spaces in the Orbit

There are four surgical spaces in the orbit. These are of clinical importance as the inflammatory process remains localized in any one of them and each space may be opened separately.
  i. *Subperiosteal space*: It lies between the periosteum and the bone.
  ii. *Peripheral orbital space*: It lies between the periosteum and the extraocular muscles. It is a continuous circular space.

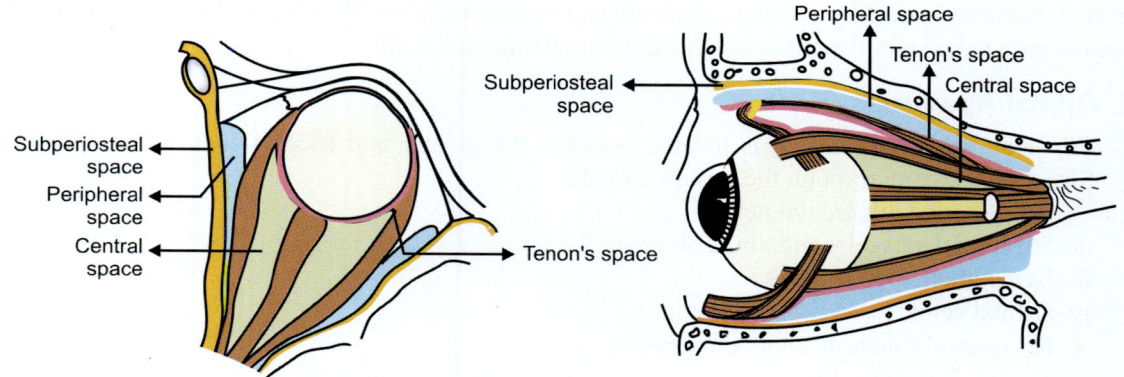

Surgical spaces in the orbit

  iii. *Central space*: It is a cone-shaped space enclosed by the extraocular muscles. It is known as the 'muscle cone'.
  iv. *Tenon's space*: It is situated around the globe underneath the Tenon's capsule.

Normal Position of the Eye in the Orbit

When a straight ruler is applied vertically to the middle of upper and lower margins of the orbit, it just touches the closed lids over the apex of the cornea.

Diseases of the Orbit

1. Orbital cellulitis
2. Cavernous sinus thrombosis
3. Exophthalmos
4. Enophthalmos.

Normal position of the eye in the orbit

ORBITAL CELLULITIS

It is the purulent inflammation of the cellular tissues of the orbit. It is a serious condition of the eye which may endanger the vision and life as well.

Etiology

Any age or any sex may be affected. It is unilateral usually.
1. It is often due to extension of infection from the neighbouring parts such as nasal sinuses, teeth, face, lips, etc.
2. Penetrating injury of the eye with or without retention of a foreign body.
3. It may occur following septic operations and panophthalmitis.
4. Metastasis from septicemia may also cause orbital cellulitis.

Symptoms

1. There is severe excruciating pain particularly on movement of the eyeball.
2. There is inability to open the eyes due to chemosis and swelling of lids.
3. Diplopia may be present due to impaired movement of the eye.

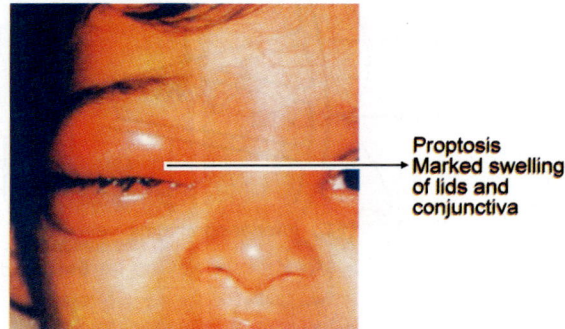

Orbital cellulitis

Signs

1. There is swelling of the lids and conjunctiva along with marked congestion.
2. Mild proptosis and impaired mobility may cause diplopia.
3. Pain is increased by pressure or on movement of the eyeball.
4. Vision is not affected. However, it may be reduced in associated retrobulbar neuritis.
5. Fever and cerebral signs may be present due to central nervous system involvement.
6. Fundus examination—It is difficult to examine the fundus. It may be normal or signs of optic neuritis are seen with engorgement of veins. Eventually optic atrophy sets in.

Complications

1. Abscess—It points in the skin of the lid near the orbital margin or may empty into the conjunctival fornix.
2. Panophthalmitis is a serious condition.
3. Purulent meningitis and cerebral abscess may occur occasionally.
4. Optic atrophy results in permanent loss of vision.
5. Thrombosis of cavernous sinus can even cause death.

Treatment

1. Hot compress relieves pain and prevents stasis.
2. Modern broad-spectrum antibiotics are given parenterally in high doses.

3. Analgesics and anti-inflammatory drugs are helpful in controlling pain and fever.
4. If an abscess is formed, incision and drainage is done promptly.

THROMBOSIS OF CAVERNOUS SINUS

It is due to the extension of thrombosis from various sources which communicate with the cavernous sinus.

Anatomy of Communication of Cavernous Sinus

It is of great clinical importance as infection may travel from face, lips orbit, mouth, pharynx, ear, nose, accessory sinuses or as a metastasis in infectious diseases or septicaemia.

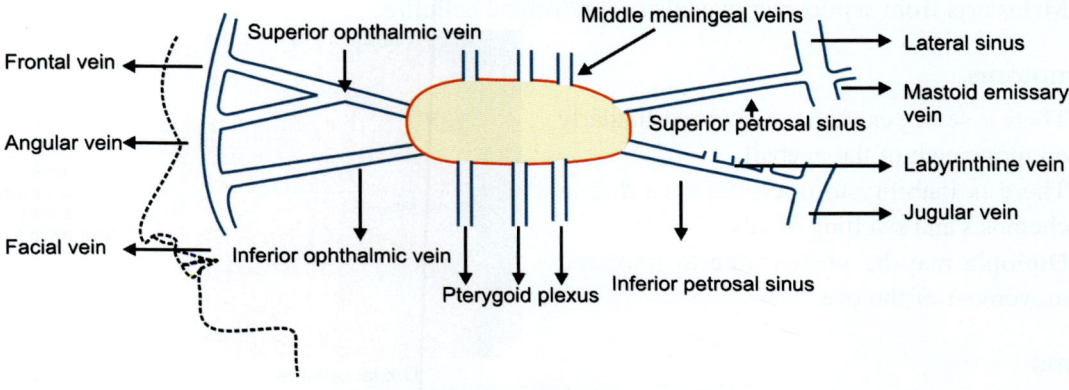

Communications of cavernous sinus—lateral view

i. The superior and inferior ophthalmic veins enter the sinus anteriorly.
ii. The superior and inferior petrosal sinus leave the sinus posteriorly.
iii. It communicates directly and indirectly with the pterygoid plexus, cerebrum and middle ear. *Therefore the swelling behind the ear is diagnostic of cavernous sinus thrombosis.*
iv. The sinus of one side communicates with the other by two or three transverse sinuses which surround the pituitary body.

Symptoms

They are same as for orbital cellulitis.
1. There is severe supraorbital pain due to involvement of ophthalmic division of the 5th nerve which is situated on the lateral side of cavernous sinus.
2. High-grade fever, rigor and vomiting are present usually.

Signs

1. Oedema over the mastoid process of the temporal bone of the affected side, i.e. behind the ear is the most important early diagnostic sign.
2. Transference of symptoms to opposite eye in 50% cases is seen. Paralysis of opposite lateral rectus muscle is suspicious of bilateral involvement.

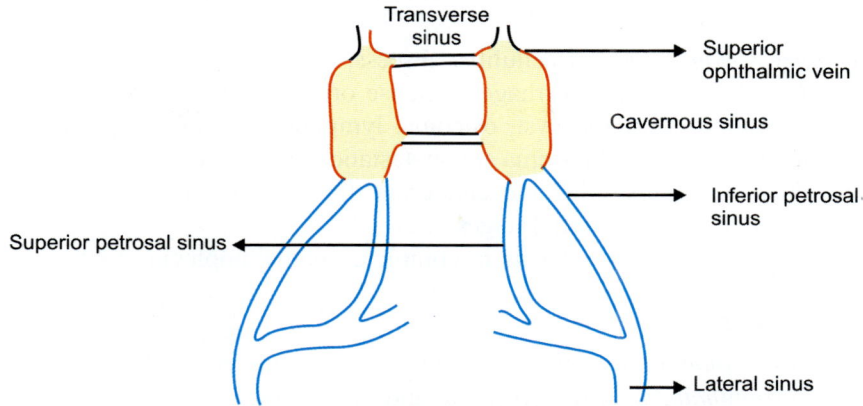
Communications of cavernous sinus—looking from above

3. Paralysis of extraocular muscles may be present.
4. Corneal anesthesia and dilated pupil are seen in later stages due to involvement of 5th nerve.
5. Proptosis occurs in almost all cases but is of late onset.
6. Fundus examination
   - Retinal veins are dilated and engorged
   - There may be pronounced papillitis
   - Papilloedema may be present.

Complication
Meningitis and cerebral abscess may occur which may lead to death.

Treatment
1. Modern potent third generation broad-spectrum antibiotic should be started immediately by intravenous route in massive doses.
2. Anticoagulant therapy may be helpful in dissolving the clot.

PROPTOSIS OR EXOPHTHALMOS

It is a condition where there is forward displacement of the eyeball beyond the orbital margin with the patient looking straight ahead. The term proptosis is synonymous with exophthalmos for practical purpose but they connote different meaning.

Proptosis
It is defined as the passive or mechanical protrusion of the eyeball.

Exophthalmos
It is defined as the active protrusion of the eyeball forwards.

Classification
It may be classified as follows:

1. Unilateral Proptosis
   i. *Inflammatory lesions*—Orbital cellulitis, abscess, etc.
   ii. *Vascular disturbances*—Haemorrhage, varicose orbital veins, haemangioma, etc.
   iii. *Cysts and tumours*—Dermoid cyst, osteoma, lymphoma, lymphosarcoma, glioma, meningioma of optic nerve, retinoblastoma and metastatic deposits in orbit.
   iv. *Systemic diseases*—Leukemias and endocrine disturbances such as Graves' disease and thyrotropic exophthalmos in initial stages.
   v. *Paralysis of extraocular muscles* as in complete ophthalmoplegia.

2. Bilateral Proptosis
   i. *Developmental anomalies of the skull*—Oxycephaly (tower skull).
   ii. *Endocrine exophthalmos*, both thyrotoxic and thyrotropic.
   iii. *Inflammatory lesions*—Cavernous sinus thrombosis.
   iv. *Tumours*—lymphosarcoma, lymphoma, pseudotumour, etc.
   v. *Lipodystrophies*—Xanthomatosis, diabetic exophthalmic dysostosis (Hand-Schüller-Christian disease).

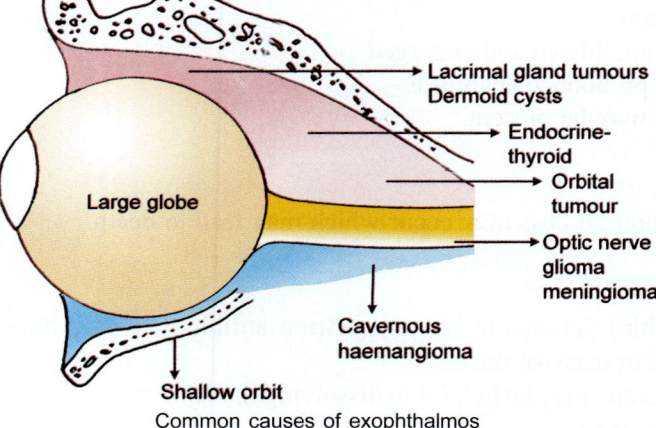

Common causes of exophthalmos

3. Intermittent Proptosis
It is usually caused by the orbital varicose veins particularly on looking down.

4. Pulsating Proptosis
It is caused by the arteriovenous aneurysm as a result of communication between the internal carotid artery and the cavernous sinus.

Clinical Evaluation
Clinical evaluation of the patient is done by taking a careful history, clinical examination, radiological and laboratory investigations.
1. **History**—Mode of onset—Whether sudden, gradual or chronic?
   - Presence and duration of pain is important.
   - Past history of thyroid dysfunction, orbital trauma, sinus disease and malignancy.

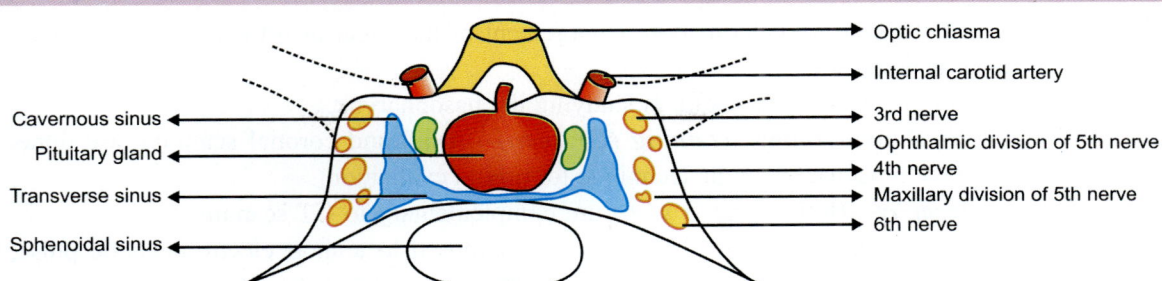

Sagittal section of cavernous sinus and adjacent structures

2. **Clinical examination**
   a. ***It is important to rule out the possibility of pseudoproptosis***. Pseudoproptosis is a condition in which the eyeball appears to be proptosed but actually there is no forward displacement. The important causes of pseudoproptosis are:
      i. *Buphthalmos*
      ii. *High axial myopia*
      iii. *Retraction of the upper eyelid*
      iv. *Shallow orbit as in craniofacial dysostosis.*

   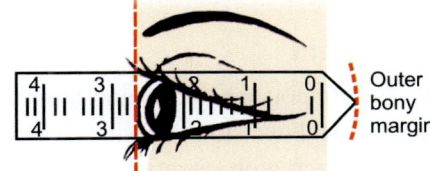
   Exophthalmometer

   b. ***Measurement of proptosis***
      i. *By clinical observation*—The patient is made to sit in front of the surgeon. His head is tilted slightly backwards and the position of the apex of each cornea is compared on both sides.
      ii. *Exophthalmometer*—It consists of a transparent plastic ruler with a groove which fits into the outer bony margin of the orbit. The scale is engraved on both sides. The level of the apex of the cornea is measured on both sides.
         • Normally the distance between the apex of the cornea and the lateral orbital margin is less than 20 mm. A reading of 21 mm or more is regarded as abnormal.
         • A difference of more than 2 mm between the two eyes is abnormal.
      iii. *Hertel exophthalmometer*—It is a more sophisticated instrument.
   c. ***There is limitations of ocular movements*** due to oedema, infiltration and fibrosis.
   d. ***Visual acuity*** may be reduced as a result of exposure keratitis and optic nerve involvement due to infiltration, pressure by swollen muscle and reduced blood supply.
   e. ***Pupillary reactions are affected*** due to optic nerve involvement.
   f. ***Fundus examination***—The disc may be normal or show features of optic atrophy, papillitis or papilloedema.
   g. ***Transillumination and auscultation*** are done for tumour and pulsating proptosis.

3. **Radiological investigation**
   a. ***Plain X-rays***
      i. *The Caldwell view (PA view)*—This view is taken with the patient's nose and forehead touching the film. It is useful in the diagnosis of orbital lesions. The enlargement of the

orbit bone density, calcification, enlargement of the superior orbital fissure and optic canal is noted.

    ii. *The lateral view*—It is useful is studying the nasopharynx.

  b. ***Computerized tomography scanning (CT scan)***—Axial and coronal scanning are done. CT scan is the most useful single technique for orbital evaluation.

  c. ***Ultrasonography***—Both A and B scans are complementary to CT scanning.

  d. ***Magnetic resonance imaging***—The tissues are exposed to a short electromagnetic pulse, and the sensitive receivers pick up this electromagnetic echo. It has the advantage of not being hampered by bone and there is no effect of ionizing irradiation on the patient.

4. **Laboratory investigation**

  i. Routine blood picture, haemoglobin, WBC total and differential count, ESR, blood sugar and cholesterol, urine examination are useful investigations.

  ii. Special tests like T3, T4, TSH level of blood, orbital venography may be done.

Treatment

1. Exploratory operation and biopsy are done.
2. Surgical excision—It is done in case of benign tumours and dermoid cysts. There are 3 routes of approach with retention of the eye:
   i. Anterior orbitotomy,
   ii. Lateral orbitotomy,
   iii. Transfrontal (intracranial).
3. Exenteration—Removal of all the structures of the orbit including the eye and periosteum is done in case of extraocular extension of malignancy as in retinoblastoma.
4. Radiation—It is recommended in cases of recurrence and metastasis of tumour.

ENDOCRINE EXOPHTHALMOS

Exophthalmos in thyroid disorders is an active process.

Etiology

The exact cause is obscure as it may be present in hyperthyroidism, hypothyroidism and elithyroid states. It may be associated with:

  i. Generalised disturbance of the endocrine system.

  ii. Increased secretion of thyrotropic hormone (TTH) from the anterior lobe of pituitary gland in response to low thyroxin level.

  iii. Increased secretion of exophthalmos producing substance (EPS) and long acting thyroid stimulators (LATS).

Pathogenesis

There is delayed hypersensitivity or autoimmune reaction to thyroglobulin leading to oedema, infiltration, deposition of fat and mucopolysaccharide substances and fibrosis of the orbital tissue.

Types

1. In hyperthyroidism (thyrotoxicosis, Graves' disease, exophthalmic goitre)—There is mild exophthalmos.
2. In hypothyroidism (thyrotropic exophthalmos, exophthalmic ophthalmoplegia)—An extreme exophthalmos occurs in hypothyroidism (after thyroid gland removal usually).

Symptoms

There is anterior protrusion of the eyeballs with inability to close the lids.

Signs

1. Features of thyrotoxicosis include tachycardia, fine muscular tremors and weight loss due to raised basal metabolic rate.
2. Ocular signs
    i. Bilateral exophthalmos with associated exposure keratitis.
    ii. Dalrymple's sign—There is peculiar stare due to retraction of the upper lid
    iii. von Graefe's sign—Upper lid lags on downward movements of the eyeball.
    iv. Stellwag's sign—There is infrequent and incomplete blinking.
    v. Mobius's sign—There is weakness of convergence
    vi. Jellinek's sign—There is increased pigmentation of lids.
    vii. Joffroy's sign—There is poor forehead wrinkling on looking up.

Treatment

1. Systemic iodide and antithyroid drugs are given in mild type.
2. Systemic corticosteroids help to reduce the oedema and infiltration.
3. Exposed cornea is protected by lubricants and lateral tarsorrhaphy.
4. Orbital decompression is indicated in rapidly progressing proptosis with optic nerve involvement.

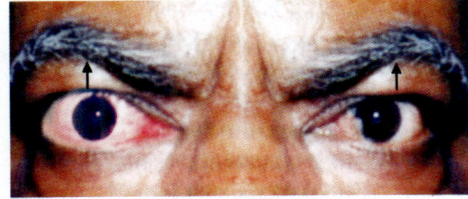

Thyrotoxicosis

ENOPHTHALMOS

It is a rare condition in which the eyeball is displaced inwards.

Etiology

1. *Structural abnormality*: It is seen in blow-out fracture of the orbital floor, phthisis bulbi and microphthalmos and other congenital defects.
2. *Atrophy of orbital content*: It is seen in orbital varicose veins, in old age and after irradiation for malignant tumour.
3. *Traction*: It occurs due to post-inflammatory cicatrization of extraocular muscles as in pseudotumour syndrome and after excessive shortening of extraocular muscles.

MULTIPLE CHOICE QUESTIONS

1. Complete paralysis of extraocular muscles occur in
   a. orbital cellulitis
   b. panophthalmitis
   c. cavernous sinus thrombosis
   d. none of the above
2. The condition which is first unilateral but soon becomes bilateral
   a. orbital cellulitis
   b. panophthalmitis
   c. cavernous sinus thrombosis
   d. all of the above
3. The common cause of unilateral proptosis in a child is
   a. retinoblastoma
   b. varicose orbital vein
   c. hyperthyroidism
   d. none of the above
4. The causes of pseudoproptosis include
   a. buphthalmos
   b. high axial myopia
   c. retraction of the upper lid
   d. all of the above
5. The term enophthalmos means
   a. absence of eyeball
   b. forward displacement of eyeball
   c. inward displacement of eyeball
   d. atrophic bulbi
6. Orbital cellulitis may occurs in
   a. penetrating injuries of orbit
   b. facial erysipelas
   c. septicaemia
   d. all of the above
7. The most dangerous complication of orbital cellulitis is
   a. abscess formation
   b. proptosis
   c. diplopia
   d. cerebral involvement
8. Swelling behind the ear is diagnostic of
   a. cavernous sinus thrombosis
   b. orbital cellulitis
   c. unilateral proptosis
   d. bilateral proptosis
9. Pulsating proptosis is seen in
   a. orbital varicose vein
   b. arteriovenous aneurysm
   c. cavernous sinus thrombosis
   d. thyrotoxicosis
10. The important investigations of proptosis include all EXCEPT
    a. CT scan
    b. exophthalmometer
    c. magnetic resonance imaging
    d. electroretinogram
11. The average volume of the orbit is
    a. 6 cc
    b. 12 cc
    c. 18 cc
    d. 24 cc
12. All the following structures are located in the lateral wall of cavernous sinus EXCEPT
    a. oculomotor nerve
    b. trochlear nerve
    c. optic nerve
    d. abducens nerve
13. Chondrosarcoma of the orbit
    a. mainly affects patients under 20 and over 50 years of age
    b. causes nasal obstruction and exophthalmos

c. spreads by local extension
   d. all of the above
14. Superior orbital fissure syndrome is frequently caused by
    a. carotid aneurysm
    b. arachnoiditis
    c. meningioma
    d. all of the above
15. Joffroy's sign is found in cases of
    a. diabetics
    b. Tay-Sachs disease
    c. thyrotoxicosis
    d. hypothyroidism

ANSWERS

1—c	2—c	3—a	4—d	5—c
6—d	7—d	8—a	9—b	10—d
11—d	12—c	13—d	14—d	15—c

CHAPTER 20
General Therapeutics

There are several therapeutic substances available which are useful in treating ocular diseases. Therapeutic agents can be introduced into the eye, mainly by four methods namely:
1. Topical instillation
2. Periocular injections
3. Intraocular injections
4. Systemic administration.

1. Instillation of the Drug into the Conjunctival Sac

This is done in the form of eyedrops, ointment, gels, soft contact lens or membrane delivery. The passage of drug through the corneal epithelium is determined by its fat solubility and the degree of dissociation of the electrolytes.

a. Eyedrops
It achieves a high concentration and is quickly washed away. More than 80% of the drug enters the lacrimal drainage system after 5 minutes. It is convenient for daytime use as it causes minimum blurring of vision.

b. Ointment
It has longer contact time but there is lower drug concentration in tears. It causes blurring of vision therefore it is applied at bedtime.

c. Gels
It also has prolong contact time and may cause less blurring of vision than ointment.

d. Soft contact lens
It absorbs small molecules of drugs when soaked in the drug. It delivers high concentrations for over about 4 hours.

e. Membrane delivery
By 'ocuserts' there is relatively constant rate of drug delivery thus reducing the side effects. Pilocarpine ocuserts cause less fluctuation in intraocular pressure as it delivers drug over a longer duration.

f. Iontophoresis
An electrolyte is given into the eye with the passage of a galvanic current which increases the permeability of the cornea. It is rarely used nowadays.

2. Periocular Injection

These include subconjunctival, sub-Tenon, retrobulbar and peribulbar routes.
  a. *Subconjunctival injections*: They achieve high concentration of drugs and are useful in acute anterior segment infections and inflammations. The drugs which cannot penetrate the cornea

owing to large-sized molecules can easily pass through the sclera. Hence a wider range of substances can be introduced into the eye.
b. *Sub-Tenon injections*: Anterior sub-Tenon injections are used mainly to administer steroids in the treatment of severe or resistant anterior uveitis. Posterior sub-Tenon injections are indicated in patients with intermediate and posterior uveitis. Depots of crystalline suspensions of corticosteroids lead to high intraocular levels of steroids without systemic side-effects.
c. *Retrobulbar injections*: These are used to deliver drugs for optic neuritis, papillitis and posterior uveitis. They are also used for administering retrobulbar block anaesthesia.

3. Injection into the Eyeball

It can be given in the anterior chamber or in the vitreous. It is reserved for desperate cases such as panophthalmitis to flood the ocular tissues.

4. Systemic Administration

Therapeutic substances can be given by mouth or parenterally by intramuscular and intravenous injections. The main factor influencing the intraocular penetration of the drug is the blood-aqueous barrier. It depends mainly on two characteristics of the drug namely:
  i. *Molecular weight*: Low molecular weight substances penetrate easily. However, most antibiotics such as penicillin are large-sized molecules and are impermeable.
  ii. *Lipid solubility*: A lipid soluble substance such as sulphonamide is 16 times more permeable than sucrose having almost same molecular weight. Similarly chloramphenicol, a lipid soluble antibiotic enters the eye freely.

ANTIMICROBIAL THERAPY

Antimicrobial agents fall into two general category:
1. Antibiotics are compounds produced by micro-organisms, e.g. penicillin, tetracycline, etc.
2. Synthetic chemicals, e.g. sulphonamides, ethambutol, rifampicin, etc. Chemotherapeutic and antibiotic drugs are bacteriostatic (inhibitory) rather than bactericidal (lethal) agents. They act by competing for the raw materials necessary for the existence of the organisms. As these drugs are rapidly excreted from the body or diffuse from local application, their repeated or continuous administration is essential. They are particularly effective in the treatment of acute infections.

1. ANTIBIOTICS

These are substances derived from fungi or other bacterias. Fleming discovered "Penicillin" in the year 1929. In the last few years many such drugs have been discovered such as cephalosporins, aminoglycosides and the various tetracyclines.
  i. *Penicillins*: These are effective against gram-positive organisms and certain spirochaetes.
  ii. *Cephalosporins*: These are broad-spectrum antibiotics which are relatively resistant to staphylococcal penicillinase.
  iii. *Aminoglycosides*: These are effective against gram-negative organisms and certain acid-fast species.

iv. *The "broad-spectrum" antibiotics*: These are effective against both gram-positive and gram-negative organisms, the rickettsiae, the Chlamydia, certain spirochaetes and protozoa.

1. Penicillins

In general penicillins act by interfering with cell wall synthesis and are all bactericidal. The optimum blood level depends on the sensitivity of the organism. It does not cross the blood-aqueous barrier due to its large molecular weight. It can cause hypersensitivity reactions such as urticaria and anaphylactic shock. It shows a synergistic action with antibiotics of the aminoglycoside group. Penicillin eyedrops are useful in superficial inflammation of conjunctiva and cornea. Penicillin is given parenterally in deep-seated inflammation of the orbit or lids.

Penicillins may be classified as follows:

a. *Penicillins effective against coccal infection and gram-positive bacilli*: Benzylpenicillin is not acid-stable and is given only parenterally.
b. *Enzyme:* Penicillinase resistant penicillins are cloxacillin, methicillin and flucloxacillin.
c. *Ampicillin*: It can be given both orally or parenterally. It is a broad-spectrum antibiotic as it is effective against most cocci except penicillinase-producing staphylococci.
d. *Amoxicillin*: It is same as ampicillin in structure and mode of action but has the advantage of rapid absorption. It produces higher and more sustained blood levels. Incidence of diarrhoea is less than with ampicillin and is thus better tolerated orally.
e. *Carbenicillin*: It is given only parenterally and is effective against *Pseudomonas aeruginosa* particularly.

2. Cephalosporins

These drugs have a similar structure and mode of action as penicillin. Allergy may develop in patients already allergic to penicillin. All the cephalosporins have a bactericidal action against a wide range of organisms.

The cephalosporins have been classified into generations, which indicate improvement in their antibacterial spectrum, stability to β-lactamase and potency.

a. *The first-generation cephalosporins* have a range of activity similar to that of broad-spectrum penicillins but are more resistant to the effect of β-lactamase. They are relatively ineffective against bacteroides species, enterococci, e.g. cephalexin 250-500 mg capsules.
b. *The second-generation cephalosporins* have greater stability against β-lactamase inactivation. They possess a broader spectrum of activity to include gram-negative rods and anaerobic organisms, e.g. cefoxitin 1-2-10 gm powder.
c. *The third-generation cephalosporins* or extended spectrum possess a high degree of *in vitro* potency, β-lactamase stability and a broader spectrum of action against many gram-negative enteric bacteria and anaerobes. They are highly active against *Neisseria* and *H. influenzae*. They retain good activity against *Streptococcus* and pneumococcus, e.g. cefotaxime sodium (Claforan) 1-2-10 gm vial for intravenous and intramuscular use.

3. Aminoglycosides

This group of drugs include streptomycin, kanamycin, neomycin, gentamicin, netilmycin and tobramycin. They are bactericidal in action and are all toxic to the eighth nerve and kidneys. They show a broad-spectrum activity but may cause allergy and bacterial resistance.

Streptomycin: It is used in the treatment of *Mycobacterium tuberculosis* in combination with a second drug to prevent the development of resistance.

Gentamicin and kanamycin: These drugs may be used parenterally in cases of serious infections by gram-positive and gram-negative organisms. It is particularly effective against penicillin-resistant strains of staphylococci and *Pseudomonas pyocyanea*. Gentamicin when injected intraocularly may cause severe retinal ischaemia. Topical and subconjunctival administration causes its penetration in the aqueous.

Tobramycin: It is 2-4 times more active against *Pseudomonas aeruginosa* and Proteus as compared to gentamicin. Topically it is used as 1% eyedrops. Fortified drops enhance bioavailability and it can also be given subconjunctivally or intravitreally.

Amikacin: It acts against many gram-positive and gram-negative organisms. It is less retinotoxic than gentamicin, but more retinotoxic than ceftazidime. For the treatment of endophthalmitis, 0.4 mg amikacin is injected intravitreally along with vancomycin, which acts synergistically.

4. Broad-spectrum Antibiotics

Tetracyclines are active against both gram-positive and gram-negative organisms, fungi, rickettsiae and the *Chlamydia* including trachoma. They are applied as eyedrops and ointments for superficial ocular infections. They may be used orally in staphylococcal or other pyogenic infections of the lids and conjunctiva.

Other Antibiotics

a. *The macrolides and the lincomycin group* include erythromycin, lincomycin and clindamycin. They are effective against gram-positive organisms having resistance or allergy to penicillin. They are given orally.
b. *Chloramphenicol*: It was originally derived from a streptomyces but it is now synthesized as chloramphenicol. It is a small molecular weight substance and lipid soluble so it enters the eye easily.
c. *Polymyxin*: It is isolated from Bacillus polymyxa. It is active against gram-negative bacteria, e.g. *Pseudomonas pyocyanea*, etc.

2. SYNTHETIC CHEMICALS

1. Sulphonamides

Sulphonamides are bacteriostatic. They prevent the synthesis of folic acid which is necessary for bacterial cell nutrition. They can be applied topically or systemically in the treatment of *Chlamydia* infections such as trachoma, inclusion conjunctivitis and lymphogranuloma venereum. They are also useful in the treatment of toxoplasmosis along with pyrimethamine. They can cross the blood-aqueous barrier being lipid soluble. The commonly used sulphonamides are sulpha-acetamide, sulphadiazine, sulphamerazine, sulphathiazole, sulphadimidine and cotrimoxazole. Cotrimoxazole is a preparation of combination of trimethoprim and sulphamethoxazole.

2. Sulphones

Oral dapsone is widely used in the treatment of leprosy.

3. Para-aminosalicylic Acid (PAS)

It may be given by mouth along with isoniazid in the treatment of tuberculosis. The standard treatment of pulmonary tuberculosis now consists of two drugs given together—rifampicin along with either isoniazid or ethambutol.

4. Rifampicin

It is a bactericidal drug interfering with the metabolism of bacterial nucleic acid. It is given by mouth 450-600 mg daily in a single dose before breakfast.

5. Ethambutol

It is given in daily dose of 15-25 mg per kg of bodyweight. The main danger is the onset of optic neuropathy, i.e. loss of visual acuity and colour vision which is not reversible even on stopping the drug.

6. Fluoroquinolones

These are potent synthetic agents, derivatives of nalidixic acid, having broad spectrum of activity against gram-positive and gram-negative organisms.

Mechanism of action: These are bactericidal drugs. These inhibit bacterial DNA synthesis.

Preparations: They are grouped into four generations:
a. **The first-generation:** Ciprofloxacin and Norfloxacin—These are used topically as 0.3% drops 1-4 hourly.
b. **The second-generation:** Ofloxacin and Lomefloxacin are the commonly used drugs of this generation, used as 0.3% drops topically.
c. **The third-generation:** Sparfloxacin is sometimes used in the same concentration.
d. **The fourth-generation:** Gatifloxacin 0.3% and Moxifloxacin 0.5% have been introduced in this group. For gram-positive infections moxifloxacin is slightly more effective than gatifloxacin but against gram-negative and atypical bacteria, gatifloxacin is more effective. Both achieve high intraocular concentration after topical administration, but none of the two effectively penetrate the vitreous. Oral gatifloxacin has been shown to achieve extremely high levels in the vitreous.

ANTIVIRAL DRUGS

1. *5-iodo-2-deoxyuridine (IDU)*: 0.1% eyedrops and 0.5% eye ointment. It inhibits the synthesis of DNA and thus prevents the replication of herpes virus. It is applied 5 times a day and at bedtime for 10-21 days. Important side effects are superficial punctate keratopathy and punctal stenosis.

2. *Acycloguanosine* is a potent antiviral drug with no toxic side effects. It is effective in treating herpetic stromal infection along with Ara-A.
   Acyclovir: 3% eye ointment, 200 mg tablets, Acyclovir IV. It is most useful in treating common herpes infections such as herpes labialis, genital herpes, herpes zoster. It can be used prophylactically to suppress recurrences. Acyclovir ointment is applied 5 times/day for 10-21 days. It is more potent than IDU and less toxic.
3. *Trifluorothimidine (F_3T)*: 1% eyedrops are applied 5-9 times/day for 14 days. It heals 90% of herpetic ulcers in a period of two weeks. It has greater potency, less toxicity and greater effectiveness in resistant cases.
4. *Adenine arabinoside (Ara-A) and Vidarabine (Vira-A)*: 3% eye ointment. They block the synthesis of nucleic acids. They are not active against stromal disease. Eye ointment is applied 5 times/day for 14- 21 days.
5. *Ganciclovir (cytovene)*: It is a new compound which is at least 10-100 times more potent than acyclovir. The usual dose is 2.5 mg/kg IV 8 hourly for 10 days and then it is reduced to 5 mg/kg/day.
6. *Zidovudine (Azidothymidine, AZT, Retrovir)*: It inhibits the virus—induced reverse transcriptase which is essential for virus replication. It is combined with immunomodulators in treating HIV infection (AIDS). The usual dose is 100-200 mg PO four to eight hourly.
7. *Foscarnet*: Foscarnet 60 mg/kg is given every 12 hours for 14 days, followed by lifelong maintenance therapy. Both ganciclovir and foscarnet act as virostatic agents.
8. A newer drug BW 256-U87, a prodrug for acyclovir is currently undergoing clinical and therapeutic trial for CMV disease.

COMMON ANTIVIRAL AGENTS

DRUGS	PRESENTATION	DOSE
1. Idoxuridine (IDU) 5-iodo-2-dioxuridine	0.5% and 0.1% eye drops	1 drop hourly in the day and 2 hourly at night
2. Trifluorothymidine (TFT)	0.5% ointment 1% solution	5 times/day. One drop 2 hourly (maximum 9 drops/day)
3. Adenine arabinoside (Ara-A) Vidarabine (Vira-A)	3% ointment 200 mg/ml IV	5 times a day
4. Acyclovir Acycloguanosine	3% ointment 20 mg/ml IV 200 mg capsule	5 times a day
5. Ganciclovir	IV	2.5-5 mg/kg IV over a period of 1 hour. Repeated every 12 hours for 14-21 days
6. Zidovudine (AZT) Azidothymidine	Oral	100-200 mg every 4-8 hourly
7. Foscarnet Trisodium salt of phosphono-formic acid	IV or intravitreal	60 mg/kg 12 hourly for 2-3 weeks

ANTIFUNGAL AGENTS

The available antifungal drugs are mainly fungistatic. They are mainly used in keratomycosis and fungal endophthalmitis. Three groups of agents are used:
1. *Polyenes*: Amphotericin-B, nystatin, natamycin.
2. *Imidazoles*: Ketoconazole, miconazole, econazole, fluconazole.
3. *Flucytosin*: 5-fluorocytosine.

Amphotericin-B
It is too toxic for systemic use, but may be used locally as 0.25% solution (made with 5% glucose) as eye drop at 1 hour interval.

Nystatin
It is used topically (as 100,000 units/ml) in fungal keratitis. It is particularly effective against *Candida*.

Natamycin (Pimafucin)
It is used topically as 5% suspension. It has a fairly broad-spectrum effect, e.g. *Candida, Aspergillus, Fusarium*. It is used most commonly.

Ketoconazole
It is a well-tolerated oral antifungal drug. Daily dose is 200-400 mg for at least 14 days.

Miconazole
It is used topically as 1% ointment " 5 times daily. It is not effective against *Fusarium*.

Fluconazole
It is also a well-tolerated oral drug and has broader spectrum of antifungal activity. It is used as 200 mg daily for 3-4 weeks.

Itraconazole
This drug is similar to ketoconazole. It is prescribed for treatment of fungal infections caused primarily by Aspergillus and has moderate effect against Candida and Fusarium infections. It is available for oral and topical use. Oral dose is 200 mg twice daily for a week. Topically it is used as 1% eye drops.

Flucytosine
It is a less effective agent and used systemically. It is not useful in oculomycosis.

HORMONE THERAPY

Hormone therapy by corticosteroids such as cortisone, prednisolone, ACTH, dexamethasone is not curative. Its main action is to keep the acute phase of inflammation under control while the cure is obtained by other methods. Thus, in infective conditions, cure can be achieved only by antibiotics.

COMMON ANTIFUNGAL DRUGS

DRUGS	PRESENTATION AND APPLICATION	ACTION	SPECTRUM IN ORDER OF SENSITIVITY
1. Nystatin	Ointment 100,000 units/g, 3.5% ointment 2 hourly	Fungistatic	Candida, Aspergillus
2. Natamycin	5% suspension 5 times/day	Fungicidal	Candida, Aspergillus, Cephalosporium
3. Miconazol	1% suspension every 2 hourly 1% ointment 5 times/day	Fungicidal	Candida, Aspergillus
4. Econazole	1% ointment, 3times/day	Fungicidal	Fusarium, Aspergillus, Penicillium
5. Ketoconazol	Oral 200-400/mg/day	Fungicidal	Candida, Aspergillus
6. Clotrimazol	1% suspension every hour	Fungistatic	Aspergillus, Candida
7. Fluconazole	0.2% drops 5 times/day	Fungicidal	Aspergillus, Candida
8. Flucytosine	1.5% drops every 2 hours Oral 200 mg/day	Fungicidal	Aspergillus
9. Silver sulphadiazine	1% suspension every 2 hourly	Fungicidal	Candida, Aspergillus, Fusarium
10. Amphotericin B	Topical 2.5-10 mg/ml 5 times a day subconjunctival 2.5 mg	Fungicidal or Fungistatic	Candida, Aspergillus,

The main effect of hormone therapy in ocular diseases is of temporary blockage of the exudative phase of inflammation and inhibition of fibrosis in tissue repair whether the disease is bacterial, allergic, anaphylactic or traumatic. It is ineffective in the removal of structural damage caused by chronic inflammations or degenerations. In ophthalmology the steroids can be used locally or systemically.

a. *Local*: Drops, ointments, subconjunctival and retrobulbar injections.
b. *Systemic*: By mouth, intramuscular or intravenous injection.

Cataract and steroid-induced glaucoma may occur after prolonged use of corticosteroids

VITAMINS

The role of vitamins is important in ophthalmology.

Vitamin A

It is a higher alcohol synthesized in the liver from carotene.

Source: Fish fat or cod-liver, halibut and shark liver oils, egg yolk, milk, butter, green leafy and yellow vegetables such as spinach, drumsticks, ripe mango, cabbage, carrot, etc.

Daily requirement: Carotene 3 mg, vitamin A 3000 units.

Function: It is necessary for the maintenance of healthy ectodermal structures such as conjunctival, corneal, retinal, respiratory, alimentary and urinary systems.

Deficiency effects: Xerosis, xerophthalmia, keratomalacia, night-blindness, dermatosis, demyelination, decreased resistance to infections.

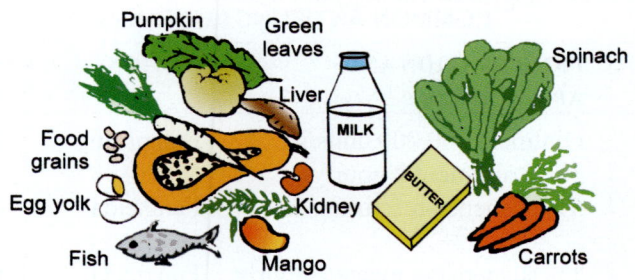

Sources of vitamin A

Vitamin D

It is calcicerol, an isomer of ergosterol formed by the action of ultraviolet light on skin.
Source: It is derived from animal fats specially cod liver oil, halibut oil, egg, milk, butter and sunshine.
Daily requirement: 1000 units.
Function: It is essential for calcium and phosphorus metablolism.
Deficiency effects: Cataract, rickets, osteomalacia, dental caries, tetany.

Vitamin K (Dimethylnaphthoqunone)

It is essential for prothrombin formation.

Vitamin C (Ascorbic Acid)

Source: It is drived from fresh citrus fruits such as orange, lemon, amla (gooseberry) and vegetables. It is destroyed by heating as it is a water soluble vitamin.
Daily requirment: 50 mg.
Function: It is required for lens metabolism, blood formation, osteogenesis, healing of wounds.
Deficiency effects: Conjunctival and retinal haemorrhages, scurvy, anaemia, osteoplasia.

Vitamin B_1 (Thiamine)

Source: Yeast, sprouted beans, peas, nuts, whole grain, flour, lean pork.
Daily requirement: 1 mg yeast.
Function: It helps in carbohydrate metabolism.
Deficiency effects: Corneal and conjunctival dystrophy, retrobulbar neuritis, beri-beri, peripheral neuritis.

Vitamin B_2 or G (Riboflavin)

Source: It is same as for vitamin B_1.
Function: It is essential for oxygenation.
Deficiency effects: Vascularizing keratitis, glossitis, cheilosis.

Vitamin B_6 and Vitamin B_{12}

Deficiency effects: Retrobulbar and optic neuritis.

SUMMARY OF MEDICAL TREATMENT OF IMPORTANT OCULAR DISEASES

The basic guidelines for the medical treatment of important ocular diseases can be summarized as follows:

1. CONJUNCTIVAL DISEASES
i. *Infective*: Broad-spectrum antibiotics are started initially. Later on specific antibiotics are given after culture and sensitivity.
ii. *Allergic*: Corticosteroid eyedrops are instilled during day time and ointment is applied at night. Non-steroidal anti-inflammatory drugs (NSAIDs) and antihistamine drugs can be given.

2. CORNEAL ULCER
i. *Bacterial:*
   a. Topical application of broad-spectrum antibiotics are started initially. Specific antibiotics are given after culture and sensitivity.
   b. Atropine drops or ointment.
   Corticosteroids are not given as they prevent healing.
ii. *Viral:*
   a. Antiviral drugs, e.g. acyclovir, iodo-deoxy-uridine, etc. are given.
   b. Corticosteroids are given only in disciform keratitis (deep keratitis).
iii. *Fungal*: Amphotericin B, nystatin, natamycin, clotrimazole, flucytosine, etc. are given topically. Corticosteroids are not given as they favour fungal growth.

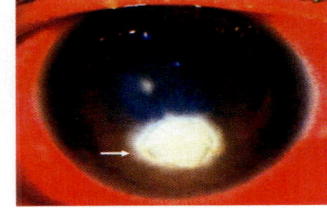

Corneal ulcer

3. EPISCLERITIS AND SCLERITIS
Corticosteroids, analgesics and anti-inflammatory drugs are given.

4. IRIDOCYCLITIS
i. Corticosteroids are given by topical, subconjunctival and systemic routes.
ii. Atropine drops and ointment are applied daily to paralyse the ciliary muscle.
iii. Potent broad-spectrum antibiotics which cross the blood aqueous barrier are given in bacterial infection (eye drops, ointment and subconjunctivally).
iv. Analgesic and anti-inflammatory drugs are given to relieve pain. *Pilocarpine* is not given as it may result in formation of posterior synechiae.

5. GLAUCOMA
i. *Local:*
   a. Pilocarpine: It increases aqueous outflow.
   b. Timolol maleate: It reduces the formation of aqueous.
ii. *Systemic:*
   a. Oral acetazolamide and glycerol: These reduce the formation of aqueous.
   b. IV mannitol and urea. These are hyperosmotic agents.
   Corticosteroids and atropine are not given as they further increase the IOP.

Iridocyclitis

CHAPTER 21
The Causes and Prevention of Blindness

In ophthalmology, the term 'blindness' strictly means 'the inability to perceive light' but from a practical point of view a person is said to be 'blind' or 'visually handicapped' when he is too blind to perform work for which eye sight is essential. The WHO has proposed a uniform criterion and defined blindness as, 'Visual acuity of less than 3/60 (Snellen) or its equivalent'. In the absence of appropriate vision charts, the WHO has added, "Inability to count fingers in daylight at a distance of 3 meters" to indicate less than 3/60 or its equivalent.

Incidence

In India, there are approximately 1.20 crore blind people which is about one-fourth of the total blind population of the world. This means that 14.9 out of every 1000 Indians are blind, compared to about 3 per thousand in most developed countries. Throughout the developing countries, two-third of the blindness is estimated to be preventable or curable if efforts are made in this direction.

CAUSES OF BLINDNESS

1. In India

The three great eye health problems are cataract, corneal opacity and malnutrition. The main diseases responsible for visual impairment and blindness in India are as follows:

The last group includes congenital anomalies, uveitis, posterior segment diseases, tumours, diabetes, hypertension and diseases of nervous system. At present there are more than 22 million cataract cases waiting to be operated in India. About 2 million new cases are being added each

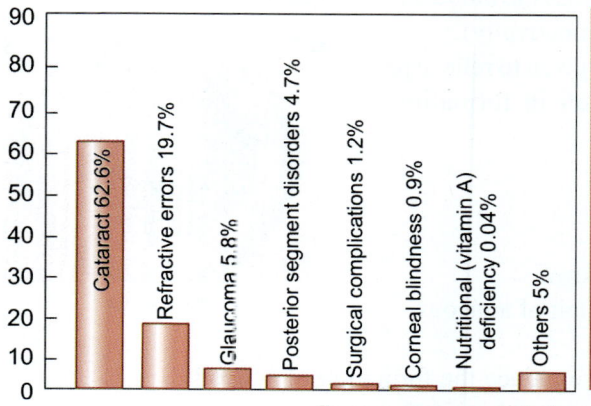

Common causes of blindness	
1. Cataract	62.6%
2. Refractive error	19.7%
3. Glaucoma	5.8%
4. Posterior segment disorders	4.7%
5. Surgical complications	1.2%
6. Corneal blindness	0.9%
7. Nutritional (vitamin A) deficiency	0.04%
8. Others	5.0%

Common causes of blindness (NPCB Survey (2001-02)

year. Majority of curable cataract blind people live in rural areas. 'Eye camps', i.e. 'doctor at the door' is the only way for providing surgical treatment.

Magnitude of Blindness in India

India accounts for 12 million blind people of the total estimated 37 million blind people globally.

Prevalence of blindness in India at present is 1.1% (NPCB Survey 2001-2002). It was 0.7% in 1996 (WHO Regional Health report), 1% in 1995 (WHO, 1995) and 1.49% in 1986-1989 (WHO - NPCB).

2. In Developed Countries

The most frequent causes of blindness are cataract, accident, glaucoma, diabetes, hypertension and other vascular diseases, hereditary and congenital conditions and degenerations of retina.

CAUSES OF WORLDWIDE BLINDNESS (2002)

1. Cataract	47.8%
2. Glaucoma	12.3%
3. ARMD (Age related macular degeneration)	8.7%
4. Corneal opacity	5.1%
5. Diabetic retinopathy	4.8%
6. Childhood blindness (including vitamin A deficiency, refractive errors)	3.9%
7. Trachoma	3.6%
8. Onchocerciasis	0.8%
9. Others	13%

3. Global Magnitude of Blindness

It is estimated that there are 161 million visually impaired persons all over the world. Out of these 37 million are blind and 124 million persons have low vision. Major causes of global blindness and the estimated number of blind persons are as follows,

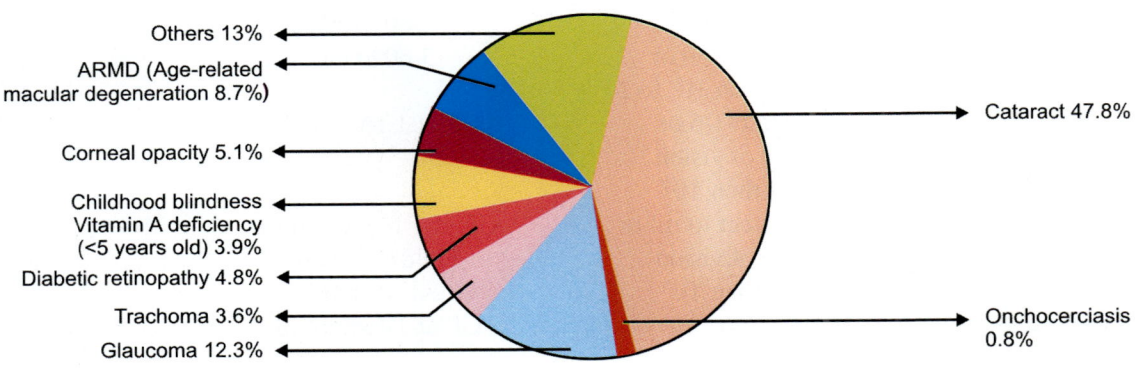

Causes of blindness, 2002 worldwide
(The World Health Report, 2002)

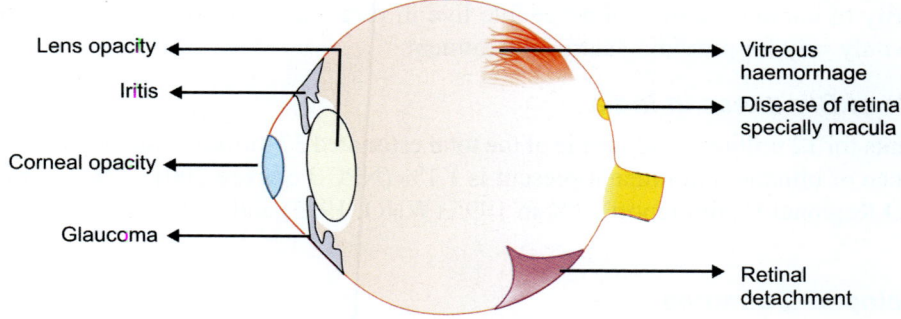

Common causes of blindness

The pattern of blindness in India has changed a lot in the last 4-5 decades. The smallpox has been completely eradicated. Ophthalmia neonatorum, interstitial keratitis and tabes optic atrophy are no longer prevalent. Trachoma blindness is on the decline. However, the blindness from cataract has increased due to the increased longevity of the population. As the diabetics are living longer, the blindness due to diabetic retinopathy is also increasing.

Rapid industrialization may cause blindness by specific diseases such as poisoning by lead and benzene derivatives in glass and iron workers, cataract and miner's nystagmus. Factory accidents and injury by foreign body can be prevented by appropriated guards, screens and goggles. There are frequent episodes of blindness seen nowadays due to liquor (methanol) poisoning. The iatrogenic blindness is also increasing due to the indiscriminate use of the sulphonamides, ethambutol, chloroquine, oral contraceptives, etc.

VISUAL IMPAIRMENT DISABILITY CATEGORIES BASED ON ITS SEVERITY AND PROPOSED DISABILITY PERCENTAGES (GOVT. OF INDIA)

CATEGORIES	ALL WITH CORRECTIONS		PERCENTAGE IMPAIRMENT
	BETTER EYE	WORSE EYE	
Category 0	6/9 to 6/18	6/24 to 6/36	20%
Category I	6/18 to 6/36	6/60 to nil	40%
Category II	6/60 to 4/60 or Field of vision 10° to 20°	3/60 to nil	75%
Category III	3/60 to 1/6 or Field of vision less then 10°	CF at 1 feet to nil	100%
Category IV	CF at 1 feet to nil or Field of vision less than 10°	CF at 1 feet to nil or Field of vision less than 10°	100%
One-eyed person	6/6	CF at 1 feet to nil	30%
CF = counting finger			

The central coordination committee under national programme for control of blindness in its 3rd meeting held on 12th March 1978 suggested that uniform definition for the purpose of categorising blindness be adopted. The following definition has accordingly being adopted in June 1978.
1. Vision 6/60 or less with the best possible spectacle correction in the better eye.
2. Diminution of field of vision to 20° or less in the better eye.
3. One eye has vision of 6/60 or less with best possible spectacle correction and the other eye has a visual field of 20° or less.

CLASSIFICATION OF BLINDNESS IN INDIA

CATEGORY OF VISUAL IMPAIRMENT	CANNOT SEE	CAN SEE
Normal vision		6/18 on Snellen's chart
Low vision	6/18 line on Snellen's chart	6/60 on Snellen's chart
Economic blindness	6/60 line on Snellen's chart	3/60 (by finger counting)
Social blindness	3/60 (by finger counting)	1/60 (by finger counting)
Manifest blindness	1/60 (by finger counting)	Perception of light present
Absolute blindness	No perception of light	No perception of light

Prevention of Blindness

The concept of avoidable blindness, i.e. preventable or curable blindness has gained increasing recognition during recent years.

The government of India has launched the National Programme for Control of Blindness in the year 1976. The ultimate aim of the national programme is:
1. To reduce blindness in the country from 1.49 to 0.3 per cent by 2000 AD.
2. To provide comprehensive eye care through primary, secondary and tertiary level health care.

At the apex, a National Institute of Ophthalmology (Dr Rajendra Prasad Centre for Ophthalmic Sciences, AIIMS, New Delhi) has been established for training personnels, research and referral services. The primary health centre, district hospital (secondary) and medical colleges (tertiary) are upgraded to render better and advanced eye health care and manpower development. The mobile eye units are extremely useful in arranging eye camps for cataract operations in remote areas with the cooperation of local voluntary organisation. The establishment of eye banks is of great value in corneal grafting.

Blindness can be prevented by the following principles:
1. Eye health education through mass communication media
2. Improving nutrition and preventing dietery vitamin A deficiency.
3. Treating and controlling the organisms which cause ocular infection.
4. Improving safety conditions on roads, factories and at home.
5. Training and rehabilitation of visually handicapped.

Eye health education is done through mass communication media, e.g. television, radio, film, books, etc. teachers, social workers, community leaders, mobile eye unit, medical and paramedical staff.

3. Refresher training to district ophthalmologists and ophthalmic assistants.
4. Fellowship training to ophthalmologists and teachers of medical college under the prevention of blindness programme.

VOLUNTARY ORGANISATIONS

Voluntary or Non-Government Organisations (NGOs) have played a vital role in the control of blindness in India. They are active in the field of educative, preventive, rehabilitative and surgical services to control blindness.

Some of the active organisations are

1. National Society for Prevention of Blindness (NSPB), India, located at Dr RP Centre for Ophthalmic Sciences, with its branches all over the country.
2. Lions International and its branches (Sight First).
3. The Royal Commonwealth Society for the Blind (Sight Savers).
4. Rotary International and its branches.
5. International Agency for Prevention of Blindness (IAPB).
6. Helen Keller International.
7. Helpage India, etc.

Other Assistance

1. WHO assistance
2. World Bank assistance
3. Danish assistance
4. Indo-UK collaboration.

World Bank assisted cataract blindness control project. It was launched in 1994 to reduce the cataract backlog in 7 states which were identified to have the highest prevalence of cataract blindness by WHO-NPCB survey namely, Uttar Pradesh, Tamil Nadu, Madhya Pradesh (Chhattisgarh), Maharashtra, Andhra Pradesh, Rajasthan and Orrissa.

GLOBAL INITIATIVE -VISION 2020
(The Right to Sight)

The current global magnitude of blindness of 45 million is likely to increase to 75 million by the year 2020; if our efforts are not intensified to control the problem. Therefore the global initiative - vision 2020; "The Right to Sight" was officially launched on 18th Feb. 1999 by World Health Organisation (WHO) and International agency for the prevention of blindness along with their constituent members.

Aim

The aim of Vision 2020 is to eliminate the main causes of avoidable blindness in order to give all the people of the world, particularly the millions of preventable blind, the right of sight by the year 2020.

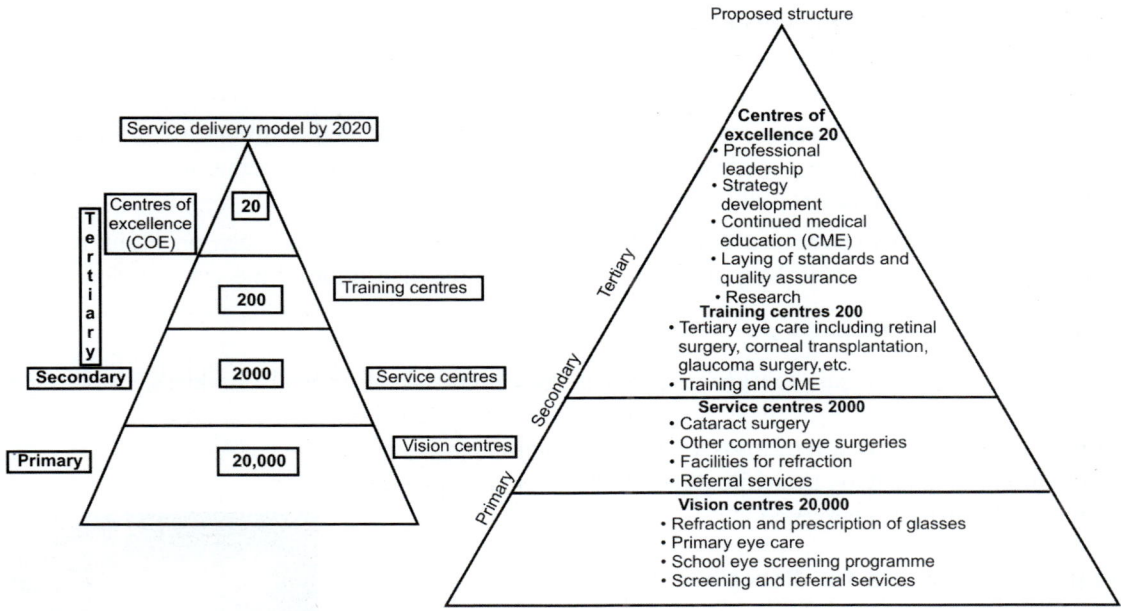

NUTRITIONAL BLINDNESS: VITAMIN A DEFICIENCY

Vitamin A deficiency along with protein energy malnutrition (PEM) results in corneal blindness. Most of the time, vitamin A deficiency is precipitated by PEM and other diseases which precipitate malnutrition (e.g. measles, diarrhoea, or other acute illnesses in children). Together this blindness is termed as 'nutritional blindness', though the main factor is vitamin A deficiency.

Vitamin A deficiency is a systemic disease that affects cells and organs throughout the body. The resultant changes in epithelial architecture are termed as "keratinizing metaplasia". The characteristic ocular manifestations of vitamin A deficiency ranging from night blindness to corneal softening are termed as 'xerophthalmia' or 'dry eye'.

Night blindness: It is usually the earliest manifestation of vitamin A deficiency. Night blindness responds rapidly (within 24-48 hours) to vitamin A therapy.

Conjunctival xerosis and Bitot's spot: The conjunctival epithelium in vitamin A deficiency is transformed from normal columnar to stratified squamous cells with a resultant loss of goblet cells, formation of a granular cell layer and keratinization of the surface.

Conjunctival xerosis first appears at the temporal side as an isolated oval or triangular patch near the limbus in the inter palpebral fissure. It is almost always present in both eyes. In some cases keratin and saprophytic bacilli accumulate on the xerotic surface, giving it a foamy or cheesy appearance. These lesions are known as Bitot's spots.

Corneal xerosis: A hazy, lustreless dry appearance of the cornea is first seen near the inferior limbus. Thick keratinized plaques may form on the corneal surface and are often more dense in the interpalbebral zone.

Corneal ulceration/ Keratomalacia: They indicate permanent destruction of a part or full thickness of corneal stroma, resulting in permanent structural alteration.

An emergency vitamin A therapy may still save the child's eye to some extent.

Xerophthalmic scar: They are usually bilateral and indicate healed sequelae of prior corneal involvement related to vitamin A deficiency. They include nebula, macula, leucoma, adherent leucoma, anterior staphyloma or phthisis bulbi.

Xerophthalmic fundus (Uyemura's fundus): Small white lesions may be seen on retina in some cases of vitamin A deficiency. They may be associated with constriction of the visual fields.

Treatment

Xerophthalmia is a medical emergency as it carries a high-risk of corneal blindness. Principle of treatment:
1. Immediate administration of massive doses of vitamin A.
2. Treatment of underlying systemic illness and protein energy malnutrition.
3. Prevention of any recurrence.

Treatment Schedule for Xerophthalmia

Vitamin A: (WHO recommendation)
1. *Immediately upon diagnosis*: 200,000 IU vitamin A is given orally.
2. *Next day*: 200,000 IU vitamin A orally.
3. *Within 1-4 weeks*: 200,000 IU vitamin A orally.
    i. Children 6-11 months old or less than 8 kg = half the above dose
    ii. Children less then 6 months old = one-quarter of the above dose.
        Oral administration is preferred, as it is safe, cheap and highly effective even in presence of mild diarrhoea (as it is also helpful for intestinal epithelium).
    Intramuscular injection of vitamin A (water-soluble) 100,000 IU is usually given when:
    i. The children cannot swallow
    ii. In case of persistent vomiting
    iii. In severe malabsorption
    iv. Where the compliance is poor.

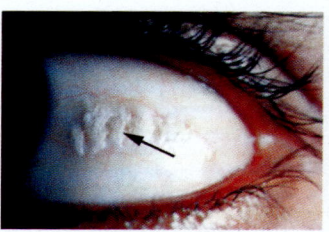

Bitot's spot

Diet and medical care: Proper treatment includes rehydration, frequent feeding with easily digestible and protein-rich food and general supportive care. Recurrent illnesses, e.g. respiratory infection, diarrhoea, and worm infestation should also be treated.

Eye care: In case of corneal involvement:
1. Broad-spectrum antibiotic eyedrops and ointment.
2. Atropine ointment.

Vitamin A Prophylaxis

It can be done by:
1. Increasing the dietary intake of foods rich in vitamin A and provitamin A.
2. Periodic administration of large doses of vitamin A.

3. Administration of fortified commonly consumed food items (vitamin A fortification).
4. *Prophylaxis*: Vitamin A is given to expecting and nursing mothers. All infants should be breastfed from the first day of birth. The schedule for children is as follows:

Doses	Age
1st dose	9th month with measles vaccine
2nd dose	1.5 years with DPT booster dose
3rd dose	2 years of age
4th dose	2.5 years of age
5th dose	3 years of age

1. Increased Intake of Dietary Sources of Vitamin A

Dark-green leafy vegetables are usually the least expensive and most widely available source of vitamin A. The dark-geen leafy vegetables should be boiled, shredded (mashed or sieved for infants) and should be combined with a small amount of edible oil to improve vitamin A absorption.

Sources of Vitamin A

1. *Vegetables sources*: Dark green leafy vegetables, spinach, carrot, drumsticks, tomato, pumpkin, papaya, mango, etc.
2. *Animal sources*: Liver, meat, cod liver oil, shark liver oil, egg yolk, etc.
3. *Fortified food items*: Vitamin A rich commercially available food items.

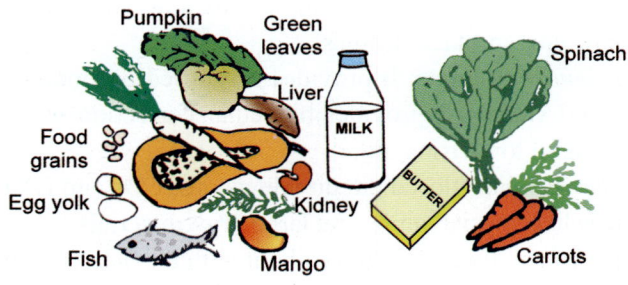

Sources of vitamin A

Daily Requirements

Children (0-4 years): 1000-1200 IU School children, adolescent and adults—3000 IU
Pregnancy and lactation: 3000-3500 IU.

The high-risk conditions are:
  i. Children with severe PEM.
  ii. Children with measles and upper respiratory tract infection.
  iii. Children with diarrhoea, lower respiratory tract infection or other acute infections, e.g. malaria, chickenpox, etc.

Fortification of Dietary Items

Fortification, i.e. the addition of vitamin A and D to common dietary items such as the vanaspati ghee, cereal grains, butter, margarine, etc. is recommended.

REHABILITATION OF THE INCURABLE BLINDS

The incurable blind persons need rehabilitation in a special way so that they can earn their livelihood and live as useful citizens. Rehabilitation can be done by the following methods:

1. ***Braille system of education***: This system was invented by Louis Braille a 16-year-old blind French. It is a system of teaching for the blind. The Braille characters are made up of raised dots arranged in 2 columns of three. There are several blind schools where facilities for Braille system of education is available. Partially blind persons may use large print books.
2. ***Low vision aids***: The term 'low-vision' denotes visual acuity between 3/60 and 6/24. The visually handicapped people can achieve improved useful vision by several special aids specially designed for near vision. The low vision aids are based on the principle of simple magnification.
   a. *Ordinary magnifying lens*: It is a biconvex, circular lens.
   b. *Rectangular magnifying lens*: It is more useful for reading.
   c. *Stand magnifier*: The size of retinal image is relatively constant.
   d. *Binocular magnifier (Head-band loupe)*: It requires the incorporation of base in prisms.
   e. *Stepped lens (Fresnel lens)*: It consists of a plastic sheet with concentric ridges (series of prisms). It is thin and devoid of aberrations.
   f. *Spectacle—born visual aid*: Single or multiple lens units, both microscopic and telescopic devices can be built into spectacle frames.
   g. *Jeweller's or watchmaker's loupe*: It provides magnified but monocular vision.
   h. *Telescopic (Galilean) system*: It provides binocular correction with large field and greater depth. It is a very useful low vision aid.
   i. Computer added devices like closed circuit televisions, CDs and DVDs for education.
   j. Non-optical devices like special lamps and large print materials.
3. ***Mobility***: Blind people can be trained to move about with the help of a stick, perform household work and look after themselves independently, i.e. without anybody's help and by using a cane.
4. ***Vocational rehabilitation***: Blind persons can be trained in making handicrafts, cane binding, book binding, candle and chalk making, cottage industries and as telephone operators. The blind workers are in no ways inferior to the sighted persons, as far as skill is concerned. They need encouragement and job opportunities rather than pity.
5. ***Reservation of jobs***: The job opportunities should be made available to blind persons in various institutions.

   In conclusion, blindness is a worldwide problem. It is preventable and curable in most of the cases—if only existing knowledge and technology could be systematically applied. It needs a conscious and constant effort from the individuals and the society.

CHAPTER 22
Ophthalmic Instruments

Ophthalmic instruments can be classified according to their function and shape as follows:
1. Knives.
2. Forceps.
3. Scissors.
4. Holders.
5. Cataract surgery instruments.
6. Lid surgery instruments.
7. Lacrimal sac surgery.
8. Squint surgery instruments.
9. Miscellaneous.

KNIVES

These are long, narrow, straight instruments.

1. von Graefe's Knife

It has a long, narrow, thin blade with a sharp tip and cutting edge only on one side.

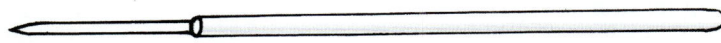

Uses
- It is used for making ab-interno corneoscleral incision during cataract surgery.
- It is also used for making incision for iridectomy and four dot iridotomy.

2. Zeigler's Knife

It has a fine hook-shaped blade with a sharp pointed tip.

Uses
- It is used for incising the after cataract.
- It may be used for doing capsulotomy during discission and extracapsular lens extraction.

3. Cystitome or Capsulotome

It is a small needle-knife with a bent sharp tip.

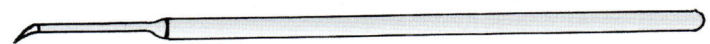

Use

It is used for doing capsulotomy during extracapsular lens extraction.

4. Keratome

It has a thin diamond-shaped blade with a sharp apex and two cutting edges. Straight as well as curved keratomes are available in various sizes (2.8 mm, 3 mm, 5.5 mm).

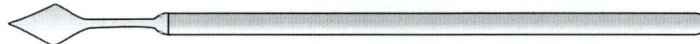

Uses

- Keratomes are used to make valvular (self sealing) corneal incisions for entry into the anterior chamber for all modern cataract surgeries like manual small incision cataract surgery (SICS) and phacoemulsification.
- It is used to make ab-externo corneal incision and for paracentesis.

5. Paracentesis Needle

It is a lancet-shaped needle with sharp cutting edges. It has a guard to prevent injury to deeper structures. It resembles a small keratome.

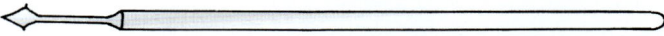

Use

It is used for paracentesis in cases of non-healing corneal ulcer, hyphaema and hypopyon associated with raised intraocular tension.

6. Foreign-body Spud

It has a blunt tip and edges on both sides.

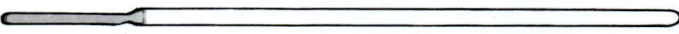

Use

It is used for removing superficial corneal foreign body.

7. 15° Side Port Entry Blade

It is a fine straight knife with a sharp pointed tip and cutting edge only on one side.

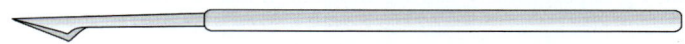

Use

It is used to make a small valvular clear corneal incision (side-port incision) in phacoemulsification SICS and other intraocular surgeries including pars plana vitrectomy.

8. MVR or V Lance Blade

It is a fine straight but triangular knife similar to 15° side port entry blade but with cutting edges on both sides.

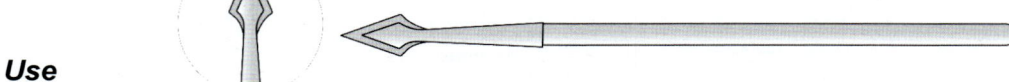

Use

Its uses are similar to 15° side port entry blade.

9. Crescent Knife

It is a blunt-tipped bevel up knife having cut-splitting action at the tip and both the sides. Its blade is curved and is mounted on a plastic handle (disposable) or fixed to a metallic handle.

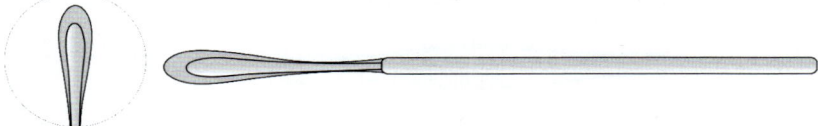

Use

It is used to make tunnel shaped incision in the sclera and cornea for phacoemulsification, manual SICS and sutureless trabeculectomy.

10. Tooke's Knife

It has a short flat blade with semicircular blunt edge on one side.

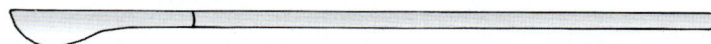

Use

It is used to separate the conjunctiva at limbus during trabeculectomy.

11. Iris Repositor

It consists of a delicate flat or bent blade with blunt edges and tip attached to a handle. It is curved at an angle of 45° (approximately) to facilitate its intraocular manoeuvring.

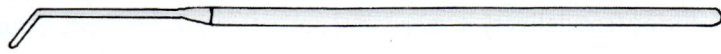

Uses

- It is used to replace or reposit the iris in the anterior chamber after an iridectomy.
- It also helps to free the iris from the lips of the section.
- It is useful in breaking the posterior synechia at the pupillary margin.

FORCEPS

Forceps consists of two limbs joined together at one end.

1. STRAIGHT FORCEPS

1. Plane Forceps

It is a simple straight forceps without any teeth.

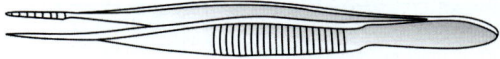

Uses

- It is used to hold the conjunctiva or skin during blunt dissection.
- It helps in tying corneoscleral sutures.

2. Corneal or One Tooth Forceps

The corneal forceps has 1 × 2 tiny fine teeth at the narrow pointed tip.

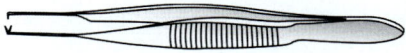

Uses

- It is used to hold the cornea while passing corneoscleral sutures.
- It may be also used to lift the cornea during lens delivery by a cryoprobe.

3. Fixation Forceps

The fixation forceps may have a narrow or wide jaws. There may be 2 × 3 or 4 × 5 teeth at the tip.

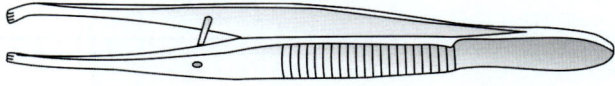

Use

It is used to fix the eyeball by holding conjunctiva and episcleral tissue at 6 O'clock position while making corneoscleral incision during cataract surgery.

2. SINGLE CURVE FORCEPS

1. Intracapsular Forceps (Arruga's)

It has a cup on the inner side of the tip of each limb. The margins of the cups are smooth. It holds the anterior lens capsule during lens delivery. Cryoprobe application is a better procedure for intracapsular lens extraction.

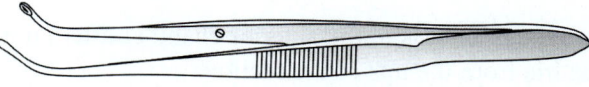

Use

It is used for intracapsular lens extraction. Which has become obsolete nowadays.

2. Extracapsular Forceps

It has 3 × 4 teeth on the inner side of the tip of each limb which tear the anterior lens capsule.

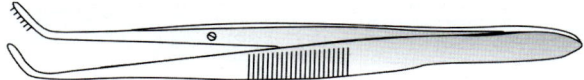

Use
It was used for extracapsular lens extraction.

3. MC Pherson Iris Forceps
It is a small delicate forceps with fine limbs having 1 × 2 teeth.

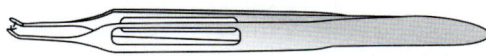

Use
It is used to hold the iris while doing iridectomy for glaucoma, cataract surgery or optical purpose.

4. Intraocular Lens Implant Forceps
It is a small delicate forceps with fine limbs and curved blunt ends.

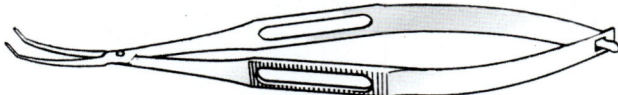

Use
It is used to hold the intraocular lens implant (IOL) and also the capsule.

5. Lens Holding Forceps for Foldable Intraocular Lenses
They may be direct action or cross action forceps and are used to evenly hold acrylic and silicone lenses.

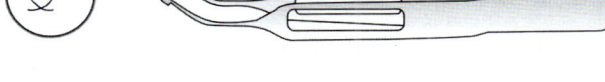

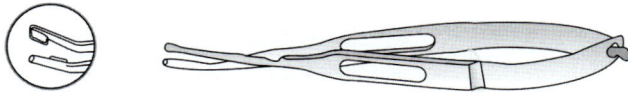

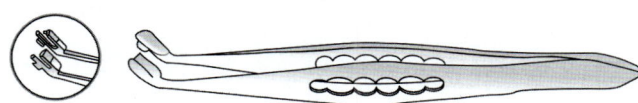

3. DOUBLE CURVE FORCEPS

1. Superior Rectus Forceps
It is a strong forceps with S-shaped tip having 1 × 2 teeth.

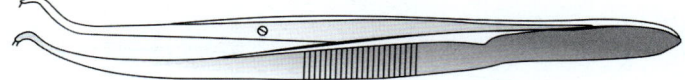

Use
It is used to hold the superior rectus muscle while passing a stay suture to fix the eyeball in downwards gaze in intraocular operations, e.g. cataract and glaucoma surgery, keratoplasty, etc.

2. Iris Forceps
It is a small and delicate forceps with fine limbs having 1 × 2 teeth.

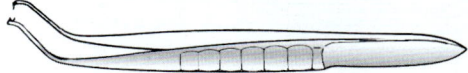

Use
It is used to hold the iris while doing iridectomy for glaucoma, cataract surgery or optical purpose.

3. Utrata Capsulorhexis Forceps
It has very delicate grasping tips and extremely thin long straight shanks.

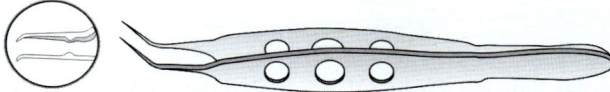

Use
It is used for holding the lens capsule after a flap has been raised with a cystitome or bent 26 gauge needle to perform a continuous curvilinear capsulotomy.

SCISSORS

1. Plane Straight Scissors
It is a fine pointed scissors with straight cutting sharp blades.

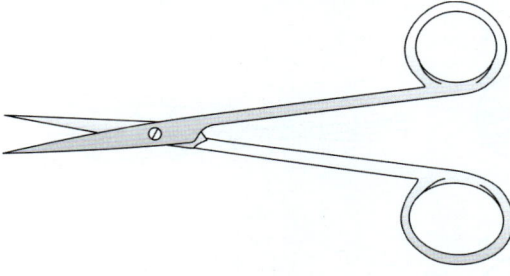

Use
It is used to cut the conjunctiva, skin and sutures.

2. Plane Curved Scissors
It is a fine pointed scissors with curved sharp cutting blades.

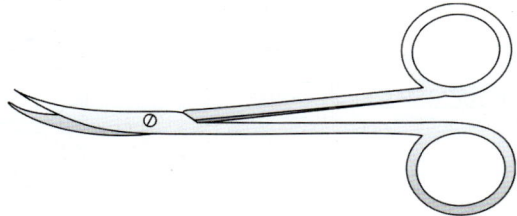

Use
It is used to cut the conjunctiva while making conjunctival flap in cataract and glaucoma surgery.

3. Corneal Scissors or Section Enlarging Scissors
It is a very fine and delicate scissors. The curved cutting blades are kept apart by spring action.

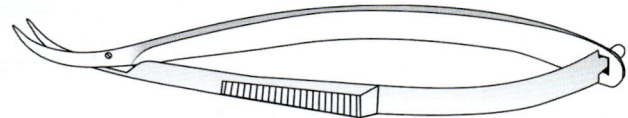

Use
It is used to enlarge the corneal or corneoscleral section in cataract surgery.

4. De-Wecker's Scissors or Iridectomy Scissors
It is a strong scissors with small V-shaped blades directed at right angles to the arms.

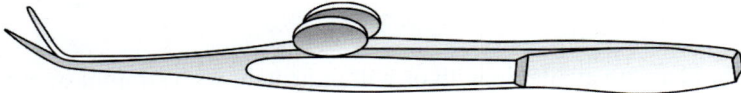

Use
It is used to perform peripheral buttonhole iridectomy.

5. Vannas Scissors
It is a fine delicate scissor with sharp edges.

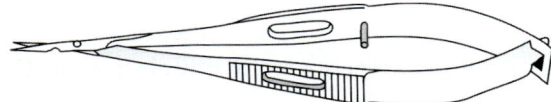

Use
It is used to cut the vitreous during vitreous prolapse.

6. Artery Forceps
It is a blunt forceps which looks like a plane straight scissors. It has multiple straight grooves (at right angle to the limbs) near the tip.

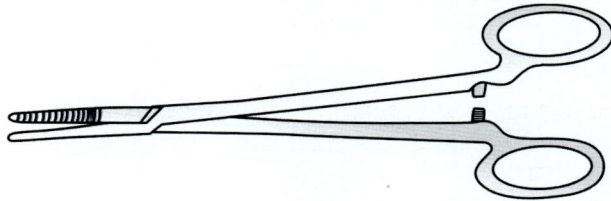

Uses
- It is used to hold the skin suture.
- It is used to catch the bleeding arteries during lacrimal sac surgery.

7. Enucleation Scissors
It is a stout strong scissors having curved sharp blades with blunt ends or tips.

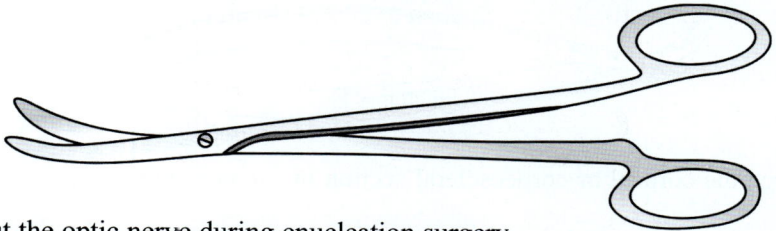

Use
It is used to cut the optic nerve during enucleation surgery.

HOLDERS

1. Needle Holder
A variety of needle holders are available with or without catch, with straight or curved tips. It holds the needle firmly.

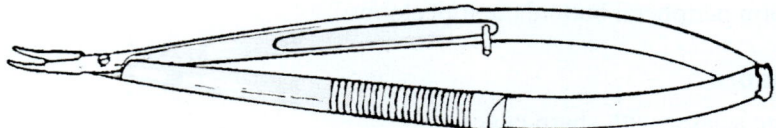

Use
It is used for passing sutures in the lids, superior rectus muscle, conjunctiva, cornea, sclera or muscle.

2. Blade Holding Forceps
It is designed to hold the razor blade firmly.

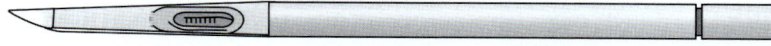

Uses
- It is used to make ab-externo incision for cataract surgery.
- It is also used for performing trabeculectomy.

CATARACT SURGERY INSTRUMENTS

1. Vectis

It is a wire loop attached to a metallic handle.

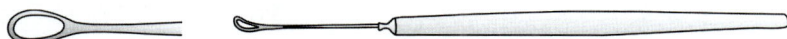

Uses

- It is used to remove the dislocated or subluxated lens.
- It was used to help in intracapsular lens extraction which is not being done at present.

2. Irrigating Vectis

It is a modified vectis with a hollow interior and multiple ports to allow the flow from the leading edge or posterior surface of the vectis. This is attached to an infusion line to assist in hydraulic separation of the nucleus.

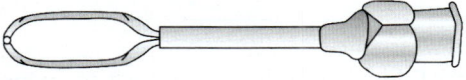

Use

It facilitates easy nucleus delivery by providing additional hydrostatic pressure to push the nucleus out of the anterior chamber through the surgical incision.

3. Lens Expressor

It is a flat metal handle with rounded curved ends.

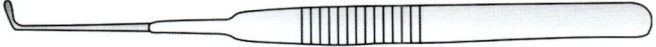

Use

It was used for intracapsular lens extraction to break the zonule and express the lens.

4. Irrigation Cannula and Air Cannula

It is attached to a syringe with saline or air. The air cannula is thinner than irrigation cannula.

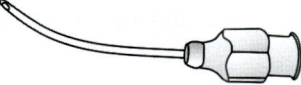

Uses

- Irrigation cannula is used in extracapsular lens extraction for irrigating the lens matter present in the anterior chamber.
- Air cannula is used to inject air into the anterior chamber after cataract surgery.

5. Suction Irrigation Cannula (Simcoe's Cannula)

It consists of two cannulas and a long rubber tubing.

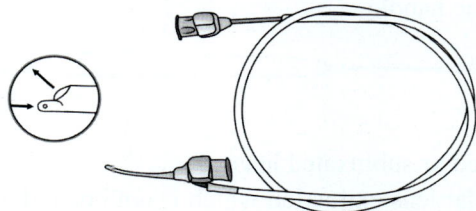

Use

It is used for suction and irrigation of lens matter in extracapsular lens extraction.

6. Sinskey Hook or IOL Dialer

It is a fine but stout instrument with a bent tip. The tip engages the dialing holes of the IOL.

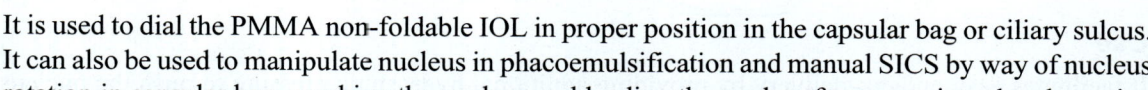

Use

It is used to dial the PMMA non-foldable IOL in proper position in the capsular bag or ciliary sulcus. It can also be used to manipulate nucleus in phacoemulsification and manual SICS by way of nucleus rotation in capsular bag, cracking the nucleus and leading the nuclear fragments into the phaco tip.

7. Chopper

It is a fine instrument resembling Sinskey hook in shape. The inner edge of the bent tip is cutting and may have different angles.

Use

It is used to split or chop the nucleus into smaller pieces and also for nuclear manipulation in phacoemulsification surgery.

8. Hydrodissection Cannula

It is a single bore 25 gauge, 27 gauge or 30 gauge cannula with a 45° angulation at about 10-12 mm from the free end. The tip at the free end can be flattened or bevelled. The tip is introduced beneath the anterior capsular margin after capsulorhexis and the fluid is injected to obtain subcapsular dissection.

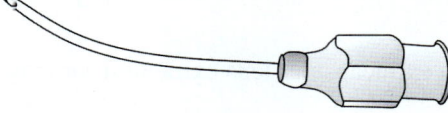

Use

It is used to perform hydrodissection (separation of capsule from the cortex) and hydrodelineation (separation of cortex from the nucleus), in phacoemulsification and manual SICS. It is attached to a syringe carrying irrigating fluid.

LID SURGERY INSTRUMENTS

1. Chalazion Clamp

It is a forceps having a screw in the centre for fixing it tightly. One arm has a round flat disc which is applied on the skin surface. The other arm has a small circular ring which is applied on the conjunctival surface over the chalazion.

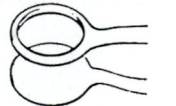 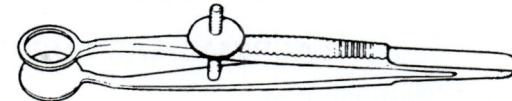

Use

It is used to fix the chalazion during incision and to obtain haemostasis.

2. Chalazion Scoop

It has a small cup with sharp margins attached to a narrow handle.

Use

It is used to thoroughly scoop out the contents of the chalazion.

3. Lid Clamp

It consists of a D-shaped plate opposed by a rim on the other side. The plate is towards the conjunctival side so it protects the eye during lid surgery on the skin side. The screw faces the outer side and the handle is always situated on the temporal side.

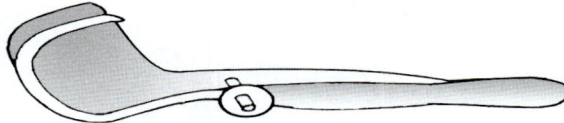

Uses

- It acts as a haemostat while doing lid surgery.
- It protects the underlying eye structures.

4. Lid Spatula

It is a plane and simple metal plate having mild convex surfaces on either side.

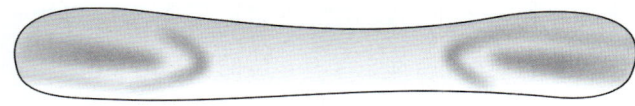

Use

It is used to support the lid and protect the cornea in entropion, ectropion and ptosis surgery.

5. Lid Retractor (Desmarres' Retractor)

It is a saddle-shaped instrument folded on itself at one end. It is attached to a metal handle.

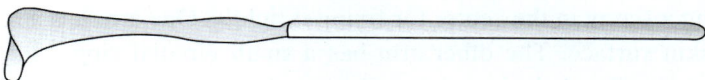

Use

It is used to examine the eyeball in cases of marked blepharospasm and in children.

LACRIMAL SAC SURGERY

1. Punctum Dilator (Nettleship's)

It has a cylindrical metal handle with a conical pointed tip.

Use

It is used to dilate the lacrimal punctum before syringing or probing.

2. Lacrimal Probes

These are a set of straight metal wires of varying thickness with blunt rounded ends.

Use

It is used to probe the nasolacrimal duct in children usually.

3. Muller's Skin-Muscle Retractor

It is a self-retaining retractor made up of two limbs with a screw to fix the limbs. Each limb has three curved pins for engaging the edges of skin and muscle.

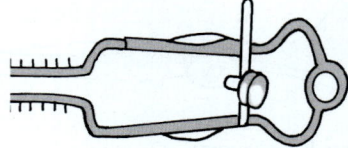

Uses

- It is used during lacrimal sac surgery as a haemostat.
- It helps to provide a good field without the help of an assistant.

4. Chisel and Hammer

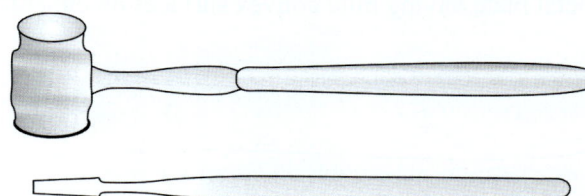

Use

It is used to cut the bone during dacryocystorhinostomy (nasal drainage operation).

5. Bone Punch

It consists of a spring handle and two blades. The upper blade has a small hole with cutting edges. The lower blade has a cup-like depression.

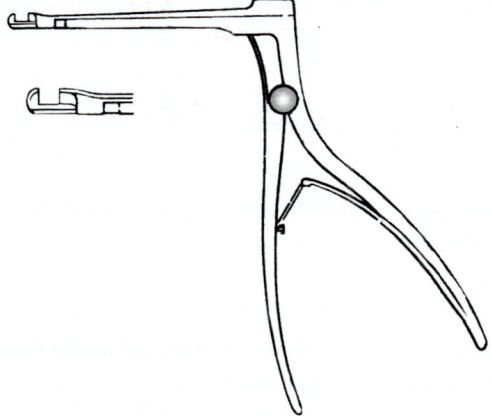

Use

It is used to cut the nasal bone during dacryocystorhinostomy.

SQUINT SURGERY INSTRUMENTS

1. Muscle Hook or Strabismus Hook

This instrument is like the lens expressor but without the blunt round knob.

Use

It is used to engage the muscle during squint surgery, enucleation and retinal detachment surgery.

2. Caliper and Rule

It is a divider-like instrument to which a graduated scale is attached to one arm. The other arm can be moved by a screw over the scale.

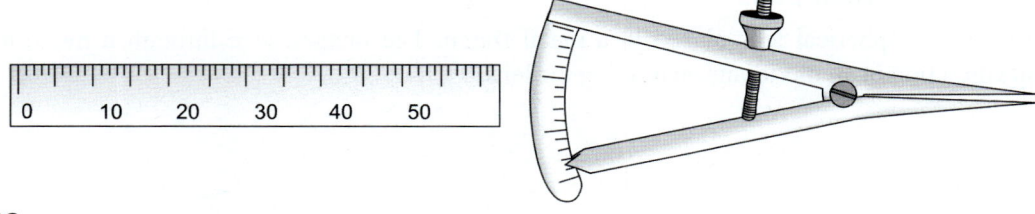

Uses

- It is used to take measurement during squint, ptosis and retinal detachment surgery.
- It is also used in localization of the foreign body in X-ray films.

MISCELLANEOUS

1. Wire Speculum

It is made up of wire and has two limbs attached at one end.

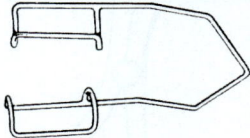

Uses
- It is used to keep the eyelids separate during any operation on the eyeball.
- It protects the underlying eye structures.

2. Trephine

Trephines are calibrated in various sizes. It has a corrugated metal handle which can be fixed into different sized circular blades having sharp cutting edges.

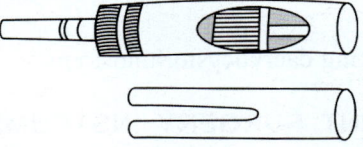

Use
It is used for cutting the corneal disc from the donor's and recipient's cornea in corneal grafting.

3. Evisceration Scoop

It is an oval shallow scoop attached to a thick metallic handle.

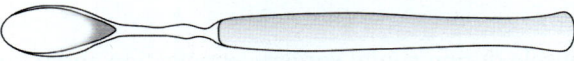

Use
It is used to scoop out the contents of the eyeball during evisceration.

DARK ROOM APPLIANCES

1. Convex Spherical Lens

It is a biconvex spherical lens placed in a metal frame. The images seen through it move in the opposite direction in all meridians on moving the lens.

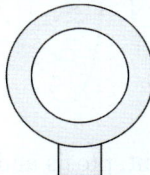

Use
It is used in hypermetropia, presbyopia, aphakia and in various ophthalmic instruments, e.g. retinoscope, Placido's disc, slit-lamp, etc.

2. Concave Spherical Lens

It is a biconcave spherical lens placed in a metal frame. The images seen through it move in the same direction in all meridians on moving the lens.

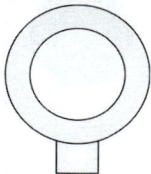

Use

It is used in myopia and Hruby's lens.

3. Convex Cylindrical Lens

The images seen through it move in the opposite direction on moving the lens but at the axis of the cylinder there is no movement.

Use

It is used in hypermetropic astigmatism whether simple, compound or mixed.

4. Concave Cylindrical Lens

The images seen through it move in the same direction on moving the lens but at the axis of the cylinder there is no movement.

Use

It is used in myopic astigmatism whether simple, compund or mixed.

5. Red and Green Glasses or Filters

Red glass is kept in front of the right eye and green glass is kept in front of the left eye.

Uses

- It is used for diplopia charting.
- It is used to test binocular vision in Worths' four dot test.
- It is also used for malingering test.

6. Occluder

It is a black coloured opaque disc.

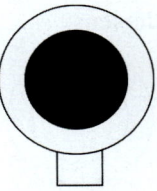

Use
It is used to occlude one eye while testing and correcting the visual acuity of the other.

7. Pin Hole

It is a black coloured opaque disc with a small central hole.

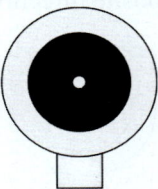

Use
It is used to find out if the impaired vision is due to refractive error or any other ocular pathology. The vision improves in cases of refractive error as the central rays passing through the pin hole are straight. The vision may remain the same or deteriorate in ocular pathology, e.g. opacity in the media, retinopathy, etc.

8. Stenopic Slit

It is a black coloured opaque disc with a vertical or horizontal straight slit in the centre.

Use
It is used for differentiating the cause of coloured halos. When a stenopic slit is moved in front of the eye,
- The halos are intact in acute congestive glaucoma.
- The halos are broken in immature cataract.

9. Maddox Rod

It consists of 4-5 cylinders of red glass prisms fused side by side in a supporting disc. The same effect is given by a disc of deeply grooved red glasses (Maddox groove).

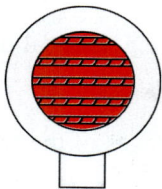

Uses
- It is used to detect heterophoria by dissociating the two retinal images.
- It is used for testing macular function.

10. Retinoscope

It consists of plane mirror on one side and concave mirror on the other. There is a small hole in the centre of each mirror having +2 D lens to exclude accommodative error.

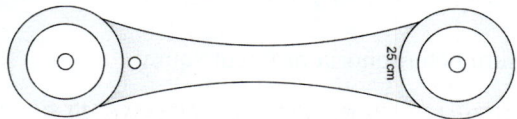

Use
It is used to determine error of refraction and opacities of the media by parallax.

11. Trial Frame

The trial frame has three compartments namely,
    Inner compartment—For keeping occluder, pin hole, stenopic slit, etc.
    Middle compartment—For placing spherical lens.
    Outer compartment—For keeping cylindrical lens.

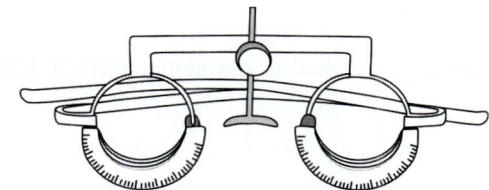

Use
It is used to test and correct errors of refraction, e.g. myopia, hypermetropia, aphakia, presbyopia.

12. Placido's Disc

It consists of alternate concentric dark and light rings. There is a spherical convex lens in the centre of the disc, having a dioptric strength of +2 D.

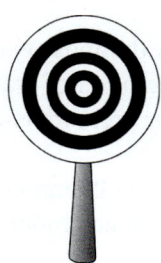

Use
It is used to diagnose irregular corneal surface, e.g. corneal ulcer, keratoconus etc.

13. Maddox Wing
It is an instrument that dissociates the retinal images of the two eyes for near fixation.

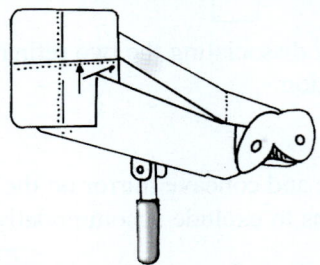

Use
It is used to diagnose and measure heterophoria or latent squint.

STERILIZATION OF INSTRUMENTS

It is essential to sterilize ophthalmic instruments before using them to prevent ocular infection.

Sterilization is a process which destroys all micro-organisms including bacteria and spores.

Disinfection is a process which kills pathogenic micro-organisms but has no effect on bacteria and spores.

METHODS
Sterilization can be achieved by,
1. *Physical agents*: Heat, filtration, radiation, etc.
2. *Chemical agents*: Alcohols, aldehydes, phenol, halogens, surface acting agents, gases, etc.

1. Heat Sterilization
Dry heat sterilization
  i. *Hot air oven*: It is the most commonly used method of sterilization by dry heat. It kills the bacteria, spores and viruses. It is used to sterilize instruments like forceps, scissors, scalpels, etc. The articles should be double wrapped and kept at 150°C for 2 hours in an oven.
  ii. *Flame*: It can be used to sterilize, tips of forceps, air way cannula, spatulas etc.
  iii. *Incineration*: It is used to destroy soiled dressings and pathological materials.

Moist heat sterilization
  i. *Autoclave (Steam under pressure)*: It is the most widely used method of sterilization. It is based on the principle that at the boiling point of water, the vapour pressure is equal to the atmospheric pressure. Thus if the vapour pressure is increased, the penetrating power of the steam also increases.
  Autoclaving at 121°C under 15 lb/in^2 for 20 minutes kills the bacteria, spores and viruses. This is useful in sterilizing various instruments, rubber articles, towels, gowns, dressing pads, swabs and eye drops.

ii. *Steaming*: It kills most bacteria and viruses but not spores. The instruments are placed on a shelf above the level of boiling water. Sharp edged instruments like knives and scissors can be sterilized by steam for approximately 30 minutes.
   iii. *Boiling*: It kills bacteria and viruses. Heavy metallic instruments can be sterilized by boiling for about 30 minutes. This methods, however, blunts the cutting edges of the instruments.

2. Chemical Sterilization

   i. *Spirit (95% alcohol)*: It kills the bacteria and spores but not viruses.
   ii. *Methylated spirit (70% isopropyl alcohol)*: Schiotz tonometer can be sterilized by it.
   iii. *Formaldehyde*:
       a. *Formalin (10%)*: It has marked bactericidal, sporicidal and some viricidal action. It is useful for cryoextractor probes and heat sensitive instruments.
       b. *Formaldehyde gas*: It is used to fumigate and to sterilize the operating room. Formaldehyde fumigation is recommended fortnightly as a routine for optimum disinfection. 500 ml of 40% formaldehyde is added to one litre of water and kept in an electric boiler or in a large bowl placed on a hot plate with safety cut-out till dry.
   iv. *Savlon*: It is a combination of cetavlon or cetrimide and chlorhexidine. Cetavlon is a surface active agent and chlorhexidine is a phenol. It is effective against most gram - positive organisms. It is commonly used for cleaning the skin. Scissors, knives, etc. may also be sterilized with it.
   v. *Glutaraldehyde (2%)*: It is commercially available as 'Cidex' solution. It is specially used to sterilize sharp instruments as their sharpness is not affected. The instruments are free from pathogens and spores in about three hours. However, instruments should be washed thoroughly with sterile water prior to use.
   vi. *Hydrogen peroxide (3%)*: It is used for sterilizing of applanation tonometer, prisms and ophthalmoscopy lenses. It is active particularly against AIDS and herpes virus.
   vii. *Ethylene oxide gas*: It is highly inflammable gas. It is mixed with an inert gas like carbon dioxide or nitrogen. It is effective against all bacterias, spores and viruses. Indirect ophthalmoscopy lenses, gonioscopy lenses and cryoprobes can be sterilized with it.
   viii. *Acetone*: It is a quick and cheap method of sterilizing instruments. Instruments are kept in acetone for 5 minutes and thereafter are thoroughly washed with sterile water before use.

3. Radiation Sterilization

   i. *Ionizing radiations:* These include gamma rays, cosmic rays, X-rays which are lethal to DNA and thus kill all types of micro-organisms. The rays can penetrate both solids and liquids without raising the temperature significantly (cold sterilization). They are used for sterilizing swabs, dressing pads, tubings, plastic syringes, etc.
   ii. *Non-ionizing radiations:* They act as a type of hot air sterilization because they are absorbed as heat. Infrared rays are useful for rapid mass sterilization of instruments.

Index

A

Absolute primary angle-closure
glaucoma 291
  complications 292
    atrophic bulbi 292
    phthisis bulbi 292
    rupture of the eyeball 292
    staphyloma 292
  signs 292
  symptom 292
  treatment 293
Acanthamoeba keratitis 132
  diagnosis 132
    clinical diagnosis 132
    confocal microscopy 133
    laboratory diagnosis 132
  etiology 132
  predisposing factors 132
  signs 132
  symptoms 132
  treatment 133
Accessory structure of the eye 5
  extraocular muscles of the eye 7
  eyebrows 6
  eyelids and eyelashes 6
  lacrimal apparatus 6
Acne rosacea 134
  etiology 134
  signs 134
  treatment 134
Acute conjunctivitis 74
  acute mucopurulent conjunctivitis 74
    complications 75
    etiology 74
    incidence 74
    signs 75
    symptoms 74
    treatment 75
  purulent conjunctivitis (acute blenorrhea) 75
    complications 76
    etiology 75
    incidence 76
    prognosis 76
    prophylaxis 76
    signs 76
    symptoms 76
    treatment 76
    types 75
Acute dacryo-adenitis 427
  complications 427
  differential diagnosis 427
  etiology 427
  signs 427
  symptom 427
  treatment 427
Acute dacryocystitis 430
  complication 430
  etiology 430
  symptoms 430
  treatment 430
Acute iridocyclitis 167
  complications and sequelae 171
    band-shaped keratopathy 171
    choroiditis 171
    complicated cataract 171
    cyclitic membrane 171
    phthisis bulbi 171
    retinal complications 171
    secondary glaucoma 171
  diagnosis 172
  investigations 172
  signs 168
    anterior chamber 168
    circumciliary congestion 168
    iris 169
    lens 171
    pupil 169
    synechiae 169
  symptoms 167
  treatment 172
    principles 172
  treatment of complications 175
    complicated cataract 175
    phthisis bulbi 175
    post-inflammatory glaucoma 175
    retinal detachment 175
    secondary glaucoma 175
Acute primary angle-closure glaucoma 284
  complications 286
  course 286
  pathogenesis 285
  signs 285
  symptoms 285
  treatment 286
    medical 286
    surgical 288
Adie pupil 31
After or secondary cataract 240
  clinical types 240
    ring of Sommerring 241
    thin membrane 240
  treatment 241
Age-related macular degeneration (ARMD) 322
  etiology 322
  signs 322
  symptoms 322
  treatment 322
  types 322
Allergic conjunctivitis 86
  acute or subacute catarrhal conjunctivitis 86
    differential diagnosis 86
    etiology 86
    signs 86
    symptoms 86
    treatment 86
  phlyctenular conjunctivitis 87
    clinical types 87
    complications 88
    etiology 87
    histopathology 87
    incidence 87
    signs 87
    symptoms 87
    treatment 88
  spring catarrh 89
    complications 90
    differential diagnosis 90

etiology 89
histopathology 89
incidence 89
keratopathy 90
prophylaxis 91
symptoms 89
treatment 91
types 89
Anatomy of the retinal nerve fibres 268
   macular fibres 268
   nasal fibres 268
   temporal fibres 269
Angle of anterior chamber 1
Anisometropia 57
   signs 58
   symptoms 57
   treatment 58
   types 57
     acquired 57
     congenital 57
Ankyloblepharon 414
   etiology 414
   treatment 414
Anomalies in the position of lids 409
   trichiasis 409
     complications 410
     etiology 410
     signs 410
     symptoms 410
     treatment 410
Anterior ischaemic optic neuropathy (Aion) 345
   classification 346
   etiology 345
   signs 346
   symptom 346
Anterior uveitis 167
   clinical forms 167
     allergic 167
     infective 167
Aphakia 55
   optical condition 55
   signs 55
   symptom 55
   treatment 55
     contact lens 56
     correction by spectacles 55
     intraocular lens implantation 57

Aphakic glaucoma 294
   etiology 295
   signs 295
   symptoms 295
   treatment 295
Applanation tonometer 32
Argon laser trabeculoplasty (ALT) 276
   contraindication 276
   indications 276
Argyll Robertson pupil 29
Astigmatism 53
   etiology 53
   prognosis 55
   symptoms 54
   treatment 54
   types 53
     irregular astigmatism 54
     regular astigmatism 53

B

Behcet's syndrome 166
Binocular single vision 380
Binocular vision 14
   mechanisms 14
     fusion 14
     simultaneous macular perception 14
     stereopsis 14
Bitot's spots 99
Bjerrum's scotoma 269
Blepharophimosis 414
   etiology 414
   treatment 415
Blood supply of the eye 7
   arterial supply 7
   venous drainage 7
Blue sclerotics 157
Bruch's membrane 2

C

Cardinal positions of gaze 380
Cataract 207
   complicated cataract 217
     etiology 217
     signs 217
     symptoms 217
   congenital cataract 207

     clinical types 208
     etiology 207
     incidence 207
     investigations 209
     signs 208
     symptoms 208
     treatment 209
   cupuliform cataract 216
     signs 216
     symptoms 216
   lens aspiration 210
     contraindications 210
     indications 210
     postoperative complications 211
     technique 210
   lensectomy 211
     indication 211
     technique 211
     visual rehabilitation 212
   senile cataract 212
     classification 213
     etiopathogenesis 212
   senile cortical cataract 213
     clinical stages 214
     etiology 213
     incidence 213
     morphological types 214
     symptoms 213
   senile nuclear cataract 216
     clinical stages 216
     etiology 216
     incidence 216
     signs 217
     symptoms 217
Causes of blindness 458
Causes of worldwide blindness (2002) 459
Central retinal artery occlusion 307
   complication 309
   etiology 307
   pathogenesis 307
   signs 308
     fundus examination 308
     pupil 308
   site of occlusion 307
   symptoms 308
   treatment 309
Central serous retinopathy (CSR) 304
   complications 304

Index

diagnosis 304
etiology 304
incidence 304
prognosis 305
signs 304
symptoms 304
treatment 305
Chalazion (tarsal or meibomian cyst) 407
   course 408
   etiology 407
   signs 408
   symptoms 408
   treatment 408
Chronic conjunctivitis 79
   angular conjunctivitis 79
      complications 80
      etiology 80
      signs 80
      symptoms 80
      treatment 80
   follicular conjunctivitis 80
      complications 81
      etiology 80
      signs 81
      symptoms 80
      treatment 81
      types 81
   simple chronic conjunctivitis 79
      etiology 79
      signs 79
      symptoms 79
      treatment 79
   trachoma 81
      diagnosis 84
      etiology 81
      incidence 82
      prophylaxis 86
      signs 82
      symptoms 82
      treatment 85
Chronic dacryocystitis 430
   etiology 430
   incidence 431
   investigations 432
   pathogenesis 431
   sequela 431
   signs 431
   symptoms 431
   treatment 432
   types 431

Chronic iridocyclitis 179
   complications 179
   signs 179
   slit-lamp examination 179
   symptoms 179
Chronic primary angle-closure glaucoma 291
   clinical features 291
   diagnosis 291
      fundus examination 291
      gonioscopy 291
   pathogenesis 291
   treatment 291
Chronic serpiginous ulcer 124
   complications 124
   etiology 124
   incidence 124
   signs 124
   symptoms 124
   treatment 125
Ciliary body 1
Classification of blindness in India 461
Coloboma of retina and choroid 331
   fundus examination 332
   symptoms 331
Colour blindness 13
   etiology 13
      acquired 13
      congenital 13
   types 14
Common causes of loss or diminished corneal sensation 27
Comparative study of intra-and extracapsular cataract extraction 230
Congenital abnormalities of lens 242
Congenital abnormality of lids 420
   coloboma 420
   distichiasis 420
   epicanthus 420
Congenital anomalies 193
   albinism 196
      signs 196
      symptoms 196
      treatment 196
      types 196
   aniridia 194
   colobomata 195
      clinical features 195
      etiology 195

corectopia 194
cysts 196
   cyst of posterior epithelium 196
   implanation cyst 196
   serous cyst 196
heterochromia iridis 194
heterochromia iridum 193
persistant pupillary membrane 194
   clinical features 195
   differential diagnosis 195
   etiology 194
   incidence 194
polycoria 194
Congenital anomalies 356
   coloboma of the optic disc 356
   medullated (opaque) nerve fibres 357
Congenital anomalies of cornea 135
   cornea plana 135
   keratoglobus 135
   megalocornea 135
      differential diagnosis 135
   microcornea 135
   posterior embryotoxon 135
Congenital anomalies of the puncta and canaliculi 428
Congenital dacryocystitis 429
   etiology 429
   signs 429
   symptom 429
   treatment 429
Congenital or infantile glaucoma 262
   diagnosis 263
      fundus examination 263
      gonioscopy 263
      measurement of corneal diameter 263
      raised intraocular pressure 263
   differential diagnosis 263
   etiology 262
   incidence 262
   signs 262
   symptoms 262
   syndromes associated with infantile glaucoma 262
   treatment 263
      medical 264
      operative 264

492 Basic Ophthalmology

types 262
    congenital glaucoma 262
    infantile glaucoma 262
    juvenile glaucoma 262
Conjugated movements of the eyeball 379
    action of extraocular muscles in binocular movements 379
    antagonist muscles 379
    synergist muscles 379
Conjunctival epithelium 1
Cornea 107
    applied anatomy 107
    functions 108
    nerve supply 108
    nutrition of the cornea 107
    structure 107
        Bowman's membrane 107
        Descemet's membrane 107
        endothelium 107
        epithelium 107
        substantia propria or stroma 107
Corneal degenerations 136
    amyloid degeneration 137
    arcus juvenilis 137
    arcus senilis 136
    band-shaped keratopathy 137
    corneal degenerations 136
    corneal dystrophies 136
    pigmentary degeneration 137
    white limbal girdle of Vogt 137
Correction of ametropia with lenses 61
    contact lenses 62
        complications 64
        disadvantages 63
        indications 63
        method of calculating the power 63
        principle 62
        types 62
    lenses 61
        cylindrical lens 62
        prism 62
        spherical lens 61
Cryosurgery in ophthalmology (cryopexy) 334
    method 334

principle 334
uses 334
Cysts 102

D

Dacryocystitis 428
Dacryops 428
Deep keratitis 135
    etiology 135
        congenital syphilis 135
        sclerosing keratitis 135
        tuberculosis 135
        viral infections 135
    treatment 135
Degenerations 92
    concretions 92
        incidence 92
        signs 92
        symptoms 92
        treatment 92
    pinguecula 92
        etiology 92
        pathology 93
        signs 92
        treatment 93
    pterygium 93
        complications 94
        course 94
        differential diagnosis 94
        etiology 93
        incidence 93
        parts 94
        pathology 93
        signs 93
        symptoms 93
        treatment 95
Detachment of choroids 193
    complications 193
    etiology 193
    prognosis 193
    signs 193
    treatment 193
Determination of refraction 59
    objective methods 59
        auto-refractometer 59
        keratometer 59
        retinoscopy 59
    subjective methods 59
        postmydriatic test 59

Diabetic retinopathy 316
    classification 317
        early treatment for diabetic retinopathy study (ETDRS) classification 319
        Eva Kohner's classification 317
    investigations 321
    pathogenesis 317
    predisposing factors
        duration of diabetes 316
        heredity 316
        hypertension/pregnancy 316
        severity of diabetic retinopathy 316
    prognosis 321
    treatment 321
Differences between congenital glaucoma and keratoglobus 263
Differences between conjunctival and ciliary congestion 26
Differences between normal physiological cup and glaucomatous cup 267
Differential diagnosis of nodule at the limbus 88
Diode laser trabeculoplasty (DLT) 277
Diseases of the conjunctiva 72
    cysts and tumours 72
    degenerative conditions 72
    inflammation (conjunctivitis) 72
        allergic types 72
        infective types 72
    symptomatic conditions 72
Diseases of the cornea 108
    degenerations 108
    ectasias 108
    inflammations (keratitis) 108
    pigmentations 108
Diseases of the lens 206
    cataract 206
        acquired cataract 206
        congenital or development cataract 206
Diseases of the retina 302
    congenital anomaly 302
    degenerations 302
    inflammations 302

retinal detachment 302
retinopathies due to systemic
 diseases 302
tumour 302
vascular lesions 302
Diseases of the uveal tract 163
congenital anomalies 164
degenerations 164
inflammation 163
syndromes associated with uveitis
 164
tumours 164
vascular disturbances 164
Dislocation of lens 241
complications 242
etiology 241
signs 242
symptoms 242
treatment 242
types 242
 complete dislocation 242
 partial dislocation 242
Down syndrome 219
Dystrophies of cornea 138
anterior dystrophies 138
 Cogan's microcystic
  dystrophy 138
 Messman's juvenile epithelial
  dystrophy 139
 Reis-Buckler's dystrophy
  138
ectatic conditions of cornea 140
endothelial dystrophies 139
 cornea guttata 140
 Fuch's endothelial dystrophy
  139
stromal dystrophies 139
 granular dystrophy 139
 lattice dystrophy 139
 macular dystrophy 139

E

Ectropion 412
signs 412
symptom 412
treatment 412
types 412
Edinger-Westphal nucleus 30
Embryonic fissure 1

Emmetropia 47
Endophthalmitis 180
clinical features 181
 bacterial endophthalmitis 181
 fungal endophthalmitis 181
complications 182
differential diagnosis 181
etiology 181
investigation 182
prevention 183
treatment 182
Entropion 410
etiology 410
symptoms and signs 411
treatment 411
types 410
Epikeratophakia 67
complications 67
indications 67
method 67
principle 67
Errors of refraction ametropia 48
etiology 48
 abnormal position of lens 48
 axial ametropia 48
 curvature ametropia 48
 index ametropia 48
Examination of the eye 23
examination of the anterior
  segment of the eye 24
 inspection 24
examination of the posterior
  segment of the eye 24
examination of the fundus
  oculi 24
examination of the retinal
  functions 24
Examination of the fundus by focal
 illumination 43
Goldmann three mirror contact
  lens 43
Hruby's lens 43
indirect slit-lamp biomicroscopy
  43
posterior fundus contact lens 43
Examination of the fundus oculi 41
general fundus 43
macula lutea 43
media 41
 direct ophthalmoscopy 41

indirect ophthalmoscopy 42
plane mirror examination at a
 distance of 1 m 41
plane mirror examination at a
 distance of 22 cm 41
optic disc 42
retinal vessels 43
Examination of the posterior segment
 of the eye 35
objective examination of retinal
  functions 40
 electro-oculogram (EOG) 41
 electroretinogram (ERG) 40
subjective examination of retinal
  functions 35
 central field 40
 colour vision 40
 field of vision 37
 peripheral field 39
 recording of visual acuity for
  distance 36
 recording of visual acuity for
  near 36
 visual acuity 35
Excision of the eyeball 200
enucleation 200
 indications 200
 technique 200
evisceration 200
 indications 200
 technique 201
frill excision 201
 technique 201
Exposure keratitis 125
etiology 125
sign 125
treatment 125
Extracapsular cataract extraction
 (ECCE) 228
indications 228
sterilization 228
technique 228
Exudative retinopathy of coats 305
complications 305
etiology 305
incidence 305
signs 305
symptoms 305
Eye bank 146

contraindications for collection of donor eyes 148
    ocular causes 148
enucletion 147
equipments 147
evaluation of donor tissue 148
    systemic causes 148
objective 146
preservation of the donor eye 148
    intermediate-term preservation 149
    long-term preservation 149
    short-term preservation 148
promotion and awareness about eye donation 149
    grief counseling 149
    publicity 149

F

Fluorescein angiography 332
Focal interval of sturm 54
Functions of the retina 12

G

Galactosaemia 219
General therapeutics 448
    antimicrobial therapy 449
        antibiotics 429
        other antibiotics 451
        synthetic chemicals 451
    antiviral drugs 452
    hormone therapy 454
    vitamins 455
Glaucoma 261
    classification 261
        acquired 261
        congenital 261
    etiology 261
    pathogenesis 261
        mechanical changes 261
        vascular factors 261
Global magnitude of blindness 459
Goldmann applanation tonometer 32
Gonioscope examination 34

H

Herbert's pits 82
Holmgren's wools 13
Horner's syndrome 29, 31

Hypermetropia 51
    etiology 52
        absence of lens or aphakia 52
        axial 52
        backward displacement of the lens 52
        curvature 52
        index 52
    incidence 51
    signs 52
    symptoms 52
    treatment 52
    types 52
        latent hypermetropia 52
        manifest hypermetropia 52
Hypertensive retinopathy 311
    classification 312
        Keith Wagner and Barker 312
        Scheie's classification 314
    clinical types 315
        hypertension with arteriolar sclerosis (diffuse hyperplastic) 315
        hypertension with involutionary sclerosis 315
        malignant hypertension 315
        simple hypertension without sclerosis 315
    pathogenesis 311
        hypertensive choroidopathy 312
        hypertensive retinopathy 311
    predisposing factors 311
    treatment 315
Hypertensive uveitis 179
    differential diagnosis 180
    signs 180
    symptoms 179
    treatment 180
Hypopyon ulcer 118
    etiology 118
    predisposing factors 119
    pathogenesis 119
    types 119

I

Indications for cataract extraction 223
Indocyanine green angiography 333

Inflammation (conjunctivitis) 73
    diagnosis 74
    evaluation 73
        conjunctival reactions 73
        discharge 73
        lymphadenopathy 74
    treatment 74
        antibiotic drops 74
        antibiotic ointments 74
Inflammation of the sclera 154
    episcleritis 154
        complication 155
        etiology 154
        incidence 154
        pathology 154
        signs 154
        symptoms 154
        treatment 155
        types 154
    scleritis 155
        complications 157
        etiology 155
        incidence 155
        investigations 156
        pathology 155
        signs 156
        symptoms 156
        treatment 157
        types 156
Inflammation of the uveal tract (uveitis) 164
    classification 165
        anatomical classification 165
        clinical classification 165
        etiological classification 166
        pathological classification 166
    etiology 166
        allergic inflammation 166
        endogenous infection 166
        exogenous infection 166
        hypersensitivity reaction 166
        secondary infection 166
Inflammations blepharitis 405
    etiology 405
    sequelae 406
    symptoms 406
    treatment 406
    types 405
Inflammations of the cornea 109

Inflammations of the retina 303
    complications 303
    Eale's disease 303
    etiology 303
    incidence 303
    prognosis 304
    signs 303
    symptom 303
    treatment 303
Injuries to the eye 361
    blunt injury (contusions) 363
        choroid 366
        cornea 364
        iris and ciliary body 364
        lens 365
        optic nerve 366
        retina 366
        sclera 364
        vitreous 365
    chemical injuries and burns 362
        complication 363
        etiology 362
        signs 363
        symptoms 363
        treatment 363
    extraocular foreign body 361
        complications 361
        etiology 361
        prophylaxis 362
        signs 361
        symptoms 361
        treatment 362
    penetrating and perforating injury 367
        aim of treatment 367
        signs of perforation of the eyeball 367
    perforating injury with retained foreign body 368
        diagnosis and localization of intraocular foreign body 369
        effects of retained foreign body 368
        methods of removal 370
        organic materials 369
        treatment 370
Interior of the eyeball 5
    aqueous humour 5
    lens 5
    vitreous 5

Intermediate uveitis 176
    complications 176
    differential diagnosis 176
    etiology 176
    incidence 176
    signs 176
    symptoms 176
    treatment 176
Internal hordeolum 409
    etiology 409
    signs 409
    symptoms 409
    treatment 409
Intracapsular cataract extraction (ICCE) 226
    complications 226
        delayed 227
        immediate 226
        late 227
    indications 226
    intracapsular lens extraction with cryoprobe 226
    technique 226

K

Kayser-Fleisher's ring 108
Keratoconus 140
    classification 140
        keratoconus 140
        morphological classification 141
    etiology 140
    incidence 140
    signs 141
        early signs 141
        late signs 141
    symptoms 141
    treatment 141
Keratoglobus 142
    differential diagnosis 142
    etiology 142
Keratomileusis 67
Keratoplasty 144
    types 144
        full thickness 144
Koeppe's nodules 186

L

Lacrimal apparatus 424
    applied anatomy 424
    accessory lacrimal glands 424
    blood supply of the lacrimal gland 425
    lacrimal canaliculi 424
    lacrimal glands 424
    lacrimal puncta 424
    lacrimal sac 425
    lymphatic drainage 425
    nasolacrimal duct 425
    nerve supply 426
Lagophthalmos 415
    complication 415
    etiology 415
Laser phacolysis 237
Lasers in ophthalmology 335
    principle 335
    production of laser beam 335
    types 335
Lens 205
    applied anatomy 205
    functions 206
    parts 206
        cortex 206
        lens capsule 206
        nucleus 206
    structure 205
        lenticular capsule 205
        lenticular epithelium 205
        lenticular fibres 205
        suspensory ligament or zonule of Zinn 205
Lesions of the visual pathway 16
    amaurosis (dark) 18
        bilateral amaurosis 18
        unilateral amaurosis 18
    amblyopia (blunt) 18
        bilateral amblyopia 18
        unilateral amblyopia 18
    hemianopia 16
        etiology 16
        types 17
Lids 403
    diseases of the lids 404

M

MacKay-Marg tonometer 32
Malignant glaucoma 296
    etiology 296
    pathogenesis 296
    signs 296

treatment 296
    medical therapy 296
    surgical therapy 296
Manual small incision cataract surgery 230
Marcus-Gunn pupil 31
Marginal ulcer 123
  complications 124
  etiology 123
  incidence 123
  signs 124
  symptoms 124
  treatment 124
McReynoids' method 96
Mechanism of laser effects and their therapeutic uses 336
  photoblation 337
    uses 337
  photocoagulation 336
    complications 337
    mode of action 336
    therapeutic uses 336
  photodisruption 337
    uses 337
Meibomian glands 403
Membranous conjunctivitis (diphtheritic conjunctivitis) 78
  complications 78
  diagnosis 78
  differential diagnosis 78
  etiology 78
  incidence 78
  prophylaxis 79
  signs 78
  symptoms 78
  treatment 79
Mikulicz's syndrome 428
Moll's glands 403
Mooren's ulcer 124
Munson's sign 141
Mycotic hypopyon ulcer 121
  diagnosis 122
  etiology 121
  incidence 121
  predisposing factors 121
  signs 121
  symptoms 121
  treatment 122
    medical therapy 122
    surgical treatment 123

Mydriasis 29
  etiology 29
    digital tension 32
    intraocular pressure 32
    palpation 32
Myopia (short sight) 48
  complications 50
  etiology 48
  prognosis 50
  signs 49
    macula 50
    optic disc 49
    peripheral fundus 50
  symptoms 49
  treatment 50
  types 49
    congenital myopia 49
    pathological myopia 49
    simple myopia 49

N

Nagel's anomaloscope 13
National programme for the control of blindness (NPCB) 462
Nerve supply to the eye 8
  autonomic nerves 8
  motor nerves 8
  sensory nerve 8
Nervous control of ocular movements 380
Neuroparalytic keratitis 125
  etiology 125
  signs 125
  symptom 125
  treatment 126
Nonpurulent keratitis 126
  herpes simplex 126
    complications 127
    diagnosis 128
    etiology 126
    incidence 126
    signs 127
    symptoms 127
    treatment 128
    types 127
  herpes zoster 129
    clinical stages 129
    complications 131
    etiology 129
    incidence 129

    signs 129
    symptoms 129
    treatment 131
Normal tension glaucoma (NTG) 278
  diagnosis 278
  etiology 278
  incidence 278
  investigation 279
  treatment 279
Nutritional blindness: vitamin a deficiency 465
Nystagmus 397
  etiology 397
    central nystagmus 399
    congenital hereditary 399
    ocular nystagmus 397
    vestibular nystagmus 399
  prognosis 399
  treatment 399

O

Ocular motility 375
  extraocular muscles 375
    horizontal recti 377
    oblique muscles 375
    recti muscles 375
    vertical recti 377
Ombrain's method 96
Opacities in the vitreous 247
  etiology 247
    degenerative causes 247
    developmental causes 247
Operation upon the iris 198
  iridectomy 198
    indications 198
    technique 198
  iridotomy 198
    choice of laser for iridotomy 199
    laser peripheral iridotomy 198
    post laser 199
Operations on the cornea 142
  indications 143
  method 143
Ophthalmia neonatorum 77
  complications 77
  etiology 77
  incidence 77

prophylaxis 78
signs 77
symptoms 77
treatment 77
Ophthalmic instruments 469
   cataract surgery instruments 477
      chopper 478
      hydrodissection cannula 478
      irrigating vectis 477
      irrigation cannula and air cannula 477
      lens expressor 477
      Sinskey hook or IOL dialer 478
      suction irrigation cannula (Simcoe's cannula) 478
      vectis 477
   dark room appliances 482
      concave cylindrical lens 483
      concave spherical lens 483
      convex cylindrical lens 483
      convex spherical lens 482
      Maddox rod 484
      Maddox wing 486
      occluder 484
      pin hole 484
      placido's disc 485
      red and green glasses or filters 483
      retinoscope 485
      stenopic slit 484
      trial frame 485
   forceps 471
      double curve forceps 473
      extracapsular forceps 472
      straight forceps 472
   holders 476
      blade holding forceps 476
      needle holder 476
   knives 469
      15° side port entry blade 470
      crescent knife 471
      cystitome or capsulotome 469
      foreign-body spud 470
      iris repositor 471
      keratome 470
      MVR or V lance blade 471
      paracentesis needle 470
      von Graefe's knife 469
      Zeigler's knife 469
   lacrimal sac surgery 480
      bone punch 481
      chisel and hammer 480
      lacrimal probes 480
      Muller's skin-muscle retractor 480
      punctum dilator (nettleship's) 480
   lid surgery instruments 479
      chalazion clamp 479
      chalazion scoop 479
      lid retractor (Desmarres' retractor) 480
      lid spatula 479
   scissors 474
      artery forceps 475
      corneal scissors or section enlarging scissors 475
      De-Wecker's scissors or iridectomy scissors 475
      enucleation scissors 476
      plane curved scissors 474
      plane straight scissors 474
      Vannas scissors 475
   squint surgery instruments 481
      caliper and rule 481
      muscle hook or strabismus hook 481
Optic atrophy 354
   pathogenesis 354
      consecutive optic atrophy 355
      glaucomatous optic atrophy 356
      ischaemic optic atrophy 355
      postneuritic optic atrophy 355
      primary (simple) optic atrophy 354
      secondary optic atrophy 355
      toxic optic atrophy 356
   types 354
Optic nerve 341
   diseases of the optic nerve 342
Optic plate 1
Optic vesicle 1
Orbit 437
   diseases of the orbit 438
      endocrine exophthalmos 444
      enophthalmos 445
      orbital cellulitis 439
      proptosis or exophthalmos 441
      thrombosis of cavernous sinus 440

P

Palpebral fissure 403
Panophthalmitis 183
   clinical features 183
   complications 183
   etiology 183
      endogenous 183
      exogenous 183
   treatment 183
      medical 183
      surgical 184
Papillitis 347
   etiology 347
   pathogenesis 347
   signs 348
   symptoms 347
   treatment 348
Papilloedema (chocked disc) 342
   complications 145
      early 145
      late 145
   contraindications 144
   differential diagnosis 345
   etiology 342
   indications 144
      cosmetic 144
      optical 144
      structural 144
      therapeutic 144
   method 145
      excision of diseased host cornea 145
      excision of the donor eye 145
      excision of the donor's cornea 145
      fixation of donor's clear graft 145
   pathogenesis 343
   signs 344
   symptoms 343
   treatment 345
      partial thickness 144

unilateral versus bilateral papilloedema 343
Pathway of the pupillary light reflex 30
Perkins tonometer 32
Persistent hyperplastic vitreous 248
    diagnosis 248
    etiology 248
    symptoms 248
    treatment 248
Phacoemulsification 231
    advantages 237
    complications 234
        immediate 234
        postoperative 235
    disadvantages 237
    technique 232
        anterior capsulotomy 232
        aspiration of the residual cortex 233
        hydroprocedures 233
        intraocular lens implantation 234
        nucleus emulsification 233
        phaco incision 232
Phakonit 237
Phlyctenular keratitis 133
    signs 133
    symptoms 133
    treatment 134
Photophthalmia 134
    etiology 134
    prophylaxis 134
    signs 134
    symptoms 134
    treatment 134
Photoretinitis 306
    prophylaxis 306
    signs 306
    symptoms 306
    treatment 306
Phthisis bulbi 184
    clinical features 184
    differential diagnosis 184
    etiology 184
    treatment 184
Physiology of vision 10
    accommodation of the eyes to light 11

movements of the eyeballs-convergence 11
size of the pupil 11
refraction of the light rays 10
lens 10
Pigment deposition in the cornea 142
Pigment epithelium 1
Pigmentary retinal dystrophy 323
    complications 324
    differential diagnosis 324
        congenital syphilis 324
        night blindness 324
    incidence 323
    prognosis 325
    signs 323
    symptoms 323
    treatment 325
    types 324
        central or inverse pigmentary degeneration 325
        retinitis pigmentosa sine pigmento 324
        retinitis punctata albescens 324
        uniocular and atypical form 325
Pigmentations of the cornea 142
    argyrosis 142
    blood staining 142
    Kayser-Fleischer ring 142
Placido's disc 27
Posterior uveitis 177
    clinical forms 177
    clinical types 178
    complications 178
    differential diagnosis 178
    signs 177
        fundus examination 177
    symptoms 177
    treatment 178
Postmydriatic test (PMT) 60
Presbyopia 58
    etiology 58
    sign 58
    symptoms 58
    treatment 58
Prevention of blindness 461
Primary angle-closure glaucoma (PACG) 279
    etiology 279

    incidence 279
    mechanism of angle-closure glaucoma 279
        irido-trabecular contact 280
        physiological iris bombe 280
        relative pupil block 279
    stages 280
Primary angle-closure glaucoma
    suspect (latent) 281
    clinical feature 281
    course 282
    diagnosis 281
    investigations 281
    treatment 282
Primary open angle glaucoma (POAG) 265
    associated ocular pathology 265
    diagnosis 266
    etiology 265
    incidence 265
    mechanism of primary open angle glaucoma 265
        sclerosed endothelium lining of canal of Schlemm 265
        sclerosed trabecular meshwork 265
    signs 266
    symptoms 266
Primordia of ocular structures 2
    mesoderm 2
    neural ectoderm 2
    surface ectoderm 2
Ptosis 415
    etiology 415
    signs 416
    symptoms 416
    treatment 418
    types 416
Purkinje-Sanson images 31
Purulent keratitis corneal ulcer 109
    complications 111
        corneal opacity 111
        descemetocele 112
        ectatic cicatrix 111
        perforation 112
    diagnosis 110
    etiology 109
    predisposing factors 109
        epithelial damage 109

poor resistance 109
virulent organisms 109
signs 110
stages of corneal ulcer 110
healing stage 110
progressive stage 110
regressive stage 110
symptoms 110
treatment 113
principles 113
procedure 115

R

Refractive corneal surgery 64
astigmatic keratotomy 65
clear lens extraction (Fucala's operation) and PC IOL 67
advantage 67
laser-assisted *in situ* keratomileusis (lasik) 66
advantages 66
disadvantages 66
method 66
photorefractive keratectomy (PRK) by excimer laser 65
advantages 66
disadvantages 66
indications 65
method 65
principle 64
advantages 64
disadvantages 65
indication 64
method 64
radial keratotomy (RK) 64
Rehabilitation of the incurable blinds 468
Reiter's disease 166
Retina 300
applied anatomy 300
ora serrata 300
structure 300
blood supply 301
functions 302
venous drainage 301
Retinal detachment 328
classification 328

secondary 329
simple detachment 328
complications 330
differential diagnosis 330
prognosis 331
signs 330
symptoms 329
treatment 331
Retinal vein occlusion 309
complications 310
etiology 309
pathogenesis 309
signs 310
site of occlusion 309
symptom 310
treatment 311
Retinoscopy 59
method 59
mydriatics in refraction 59
neutralisation 60
observations and inferences 60
optical principle 59
Retrobulbar neuritis 349
complications 350
differential diagnosis 350
signs 349
symptoms 349
treatment 350

S

Schiotz tonometer 32
Sclera 153
applied anatomy 153
apertures 153
functions 153
Secondary glaucoma 293
etiology 293
inflammatory glaucoma 293
intraocular tumour 294
lens 293
massive intraocular haemorrhage 293
obstructive glaucoma 294
perforation of cornea 293
postinflammatory 293
venous obstruction 294
treatment 294
Seidel's sign 269
Sjögren's syndrome 98

Snellen's test type 35
Specific national programmes of blindness 463
Specific types of uveitis 185
gonorrhoea 185
clinical features 185
incidence 185
treatment 185
leprosy 186
incidence 186
treatment 186
types 186
sarcoidosis 187
syphilis 185
clinical features 185
incidence 185
treatment 185
toxoplasmosis 187
clinical features 187
etiology 187
treatment 187
tuberculosis 185
clinical features 185
incidence 185
treatment 186
Squint strabismus 381
apparent squint 381
latent squint (heterophoria) 381
diagnosis 382
etiology 382
symptoms 382
types 381
manifest squint (heterotropia) 385
concomitant squint 385
paralytic squint 391
Staphyloma 158
clinical types 158
anterior staphyloma 158
ciliary staphyloma 158
equatorial staphyloma 158
intercalary staphyloma 158
posterior staphyloma 158
etiology 158
treatment 158
Stem cell transplant 145
indications 145
procedure 146
Sterilization of instruments 486
chemical sterilization 487

heart sterilization 486
radiation sterilization 487
Stocker's line pterygium 96
Structure of the eye 4
    inner nervous tissue layer 4
        optic disc 5
        optic nerve 5
        retina 4
    middle vascular layer 4
        choroids 4
        ciliary body 4
        iris 4
    outer fibrous layer 4
        cornea 4
        limbus 4
        sclera 4
Sturm's conoid 53
Stye (Hordeolum) 407
    etiology 407
    signs 407
    symptoms 407
    treatment 407
Subacute (intermittent) primary angle-closure glaucoma 282
    course 283
    diagnosis 283
    differential diagnosis 284
        halo in conjunctivitis 284
        iritis 284
        lenticular halos 284
    symptoms 282
        blurring of vision 282
        coloured halos around lights 283
        in between the recurrent attacks 283
        mild headache and browache 283
    treatment 284
Summary of medical treatment of important ocular diseases 457
    conjunctival diseases 457
    corneal ulcer 457
    episcleritis and scleritis 457
    glaucoma 457
    iridocyclitis 457
Symblepharon 413
    etiology 413
    signs 414
    symptoms 414
    treatment 414
    types 413
Sympathetic ophthalmitis 371
    etiology 371
    pathology 372
    prognosis 372
    signs 372
    symptoms 372
    treatment 372
Symptomatic conditions 96
    argyrosis 102
    chemosis 102
        etiology 102
    subconjunctival haemorrhage 96
        course 96
        etiology 96
        sign 96
        symptom 96
        treatment 97
    xerosis (dry eye) 97
        complications 98
        etiology 97
        investigation 99
        prophylaxis 101
        signs 98
        symptoms 98
        treatment 100
        visual display terminal syndrome 98
Symptoms of acquired cataract 219
    early 219
        black spots 220
        colored halos 220
        colour value changes 220
        glare 219
        uniocular diplopia or polyopia 220
    late 220
Syndromes associated with uveitis 187
    acquired immunodeficiency syndrome (AID) 187
        clinical features 187
        etiology 187
        incidence 187
        treatment 189
    ankylosing spondylitis 190
    Behcet's syndrome 189
        clinical features 189
        treatment 190
    heterochromic iridocyclitis of Fuchs 191
        complications 191
    ocular histoplasma syndrome 191
        treatment 191
    Reiter's disease and uveitis 190
        clinical features 190
        treatment 190
    Stevens-Johnson syndrome 190
        complication 190
        etiology 190
        treatment 190
    uveoparotitis (Heerfordt's disease) 189
    Vogt-Koyanagi syndrome 190

T

Tarsorrhaphy 143
    indications 143
    method 143
    types 143
        lateral tarsorrhaphy 143
        paramedian tarsorrhaphy 143
Tears 426
    functions 426
    tear film 426
        aqueous layer 426
        lipid layer 426
        mucous layer 426
Tenon's space 438
Topical anti-glaucoma drugs 275
Toxemia of pregnancy 315
    classification 315
        stage of angiospasm 315
        stage of retinopathy 316
        stage of sclerosis of vessels 316
    complications 316
    treatment 316
Toxic amblyopias (chronic retrobular neuritis) 350
    chloroquine 353
    ethambutol 354
    ethyl alcohol 352
    lead 353
    methyl alcohol 352
        complications 353
        etiology 352

incidence 352
pathology 352
signs 352
symptoms 352
treatment 353
oral contraceptives 354
quinine 353
signs 353
tobacco amblyopia 351
etiology 351
incidence 351
pathogenesis 351
predisposing factors 351
prognosis 352
signs 351
symptoms 351
treatment 352
Transillumination 35
trans-pupillary 35
trans-scleral 35
Traumatic cataract 219
Treatment of 116
corneal abscess 117
impending perforation 117
non-healing corneal ulcer 116
perforated corneal ulcer 117
Treatment of aphakia 238
contact lens 239
advantages 239
disadvantages 239
correction by spectacles 238
advantages 238
disadvantages 238
intraocular lens (IOL) implant 239
advantages 239
biometry 239
complications 239
Treatment of associated raised tension 240
Treatment of Senile cataract 223
medical treatment 223
surgical treatment 223
Treatment of unilateral cataract 240
Tumour of the optic nerve 356
glioma 356
meningioma 356
Tumours of the lids 419
benign tumour 419

haemangioma 419
mole (naevus) 419
neurofibroma 419
xanthoma 419
malignant tumour 420
basal cell carcinoma (rodent ulcer) 420
squamous cell carcinoma 420
Tumours of the retina retinoblastoma 325
differential diagnosis 327
incidence 325
pathology 325
prognosis 328
signs 326
stages 327
symptoms 326
treatment 328
types 326
glioma endophytum 326
glioma exophytum 326
Types of gonioscopy 34
direct gonioscopy with goniolenses 34
indirect gonioscopy with gonioprisms 34

U

Ulcus serpens 119
complications 120
signs 119
symptoms 119
treatment 120
Uveal tract 161
choroid 162
blood supply 163
structure 163
ciliary body 162
functions 162
parts 162
structure 162
iris 161
parts 161
structure 161

V

Vascular disturbances 191
rubeosis iridis 191

clinical features 191
etiology 191
prophylaxis 192
treatment 192
Vascular lesions of the retina 306
course 307
etiology 306
types 307
intraretinal haemorrhage 307
preretinal or subhyaloid haemorrhage 307
vitreous haemorrhage 307
Visual display terminal syndrome (VDTS) 98
Visual pathway 15
lateral geniculate bodies 15
occipital cortex 16
optic chiasma 15
optic nerves 15
optic radiations 15
optic tract 15
Visual perceptions 12
colour sense 13
brightness or luminosity 13
saturation or calorimetric purity 13
wavelength 13
form sense 12
light sense 12
dark adaptation 12
light minimum 12
sense of contrast 12
Vitrectomy 252
anterior vitrectomy 253
automated vitrectomy 253
sponge vitrectomy 253
pars plana vitrectomy 254
aims 254
indications 254
technique 255
Vitreous 246
diseases of the vitreous 247
opacities in the vitreous 247
persistent hyperplastic vitreous 247
vitreous bands and membranes 247
vitreous detachment 247
vitreous haemorrhage 247

vitreous inflammation 247
vitreous loss 247
Vitreous bands and membranes 248
Vitreous detachment 251
    detachment of vitreous base and anterior vitreous 252
    posterior vitreous detachment 251
    complications 251
    incidence 251
    signs 251
    symptoms 251
Vitreous haemorrhage 248
    complications 249
    etiology 249
    investigations 249
    prognosis 250
    signs 249
    symptoms 249
    treatment 250
    types 248
        intravitreal haemorrhage 249
        preretinal or subhyaloid haemorrhage 248
Vitreous inflammation 251
Vitreous loss 250
    etiology 250
    prophylaxis 250
    signs 250
    treatment 250
Vitreous substitutes 255
Voluntary organisations in control of blindness 464
von Hippel-Lindau disease 306

W

Worth's four dot test 393

Z

Zeis's glands 403